MEDICAL RADIOLOGY

Diagnostic Imaging

Editors:
A. L. Baert, Leuven
K. Sartor, Heidelberg

Springer-Verlag Berlin Heidelberg GmbH

I. P. Arlart · G. M. Bongartz · G. Marchal (Eds.)

Magnetic Resonance Angiography

2nd Revised Edition

With Contributions by

I. P. Arlart · M. Bock · J. Bogaert · G. M. Bongartz · M. Boos · H. Bosmans · J. F. Debatin
C. Diehm · A. J. Duerinckx · S. Dymarkowski · J. Gaa · A. Gerlach · R. Hausmann
P. R. Hilfiker · G. P. Krestin · M. E. Ladd · G. Laub · G. Marchal · P. Reimer · K. Scheffler
S. Sonnet · J. Van Cleynenbreugel · R. Vosshenrich · D. Weishaupt · S. Wetzel · G. Wilms

Foreword by

A. L. Baert

With 345 Figures in 704 Separate Illustrations, Some in Color

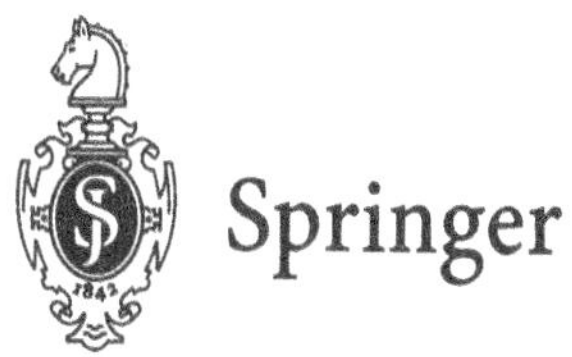

Springer

Ingolf P. Arlart, PhD, MD
Radiologisches Institut Stuttgart
Katharinenhospital
Kriegsbergstrasse 60
70174 Stuttgart
Germany

Georg M. Bongartz, PhD, MD
Department of Radiology
University Hospital
Kantonsspital
Petersgraben 4
4031 Basel
Switzerland

Guy Marchal, PhD, MD
Professor
Department of Radiology
University Hospitals K.U. Leuven
Herestraat 49
3000 Leuven
Belgium

Medical Radiology · Diagnostic Imaging and Radiation Oncology
Continuation of
Handbuch der medizinischen Radiologie
Encyclopedia of Medical Radiology

ISBN 978-3-540-65091-1

Library of Congress Cataloging-in-Publication Data
Magnetic resonance angiography / I. P. Arlart, G. M. Bongartz, G. Marchal (eds) ; with contributions by I. P. Arlart ... [et al.] ; foreword by A. L. Baert. -- 2nd rev. ed.
p. ; cm. – (Medical radiology)
Includes bibliographical references and index.
ISBN 978-3-540-65091-1 ISBN 978-3-642-56247-1 (eBook)
DOI 10.1007/978-3-642-56247-1
1. Blood-vessels--Magnetic resonance imaging. I. Arlart, I. II. Bongartz, Georg M., 1955- III. Marchal, Guy, Prof. Dr. Med. IV. Series.
[DNLM: 1. Magnetic Resonance Angiography. WN 185 M1955 2002]
RC691.6.A53 M334 2002
616.1'307548-dc21 00-067912

htp://www.springer.de

Originally published by Springer-Verlag Berlin Heidelberg New York in 2002

Cover-Design and Typesetting: Verlagsservice Teichmann, 69256 Mauer

SPIN: 106 923 70 21/3130 – 5 4 3 2 1 0 – Printed on acid-free paper

Dedicated to

Gudrun, Oliver and Tobias	I. P. Arlart
Mathieu	G. M. Bongartz
Rita, Kathleen and Paul	G. Marchal

Foreword

Since the publication of the first edition of this standard work astonishing progress has been achieved in magnetic resonance angiography, an exquisite non-invasive method for visualizing large and small arteries of the internal organs as well as of the limbs.

Indeed, important technical advances related to the introduction of more rapid gradient systems and new sequences, coupled with more efficient use of contrast media, have led to substantial improvements in the technical and image quality of MRA. This method has reliably replaced conventional X-ray angiography in many anatomic areas and is now firmly established in routine clinical radiology.

I would like to thank the editors as well as the authors of the individual chapters for their outstanding performance in the preparation of this second edition, which provides a much-needed update of the technique of MRA and offers a comprehensive overview of the current state of development of this fascinating modality.

I am convinced that this book will be of great interest to the radiologist who wants to be informed about the optimal application of MRA and about its current potential in clinical diagnosis. Non-radiological clinicians will also find this book very valuable because it clearly defines the exact position of MRA in diagnostic algorithms and clinical decision making.

I am confident that this volume will meet with the same great success as the previous edition.

Leuven

Albert L. Baert

Preface of the Second Edition

The idea to publish a book on magnetic resonance (MR) angiography was born in the early nineties when flow-sensitive non invasive imaging of vessels had become possible. Although in rapid evolution, MR angiography was readily introduced into clinical routine. The success of this noninvasive technique allowed to gather special experience in a relatively short time - and on the other hand underlined the growing demand on education and knowledge in this field. This led to the publication of the first edition of "MR ANGIOGRAPHY", which was published in January 1996. It could already be expected at that time that contrast-enhanced MR angiography prospectively would be superior to "time-of-flight" and "phase contrast" techniques in a majority of vascular disorders. This expectation was confirmed in the late nineties and led to the publication of a second edition of "MR ANGIOGRAPHY".

Whithin a period of 5 years, MR imaging has shown an immense development which could be realized following a significant technical improvement of MR hardware and MR software. High gradient fields over 20 mT/m and extremely short slew rates below 150ms allow the application of ultrashort repetiton-times and echo-times. On this basis suitable sequence protocols have been established including echo planar imaging, ultrafast gradient-echo imaging and particular k-space sampling-techniques. Recent achievements, such as spiral acquisition, enable realtime body imaging today with minimal acquisition times of 50ms to 80 ms per image.

A simultaneous development and successful introduction of dedicated phased array coils resulted in a significant improvement in signal to noise ratio and thus, of spatial resolution.

In vascular imaging, these technical innovations had a strong influence on further development of MR angiography. Traditional time-consuming sequences based on flow-sensitive signal modification such as time-of-flight or phase contrast suffered from instability of flow signal, disturbing flow voids, pulsation- and motion artifacts, and long acquisition times up to ten minutes for the examination of a single vascular area. Utilizing the newly developed technical improvements, signal acquisition of MR angiography was shortened to a breath-hold period. The coordination of such an ultrafast sequence to the arterial first pass of a contrast material bolus was the basic concept of contrast-enhanced MR angiography. Not only its speed but also the expanded application of MR angiography to nearly all vascular areas produced a second peak in the MR angiography story-of-success. Using this technique, three dimensional acquisition on the basis of gradient-echo sequences become possible and show excellent results comparable to the "gold standard", i.e. invasive intraarterial digital subtraction angiography.

The examination of thoracic and abdominal vasculature can be performed within a breath-hold, optimized localization of the maximal contrast-bolus into the center of the k-space can be realized by specific methods of automatically controlled bolus timing, and peripheral arteries of the extremities can be visualized by a single bolus of contrast agent using a table movement technique. Spatial resolution is optimized by adapted coils like the dedicated extremity coil, and time resolution is optimized by ultrashort acquisition that allows time-resolved vascular imaging with one image per second.

Up to now, similar examination techniques are recommended by many user groups. However, generally accepted examination standards of contrast-enhanced MR angiography have not been established yet and can be definitively expected only when technical development will comes to a stable status and time-resolved high-resolution MR angiography is presented in a manner that is directly comparable to conventional x-ray angiography.

Contrast agents used for angiographic MR studies have shown to be widely free from severe side-effects which are well known in x-ray contrast agents. Thus, contrast-enhanced MR angiography furthermore can be attributed as a non invasive technique, useful particular in high risk patients with diabetes mellitus, compensated renal failure, severe arterial hypertension, and compensated cardiac failure.

On the other hand, excellent image quality of contrast-enhanced MR angiography enables this method prospectively for overall diagnostic evaluation of arterial and venous disorders, so that intraarterial DSA remains reserved for interventional procedures only.

As a non invasive method, MR angiography has not only to compete with computed tomography (CT) systems for multislice spiral scanning, i.e. volume scanning, but in particular with color duplex ultrasonography (US). Under availability of recently developed techniques, i.e. tissue harmonic imaging, power Doppler imaging, vascular „panorama scanning“ and three-dimensional imaging, this method has been shown to be an excellent tool for vessel visualization and blood-flow quantification in the hands of experienced personnel. Allthogether, these three non invasive vascular imaging techniques combine the advantage of being well tolerated and giving a 3D access to the vessels due to their cross-sectional nature.

Further comparative studies including the rapid development in US-, CT- and MR- techniques may give the answer which of the systems will win the battle of non invasive vascular imaging with respect to cost-effectiveness.

Stuttgart
Basel
Leuven

Ingolf P. Arlart
Georg M. Bongartz
Guy Marchal

Introduction

Ingolf P. Arlart and Georg M. Bongratz

For vascular imaging different technical modalities have been introduced successfully in clinical practice such as conventional angiography and digital subtraction angiography (DSA), respectively, contrast-enhanced computed tomographic (CT) angiography, and color coded duplex Doppler ultrasonography (US). In particular DSA is able to visualize vascular structures with high temporal and spatial resolution and thus it is accepted as the gold standard of vascular imaging. However, because this method allows only intraluminal evaluation of vascular structures, both CT angiography and US have shown to be useful as a complementary tool in the evaluation of vessel wall structures as well as perivascular space. Moreover, US as the unique modality is able to provide not only angiomorphological but also functional information of blood flow and velocity.

There is a general consensus that for purely diagnostic purposes, invasive x-ray angiography should be replaced by non invasive techniques because of associated risks to the patients, e.g. radiation exposure, potentially nephrotoxic contrast material and invasive catheterism. Further reasons to overcome diagnostic invasive angiography are high costs of the procedure including investments for the angiographic equipment, stand-by of educated and experienced personnel, and the need to hospitalize the majority of patients.

Although only minimal invasive due to the necessity of iodinized contrast material, also CT angiography shows certain drawbacks for the patient due to potentially side effects of contrast agents and radiation exposure. Moreover, the separation of high density contrasted vessels from neighboring osseous structures limit the technique to certain areas.

Thus, as a classic non-invasive diagnostic imaging technique, US has been successfully introduced for the evaluation of vascular disorders already many years ago. US is the most rapidly growing technique of all imaging modalities. This growth results from the revolutionary development in computer technology and the increasing acceptance of the diagnostic value of US by clinicians. One among the recent and most important new applications of US is color duplex Doppler imaging. By combining high-resolution tissue imaging with simulaneous display of flow information as well as conventional Doppler spectral analysis, color Doppler has provided the opportunity for detailed non invasive assessment not only of morphology but also of function as reflected in organ blood supply and perfusion. Since its clinical introduction in the mid 1980´s it has become widely accepted as a means of evaluating the peripheral vascular system and as an adjunct to grey-scale imaging for numerous applications in the abdomen, pelvis, and neck region.

Further developments recently became available including tissue harmonic imaging in high resolution, power Doppler, panoramic imaging of long vascular structures, computer assisted three-dimensional vascular imaging, compound array scanning, and the application of specific contrast agents which markedly improves flow signal. For dynamic flow evaluation, a sound spectrum waveform analyzer shows the Doppler shift frequency of pulsatile blood flow within the sample volume. Frequency levels in kHz of the different red blood cell velocities moving through the sample volume are displayed on the vertical axis, and the duration of each cardiac cycle is given on the horizontal axis in seconds. The amplitude or volume of the Doppler signal sound at any given frequency is displayed in shades of grey on the sound spectral analysis waveform. Using spectral analysis, the pulsatile Doppler frequency can be measured and following correction of the angle between vascular axis and Doppler beam, flow velocities can be determined quantitatively.

The form of Doppler frequency and velocity curves, respectively, is influenced by the peripheral vascular resistance of the arterioles. A „low resistance flow“ can be differentiated from a „high resistance flow“. In oder to quantitate the pulsatility of Doppler frequency curves and velocity curves, two different indices exist: a) the „resistance-index“ (RI) and b) the „pulsatility index“ (PI). RI means the ratio of systolic flow velocity (Doppler frequency) minus enddiastolic flow velocity (Doppler frequency) against systolic flow velocity. PI can be expressed by the maximum velocity amplitude against mean velocity. The maximal velocity amplitude is expressed by the difference between maximum systolic and minimal diastolic velocity. To obtain maximum information, a skilled operator must perform careful sampling of all of the sites within the vessel lumen where flow disturbances are likely to be found.

With Doppler it is possible to determine the net direction of blood flow as well as brief changes in flow direction that may occur during the course of the cardiac cycle. Doppler permits the identification of vessel occlusion and may be used to infer the presence and degree of vessel narrowing. Doppler aids in the characterization of flow to organs, transplants, and tumors. Finally, the importance of Doppler information in the interference of abnormalities in the peripheral vascular bed of an organ or tissue deserves special emphasis. Changes in spectral waveform or in the appearance of flow in diastole provide insights into the resistance of the vascular bed supplied by the vessel and, although not specific, may indicate changes due to a variety of disorders.

Major advantages of US are the possibility of bed-side examinations, relatively low investment costs, and the individual investigation of selected vascular areas. The limitation of duplex Doppler US is that flow information is obtained only from the remainder of the image. A preferable approach would be a method allowing evaluation of flow characteristics throughout the entire image combined with high-resolution display of the vessel wall and surrounding tissue features. This approach is exactly what is provided by combining Doppler flow and tissue imaging. Doppler color-flow instruments are pulsed and are subject to the same limitations such as Doppler angle dependence and aliasing, as other Doppler instruments. Other existing limitations of US include the dependence of diagnostic accuracy on the experience of the operator, habitus and obesity of the patient, and areas that cannot be penetrated by US waves such as air and bone structures. Like in other sonographic investigation, the diagnostic results are not easy to document and therefore the communication of the results is inferior to other diagnostic approaches.

As an noninvasive alternative to color coded duplex Doppler US MR imaging has been introduced into clinical routine more than ten years ago revealing continuous improvements up to now. By using suitable examination sequences both angiomorphologic and perivascular informations can be obtained successfully with the MR technique promising a variety of advantages over US. Moreover, acquired functional quantitative MR based informations of blood flow allow a reliable evaluation of vascular pathologies.

Thus, this volume was planned to provide a comprehensive overview of the current state of the development in vascular MR imaging and MR angiography in order to demonstrate the clinical usefulness of this technique. In different chapters anatomic and physiologic informations of the normal arterial and venous system, a general description of different vascular diseases and its pathophysiology, the basic principles of physics in MR, flow-related and contrast-enhanced imaging techniques, informations of different MR contrast materials, display and postprocessing techniques, hardware conceptions and its recent developments, quantification of blood flow, and potential artifacts and limitations in MR angiography are presented. A well established concept of providing the clinical overview of MR angiography in different vascular areas includes chapters about the intra- and extracranial cerebral vasculature, the different arterial systems of the chest and the abdomen, and the arteries of the extremities. In addition, the venous systems of the body are presented in two chapters. Each chapter is systematically devided into a general introduction that includes alternative imaging modalities , a consideration of MR angiographic techniques, recommendations of suitable imaging protocols, a clinical part that refers to both anatomy and pathology, and a validation of the technique including the discussion of advantages and drawbacks of MR angiography, a comparison with other vascular imaging techniques, and a catalogue of generally accepted indications. A short conclusion at the end of each chapter characterizes the clinical and practical essentials for the area under consideration. A large number of representative MR angiograms based on current acquisition techniques is provided to illustrate normal and pathologic vascular findings. In two final chapters cuurent state and future of MR guided intravascular therapeutic procedures, and the evaluation of intravascular implants is provided in order to complete the topic of this volume.

In this respect, the book is primarily addressed to radiologists, angiologists, vascular surgeons, and neurosurgeons as well as to other physicians who are involved in vascular imaging and have only limited experience in vascular MR imaging.

Contents

1 The Vascular System: Normal and Pathologic Anatomy and Hemodynamic Principles

INGOLF P. ARLART and CURT DIEHM

CONTENTS

1.1 Anatomy of the Vascular System

1.1.1 Arterial System

1.1.1.1 Supraaortic Arteries

(ABRAMS et al. 1983; NETTER et al. 1989, KADIR et al. 1991, UFLACKER et al. 1997)

1.1.1.1.1 Neurovascular Extracranial Arteries (Figs. 1.1a, b)

The main extracranial arteries are the right and left vertebral arteries and the right and left common carotid arteries, which bifurcate into the external carotid artery (ECA) and the internal carotid artery (ICA) at the level of C3-C6. Major branches of the ECA are the superior thyroid artery, the ascending pharyngeal artery, the facial artery, the lingual artery, the occipital artery – with an ascending pharyngeal and posterior auricular segment – the posterior auricular artery, the superficial temporal artery, and the internal maxillary artery, including a mandibular, pterygoid and pterygopalatine segment. The ICA ascends medial and anterior to the internal jugular vein before entering the carotid canal of the petrous bone. The carotid siphon has five segments in its extradural and intradural portion:

a. Meningohypophyseal trunk
b. Inferolateral trunk
c. McConnell's capsular artery
d. Ophthalmic artery
e. Superior hypophyseal branch and posterior communicating branches

Several important extra- and intradural branches of these arteries may form anastomoses with the ECA branches.

The vertebral arteries normally ascend through the foramen tranversarium from C6 to C1 and pass intradurally medial to the capsule of the atlanto-occipital joint through the foramen magnum. The basilar artery (BA) is formed by the junction of the two vertebral arteries. Important branches of the vertebral artery are those to the anterior spinal artery (C2-C6 level), an odontoid branch (C1-C2 level), and to the origin of the anterior spinal artery.

1.1.1.1.2 Neurovascular Intracranial Arteries (Figs. 1.2–1.4)

The ICA through the posterior communicating branches, the anterior cerebral artery (ACA), the middle cerebral artery (MCA), and its perforating branches provides the arterial supply of the cerebrum. The branches of the ACA are the anterior communicating artery, perforating branches to the medial striate group, the recurrent artery of Heubner, the pericallosal artery, the frontopolar artery, the orbitofrontal artery, the callosomarginal artery, the internal parietal arteries, and the triple callosal artery. For the MCA these are perforating branches to the lateral striate group, cortical branches to the

I.P. ARLART, MD
Radiologisches Institut Stuttgart, Katharinenhospital, Kriegsbergstrasse 60, 70174 Stuttgart, Germany
C. DIEHM, MD
Klinikum Karlsbad-Langensteinbach, Guttmannstrasse 1, 76307 Karlsruhe, Germany

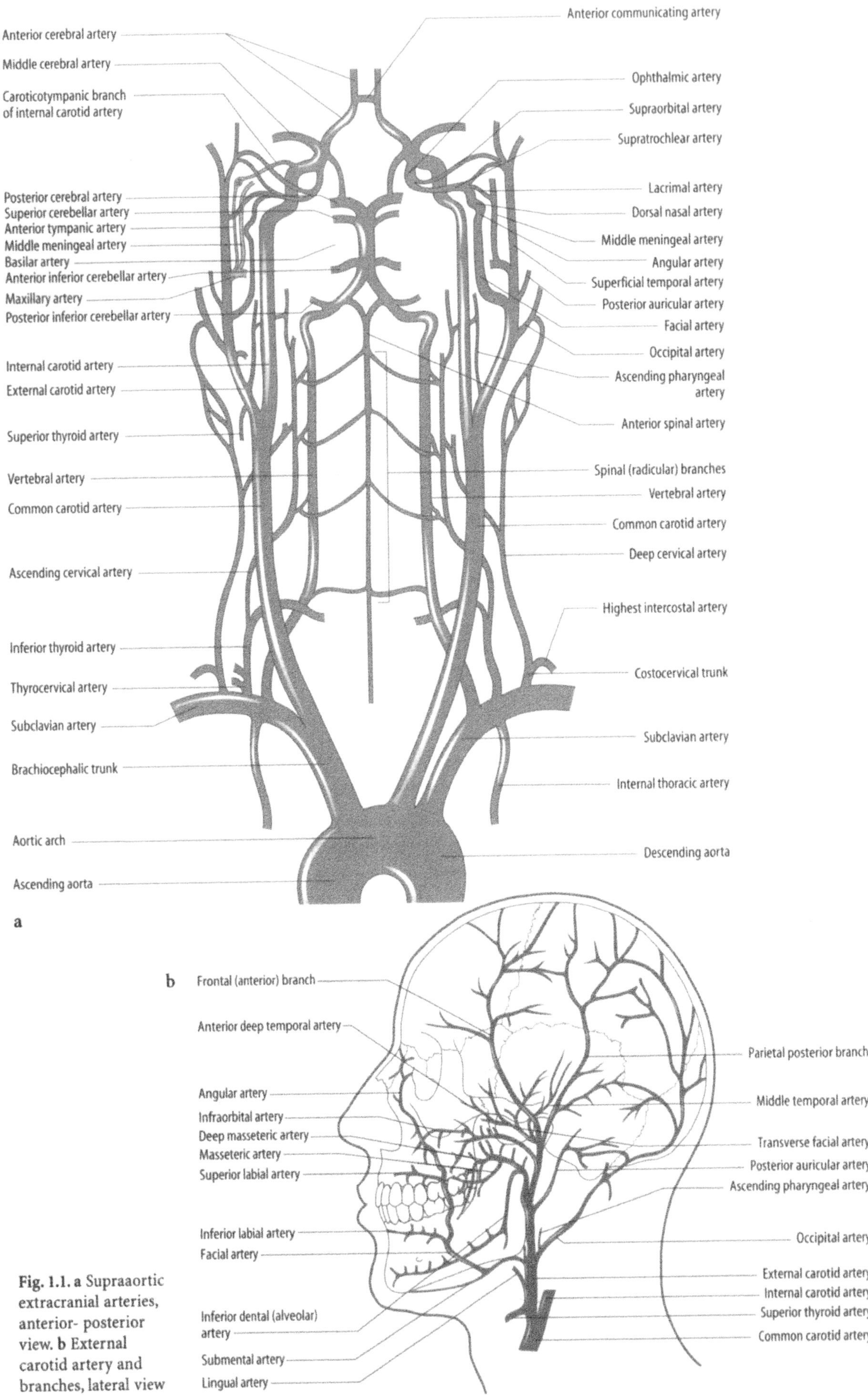

Fig. 1.1. a Supraaortic extracranial arteries, anterior- posterior view. **b** External carotid artery and branches, lateral view

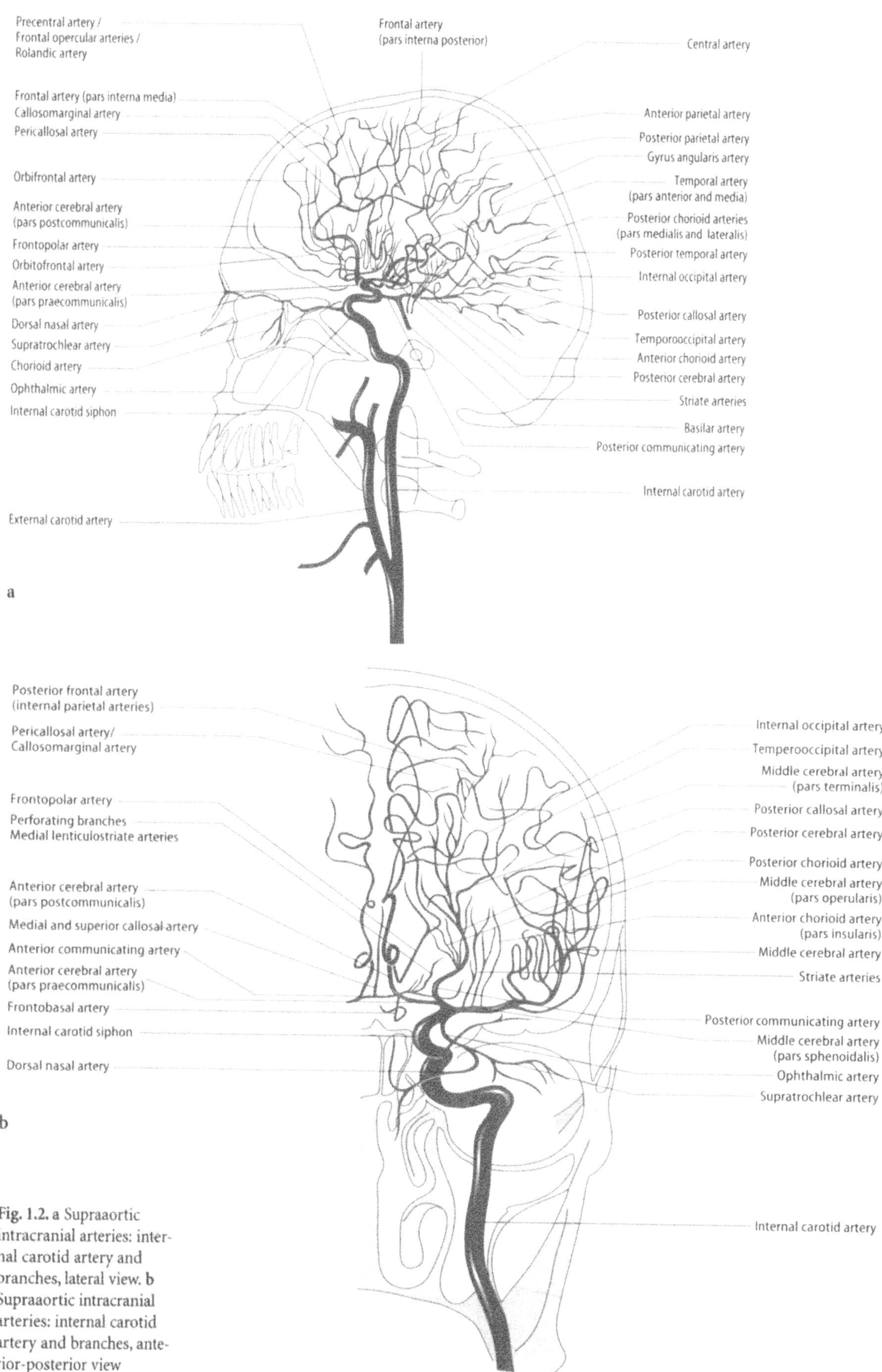

Fig. 1.2. a Supraaortic intracranial arteries: internal carotid artery and branches, lateral view. **b** Supraaortic intracranial arteries: internal carotid artery and branches, anterior-posterior view

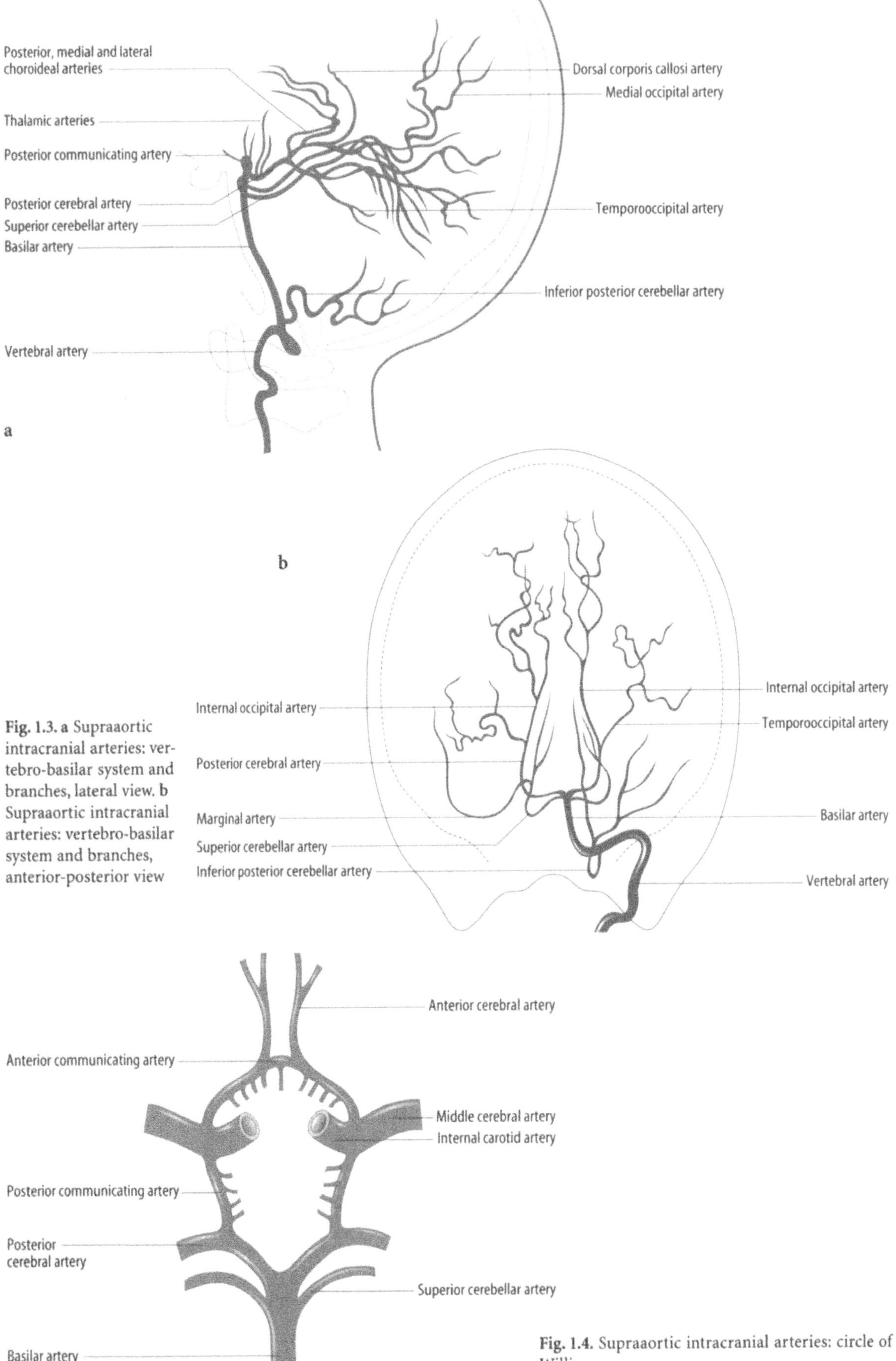

Fig. 1.3. a Supraaortic intracranial arteries: vertebro-basilar system and branches, lateral view. **b** Supraaortic intracranial arteries: vertebro-basilar system and branches, anterior-posterior view

Fig. 1.4. Supraaortic intracranial arteries: circle of Willis

orbitofrontal and temporopolar areas, orbitofrontal branches, opercular branches, pre-rolandic branches, rolandic branches, posterior parietal branches, angular branches, and posterior temporal branches.

The arterial supply of the posterior fossa via the vertebral artery includes perforating vessels to the brainstem, the anterior spinal artery, the posterior inferior cerebellar artery (PICA), and the posterior meningeal artery. Arterial supply via the BA includes perforating vessels, the posterior cerebral artery (PCA), the superior cerebellar artery, and the anterior inferior cerebellar artery (AICA). Branches of the PCA are perforating vessels to the brainstem, the medial posterior choroidal artery, meningeal branches (Davidoff-Schechter), the thalamogeniculate artery, the lateral posterior choroidal artery, and cortical trunks.

The ICA and BA have important anastomoses in the suprasellar cistern termed the circle of Willis. A complete, intact circle occurs only in less than 20% of cases. Arterial portions that comprise the circle of Willis are the left and right ACA, the anterior communicating artery, the left and right posterior communicating arteries, and the left and right PCA.

1.1.1.2 Aortic Arch (Figs. 1.1a, 1.5)

The three main branches of the aortic arch are the brachiocephalic (innominate) artery, which divides into the right subclavian and right common carotid arteries, the left common carotid artery, and the left subclavian artery. Variants include a common origin of the brachiocephalic and left common carotid arteries (22%), a left vertebral artery from the aortic arch (6%), a thyreoidea ima artery (6%), an aberrant right subclavian or brachiocephalic artery (1%), a right aortic arch, a ductus diverticulum, and other miscellaneous anomalies.

1.1.1.3 Arteries of the Upper Extremities (Fig. 1.6)

The right subclavian artery originates from the brachiocephalic artery, the left subclavian artery from the aortic arch. Branches of the subclavian artery are the vertebral artery, the thyreocervical trunk, the internal mammary artery, and the costocervical trunk. The subclavian artery continues as the axillary artery. Branches of the axillary artery are the superior thoracic artery, thoracoacromial artery, lateral thoracic artery, subscapular artery, and circumflex humeral artery. The axillary artery continues as the brachial artery which trifurcates into the radial, ulnar, and interosseous arteries. The radial and ulnar arteries feed the deep and superficial palmar arch. The deep arch is complete in 95%–97% of cases, the superficial arch in 78%. Branches of the palmar arches are the palmar metacarpal arteries and the common palmar digital arteries.

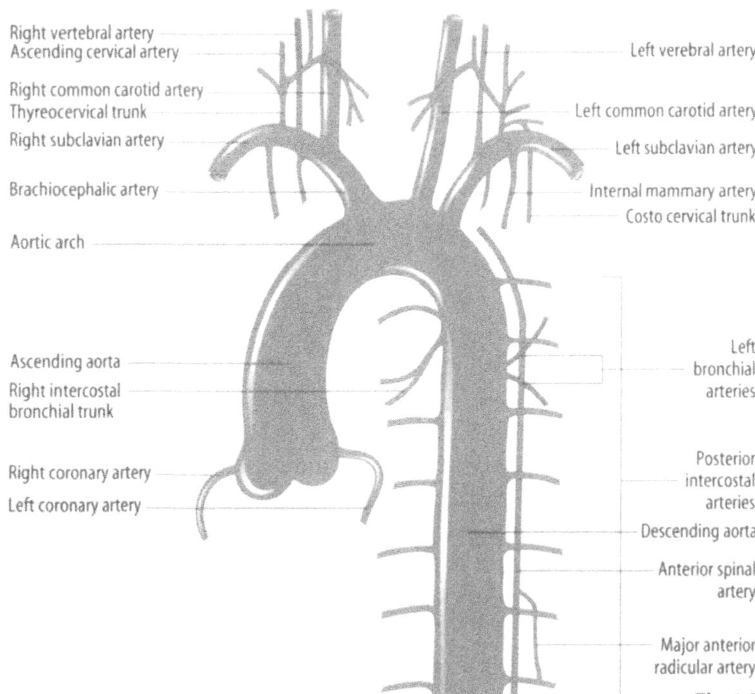

Fig. 1.5. Aortic arch and main branches, LAO view

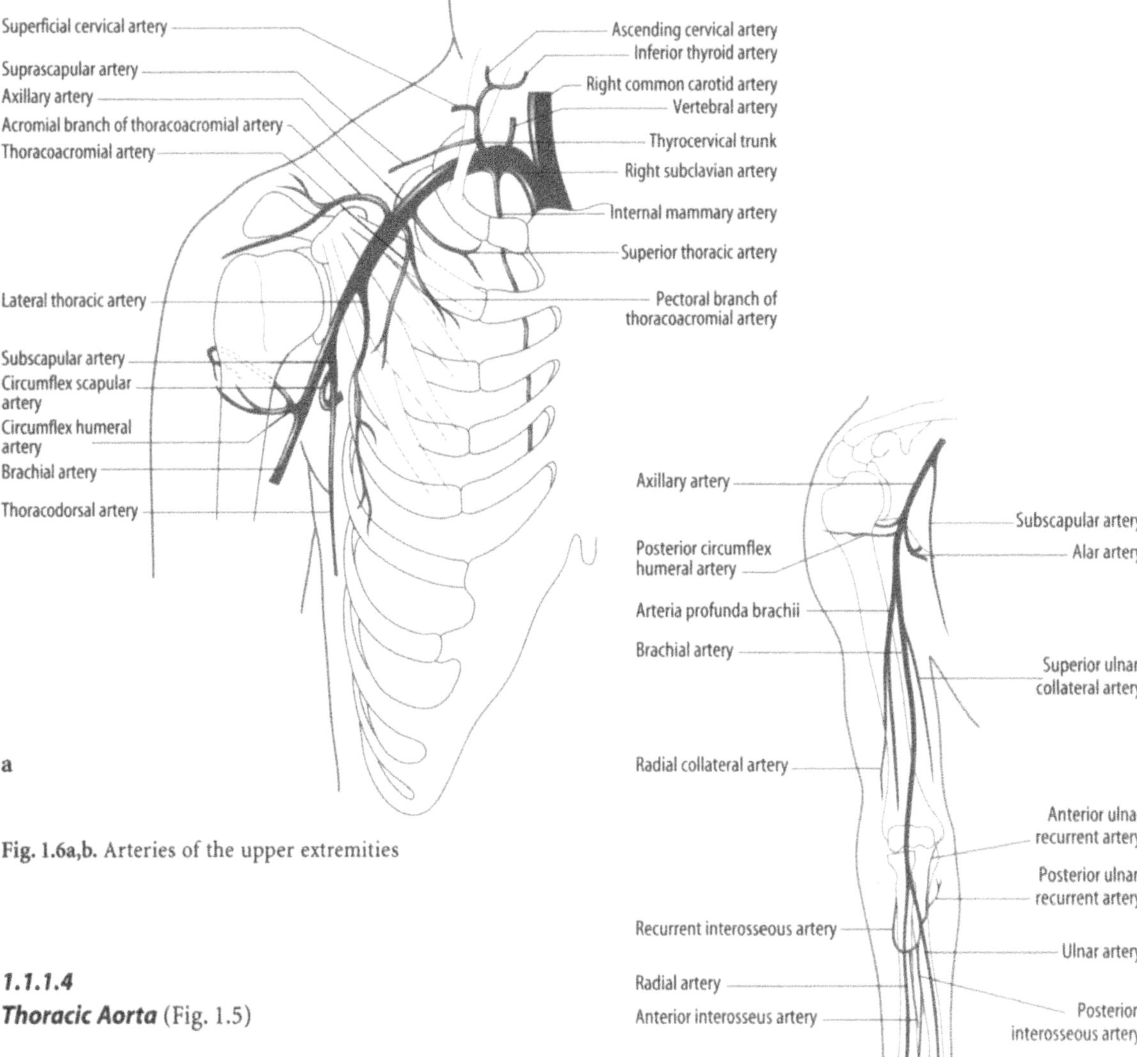

Fig. 1.6a,b. Arteries of the upper extremities

1.1.1.4
Thoracic Aorta (Fig. 1.5)

The thoracic aorta courses within the mediastinal space and separates into a right ascending portion, a left aortic arch, and a left descending portion. This condition can be observed in approx. 70% of individuals.

1.1.1.4.1
Ascending Aorta and Coronary Arteries (Fig. 1.7a, b)

The ascending aorta originates from the left ventricle of the heart and ends with the origin of the brachiocephalic artery. The normal diameter ranges from 1.5 to 2.5 cm.

The right coronary artery (RCA) arises from the right sinus of Valsalva and can be divided into a proximal portion (with a horizontal course in most cases), a middle portion, and a distal segment. The first ventricular branch of the RCA is the conus artery; marginal branches arise from the middle portion, and the distal portion divides into a posterior interventricular and posterior left ventricular artery. The left coronary artery (LCA) originates from the left sinus of Valsalva and normally bifurcates into the left anterior descending (LAD = left anterior interventricular artery) and left circumflex artery (LXA). The LAD has epicardial, septal, and atrial branches, and a terminal right and left ventricular branch. It is usually the longest artery going to the apex. The LXA runs within the left atrioventricular groove and typically branches off to the left circumflex marginal arteries. There is a great variability in the termination of the RCA, LAD, and LXA.

1.1.1.4.2
Descending Aorta

The normal diameter of the descending aorta ranges from 1.5 to 2.5 cm. The intercostal and subcostal arteries, the bronchial arteries (common origin of a right bronchial and intercostal artery in over 70%), the spinal arteries (anterior and posterior branches), the esophageal arteries (4–5 in number), and the superior phrenic arteries arise from the descending aorta.

In 75% of cases the major anterior radicular artery (artery of Adamkiewicz) arises between T9 and T12 from the left posterior intercostal artery. Its origin can vary between T5 and L2.

1.1.1.5
Pulmonary Vessels

1.1.1.5.1
Pulmonary Arteries (Fig. 1.8a)

The main pulmonary artery is located intrapericardially and divides to form the left and right pulmonary artery. The right pulmonary artery divides into an upper lobe artery with three segmental arteries (apical, posterior, and anterior), a middle lobe artery with two segmental arteries (medial and lateral), and a lower lobe artery with five segmental arteries (cardial, apical, anterior-lateral, posterior-lateral, and posterior-basal). The left pulmonary artery divides into an upper lobe artery

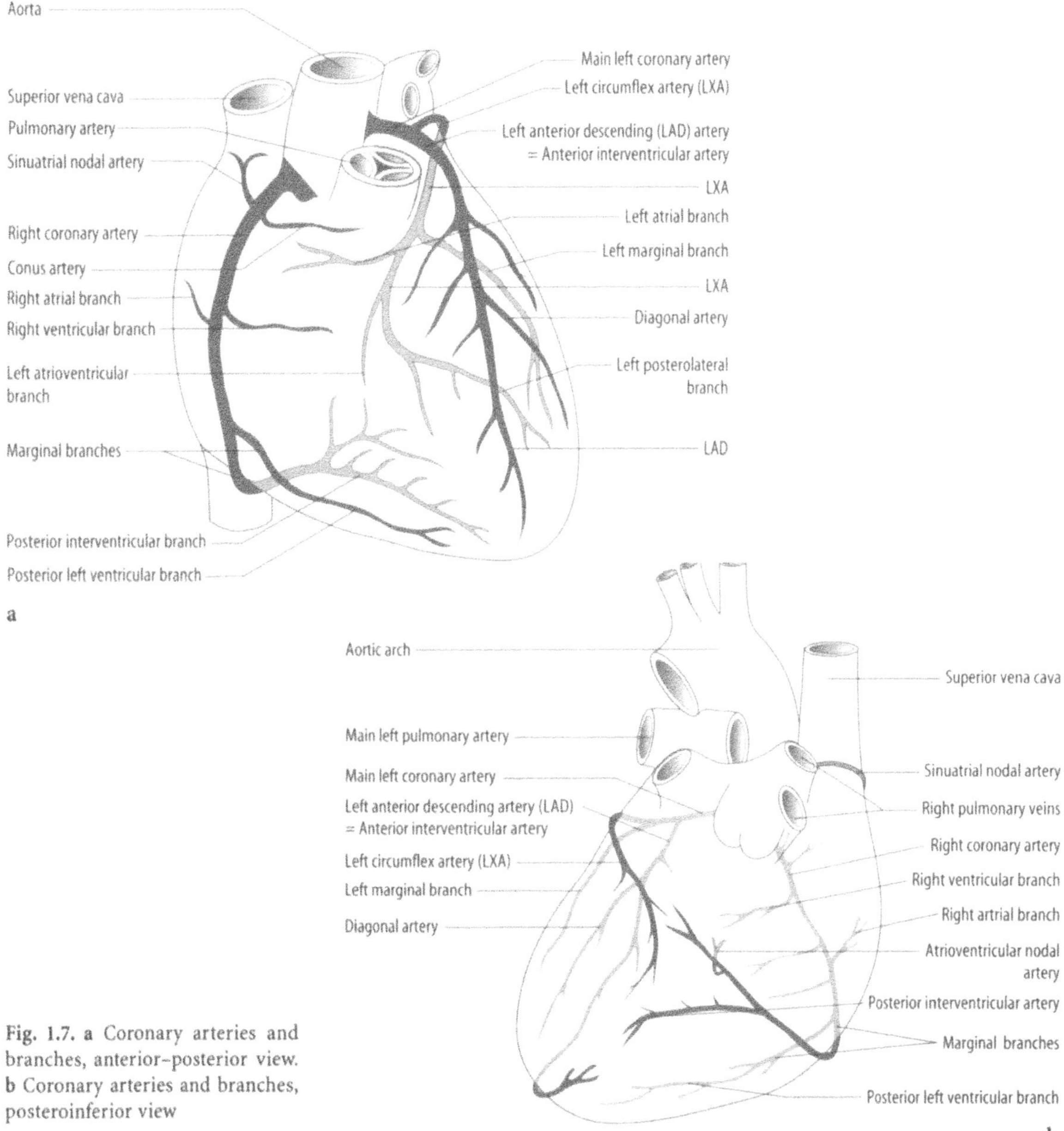

Fig. 1.7. a Coronary arteries and branches, anterior–posterior view. **b** Coronary arteries and branches, posteroinferior view

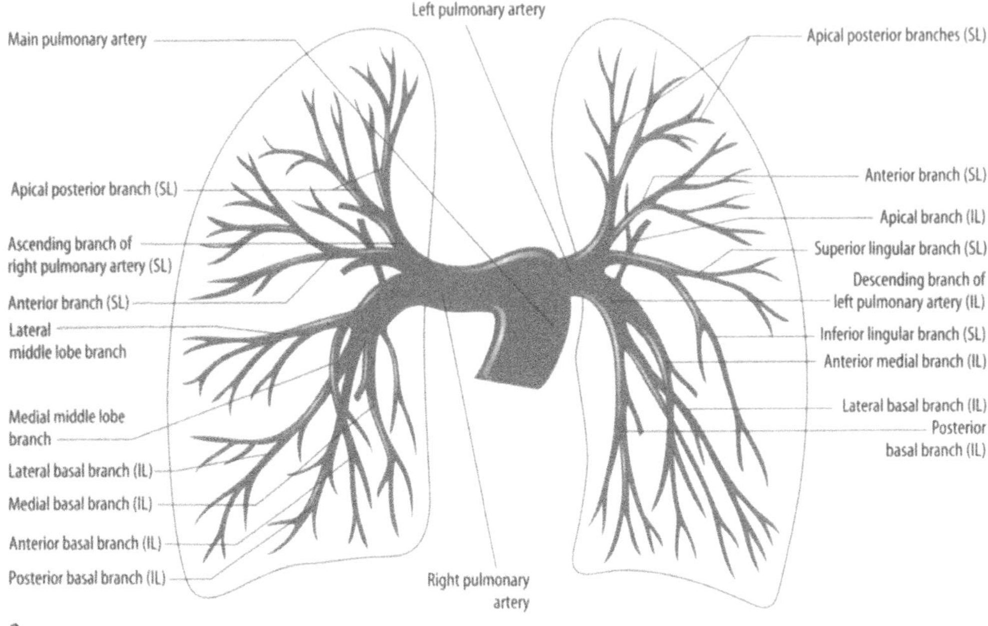

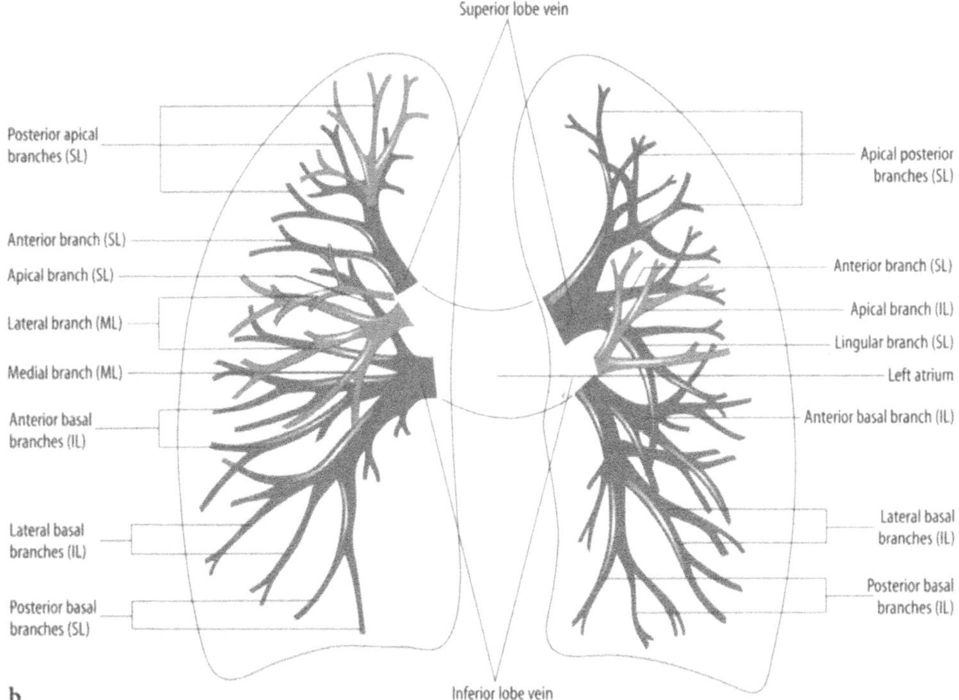

Fig. 1.8. a Pulmonary arteries and branches, anterior-posterior view. **b** Pulmonary veins and tributaries, anterior-posterior view

with five segmental branches (apical-posterior, anterior, superior lingular, and inferior lingular) and a lower lobe artery with four segmental arteries (apical, anterior-basal, posterior-lateral, and posterior-basal).

1.1.1.5.2
Pulmonary Veins (Fig. 1.8b)

The right lung is drained by four branches of the superior and three branches of the inferior pulmonary vein. The left lung is also drained by two sets of pulmonary veins. The left and right pulmonary veins drain separately into the left atrium.

1.1.1.6
Abdominal Aorta and Branches (Figs. 1.9a, b)

The abdominal aorta courses within the retroperitoneal space; the normal diameter ranges from 1.5 to 2.5 cm. The branches from proximal to distal are the inferior phrenic arteries, the celiac artery,

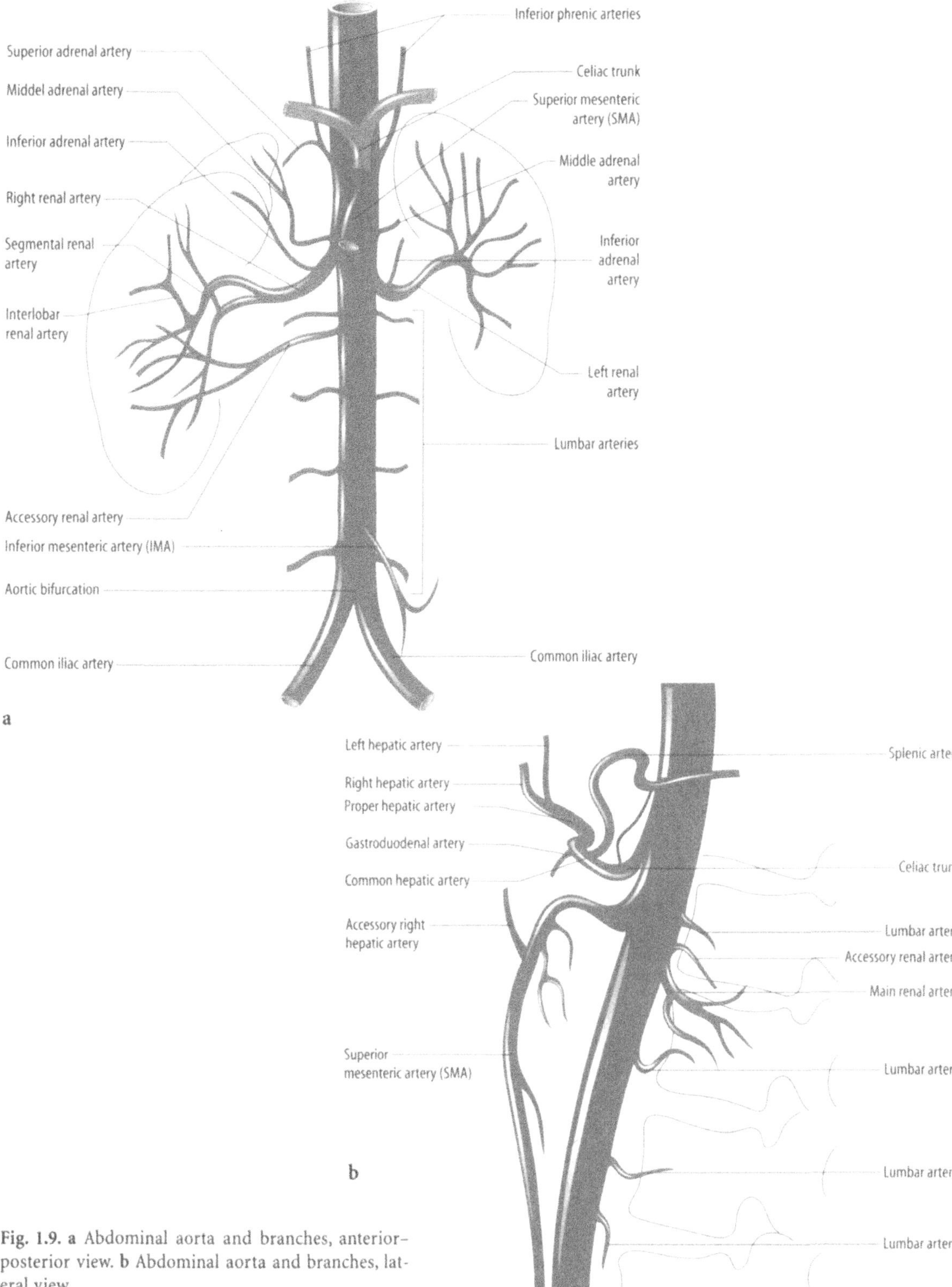

Fig. 1.9. a Abdominal aorta and branches, anterior-posterior view. **b** Abdominal aorta and branches, lateral view

the superior mesenteric artery (SMA), the renal arteries, and the inferior mesenteric artery (IMA). Lumbar arteries arise in pairs from the abdominal aorta in each of the five segments. The abdominal aorta bifurcates at the L4 or L5 level into the iliac arteries.

1.1.1.6.1 Celiac Artery (Fig. 1.10)

The celical artery arises from the T12-L1 level and typically branches in over 70% of cases into the splenic artery, left gastric artery, and common hepatic artery. In more than 55% of cases the common

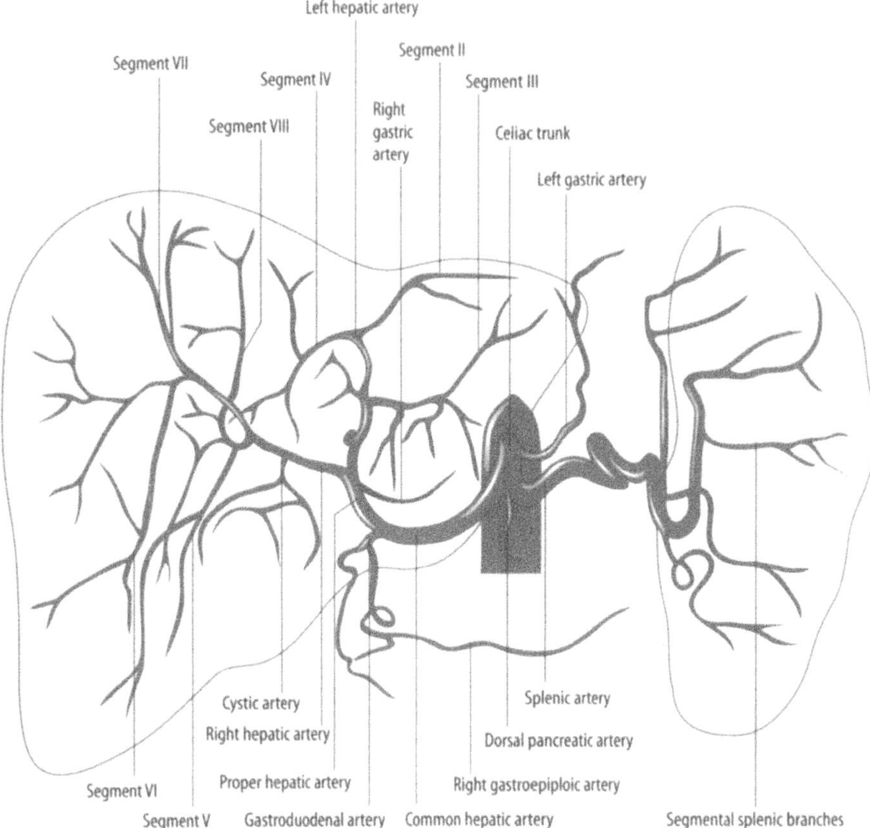

Fig. 1.10. Celiac artery and branches, anterior–posterior view

hepatic artery divides into a right and left hepatic artery, and in approx. 75% the left hepatic artery arises from the proper hepatic artery. The right hepatic artery may arise in up to 10% of cases from the SMA; the branches are the cystic and biliary arteries. The gastroduodenal artery arises from the common hepatic artery in approx. 75% of cases; the branches are the supraduodenal artery, the right gastroepiploic artery, and the anterior and posterior superior pancreatico-duodenal arteries that show pancreatico-duodenal arcades and anastomose with the inferior pancreatico-duodenal arteries, providing a connection between the celiac artery and the SMA. Major branches of the splenic artery are the pancreatic arteries, the posterior and short gastric arteries, and the left epiploic artery.

1.1.1.6.2
Mesenteric Arteries (Figs. 1.11, 1.12)

Main branches of the SMA are the inferior pancreatico-duodenal arteries, jejunal and ileal arteries, the middle and right colic artery, the ileocolic artery, and variants. The IMA commonly arises from the anterolateral aorta at L3 and divides into the left colic artery, sigmoid arteries, and the superior hemorrhoidal artery. Communications between the inferior and superior mesenteric arteries are the arc of Bühler and the arc of Riolan.

1.1.1.6.3
Renal Arteries (Fig. 1.9a)

The renal arteries originate from the aorta at the L1-L2 level in approx. 75% of individuals. In about 60% the renal arteries divide into segmental arteries at the renal hilus. Multiple renal arteries can be observed unilaterally in about 30% and bilaterally in 12% of cases. Approx. 10% are accessory vessels and 20% are aberrant arteries.

1.1.1.7
Iliac Arteries (Fig. 1.13)

The right and left common iliac arteries bifurcate into the right and left external and internal iliac arteries. The branching pattern of the internal iliac artery can vary. Commonly, an obturator artery, an inferior and superior gluteal artery, an internal pudendal artery, visceral branches, an iliolumbar artery, and lateral sacral arteries can branch off.

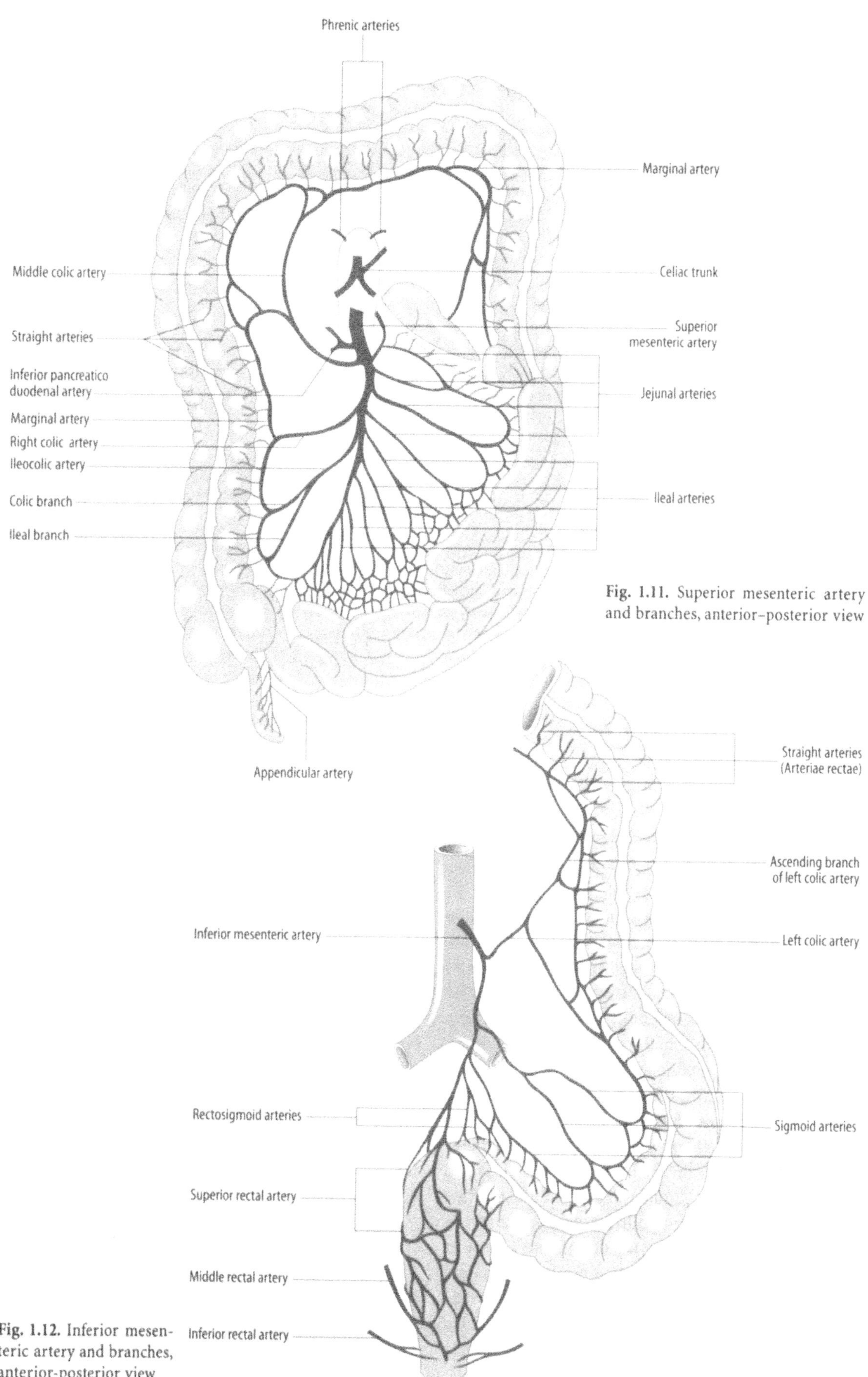

Fig. 1.11. Superior mesenteric artery and branches, anterior–posterior view

Fig. 1.12. Inferior mesenteric artery and branches, anterior-posterior view

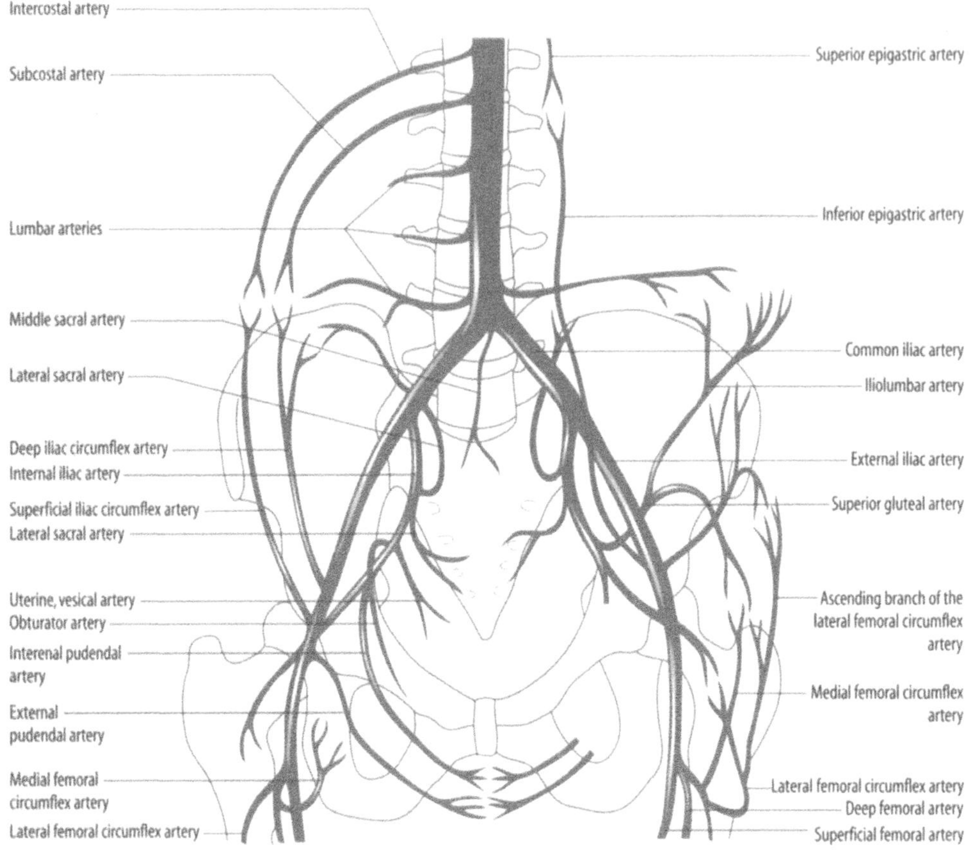

Fig. 1.13. Pelvic arteries and branches, anterior-posterior view

1.1.1.8
Arteries of the Lower Extremities (Fig. 1.14)

The external iliac artery continues as the common femoral artery below the inguinal ligament and bifurcates into the superficial and deep femoral artery. In 60% of cases the deep femoral artery exists as a single trunk; in 40% a branching pattern can be observed. Potential collaterals are present to form branches of the deep femoral artery to the distal portion of the superficial femoral artery and the popliteal artery. The popliteal artery can separate into a proximal, middle, and distal portion and divides in 95% into the lower leg arteries at the lower margin of the popliteal muscle. Typically, the distal portion of the popliteal artery bifurcates proximally into the tibiofibular trunk and the anterior tibial artery; the tibiofibular trunk divides into the fibular artery and the anterior tibial artery. The anterior tibial artery continues as the dorsal artery of foot and the arcuate artery of foot. The arcuate artery itself divides into four dorsal metatarsal arteries. The posterior tibial artery continues as the lateral plantar artery, forming the plantar arch together with two deep plantar branches from the dorsal artery of foot.

1.1.2
Venous System (Abrams 1983; Netter 1989; Kadir 1991; Uflacker et al. 1997)

1.1.2.1
Veins of the Head and Neck (Figs. 1.15a, b, 1.16)

The deep cerebral venous system drains into the inferior sagittal sinus and straight sinus. Branches of the deep venous system are the anterior caudate vein, thalamostriate vein, internal cerebral vein, inferior ventricular vein, basal vein of Rosenthal, and the vein of Galen. Veins of the posterior fossa drain into the vein of Galen, the petrosal sinuses, the straight sinus, the occipital sinus, and the transverse sinuses. Branches of the superficial cerebral venous system are the vein of Trolard, the superficial middle cerebral vein, and Labbé's vein.

The extracranial facial venous system drains via the external and internal jugular vein and has anastomoses with deep extra- and intracranial venous structures.

The brain drains into a superficial and a deep venous system. Both are drained via the dural sinuses. Commonly, ten different dural sinuses can be dis-

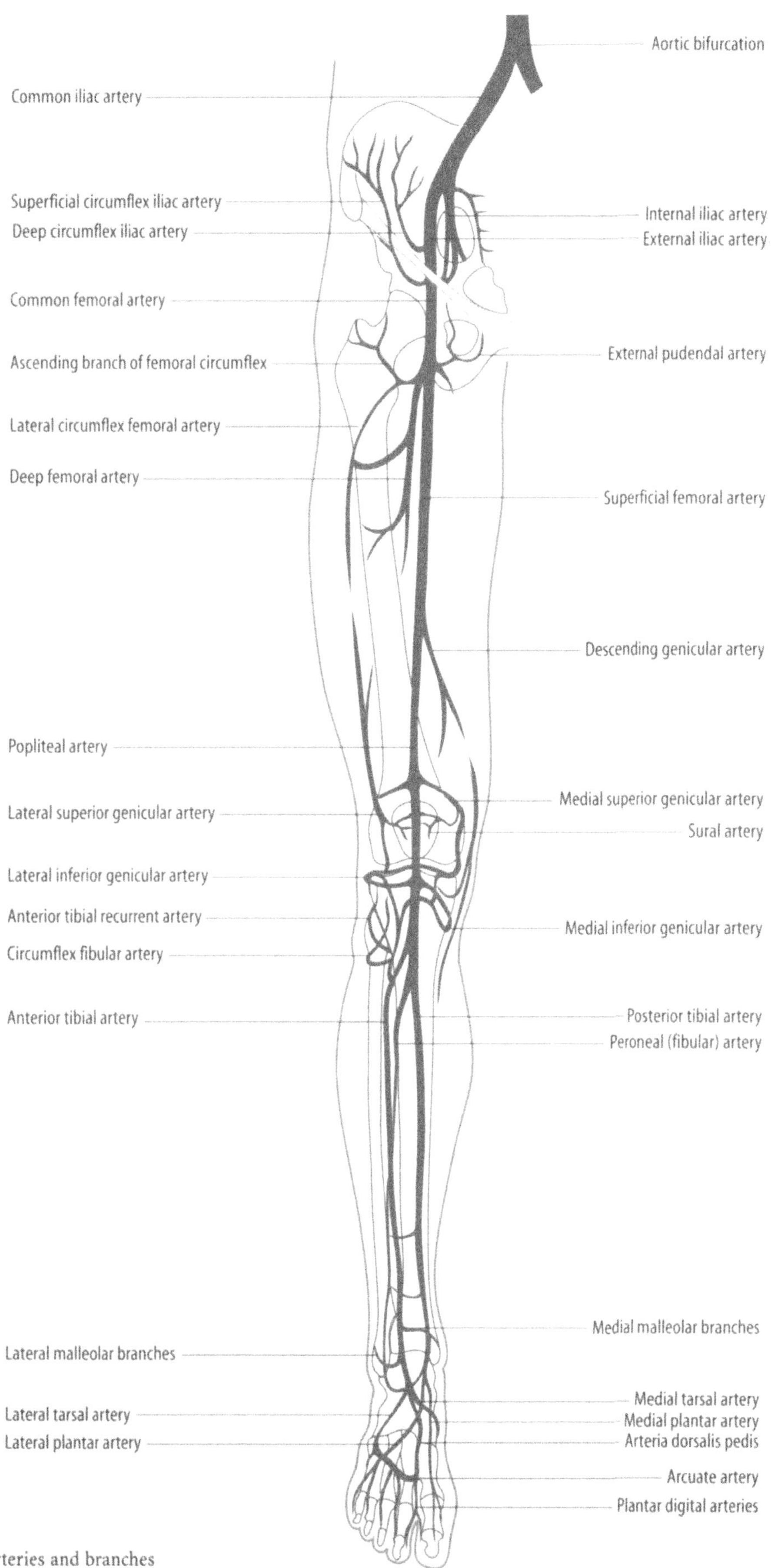

Fig. 1.14. Lower extremity arteries and branches

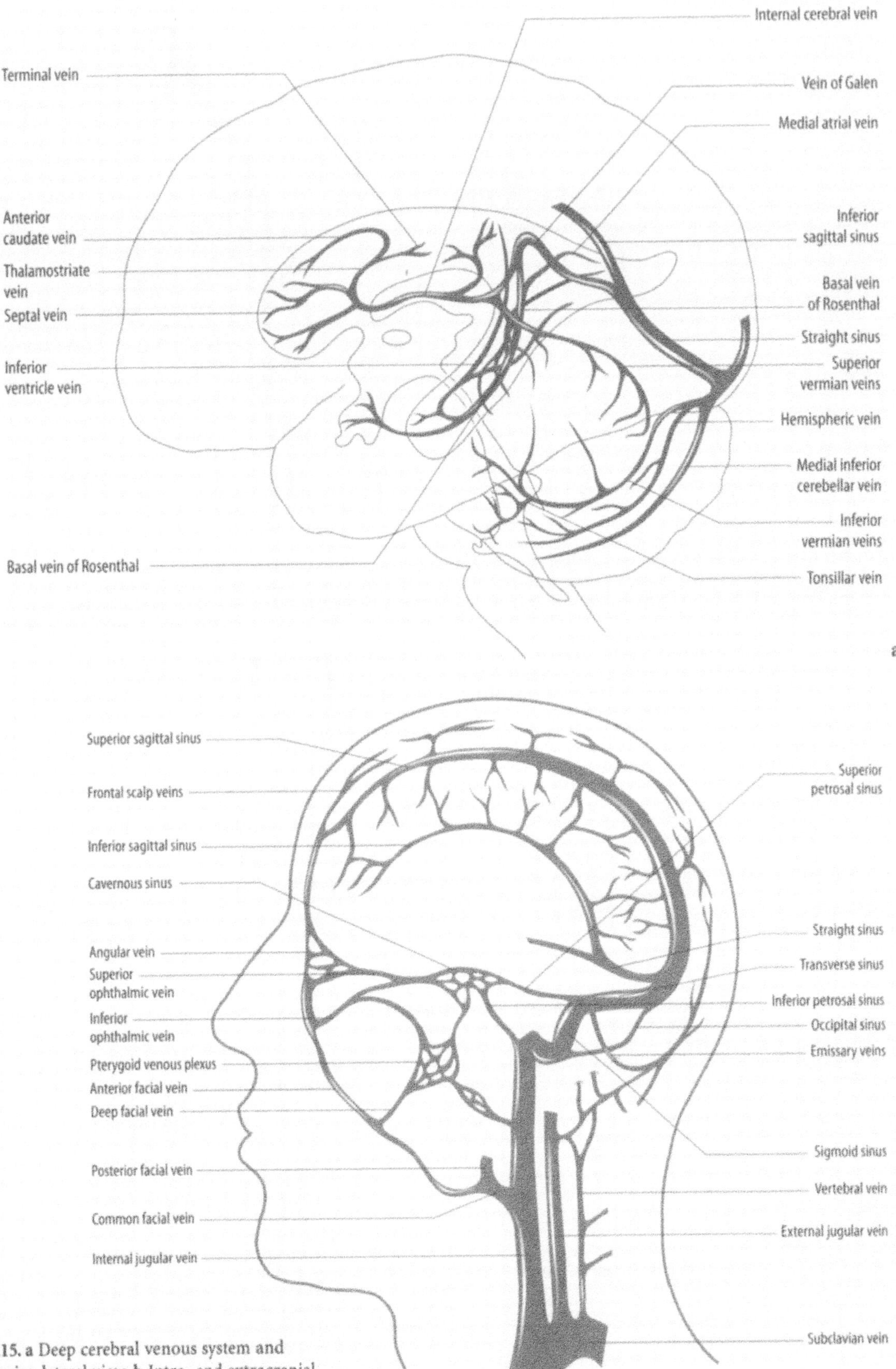

Fig. 1.15. **a** Deep cerebral venous system and tributaries, lateral view. **b** Intra- and extracranial facial venous system and tributaries, lateral view

Fig. 1.16. Central chest veins and tributaries, anterior-posterior view

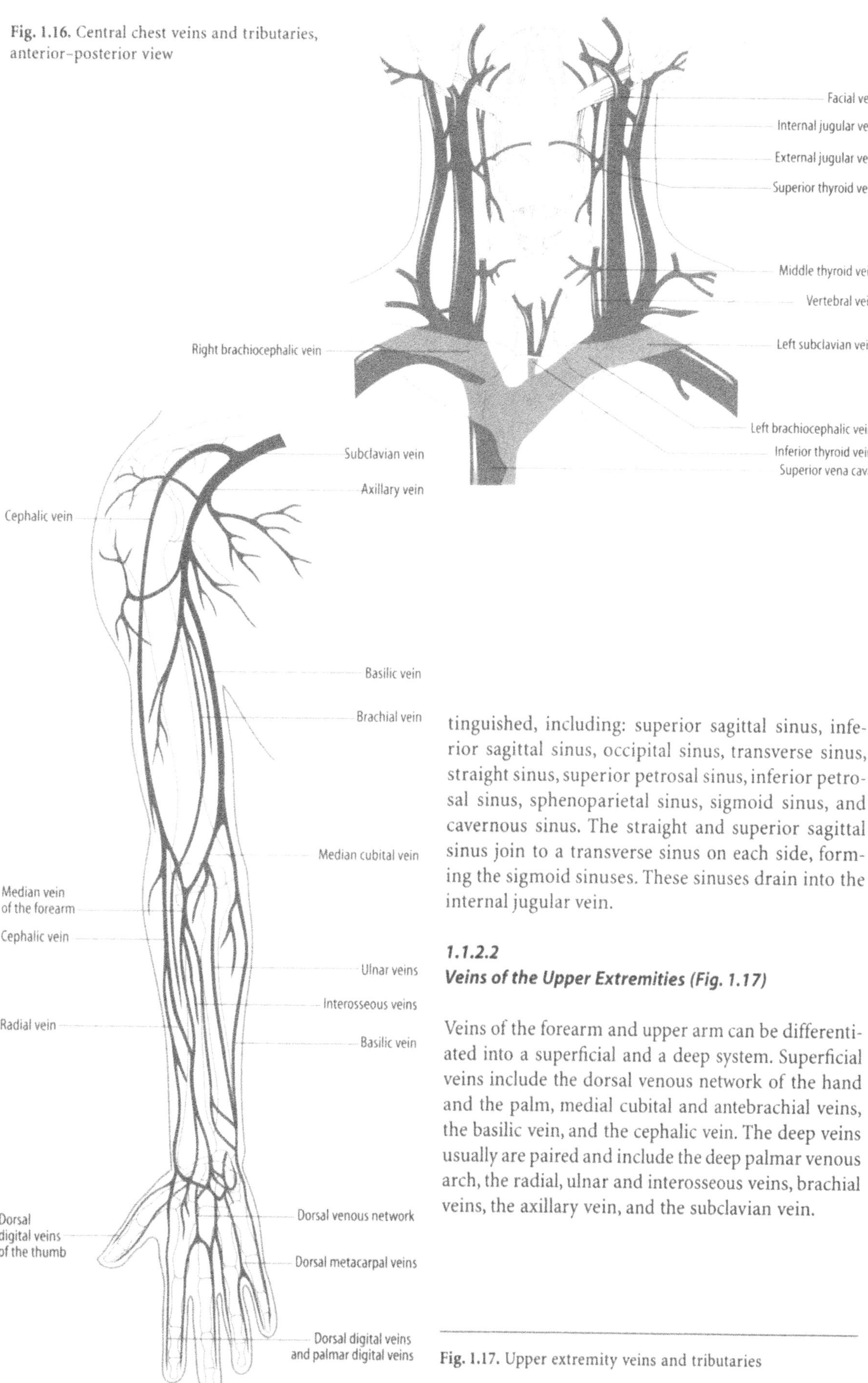

tinguished, including: superior sagittal sinus, inferior sagittal sinus, occipital sinus, transverse sinus, straight sinus, superior petrosal sinus, inferior petrosal sinus, sphenoparietal sinus, sigmoid sinus, and cavernous sinus. The straight and superior sagittal sinus join to a transverse sinus on each side, forming the sigmoid sinuses. These sinuses drain into the internal jugular vein.

1.1.2.2 Veins of the Upper Extremities (Fig. 1.17)

Veins of the forearm and upper arm can be differentiated into a superficial and a deep system. Superficial veins include the dorsal venous network of the hand and the palm, medial cubital and antebrachial veins, the basilic vein, and the cephalic vein. The deep veins usually are paired and include the deep palmar venous arch, the radial, ulnar and interosseous veins, brachial veins, the axillary vein, and the subclavian vein.

Fig. 1.17. Upper extremity veins and tributaries

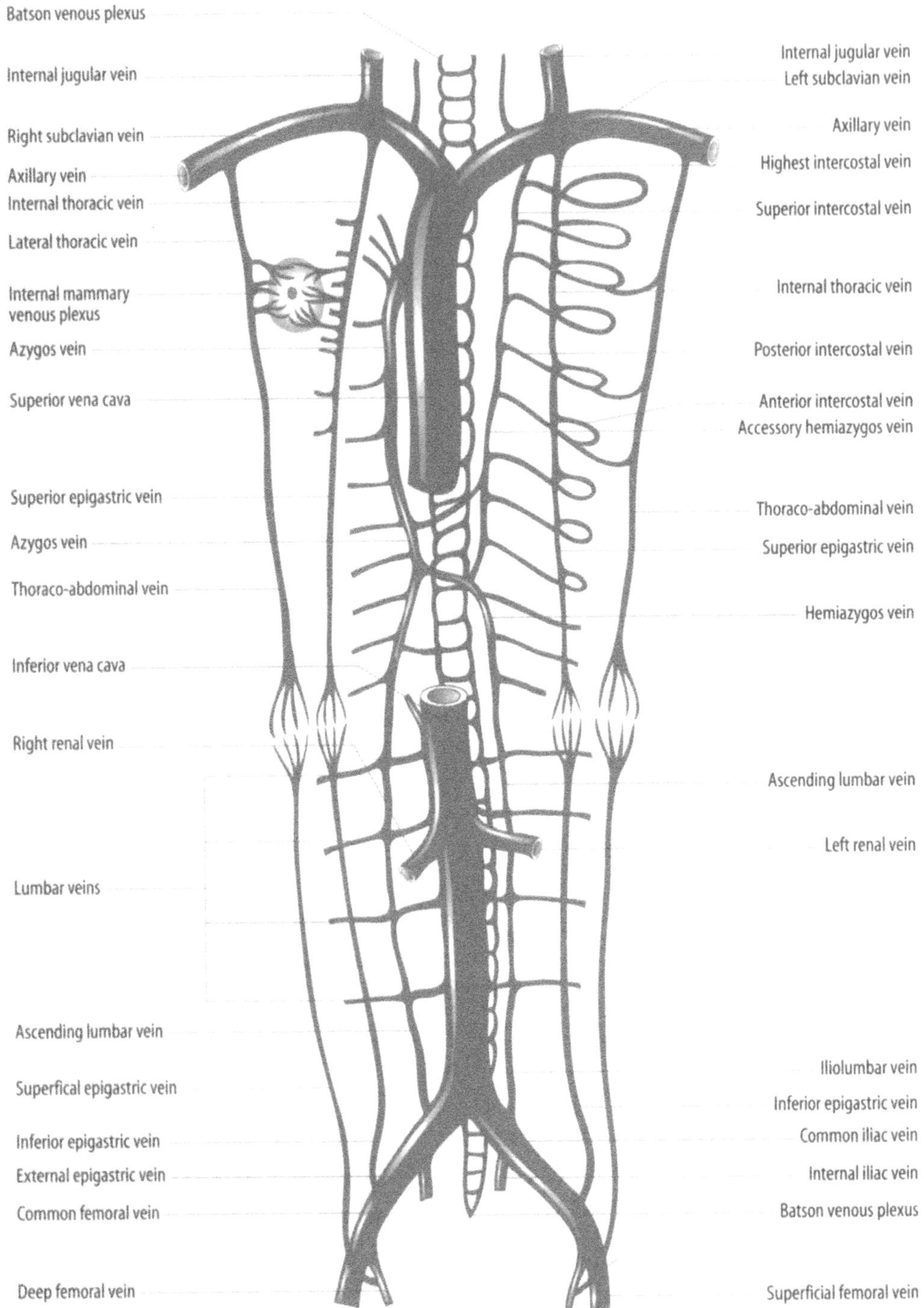

Fig. 1.18. Venae cavae, azygos-hemiazygos system, and potential collateral pathways

1.1.2.3 Central Chest Veins, Venae Cavae, and Azygos-Hemiazygos System (Figs. 1.18, 1.19)

The superior vena cava (SVC) is formed by the junction of the two brachiocephalic (innominate) veins. The lower part of the SVC lies within the pericardium. Its major tributary is the azygos vein which drains into the SVC at the level of T4-T5. Major tributaries of the azygos vein include the hemiazygos-accessory hemiazygos vein, the right superior intercostal vein (2–4), the right posterior intercostal vein (5–11), esophageal veins, mediastinal veins, pericardial veins, and right bronchial veins.

The azygos vein is formed by the right ascending lumbar vein; the hemiazygos vein is formed by the

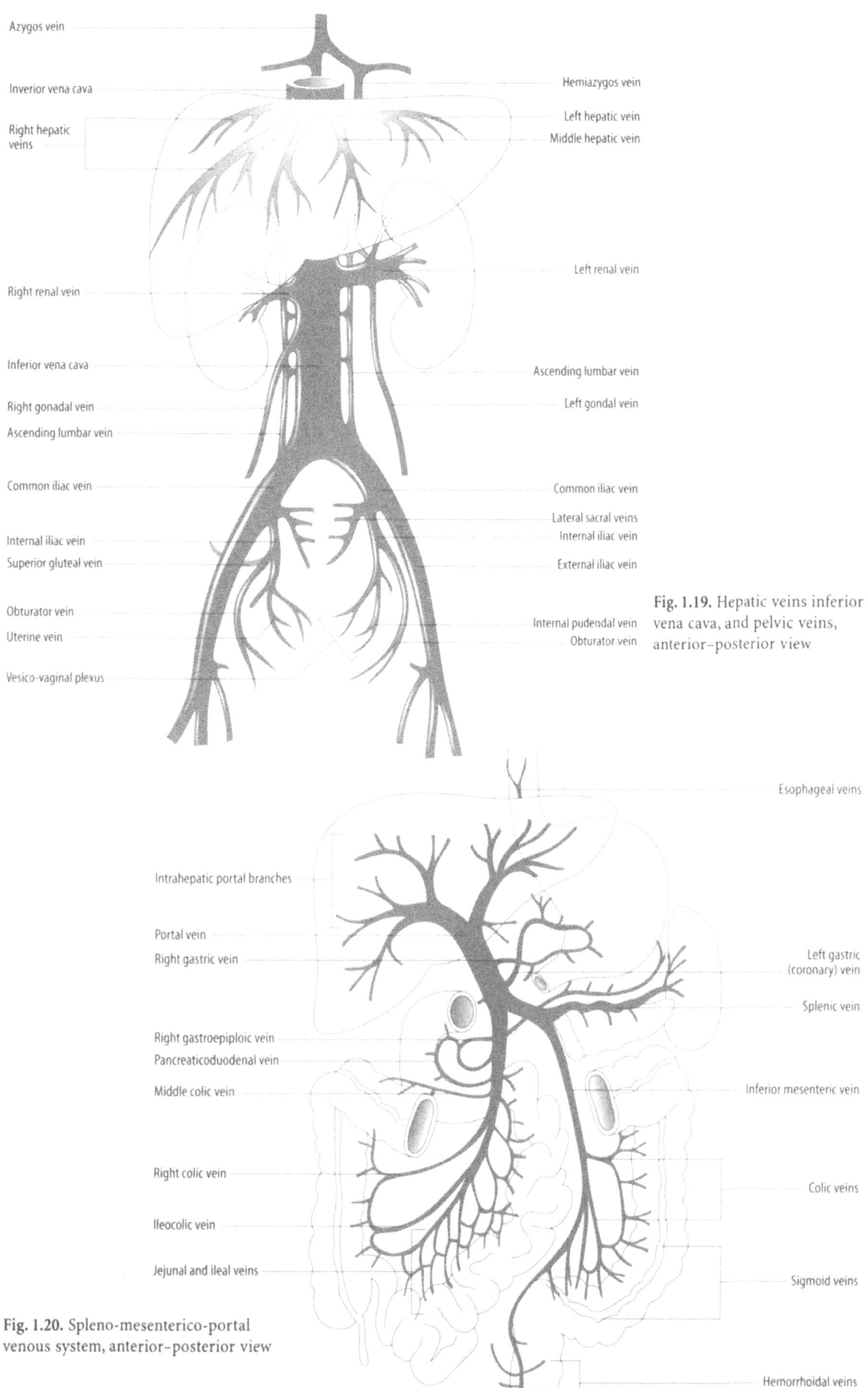

Fig. 1.19. Hepatic veins inferior vena cava, and pelvic veins, anterior–posterior view

Fig. 1.20. Spleno-mesenterico-portal venous system, anterior–posterior view

left ascending lumbar vein. The ascending lumbar veins originate from the common iliac veins and connect with the iliolumbar and lumbar veins. The lumbar veins drain the vertebral plexus. The inferior vena cava (IVC) is formed by the junction of the common iliac veins at the L5 level. At the T9 level the IVC enters the right atrium. The main tributaries of the IVC are the ascending lumbar veins, renal veins, adrenal veins, gonadal veins, inferior phrenic veins, and hepatic veins.

1.1.2.4 Spleno-mesenterico-portal System (Fig. 1.20)

The portal system collects the blood from the gastrointestinal tract. The hepatic perfusion is formed to 75%–80% by the portal venous blood; the hepatic veins provide the entire venous outflow through the IVC into the right atrium. The extrahepatic portal vein is formed by the confluence of the splenic

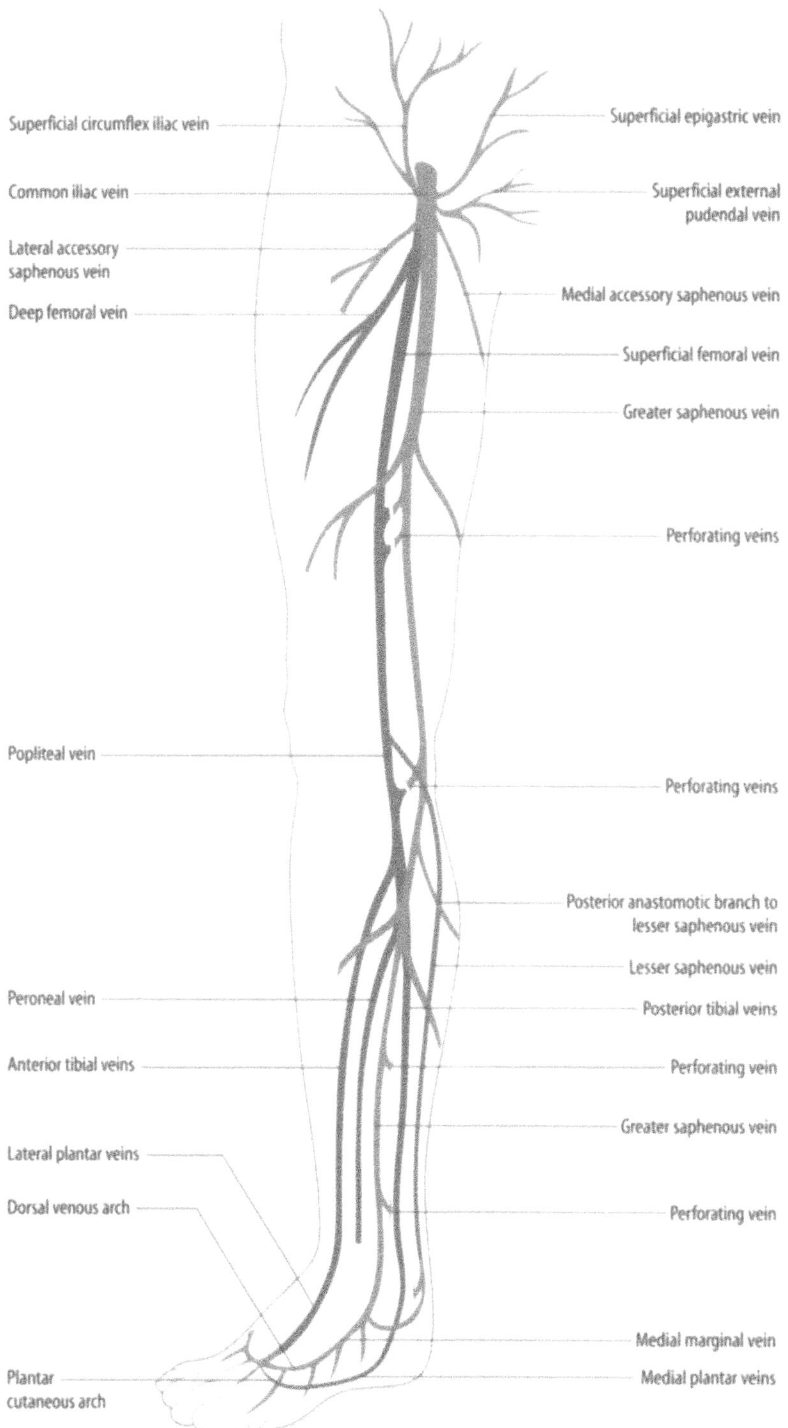

Fig. 1.21. Lower extremity venous systems

and superior mesenteric veins. The major segmental branches of the SMV drain the jejunum, ileum, right and transverse colon, and pancreaticoduodenal region. Major tributaries of the splenic vein are the inferior mesenteric vein, left gastric vein, short gastric vein, gastroepiploic vein, and pancreatic veins.

1.1.2.5
Veins of the Lower Extremities and Pelvis (Figs. 1.19, 1.21)

The veins of the lower extremity can be divided into a superficial and a deep system. The superficial system includes the four dorsal metatarsal veins and the dorsal venous arch, continuing into the greater and lesser saphenous vein. The deep system begins at the plantar metatarsal veins, forming the deep plantar venous arch, and continues into the posterior tibial veins. The anterior tibial veins are a direct continuation of the dorsal venous arch. The peroneal veins originate from multiple tributaries at the ankle. These three deep veins of the calf are mostly paired and continue via the popliteal vein and superficial femoral vein into the external iliac vein. Frequently, distal anastomoses are present between the superficial and deep femoral vein. The calf muscles drain via the soleus and gastrocnemius veins and of the thigh muscles via branches of the deep femoral vein. The venous confluence of the greater saphenous vein, the superficial and the deep femoral vein is located below the inguinal ligament.

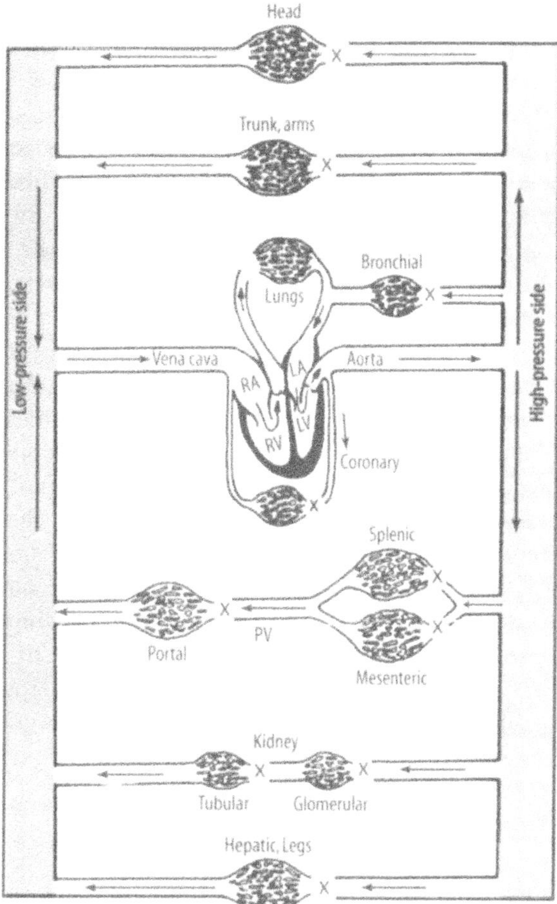

Fig. 1.22. Schematic of the circulation: through parallel routes the circulation passes from the aorta to the vena cava (*RA*, right atrium; *LA*, left atrium; *RV*, right ventricle; *LV*, left ventricle; *PV*, portal vein). From Burton AC (1972) Physiology and biophysics of the circulation, 2nd edn. Year Book, Chicago)

1.2
Physiology of Blood Flow

With respect to anatomy and function, the vascular system can be divided into a high-pressure side, which is the arterial system, including arteries of the elastic type (large central arteries), arteries of the muscular type (small arteries, and arterioles), a pre-/post capillary (resistive vessels) and capillary system, and a low-pressure side, which is the venous system, including larger venules and large veins (Fig. 1.22).

The blood circulation of the human body has two different responsibilities: to maintain the nutritive and the metabolic function of the entire organism. This is regulated by a central (neural, humoral) and a local (metabolites, hypoxia, thermal influences) mechanism (Burton 1972; Caro et al. 1978; Milnor 1982).

1.2.1
Vessel Wall and Regulatory Mechanisms of Blood Circulation

1.2.1.1
Arterial Vessel Wall

The anatomy of the arterial wall shows different morphological characteristics, depending on function, localization, and diameter, which lead to a separation into arteries of the elastic type and muscular type and arterioles. Typically, the arterial wall is compact and stiff in structure, which prevents vascular collapse. The arterial wall includes five different layers:

a, Intimal tunica
b. Internal elastic membrane
c. Medial tunica
d. External elastic membrane
e. External tunica (adventitia)

The intimal tunica is represented by a single layer of endothelium, the medial tunica by spindle-like smooth muscle cells, and the adventitia by collagen fibers and bundled smooth muscle cells. Large central arteries of the body such as the aorta, subclavian arteries, common carotid arteries, common iliac arteries, and the pulmonary trunk belong to the elastic type, in which the media consists of a network of thick, fenestrated lamellae in concentric layers. Small arteries and arterioles have the function of resistive vessels and consist of particular layers of smooth muscle fibers. In arterioles, which are called precapillary resistive vessels, the wall of arterioles contains smooth muscle bundles and shows a separate myogeneous component with spontaneous rhythmic motion, i.e., the basal tonus of the vessel wall. The tonus is regulated by vasoconstrictive and vasodilatative vegetative nerve fibers via catecholamines and acetylcholine. Arterioles in which the perfusion pressure decreases control blood flow of the different capillary areas and regulate the peripheral circulation.

1.2.1.2
Venous Vessel Walls

Similar to that of the arteries, the wall structure of veins varies, depending on location. However, compared with the arterial wall, the venous wall is thin, the layers are loose in structure, and the venous lumen may collapse under low or negative intravascular pressure conditions. Particularly in larger veins of the lower extremities, the intima shows longitudinal smooth muscle cells which may influence the vascular tonus. Venous valves are formed by intimal folds with a network of collagen fibers. The media of the venous vessel wall consists of a loose or compact ring-shaped, spiral-shaped, or longitudinal layer of smooth muscle cells and a network of collagen and elastic fibers. The loose external tunica merge into the surrounding fiber tissue. The adventitia consists of collagen fiber tissue and some smooth muscle fibers as well.

1.2.1.3
Regulatory Mechanisms

The peripheral blood circulation is controlled by a regulation system of neural and humoral factors located centrally and peripherally. The cortical and bulbar vasomotoric center regulates the distribution of blood. Baro- and chemoreceptors and both oxygen and carbon dioxide influence the activity of the vasomotoric center. Nerve fibers with a vasoconstrictor function belong to the adrenergic (norepinephrine) system, those with vasodilatating function to the cholinergic (acetylcholine) system. The two receptor types (α- and β-receptors) react differently to catecholamines: α-receptors on cutaneous vessels, β-receptors on vessels of the muscle.

Besides the central regulation of the peripheral circulation, local mechanisms exist which can dominate the central mechanisms under certain conditions. Locally produced vasoactive substances (metabolites) may cause vasodilatation by directly influencing the vessels, for instance, under conditions of physical work or stress. On the other hand, the body temperature can be maintained at a constant level by the cutaneous circulation when the surrounding temperature changes.

1.2.2
Arterial Blood Flow

The large arteries of the trunk have the exclusive function of transporting the blood, whereas the parenchymal arteries are responsible for the nutrition of organs and the maintenance of metabolic function (kidneys, lungs) and/or electromechanical function (myocardium, muscles). In the physiology of the arterial system, the status of the vascular wall and biophysical principles (such as heart rate, flow volume, pressure gradient, pulsatility etc.) play an important role in addition to the central and local regulatory mechanisms already mentioned.

1.2.2.1
The Nature of Arterial Blood Flow

(Milnor 1982; Skalak et al. 1981; Sumner 1989; Nichols and O'Rourke 1990; Turitto and Goldsmith 1992; Zierler 1994)

The oxygenated blood volume which is ejected by the left ventricle into the aorta has to circulate back via the venous system to the right atrium after passage through parenchymal organs, the gastrointestinal tract, and the musculoskeletal system. Myocardial function, left ventricular volume, and heart rate determine both the stroke volume and the cardiac output. According to the *principle of Starling*, cardiac output is controlled by venous return of blood to the heart and depends on it. Thus, an increase in venous backflow increases the heart rate, and a decrease in venous backflow reduces the heart rate.

Different types of arterial blood flow exist, such as flow through large arteries of the elastic type, flow through smaller arteries of the muscular type, flow through the capillary bed (perfusion), and flow at a molecular level (diffusion).

Arterial hemodynamics are determined by the perfusion pressure, which in turn depends on the stroke volume of the left ventricle, the local vascular resistance, and the velocity of blood flow (run off) in the peripheral arteries. A difference in pressure between two points (pressure gradient) actually causes the blood to flow. Velocity profiles show a typical behavior and are determined by pulsatile flow movement, the pressure gradient, the vascular diameter, the vascular resistance, the viscosity of blood, the viscoelastic vessel wall, and the shear forces between blood and vessel wall.

The basic consideration of blood which is flowing in the vascular system involves certain physical laws which govern the flow of liquids in cylindrical tubes. In this context the principles of Poiseuille, Ohm, Bernoulli, and Laplace are of major importance.

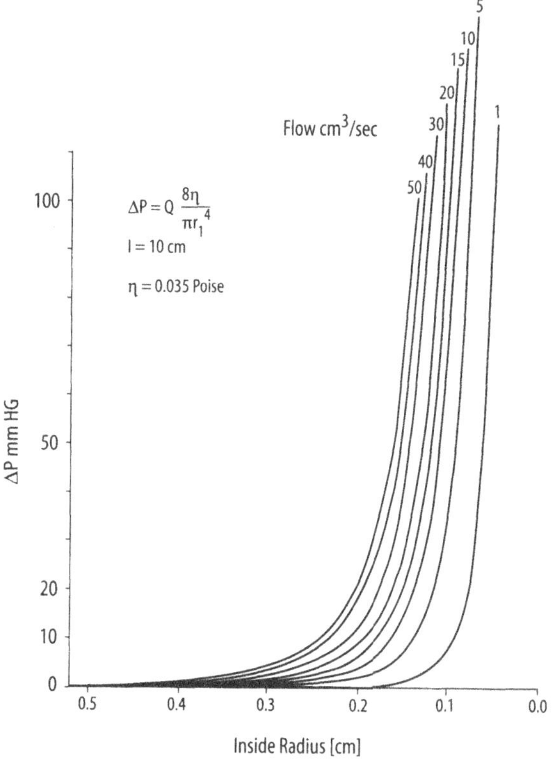

Fig. 1.23. Arterial hemodynamics: relationship between inside radius and pressure drop for various rates of steady laminar flow through a cylindric tube 10 cm in length. From Strandness DE Jr (1975) Hemodynamics for surgeons. Grune and Stratton, Orlando

1.2.2.1.1
Flow Volume and Vascular Impedance

Steady flow in a cylindrical tube is described by the *Poiseuille equation*, which states that the pressure drop along a tube between two points (P1-P2) is directly proportional to the length of the tube (L), the rate of flow volume (f), and the viscosity of the fluid (n), and inversely proportional to the fourth power of the internal radius (r). To maintain a steady flow, there must be a constant head of pressure (P) applied to the fluid because of its viscosity or internal friction. Thus, flow volume (f) at a constant rate depends on the viscosity, the vessel radius, and the vessel length according to the equation:

$$f = \frac{\Pi r^4 (P_1 - P_2)}{8\eta L}$$

The Poiseuille principle acts in vitro under conditions of steady flow rate, a homogeneous fluid, constant viscosity, no slip at the wall, laminar flow, a long and rigid tube, and a constant tube diameter (Fig. 1.23).

However, this equation is not directly applicable to the complex structure of human circulation, which shows an inhomogeneous content of blood fluid, pulsatile blood flow, elasticity of the vessel wall, and a vessel radius which decreases towards the periphery.. Under living conditions, blood can only be considered as a homogeneous fluid with a viscosity that is independent of the velocity gradient in large arteries and veins, whereas in vessels with an internal radius of less than 0.5 mm changes in apparent viscosity occur which influence flow: an increase in viscosity occurs with a decrease in vessel diameter. Only in vessels which are so small and numerous that their dimension can only roughly be measured can the Poiseulle equation be applied, whereas in vessels as large as the proximal arterioles, in which flow is still pulsatile and diameter changes with larger changes in internal pressure, it has been suggested that flow is proportional to the third (not fourth) power of radius.

The different factors which determine vascular resistance between the aorta and right atrium have to be considered specifically as do the velocity profiles and pressure/flow relationships under pulsatile flow conditions.

Flow volume (f) also can be determined by the inverse relationship between pressure gradient (P1-P2) and vascular resistance (R) (see the Ohm equation): f = (P1–P2) / R.

The relationship between pulsatile pressure and pulsatile flow in an artery feeding a particular vascular bed is determined by the vascular impedance.

Four types of impedance have been defined: longitudinal, input, characteristic, and terminal impedance. Longitudinal impedance is the ratio of pressure gradient to flow and is thus the pulsatile analog of longitudinal arterial resistance. Input impedance is the ratio of pressure and flow at a particular arterial site, which may be regarded as the input to the entire vascular tree beyond this site. Characteristic impedance is the relationship between pressure and flow in an artery in which pressure and flow waves are not influenced by wave reflection. Terminal impedance is the opposition to flow at the termination of the vascular bed immediately upstream from this termination. This termination is taken to represent the high-resistance arterioles.

By determining the heart rate (normally about 5000 ml/min and 83 ml/s, respectively), the flow volume of blood can be calculated. Of the flow volume leaving the left ventricle, approx. 25% runs to the head and upper limbs, 40% through the large abdominal branches, and 25% through the termination of the aorta. The distribution of blood flow is demonstrated in Table 1.1

Table 1.1. Distribution of blood flow in humans at rest (Nichols and O'Rourke 1990)

Circulation	Blood flow (ml/min)	(% total)
Splanchnic (liver, intestines, spleen)	1.400	24
Renal	1.100	19
Cerebral	750	13
Coronary	250	4
Skeletal muscle	1.200	21
Skin	500	9
Other organs	600	10
Total	5.800	100

1.2.2.1.2 Vascular Resistance

Throughout the vascular bed, the total fluid resistance may be regarded as the resistance of the arteries, arterioles, capillaries, and veins in a series. Depending on the number of resistive vessels in different vascular areas of the body, the regional vascular resistance is different.

The large arteries contribute approx. 10%, the arterioles 60%, the capillaries 15%, and the veins 15% to the total peripheral resistance. The vascular resistance is minimal in the cerebral and mesenteric system or the kidneys and maximal in the extremities.

Following the *Ohm principle*, the vascular resistance can be expressed by the ratio of pressure gradient (P1-P2) and flow volume (f), and is indicated by R

$$R = \frac{P_1 - P_2}{f} \text{ and } P_1 - P_2 = R \cdot f$$

Using both the Ohm equation and the Poiseuille equation, the vascular resistance can be expressed as:

$$R = \frac{8\eta L}{\Pi r^4}$$

As the resistance is proportional to the drop in mean pressure, it is apparent that the resistance of the arteries constitutes the largest proportion of the whole. When mean arterial pressure is calculated normally with 100 mmHg, it decreases little in the large arteries, up to 60 mmHg in the arterioles immediately proximal to the capillaries, 30 mmHg in the capillaries at the proximal end, and 10 mmHg at the distal end.

On the basis of the Ohm equation, the total peripheral resistance can be determined by the pressure difference between aorta and right atrium (i.e., perfusion pressure) when P1 = 100 mmHg and P2 = 5 mmHg:

$$R = P1 - P2/f = 95 \text{ mmHg}/83 \text{ ml/s} = 1.1$$

This total resistance, which acts against flowing blood on the way from the aorta to the right atrium, is a net resistance of all existing single resistances. When the organ-specific blood volumes per minute are known, each partial resistance can be determined. Normal values of total vascular resistance are presented in Table 1.2 on the basis of the Poiseuille equation. Values are calculated using the aortic and right atrium pressures and main pulmonary artery and left atrial (or wedge) pressures.

Table 1.2. Normal values of total vascular resistance (dyne-s/cm^5) at rest (Nichols and O'Rourke 1990)

Vascular bed	Total vascular resistance (Mean)	(SD)
Systemic	1344 (1268)	183 (161)
Pulmonary	194 (88)	34 (17)

1.2.2.1.3 Intravascular Pressure and Flow Velocity

The hemodynamics of the circulation can be described basically by the *Bernoulli principle* and are deduced from the principle of the conservation of energy. For steady, nonviscous, noncompressive fluid flow within a tube, the energy consists of three parts:

a. Pressure energy,
b. Kinetic energy
c. Potential energy in a gravitational field

Following the Bernoulli equation, the total of frontal and lateral pressure within a tube is constant. The lateral pressure against the wall varies inversely with the flow velocity. The energy which regulates the velocity (v) of blood flow in horizontal position can be expressed as follows:

$$e = P + 1/2\ qv^2 \quad (q = \text{density})$$

which means that the total of intravascular pressure (P) and kinetic energy (e) remains constant.

Basically, the Bernoulli principle is only valid in vitro if energy loss by friction can be neglected. However, it can also be applied to unsteady flows. The difference between impact and lateral pressure in an artery is totally dependent on the square of the linear flow velocity and can be calculated from the Bernoulli equation. The greatest differences between impact and lateral pressure occur when the flow velocity is high during exercise or when the artery is narrowed. The impact pressure includes the kinetic energy which is imported to the blood at a high flow velocity. The most important clinical use of the Bernoulli equation is in Doppler cardiography to calculate the pressure gradient across a narrowed part of the cardiovascular system.

The blood flow at a certain point is the product of average velocity (v1, v2=velocity at point 1,2) and cross sectional area (a). Following the Bernoulli principle, flow velocity in a tube is the same at any two points and can be expressed as follows:

$$v_1 \cdot a_1 = v_2 \cdot a_2 \text{ or } v_2 \left(\frac{r_2}{r_1}\right)^2 \quad (r = \text{vessel radius})$$

Blood flow velocity (v) varies directly with the flow volume (f) and inversely with the vessel diameter (d) according to the equation:

$$v = f/d$$

In the case of a constant vessel diameter, a decrease in blood flow leads to a decrease in flow velocity. That means, velocity is a function of $1/d^2$. For instance, in a 75% vessel narrowing, velocity of blood flow through the stenosis is increased fourfold. Furthermore, flow velocity is controlled by the vascular resistance and varies directly with the intravascular pressure gradient. The pressure gradient is generated by the pumping action of the heart and the elasticity of major vessels. Thus, flow velocity is maximal in large diameter vessels and less in branching vessels (Fig 1.24).

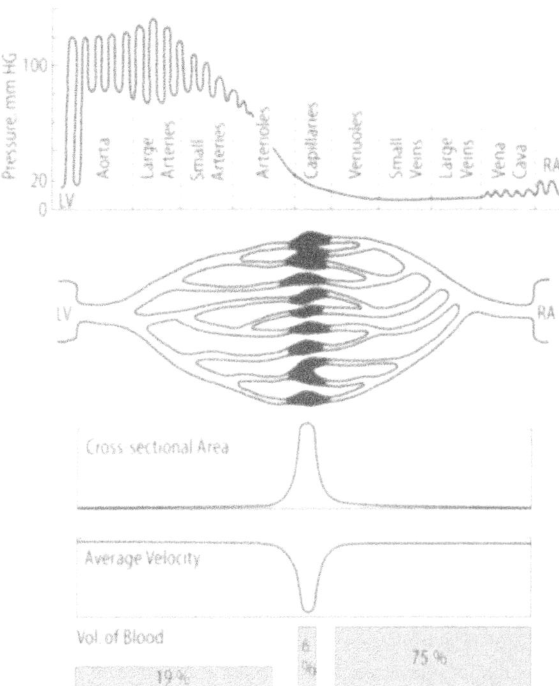

Fig. 1.24. Behavior of arterial pulsation and pressure in the cardiovascular system. From Hussain AKM (1977) Mechanics of pulsatile flows of relevance to the cardiovascular system. In: Hwang NHC, Normann NA (eds) Cardiovascular flow dynamics and measurements. University Park Press, Baltimore

1.2.2.1.4 Velocity Profiles in Pulsatile Flow

The factors involved in moving a fluid at a pressure that oscillates within a viscoelastic tube are clearly much more complex than those required for steady state flow condition according to the Poiseuille equation.

When a pressure force is applied during systole, the blood will first appear to resist movement because of its inertia. As blood accelerates, it acquires ever-increasing momentum, and it will continue to accelerate as the pressure gradient increases. With increasing velocity the viscous drag also increases. If the pressure gradient suddenly falls during diastole, the momentum of the blood will keep it moving until the opposing forces bring it slowly to rest (Fig. 1.25). The gradient reverses when the pressure has passed its peak, causing a rapid deceleration of the flow. Only if the reversal of the gradient continues after the forward flow has been brought to a halt does it lead to a reversal of flow. Whereas the forward flow is generated by the pumping function of the heart during systole, the reverse component is also generated by the reflection of pulse pressure waves during diastole at distal vessel curves or bifurcations at the resistive arteriolar level. Flow reversal occurs in particular

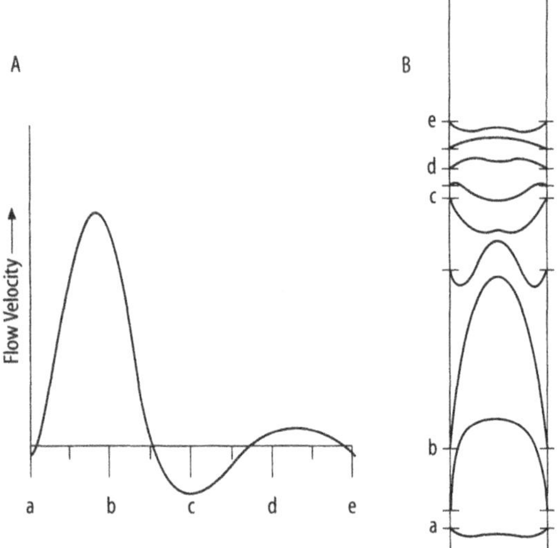

Fig. 1.25. Velocity waveform (**A**) and velocity profiles (**B**) representing normal peripheral arterial flow. *Lower-case letters* indicate corresponding points in the cardiac cycle. Maximum forward velocity occurs near point *b*, where the flow profile is parabolic. Reversed flow is most prominent at point *c*. From Sumner DS (1989) Essential hemodynamic principles. In: Rutherford RB (ed) Vascular surgery, 3rd edn. Saunders, Philadelphia, p 18

near the vessel wall where blood flow is slowest and has the least forward motion. Both flow components are influenced by high or low vascular resistance.

In the descending thoracic aorta and the large arteries of the body close to the left ventricle, blood flow is typically pulsatile. This means that the blood periodically flows forward and in reverse. In the ascending aorta, however, this reversal does not occur, owing to the presence of valves.

In the arteries of the trunk, which have a "windkessel" function, pulsatile blood flow changes to homogeneous flow. In smaller arteries flow reversal is only minimal or completely absent.

Under normal physiologic conditions pulsatile flow remains laminar. An alteration from laminar to turbulent flow is influenced by pulsatility. Flow acceleration stabilizes laminar flow and flow deceleration destabilizes the velocity and leads to dispersion of corpuscular blood elements. Whether the pulsatile character of the velocity has a stabilizing or destabilizing effect on blood flow has not yet been definitively determined.

Laminar Flow

Under steady pressure conditions the fluid in the axis of a tube moves much faster than that near the wall, assuming a parabolic shape, because the particles of liquid are flowing in a series of laminae parallel to the sides of the tube. The fluid in contact with the wall is stationary and each successive lamina slips against the viscous friction of the lamina outside it. This type of flow is called laminar or, alternatively, "Poiseuille-type" flow because it obeys the Poiseuille equation. In Fig. 1.26 the motion of the fluid is pictured as the telescopic sliding of cylinders over each other. The layer at the wall is 0 at rest and the velocity in the axial direction increases parabolically with increasing radial distance, reaching a maximum at the tube axis.

However, as blood flow in arteries is not steady but rather pulsatile, the vessel wall is apparently viscoelastic, and the viscosity of the blood is affected by corpuscular elements within the plasma; thus, the Poiseuille equation is violated. Under life conditions, the form of the velocity profile is created by a pressure gradient which oscillates sinusoidally according to the heart beat and changes the velocity profile that is formed in steady laminar flow.

Analysis of the form of the velocity profile under living conditions shows that a true parabolic profile is not formed at any time because the laminae near the wall always have a lower velocity, owing to the effect of viscosity. In contrast to the viscosity of plasma (blood without cellular elements), which behaves like a Newtonian viscous fluid, viscosity of the normal blood is significantly increased due to blood cells and depends on the cell concentration (hematocrit).

The viscosity depends on the friction between blood and vessel wall, and fluid "shear stress" is required to overcome the friction between adjacent layers of fluid sliding over each other. On the other hand, the forward motion of corpuscular elements within the blood keeps them to the center of the vessel, resulting in a plasma-poor blood towards the center of the vessel and plasma-rich blood towards the periphery. This phenomenon produces the so-called "boundary layer effect," which is maximal towards the wall and decreases towards the center

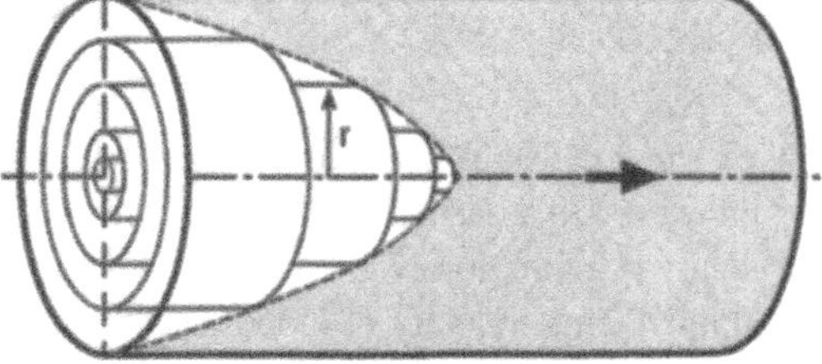

Fig. 1.26. Poiseuille or laminar viscous flow of a Newtonian liquid through a rigid circular tube demonstrating the motion of the liquid as a telescopic sliding of cylinders over each other. From Goldsmith HL (1972) The flow of model particles and blood cells and its relation to thrombosis. In: Spaet TH (ed) Progress in hemostasis and thrombosis, vol 1. Grune and Stratton, New York, pp 97–139

of the vessel. The velocity gradient perpendicular to the vessel wall is called "shear rate" and defines the change in flow velocity from the center to the vessel wall. While the linear fluid velocity decreases parabolically with increasing radius, the gradient in velocity or "shear rate" increases linearly, with increasing radius being 0 at the tube center and at a maximum at the tube wall. A "low-shear large-vessel" effect can be distinguished from a "high-shear small-vessel" effect. Both the frictional forces among fluid components and the "boundary layer effect" cause the typical parabolic shape of laminar flow in arteries.

Only in larger arteries and veins can blood, including its particles and under physiologic conditions, be considered as a homogeneous fluid with a viscosity that is independent of the velocity gradient. In smaller arteries with a diameter of less than 1.0 mm, apparent changes in viscosity occur. Table 1.3 demonstrates the mean velocity values of representative vessels in the human circulation, depending on vessel diameter, wall shear rate, and wall shear × stress.

Table 1.3. Flow parameters in the human circulation (TURITTO and GOLDSMITH 1992)

Vessel	Diameter (mm)	Mean velocity (mm/s)	Mean wall shear rate (per sec.)	Mean wall shear×stress (N/m^2)
Ascend. aorta	23–43	245–875	45–305	0.16–1.07
Femoral artery	5	188	302	1.06
Comm. carotid art.	5.9	187	253	0.89
Small arteries	0.3	50	1335	4.67
Arterioles	0.025	5	1600	5.60
Capillaries	0.0012	0.84	560	1.96
Venules	0.050	7–10		
Inferior vena cava (thoracic)	20	107–160	43–64	0.15–0.22

Plug Flow

Under normal conditions arterial blood flow is laminar with a maximum velocity in the longitudinal axis and prestasis near the vessel wall. Besides the laminar flow profile, under certain conditions plug flow can be observed which is caused by several factors, including vascular pulsation, vessel size, vessel diameter, and shape of major arteries. Plug flow profiles are predisposed by frequency and large amplitude pulsation, in which flow velocity is uniform across the vessel diameter. Plug flow is most pronounced in large diameter vessels, such as the ascending aorta, in which boundary layer effects are minimal, and occurs when fluid enters a vessel with a small diameter from one with a larger diameter , as from the left ventricle to the aorta.

Turbulent Flow

If the flow rate of a fluid through a tube continuously increases under steady pressure conditions, there comes a point when the resistance of flow increases quite sharply and the Poiseuille equation no longer applies. Under these conditions the fluid mixes across the tube and its particles are no longer moving regularly in the line of flow; instead they move across the entire diameter of the tube as well as along the tube. This is called turbulent flow. The pressure/flow relationship of turbulent flow is not linear and the decrease in pressure is more pronounced than in laminar flow. Many transitory conditions of altered flow velocity can be observed between laminar and turbulent flow patterns. A truly turbulent flow only exists when the entire spatial dimension is affected by the altered velocity and persists over the entire cardiac cycle under pulsatile flow conditions.

Flow patterns may be altered from laminar to turbulent by pulsatility, non-Newtonian fluids, artificial heart valves, regurgitation, complex vessel entrance regions, curvatures, branching, and obtuse bifurcation. At vessel curves, a higher velocity flow is tilted toward the outer wall and may produce flow turbulence at the inner wall. Near-branch ostial flow is disturbed and secondary turbulent flow patterns may develop if the stream of blood from the vessel wall separates and forms a vortex or a recirculation zone between the forward-flowing frictionless main stream and the wall (Figs. 1.27, 1.28). In addition, tur-

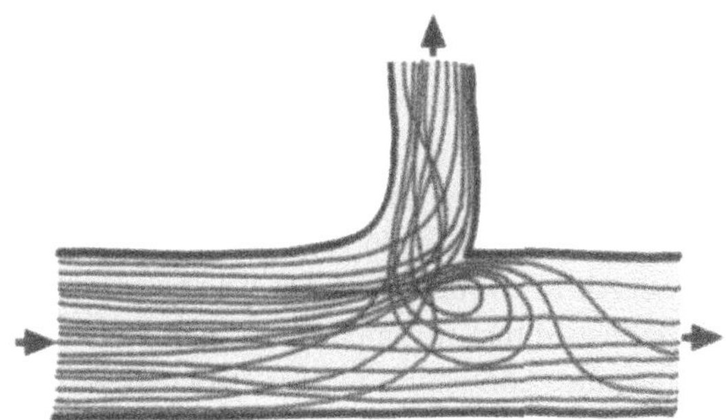

Fig. 1.27. Flow pattern at a 90° arterial branching: curvature of the wall opposite the flow divider is high, and that at the flow divider is low. This phenomenon minimizes flow disturbance and results in the formation of thin-layered recirculation zones on both sides of the common median plane, adjacent to the vessel wall wrapped around the undisturbed mainstream. From Karino T, Motomiya M, Goldsmith HL (1990) Flow patterns at the major T-junction of the dog descending aorta. J Biomech 23:537

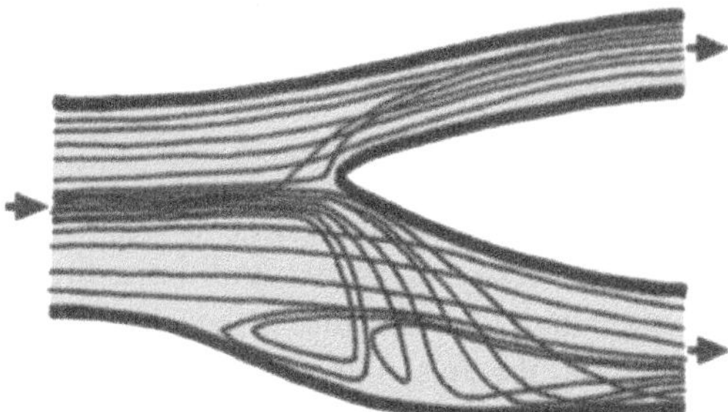

Fig. 1.28. Flow pattern at an arterial bifurcation under steady flow conditions: the formation of a recirculation zone and a counter-rotating double-helicoidal flow occur, both located symmetrically on either side of the common median plane. From Motomiya M, Karino T (1984) Flow patterns in the human carotid artery bifurcation. Stroke 15:50

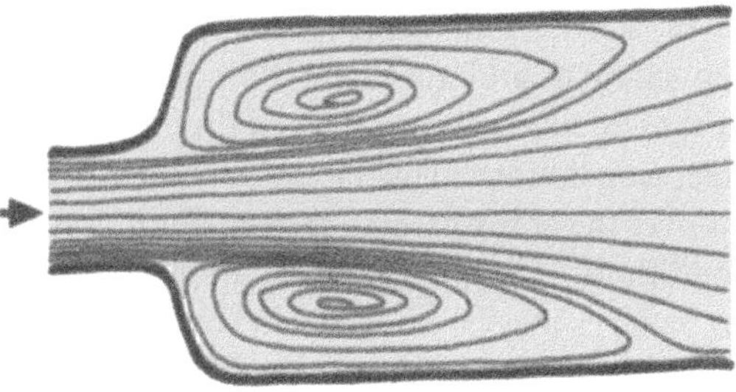

Fig. 1.29. Flow pattern at a concentric expansion of the arterial lumen: flow separation occurs following rapid deceleration, leading to a positive adverse gradient in pressure in the direction of flow. Near the wall, flow is forced to a standstill and a backward direction, leading to the formation of a vortex, the mainstream being pushed away from the wall where it is separated from the beginning of the expansion. From Karino T, Goldsmith HL (1977) Flow behaviour of blood cells and rigid spheres in an annular vortex. Philos Trans R Soc Lond B Biol Sci 279:413

bulent flow occurs in vascular lesions such as vessel wall irregularities due to thrombotic or plaque material, stenoses which produce partial obstruction to flow, and in a sudden concentric expansion of the vessel lumen (Fig. 1.29) as well as in hematological disorders such as changes in erythrocyte concentrations or erythrocytic deformability. The premise has been established that turbulence is a hemodynamic factor that may contribute to vessel dilatation and the formation of thrombi due to the effect of shear stresses on platelets.

Reynolds Number

The most frequently used fluid dynamic parameter in regard to turbulence is the *Reynolds number*. The profile of blood flow, which depends on a number of factors, can be expressed by this number. The Reynolds number is a dimensionless quantity used to describe the characteristics of steady flow through straight tubes at which a transition from laminar to turbulent flow would occur. It combines into one parameter the effects of vessel radius (r), blood density (q), viscosity (η), and average flow velocity (v) and can be expressed as:

$$R_n = v \cdot q \cdot r / \eta$$

The Reynolds number determines the mean velocity at which laminar flow ceases and is replaced by turbulent flow. The fluid stresses associated with turbulence (=Reynolds shear stresses) act tangentially on a surface of an element of the fluid and differ from pressure and viscous stresses.

However, it is important to consider that the calculation of the critical Reynolds number, at which turbulence occurs in a steady flow system, is different in the cardiovascular system in vivo.

For simple fluids, the laminar flow profile breaks down when the Reynolds number exceeds 2000 to 2300, whereas in vivo laminar flow conditions may persist even when the Reynolds number exceeds this critical value because of the pulsatility of arterial flow. The higher the velocity and vessel radius, and the lower the viscosity, the more likely turbulent flow will occur. The critical point at which laminar flow in vivo changes to turbulent flow can be calculated in large arteries with a smooth vessel wall when the Reynold number is approximately 1000, whereas in stenotic disease the number may be significantly lower.

Flow disturbances can be observed in particular near cardiac valves and in the proximal ascending aorta due to Reynolds shear stresses, whereas in other arterial areas under normal healthy conditions flow is not turbulent.

1.2.2.2 *Relationship Between Biophysical Factors and Arterial Vessel Wall* (Nichols and O'Rourke 1990)

The free vascular lumen is determined by the relationship between blood flow, transmural pressure, and vessel wall tension. Transmural pressure is the difference between pressure of the intra-and extravascular space. The relationship between these antagonistic forces of transmural pressure (P_t), wall tension (T), and vessel radius (r) is expressed by the *Laplace principle*:

$$P_t = T/r$$

Arteries develop a certain resistance to elevated intravascular pressure by both the wall tension and the wall elasticity. Wall tension is caused by two forces, the active tension of the contractile smooth musculature and the passive tension of the collagen fibers. The wall tension varies directly with respect to the vessel radius and the intravascular pressure which is directed towards the vessel wall. When the extravascular tissue pressure is higher than both intravascular pressure and wall tension, a vascular collapse may result. This phenomenon appears particularly in veins and is more prominent in smaller than in larger arteries.

Each element in the vessel wall is subject to stresses in the longitudinal, radial, and circumferential (tangential) direction. The force per unit area of the vessel wall that produces a deformation is called "stress." The deformation, described as the ratio of the deformation to its original form, is called "strain." The relationship between stress and strain is expressed as the "elastic modulus." The shear modulus or modulus of rigidity is the ratio of shear stress to angular stress. The vascular wall is attacked by both stress and strain.

Under distending pressure (P), i.e., the intravascular pressure wave, which is generated by the ejection of blood from the left ventricle, the applied force acts against the viscoelastic arterial wall and its longitudinal and circumferential elastic modulus. Each pulsating pressure wave leads to both a radial dilatation and a limited longitudinal movement, which are measurable and depend on the elastic modulus of the vessel wall. The applied force (P) corresponds to the circumferential tension (T) in the wall. For thin-walled tubes with a radius (r), the tension is given by the relation referred to as the law of Laplace: $T=P+r$. If the wall has a thickness (h), then the circumferential stress (t) is given by $t=P+r/h$ (Lamé equation). The elastic modulus of blood vessels increases as the circumferential strain increases, and this enables arteries and veins to remain stable over a wide range of pressure.

The artery as a viscoelastic tube whose diameter varies with a pulsating pressure propagates pressure and flow waves at a certain velocity, which is largely determined by the elastic properties of the arterial wall. Many of the physical conditions, such as the viscosity of blood, the elastic property of the vessel wall, the damping of propagated waves, and the presence of reflected waves, change the velocity of propagation of the pulse wave. The Moens-Koste equation can be utilized to calculate the wave velocity from the elastic modulus (Nichols and O'Rourke 1990).

1.2.3 Microcirculation in the Capillary System

(Kaley and Altura 1978; Nichols and O'Rourke 1990; Turitto and Goldsmith 1992)

The capillary bed is found between the arterial and venous system. The structure and hemodynamics are variable, depending on local function, and are different in parenchymal organs and peripheral areas of skin and muscles. Thus, we differentiate between nutritive and non-nutritive tissue flow. Precapillary sphincters and arteriovenous anastomoses allow a fast adaptation to local requirements of blood circulation. These adapting factors work passively because the capillary bed does not have its own vasomotoric activity. The capillary walls show an inner basal membrane which comprises a single layer of endothelium and an outer network of perivascular fiber tissue as well as a layer of perithelium with pericytes. The pericytes contain fine filaments of cytoplasm.

The capillary velocity depends on the morphology of the capillary bed, the vasomotoric tonus, the pressure in afferent and efferent vessels, and the rheology of the blood.

The flow behavior of capillary blood is important for rheology, which describes the viscosity and flexibility of red blood cells. In small arteries less than 1 mm in diameter, the viscosity of blood decreases significantly and is minimized in capillaries. There, red blood cells and other corpuscular elements flow one behind the other in the center of the vessel and are separated from the vessel wall by a layer of plasma, inducing a reduction of friction resistance.

The capillary walls regulate the blood volume as well as filtration, absorption, and diffusion, by which fluid exchange, including nutritive products and metabolites, occurs. The transcapillary filtration depends on the intracapillary pressure, pressure of the surrounding tissue, and the intra-/perivascular colloidosmotic pressure. By diffusion the small water-soluble and lipid-soluble molecules can be transported and the ionic concentration increases at the capillary membranes. The diffusion rate per second depends on a diffusion coefficient, the surface of the capillary bed, and the difference in substance concentration.

1.2.4 Venous Blood Flow

The main function of veins is the transport of slowly flowing and non-pulsating blood back to the right side of the heart and the lung in order to exchange carbon dioxide by oxygen during the pulmonary passage. The mesentericosplenoportal system, isolated from the general arteriovenous circulation, has the particular function of transporting metabolites to the liver, which have been resorbed in the small and large bowel.

1.2.4.1 Hemodynamic Considerations in Veins

(DONALDSON 1992; CHEATLE 1994; STRANDNESS 1994)

The venous system contains 65%–75% of the total blood volume, or about three times the volume of blood in the arterial system. Return of venous blood to the right atrium has to be guaranteed in the prone, supine, and erect positions under the particular hemodynamic conditions of each. The veins are capacitance vessels, which constrict in response to systemic hypovolemia and act to moderate the effects of gravitational shifts in blood during changes in posture. Activation of muscle contraction causes venous volume in the extremities to fall dramatically. Pressure at any particular location in the venous system represents a combination of static filling pressure, hydrostatic pressure, and cardiogenic pressure. Static pressure is determined by the elastic recoil of the vein's wall, extravascular tissue pressure, and atmospheric pressure, and is normally less than 2 cm of water. Hydrostatic pressure is determined by the vertical distance of the vein from the right atrium and changes dramatically with posture, varying between 10 mmHg in a recumbent position and 80–100 mmHg in standing. Cardiogenic pressure is determined by the pumping and siphoning action of the heart. Flow of venous blood centripetally towards the heart is caused by energy and pressure gradients which are determined by cardiac contraction, peripheral muscle contraction, respiratory action, and posture. These regulatory mechanisms maintain a pressure gradient of about 15 mmHg in the venules, 10 mmHg in the large veins, and 5 mmHg at the level of the right atrium. In contrast to the arterial system, the venous perfusion pressure is low but venous flow normally also is laminar. The venous transport capacity of blood is high due to the small flow resistance. The peripheral vascular resistance is influenced not only by the arterioles but also by the venules (postcapillary resistive vessels). The venous wall tension is defined by the relationship between intravenous pressure and volume. The quotient of pressure enhancement and volume enhancement is proportional to the venous wall tension. A small pressure enhancement causes a large increase in volume, whereas a decrease in the volume under constant intravascular pressure conditions is caused by an enhancement of venous wall tension. In order to maintain normal venous flow dynamics, the thin-walled vessels, muscle-pump, and venous valve apparatus must work together effectively.

1.2.4.1.1 Normal Venous Flow in the Extremities

The hydrostatic portion of the blood normally amounts to approx. 300–350 ml for one lower extremity and is activated when posture is changed from the supine to an erect position. In the erect position a passive dilatation of the venules, acting as resistive vessels, and an increase in tissue pressure occurs as a result of the elevated filtration of fluid within the capillary system. The deep veins of the lower extremity can be characterized as capacity vessels. They may contain varying volumes of blood with only minimal changes in pressure. Venous blood return at rest depends on small local pressure gradients, on the dynamic pressure transmitted from the arterial side, and on changes in intrathoracic pressure. The dynamics of venous flow change when the veins of the calf are compressed by the contracting muscles. Muscle contraction in the extremities in the presence of normal venous valves causes a compression of deep capacity veins, providing a strong propulsive force for venous blood, and supplying as much as 30% of the energy for overall circulation during strenuous exercise. During muscle contraction, valves in the communicating veins close to prevent flow back into the superficial system, as antegrade flow is augmented in both the deep and superficial veins. During muscle relaxation, the valves of the deep system close, minimizing retrograde flow and allowing the deep veins to refill from the superficial veins and the capillary bed (Fig. 1.30).

Normal venous flow is characterized by respiratory phases. In the proximal lower extremities, venous flow is relatively increased during expiration and decreased during inspiration. The latter effect is secondary to inspiratory descent of the diaphragm and compression of the IVC. The reverse occurs in the upper extremities, in which flow is increased during inspiration due to the effects of negative intrathoracic pressure, which is not modulated by any muscular compression. Relative venous stasis occurs in the veins of both the upper and lower extremities when patients perform a Valsalva maneuver. In addition to stasis, there is venous dilatation. Venous flow may be augmented upon cessation of the Valsalva maneu-

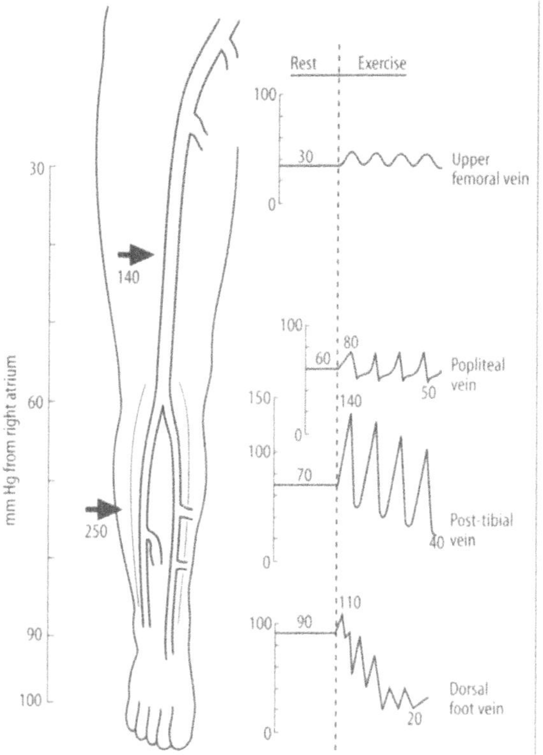

Fig. 1.30. Pressure changes in the normal deep leg veins: hydrostatic pressure is highest in the distal leg at rest, lowest in the distal leg with exercise if deep valves are intact. From Bergan JJ, Yao JST (1985) Surgery of the veins. Saunders, Orlando, p 193

ver and with distal mechanical compression of the venous system in the upper and lower extremities. Both phasic patterns and augmentation are normal flow characteristics.

1.2.4.1.2
Central Venous Flow

In central venous flow, the most important passive factors which influence venous transport back to the heart are the rhythmic alteration between the inspiratory decrease in pressure within the thorax and increase in pressure within the abdomen, evacuation of the right atrium during diastole, change of the level of the tricuspid valve during early systole, and changes in the venous wall tension as a result of reflection or which are controlled by the central nervous system. During normal respiration, an inspiratory decrease in pressure within the thorax causes suction on both the SVC and IVC near the right atrium due to temporary negative pressure. An increase in intraabdominal pressure during inspiration supports inflow of blood into the thoracic part of the IVC. This enhanced pressure is continued to the distal part of the IVC and iliac veins and causes a venous stasis of flow in the femoral vein during end-inspiration. During expiration, the pressure gradient is reversed, accelerating venous blood flow in the pelvic veins and distal IVC. This flow phenomenon can be provoked by the Valsalva maneuver, leading to a complete ceasing of orthograde flow and inducing even a slight reverse flow. Immediately after stopping the press maneuver, an acceleration in flow can be observed due to normalization of the pressure gradient which was enhanced by the stop of flow. Blood flow in the IVC near the right atrium shows a double peak velocity. The first peak is caused by the motion of the tricuspid valve followed by a short phase of inverse flow due to filling of the right atrium. The second peak occurs after the tricuspid valve has opened and the right ventricle has filled. The mean flow velocity in the vena cava can be measured at about 20 cm/s.

1.2.4.1.3
Portal Venous Flow

The portal vein drains the splanchnic circulation and carries about 75% of the afferent flow to the liver.

Physiologic flow in the portal vein is minimally pulsatile, depending on the cardiac and respiratory phase patterns without flow reversal. Normal flow is antegrade (hepatopetal); the vessel diameter ranges from 9 to 13 mm, flow volume from 600 to 1200 ml/min, and mean flow velocity from 10 to 30 cm/s. Portal venous flow can be increased by caloric meal stimulation.

1.3
Vascular Pathoanatomy and Pathophysiology of Blood Flow

1.3.1
Arterial System

1.3.1.1
Age-Dependent Changes in Arterial Hemodynamics

(Nichols and O'Rourke 1990)

An increase in arterial stiffness with age causes an increase in pulse wave velocity which is greater in the aorta than in the peripheral arteries. This change is independent of any increase in mean arterial pressure. In the aorta the greatest change appears between the ages of 10 and 50, when the wave velocity increases by approx. 60%, from 6.5 m/s to 11 m/s. In peripheral arteries (brachioradial and the femorocrural system) this change is approx. 20%. Differences in the degree of dilatation with age, with a greater increase in the thoracic than in the abdominal aortic diameter, may explain the greater propensity for atherosclerosis in this region because of the greater shear stress of the aortic wall at a region of relative narrowing. Pressure wave amplification is related to the central aortic pressure wave, which is influenced by left ventricular ejection duration. A marked decrease in pressure wave amplification has been observed with age between the central aorta and the femoral arteries, the major factor being a relative loss of elastic nonuniformity. A progressive increase in cardiac load with age is probably responsible for the gradual increase in left ventricular mass and for the progressive impairment in left ventricular function. There is a substantial change in ascending aortic impedance and pulse wave velocity with age over a range of 40 years in humans. These changes include an increase in values, suggesting that there is a greater degree of degeneration in the ascending than in the descending aorta.

1.3.1.2 *Atherosclerotic Nonocclusive Disease* (Nichols and O'Rourke 1990; Schwartz and Dilley 1992)

The most frequent cause of arterial occlusive disease is atherosclerosis. Atherosclerotic plaques are only found in the intima, suggesting a specific role of the intimal environment. Two different lesions have been proposed as initial lesions of atherosclerosis:

1. A local accumulation of fat in the vessel wall
2. A focal accumulation of intimal smooth muscle cells, termed intimal cell masses

Three hypotheses have been put forth to explain the origin of the characteristic atherosclerotic lesions: the insudation hypothesis, the platelet hypothesis, and the monoclonal hypothesis. The insudation hypothesis suggests that lipid components of the plaque derives from plasma lipoproteins. The platelet hypothesis is based on the observation that atherosclerotic plaques contain recognizable platelet products as well as fibrin. Platelets accumulate on plaque material and at sites of endothelial lesions, inducing smooth muscle proliferation. The so-called monoclonal hypothesis proposes that atherosclerosis begins as a mutation or viral event in which a single, isolated smooth muscle cell is transformed into a progenitor of a proliferative clone. Most human atherosclerotic plaques derive from cells having a single allotype, and plaques have been observed to be monoclonal. The mechanism of this monoclonal proliferation is not known. Several other lesion components such as a prominent neovascular component as well as the presence of activated T-cells initiate a response in the vessel wall.

Histologically, in arterial atherosclerotic disease the basic plaques consist mainly of fibrous tissue, cholesterol, and platelets, producing localized stenosis of the lumen with or without areas of complete arterial obstruction. Deposition of thrombus and, subsequently, progressive fibrosis occur in eccentric layers. Fragmentation of the internal elastic lamina typically occurs along the areas of intraplaque hemorrhage and calcification that characterize advanced atherosclerotic lesions.

The major adverse effects of atherosclerosis are caused by restricting mean blood flow to particular organs. An atheroma has only little effect on pressure or flow contours in the aorta or major arteries, whereas the influence of atherosclerosis is seen in flow patterns, which are changed significantly in and beyond a stenotic arterial lesion, and in the pressure pattern down stream of the lesions.

1.3.1.3 *Arterial Occlusive Disease*

(Fauci et al. 1978; Kadir 1986; Halperin and Creager 1992; Creager et al. 1992, 1992b; Pariser and Wolff 1992; Kohler 1994)

In arterial occlusive disease, stenotic patterns of the central and large arteries can be distinguished from those affecting smaller and peripheral arteries. The most important etiology of central and peripheral arterial occlusive disease is atherosclerosis, which occurs typically in the population aged above 50 years and is influenced both by genetic factors and risk factors such as nicotine use, arterial hypertension, hyperlipidemia, obesity, and others. In large arteries, stenotic disease is caused by "coral reef" atherosclerosis, congenital coarctation syndromes (neurofibromatosis, tuberous sclerosis, congenital rubella syndrome, William's syndrome), Takayasu's arteritis, fibromuscular dysplasia, and iatrogenic or posttraumatic lesions, whereas the etiology of peripheral arterial occlusive disease is mainly associated with arteriopathy in diabetes mellitus and terminal renal failure, Buerger's thrombangitis, systemic vasculitis (Table 1.4), and vasospastic disorders such as Raynaud's phenomenon (Table 1.5) and Raynaud's disease (Table 1.6), acrocyanosis, livedo reticularis, pernio, frostbite, erythromelalgia, and reflex sympathetic dystrophy. Acute embolization due to migrating

Table 1.4. Classification of vasculitis (Fauci et al. 1978)

Group 1:	Systemic necrotizing vasculitis Polyarthritis nodosa Allergic angiitis and granulomatosis (Churg-Strauss syndrome) Overlap syndromes Rheumatoid vascultis Cryoglobulinemia
Group 2:	Hypersensitivity vasculitis Henoch-Schönlein purpura Serum sickness Vasculitis associated with infectious disease Vasculitis associated with neoplasm Vasculitis associated with connective tissue diseases Vasculitis associated with other disorders Erythema elevatum diutinum Mixed cryoglobulinemia Urticarial vasculitis
Group 3:	Giant cell arteritis Temporal arteritis Takayasu's arteritis
Group 4:	Miscellaneous Wegener's granulomatosis Angiocentric immunoproliferative lesions Kawasaki syndrome Behcet's disease Cogan's syndrome Thrombangiitis obliterans Others

Table 1.5. Possible mechanisms of the Raynaud's phenomenon (Creager et al. 1992b)

1. Vasoconstrictive stimuli
   - Increased sympathetic nervous system activity
   - Digital vascular hyperreactivity to sympathetic stimuli (local fault)
   - β-Adrenoceptor blockade (loss of digital vasodilator mechanism)
   - Circulating vasoactive hormones (angiotensin II, serotonin, thromboxane A2)
   - Endothelial dysfunction
   - Exogenous administration of vasoconstrictors (Ergot alkaloids, sympathicomimetic drugs)
2. Decreased intravascular pressure
   - Low systemic blood pressure
   - Arterial occlusive disorder (arteriosclerosis, thrombangitis obliterans)
   - Digital arterial occlusions (systemic sclerosis, rheumatoid arthritis, thromboembolism)
   - Loss of potential energy (hyperviscosity syndrome, cold agglutinin disease, cryoglobulinemia)

Table 1.6. Secondary causes of Raynaud's disease (Creager et al. 1992b)

1. Collagen vascular diseases
   - Systemic sclerosis (sleroderma)
   - Systemic lupus erythematosus
   - Rheumatoid arthritis
   - Dermatomyositis and polymyositis
   - Mixed connective tissue disease
   - Sjögren's syndrome
   - Necrozing vasculitis
2. Arterial occlusive disease
   - Atherosclerosis of the extremities
   - Thrombangitis obliterans (Buerger's disease)
   - Thromboembolism
   - Thoracic outlet syndrome
3. Neurologic disorders
   - Carpal tunnel syndrome
   - Reflex sympathetic dystrophy
   - Stroke
   - Intervertebral disk disease
   - Syringomyelia
   - Poliomyelitis
4. Blood dyscrasias
   - Hyperviscosity syndrome
   - Cold agglutinin disease
   - Cryoglobulinemia
   - Cryofibrinogenemia
   - Myeloproliferative diseases
5. Trauma
   - Exposure to vibrating tools
   - Electric shock injury
   - Thermal injury
   - Percussive injury
   - Hypothenar hammer syndrome
6. Drugs and toxins
   - Ergot alkaloids
   - Methysergide
   - Vinblastine
   - Bleomycin
   - β-Adrenoceptor antagonists
   - Polyvinyl chloride
7. Miscellaneous
   - Hypothyroidism
   - Arteriovenous fistula
   - Pulmonary hypertension

thrombi mostly originating from the left atrium or left ventricle plays an additional role in arterial occlusive disease.

The initial symptoms of atherosclerotic occlusive disease develop in the majority of cases when the vascular lumen has narrowed by at least 50%. In arterial stenotic disease, under intact regulatory conditions, three factors play an important role:

1. The diameter of the stenotic segment
2. The pressure gradient
3. The arteriolar resistance

A stenosis becomes hemodynamically significant even when the resistance due to the stenosis is similar to the peripheral resistance. Under resting conditions when peripheral resistance is high, the stenosis has less effect on blood flow, whereas following further narrowing of the arterial lumen (stenosis of 70%–80%), the flow decreases distal to the stenosis. Under stress and exercise conditions, the peripheral resistance decreases and the stenotic effect is accelerated.

According to the principle of Bernoulli, flow velocity within the stenotic area increases, whereas arterial pressure increases proximal to the stenosis and decreases distal to the lesion. In significant stenosis of the arteries, velocity increases markedly with decreasing vessel diameter, inducing a velocity exceeding several meters per second. The intravascular pressure behind the arterial stenosis is reduced, and the pressure gradient correlates well with the degree of stenosis (Figs. 1.31, 1.32). Both stenotic resistive and collateral vessels are factors limiting an increase in blood flow. The stenotic effect is determined more by the lumen reduction than by the length of the lesion.

Immediately distal to the stenosis, vessel dilatation can be observed. In this vascular area, "boundary layer" separation results in the formation of a vortex with retrograde flow near the vessel wall. Poststenotic dilatation has been attributed to progressive weakening of the wall as a result of progressive turbulence. Several factors, when combined, may produce dilatation, such as the conversion of the high kinetic energy of the swiftly moving stream, the shock of the impact of alternating high and low pressure, increasing lateral pressure as a result of the lower velocity, and high frequency pressure fluctuations.

In high-grade stenosis, direct orthograde blood flow is partially interrupted and in complete arterial occlusion totally cut off, and the arterial portion distal of the occlusion can only be perfused by collateral circulation.

Collateral vessels develop from fine, preexisting anastomoses and primarily show a passive dilatation. In acute arterial occlusion, the smooth muscle tension in postocclusive arterioles decreases significantly due to ischemic vasodilatation and reduction of transmural pressure. Secondarily, these anastomoses become wide collaterals due to the enhanced collateral pressure gradient and the acceleration of flow. The pressure gradient correlates with the amount of blood volume flowing through the collaterals. A high pressure gradient exists when postocclusive blood flow is minimal and typically can lead to severe symptoms of ischemia.

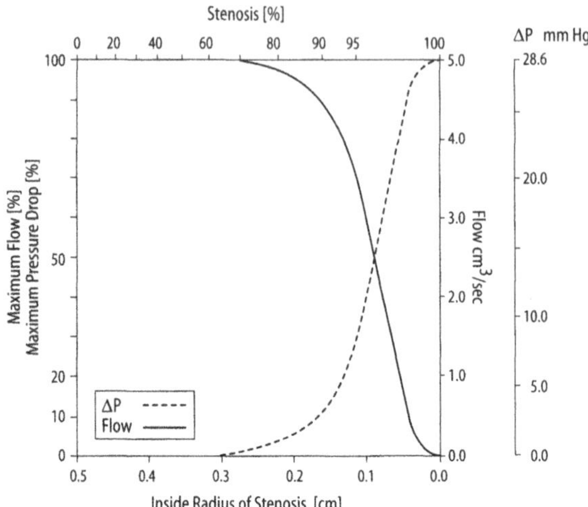

Fig. 1.31. Arterial stenosis: effect on increasing stenosis on blood flow and pressure drop across the stenotic segment. From Strandness DE Jr (1975) Hemodynamics for surgeons. Grune and Stratton, Orlando

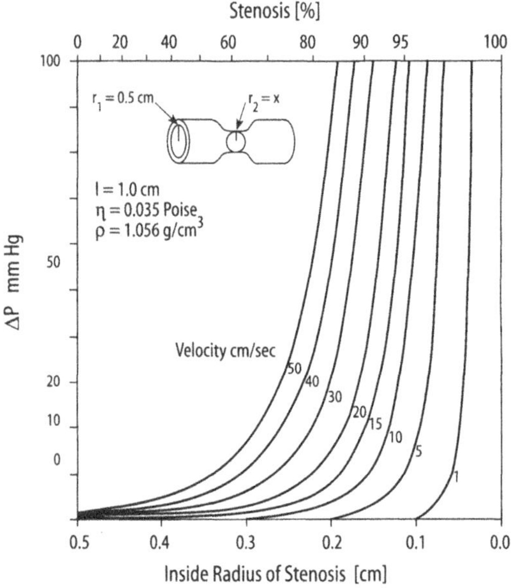

Fig. 1.32. Arterial stenosis: relationship of pressure drop across a stenosis to the radius of the stenotic segment and the flow velocity. From Strandness DE Jr (1975) Hemodynamics for surgeons. Grune and Stratton, Orlando

As collateral vessel diameter develops, both the collateral resistance and pressure gradient decrease. Thus, the number of collaterals varies with the age of the occlusion (minimal in acute embolic occlusion, moderate in progressive chronic atherosclerotic disease, and high in long-standing occlusion).

In collateral vessels inverse or reverse blood flow can be observed, depending on the pressure gradient.

In separated arterial systems which supply neighboring organs and have a close topographic relationship, flow can be changed subsequent to stenotic or occlusive disease in one of the systems. Under these conditions the organ behind the occlusion may steal the blood from the other organ. The "subclavian steal syndrome" is the best known example of this, in which the left vertebral artery by flow reversal supplies the postocclusive left arm. As a consequence cerebral symptoms of temporary ischemia can occur. Another typical "steal phenomenon" with the symptoms of "angina abdominalis" can be observed in terminal aortic occlusion or stenosis of the superior mesenteric artery when the inferior mesenteric artery acts as a collateral vessel via the Riolan's collateral.

1.3.1.4 Arterial Dissection

(Kadir 1986; O'Gara and DeSanctis 1992)

A classification of arterial dissection has been established for lesions of the thoracic aorta. The DeBakey classification was used formerly and distinguishes a type I (dissection of the ascending aorta, the aortic arch, and the descending aorta) from a type II (only dissection of the ascending aorta), and a type III (only dissection of the descending aorta without or with involvement of the abdominal aorta). The Stanford classification, mainly used today, divides dissections into type A (solitary dissection of the ascending or dissection of the ascending aorta, the aortic arch, and the descending aorta), and type B (only dissection of the descending aorta without or with an involvement of the abdominal aorta).

The vascular region in which arterial dissection occurs most commonly and typically is the thoracic aorta. The signaling event of an aortic dissection is an intimal tear through which blood surges into the middle or outer layers of the media, thereby separating the intima from the adventitia. Although retrograde dissection may occur, most commonly a dissection advances in an antegrade direction from the entry, owing to the propelling force of the blood, and creates a double lumen of the aorta with a true and false channel. Primary tears are most often located in the ascending aorta (60%) and in the descending aorta (30%) whereas the primary entry is located in the aortic arch in 7% and in the abdominal aorta in the remaining 3% of cases. The spontaneous development of reentries provides a mechanism for decompressing an intramural hematoma and may help to prevent aortic rupture and to restore flow in arteries whose origins are obstructed by the dissecting hematoma. On rare occasions, an aortic dissection can heal spontaneously, a process that leads either to the formation of a persistent double-lumen aorta or to a normal single-lumen aorta following complete thrombosis of the false channel.

Any process leading to the destruction of the supporting elements of the arterial wall can predispose to dissection. Major factors are medial degeneration, including cystic medial necrosis as described by Gsell and Erdheim, inheritable disorders of connective tissues – most notably Marfan's syndrome and Ehler's-Danlos syndrome – iatrogenic processes, external trauma, intramural hematoma subsequent to ruptured aortic vasa vasorum, and atheromatous penetrating aortic ulcers. Many other conditions have been associated with an increased risk of dissection, such as arterial hypertension, coarctation of the aorta, Turner's syndrome, Noonan's syndrome, giant cell arteritis, relapsing polychondritis, and systemic lupus erythematosus.

Hemodynamics in aortic dissection depend on the location and size of the entries and reentries as well as on the diameter of the true and false lumen. In the majority of cases, the diameter of the true lumen is smaller than that of the false lumen due to the reduced tensile strength of the aortic wall within that part of intramural extension. When not significantly compressed by the false lumen, blood flow and flow velocity in the true lumen are normal or accelerated. In the false lumen flow velocity is reduced in most of the cases, whereas blood flow is reduced or can even be reversed in particular cases.

1.3.1.5 Aneurysmal Disease in Arteries

(Kadir 1986; Creager et al. 1992a; Millis et al. 1992)

Aneurysms can be classified according to morphology, etiology, and location.

Morphologic classification distinguishes true aneurysms as fusiform or saccular from pseudoaneurysm or false aneurysms which develop in a contained arterial rupture in which the wall of the aneurysm is not the original wall of the artery but rather a mass of connective tissue and structures surrounding extravasated blood.

Under normal physiologic conditions transmural pressures react to adaptations of the vessel wall. However, under pathologic conditions (congenital dysplasia, ischemia, atherosclerotic changes including layers of lipids/cholesterol/ calcification, inflammatory disease, and others), the vessel wall cannot resist the transmural pressure, which frequently is enhanced due to arterial hypertension. Thus, an abnormal dilatation of the involved artery may occur.

The multiple causes of arterial (aortic) aneurysms are presented in Table 1.7 (CREAGER et al. 1992a).

Table 1.7. Causes of aortic aneurysms (CREAGER et al. 1992a)

1. Atheroslerosis
2. Cystic medial necrosis
   Primary (Gsell-Erdheim)
   Marfan's syndrome
   Ehlers-Danlos' syndrome
3. Vasculitis
   Takayasu's arteritis
   Giant cell arteritis
   Ankylosing spondylitis
   Rheumatoid arthritis
   Reiter's syndrome
   Relapsing polychondritis
4. Infectious aortitis, inflammation
   Syphilis
   Tuberculosis
   Mycotic infections (*Staphylococcus*, *Streptococcus*, *Salmonella*, *Pseudomonas*, mycosis)
5. Congenital infections
6. Trauma

The development of arterial vessel dilatation, vessel elongation, or aneurysmal vascular disease is caused by a pathologic interaction between hemodynamics and vessel wall. Each of the four components of the arterial (aortic) wall, i.e., elastic tissue, collagen fibers, smooth muscle cells, and basic mucoid substance, changes with age. As a result, the ratio of elastic and fibrous tissue of the arterial wall is shifted to the latter, the artery becoming less distensible with aging, and the ability of the arterial wall to absorb the forces derived from left ventricular contraction is diminished. Thereafter, the arterial wall may weaken, leading to dilatation of the lumen and elongation, i.e., ectasia.

Major locations of arterial aneurysms are the thoracic aorta, thoracoabdominal aorta, infrarenal abdominal aorta, iliac arteries, arteries of the lower-extremity (femoral, popliteal) and the proximal upper extremity (brachiocephalic, subclavian, axillary), renal arteries, and the splanchnic arteries (splenic, hepatic, mesenteric).

1.3.1.5.1
Hemodynamics

The hemodynamics in aneurysms are characterized by slow flowing blood as well as turbulent blood flow which can lead to reversed flow within the aneurysmal sac. The lower velocity caused by the widening of the vessel, according the Bernoulli equation, would itself increase lateral pressure and cause even greater dilatation. In addition, high-frequency pressure fluctuations within a turbulent field may contribute to structural fatigue and lead to further dilatation. Following the principle of Laplace, the radial pressure forces from the entire arterial lumen and the aneurysmal sac act against the arterial wall. Thus, for calculating an aneurysmal diameter, both the arterial lumen and the aneurysmal sac must be taken into account.

1.3.2
Venous System

1.3.2.1
Acute Venous Occlusive Disease (Thrombosis)

(BERGAN and YAO 1985; CHEATLE 1994a; TRETBAR 1999)

Acute venous thrombosis, in the majority of cases, occurs in the lower extremities and the iliac veins. Larger thrombi represent a potential risk for life-threatening pulmonary embolism. Though found less frequently, the subclavian vein at the level of costoclavicular narrowing is another important localization of acute thrombosis, which leads to what is know as "Paget v.Schroetter's syndrome". Rare but of high clinical relevance is acute thrombosis of the vena cava and the mesentericosplenoportal system. Virchow's triad, including venous stasis, venous injury, and hypercoagulability, provides a framework for understanding the complex problem of thrombosis.

The pathogenesis of acute deep vein thrombosis (DVT) is a multifactorial event. Altered muscular pumping as a result of paralysis, immobilization, obesity, advanced age, trauma, surgery, endothelial lesions, cancer, heart disease, stroke, oral contraceptives, hematologic and myeloproliferative disorders, paraneoblastic syndromes, heparin-induced thrombosis syndrome, and antiphospholipid syndrome are intrinsic factors which may cause DVT. Extrinsic factors may also play a role in acute DVT, being associated with venous compression due to traumatic or inflammatory disorders or tumors. The nidus of thrombosis is thought to be within a valve sinus, where eddy currents may occur when blood flow is diminished. Successive layers of fibrin accumulate into which platelets are intertwined. The early thrombus is loosely attached to the vein wall by a fibrinous strand. By collecting thrombotic material, the thrombus elongates, floats up into the vein lumen, and may obstruct blood flow.

The more proximal the deep venous outflow obstruction, the greater the venous insufficiency. It is obvious that DVT of the iliofemoral tract blocks flow more than obstruction of calf veins does. In the calf, DVT may alter the pumping capability of the muscles, with subsequent incomplete emptying and back-up of blood. When the reservoir can no longer compensate for the increasing volume, venous hypertension ensues. The size and extent of DVT is important in determining the ultimate degree of venous insufficiency. The obstructive effects include dilatation of the distal venous system by reflux and valve incompetence, with possible secondary complications. In total venous occlusion, blood flow is completely interrupted and modulation by respiration cannot be observed. In stenotic disease, an enhanced flow velocity of more than 50 cm/s can be registered at the stenotic area and flow can still be modulated by respiration. Distal to a venous occlusion, intraluminal pressure is initially more elevated than in stenosis. Blood flow is reduced in this area, may decrease to stasis, and may be diverted through side branches or collaterals. Viscosity of blood increases markedly and secondary descending thrombi may develop. The blood volume within a collateral vessel depends on the pressure gradient and the capacity of the vessel. The capacity of venous collaterals typically increases with duration of the occlusive disease. Typical venous collateral function is defined by permanent flow which cannot be modulated by respiration or Valsalva maneuver in the early phase with the patient in supine position. In excessive collaterals, however, permanent flow may be increasingly influenced by changes in abdominal pressure and respiration, respectively. As a complication, secondary ascending thrombus development is possible in the nonperfused vascular portion between the occlusion and the inflow of collaterals proximal to the occlusion.

1.3.2.2 Chronic Venous Disorders: Occlusive and Varicose Disease (Bergan and Yao 1985; Donaldson 1992)

Different clinical and morphological degrees of severity can be distinguished in postthrombotic syndrome, depending on the extent of revascularization of the veins involved, the number of collaterals which have developed following acute occlusion, and the degree of alterations of the vessel wall. Morphologic changes include destruction of the endothelium, a resulting stiff vessel wall, irreversible lesions of venous valves, and the development of intraluminal septal structures in a longitudinal direction. Blood flow through deep veins which have been altered by postthrombotic disease may be diminished when recanalization has not been complete. Isolated obstruction of the deep veins below the knee produce little hemodynamic impact on the limb, whereas obstructions at the level at or above of the knee may cause major problems in venous flow, depending on the availability of collaterals. Typical collateral systems of the lower extremity include the deep femoral vein, concomitant veins of the superficial femoral vein, and the greater saphenous vein. In the pelvic region homolateral collaterals such as branches of the internal iliac vein can be distinguished from contralateral collaterals such as suprapubic or presacral branches. Ipsi- and contralateral collateral systems of the upper extremities include suprascapular branches, the external jugular vein, thyroidal veins, lateral thoracic branches, and intercostal veins. In occlusive disease of the vena cava, the azygos/hemiazygos system may take on a collateral function, including the paravertebral venous plexus, the ascending lumbar veins, and superficial extrathoracic/-abdominal veins. In chronic venous occlusive disease, increased distal venous pressure causes increased flow through all available collaterals that lead to the proximal portions of the veins which have a lower pressure. Increased flow gradually enlarges these preexisting channels over a period of weeks following acute obstruction. If venous enlargement is sufficient to produce valvular insufficiency, the communicating veins lose their patency, resulting in collateral secondary varicosities of the superficial veins. Even in existing extensive collateral pathways, venous volume and pressure may remain elevated in rest, whereas with exercise distal venous volume and pressure increase due to an increase in arterial blood flow.

A complete recanalization of an initially occluded vein can be observed spontaneously or under therapy. The time of recanalization is estimated at 6–12 months following the initial occlusion. In the majority of cases, valvular malfunction arises after DVT following partial or complete recanalization. In the presence of valvular malfunction, the directional flow of blood and emptying of the deep veins is not efficient. With activation of the muscle pump, blood is partially forced in a retrograde directions. Pressure in the distal venous tree fails to decrease during muscle activity. Distinct valvular reflux may occur in normal subjects, whereas severe reflux due to destroyed valves of the deep leg veins may cause an insufficiency of the perforating veins, leading to severe superficial venous varicosities.

Varicose disease is a phenomenon which in the majority of cases appears in the lower extremity. In general, varicose veins are defined as tortuous, elongated, dilated or ectatic, redundant veins which have lost their valvular competence. Primary varicosis is limited to extrafascial superficial veins or to superficial and perforating veins, the deep venous system being normal, and includes saphenous dysfunction, nonpatent perforating veins, and transfascial forms of side-branch varicose veins. Suggested etiological mechanisms of primary varicose disease include defective structure and function of valves in the saphenous veins, intrinsic weakness of the veins' walls, and the presence of tiny arteriovenous connections that gradually lead to venous engorgement. In addition, an inherited defect in venous structure or function has been suggested. Regardless of the cause of varicose veins, the resulting abnormality is enlarged and nonpatent veins and reflux of blood. The disease may progress into the peripheral branches and communicating veins. The longer the engorged vein segments, the greater are the increases in hydrostatic pressure exerted by the uninterrupted column of blood. With high pressures and inefficient emptying of the leg veins, edema and extravasation occur, associated with secondary inflammatory reaction, eczema, and ulceration of the skin. Due to low flow rates or stasis of blood in ectatic varicose veins, this lesion predisposes to acute superficial thrombosis.

1.3.2.3
Hepatic Venous Outflow Obstruction
(Takayasu and Okuda 1997)

Hepatic outflow obstruction may result from microscopic veno-occlusive disease affecting the centrilobular venous radicles or secondary to the obstruction of major hepatic veins as they approach or enter the IVC. Causes of hepatic outflow obstruction are partial or complete thrombotic occlusion of the hepatic veins, congenital webs, localized phlebitis, and intrahepatic venous occlusion due to radiation therapy or chemotherapy. An occlusion of the hepatic veins and their tributaries or an outflow block to hepatic venous system at any site, including the IVC, is known as Budd-Chiari syndrome. Outflow block in "classic" Budd-Chiari syndrome can be caused not only by the hepatic venous occlusion but also obstruction of the IVC above the opening of the hepatic veins. Hepatic vein thrombosis is the most common cause of primary Budd-Chiari syndrome and is frequently associated with hypercoagulable states such as myeloproliferative disease, coagulation factor deficiency, systemic lupus erythematosus, etc. IVC obstruction within the hepatic portion of the IVC without known cause is called "idiopathic" Budd-Chiari syndrome. The IVC occlusion may be preceded by mural thrombus with incomplete obstruction developing into fibrous or membranous obstruction when it becomes organized. However, membranous obstruction due to a fibrous diaphragm or web may also be caused by congenital malformation. In secondary Budd-Chiari syndrome, occlusion of the hepatic portion of the IVC may be caused by a mass developing in the liver, by an intravascular tumor mass arising from the adrenals or kidneys, and by thrombus of the intrahepatic portion of the IVC. Intrahepatic anastomoses expedite the flow of blood into the right atrium if major hepatic veins remain patent.

Depending on the degree of obstruction in Budd-Chiari syndrome blood flow in the IVC and hepatic veins may be absent, reversed, turbulent, or show a continuous pattern. All types of hepatic outflow obstruction result in hepatomegaly, ascites, and portal hypertension. Long-standing venous thrombosis or congenital webs may produce hepatic vein collaterals, giving a "spider web" appearance.

1.3.2.4
Portal Hypertension and Portal Vein Thrombosis
(Kadir 1986; Okuda and Benhamou 1991; Takayasu and Okuda 1997)

Portal hypertension is a manifestation of obstruction of the portal venous system. It is classified according to the anatomic location of the obstruction. Suprahepatic portal hypertension results from hepatic venous outflow obstruction and is present in the Budd-Chiari syndrome, right-sided heart failure, and constrictive pericarditis. Intrahepatic portal hypertension is caused by pre- and postsinusoidal venous obstruction and may result from alcoholic or primary biliary cirrhosis and chronic active hepatitis. Less common causes include hemochromatosis and cirrhosis associated with Wilson's disease, secondary biliary cirrhosis, and α1-antitrypsin deficiency. Extrahepatic portal vein obstruction is typically due to portal vein thrombosis or obstruction by tumor. The condition of portal hypertension has been pathophysiologically graded by a combination of corrected sinusoidal pressures and recording flow direction in the portal vein. Once the pressure in the portal vein exceeds about 10 mmHg, collateral vessels develop between the high-pressure portal vessel and the low-pressure systemic veins. Four grades of portal hypertension have been established. Grades

I, II, and III show hepatopedal flow with sinusoidal pressure increasing from 10 to 25 mmHg, respectively. Grade IV portal hypertension with a corrected sinusoidal pressure greater than 30 mmHg is associated with hepatofugal flow in the portal vein. With increasing grade of portal hypertension, a decrease in flow velocity can be demonstrated. In mild to moderate portal hypertension (grades I and II) decreased flow velocities are associated with increased diameter of the portal veins so that the total hepatopetal volume flow is maintained at normal levels. Shunting via portal systemic collaterals is usually established at this phase. Flow volumes are influenced by the degree of intrahepatic resistance and the capacity of the collateral flow. Portal venous volume flow declines in moderate to severe portal hypertension (grade III), which is associated with increased diameter and flow in the hepatic artery. In more advanced grade III, portal venous flow may be balanced or bidirectional with a relatively slow flow velocity. The most common portal systemic venous collaterals include the umbilical vein, left gastric vein, and spontaneous splenorenal anastomoses. Varices can develop from the left gastric vein into the gastric fundus and the esophagus. Long-standing elevation of pressure in the splenoportal system of more than 40 mmHg causes massive dilatation of collateral vessels and may lead to life-threatening gastrointestinal bleeding via varicose veins.

The prevalence of spontaneous portal vein thrombosis in hepatic cirrhosis and portal hypertension is low. Predisposing conditions are primary or metastatic hepatic tumors, HCC in particular, sepsis, pancreatitis, pancreatic carcinoma, trauma, abdominal surgery, including portal systemic surgical shunts, and myeloproliferative disorders. In complete portal vein thrombosis intrahepatic portal venous flow may be reestablished antegradely by arterioportal shunts through the vasa vasorum between hepatic artery branches and portal vein radicles. This is in contrast to the effect of arteriosinusoidal shunts, the mechanism of portal vein flow reversal in grade IV hypertension in which sinusoidal venous flow is diverted retrogradely by hepatic vein obstruction.

1.3.3 Angiodysplasias and Vascular Malformations

(Below et al. 1989; Virmani et al. 1992)

Vascular malformations are congenital defects and can be classified into primary embryological abnormalities and secondary disorders which are consequences of the primary defects.

1.3.3.1 Etiology and Pathogenesis

Primary malformations are caused by embryologic errors in the course of formation of conduits into temporary or definitive arteries or veins which lead to truncular anomalies, dilatation, stenosis, agenesis of definitive vessels, or persistence of temporary embryologic vessels. Errors in regression of the anarchic reticulum between arteries and veins or the organization of the reticulum into a capillary network cause a persistence of arteriovenous communications by lack of involution of the reticulum or by lack of its organization, with the reticulum remaining immature and preserving its blastic potential. Errors which occur during the reticular stage of its embryonal development lead to extratruncular forms developing from the primitive vascular network.

Primary malformations or angiodysplasias have been classified according to the "Hamburg classification" (Below et al. 1989), which is presented in Table 1.8.

Table 1.8. Classification of arteriovenous malformations (Below et al. 1989)

a) Predominantly arterial defects:
- Truncular malformations
  - (agenesia, aplasia, obstruction, stenosis, dilatations)
- Extratruncular malformations
  - (angiomas, infiltrating forms)

b) Predominantly venous defects:
- Truncular malformation (aplasia, obstruction, dilatation)
- Extratruncular malformation
  - (angiomas, infiltrating forms)

c) Predominantly arteriovenous shunting defects:
- Truncular malformation
  - (deep arteriovenous fistulas, superficial arteriovenous fistulas)
- Extratruncular malformation
  - (angiomas, infiltrating forms)

d) Combined vascular defects:
- Truncular malformation (arterial, venous, hemolymphatic)
- Extratruncular malformations
  - (hemolymphatic infiltration, hemolymphatic angiomas)

Secondary malformations consequently appear as a result of hemodynamic disturbances from primary malformations with venous hypertension. Thus, the vascular lesions occur in the venous system. In superficial veins which are not protected, dilatation develops due to hypertension and reflux. Varices may appear, with trophic changes of the skin and the subcutaneous tissue. Another localization is bone, where vascular malformations can lead to hypertrophy. Other dystrophies may also be sometimes associated with vascular lesions.

1.3.3.2 Pathology and Hemodynamics

Congenital vascular malformations may affect the normal development of the body during childhood. Because every blood vessel can be affected by malformative diseases, the hemodynamic disturbances caused by the vascular defect can have an effect on the whole body (central and visceral defects), on a large part of the body (central arterial and venous defects), or each organ (visceral and peripheral vascular defects). Serious changes in hemodynamics of the affected part and severe disturbances in tissue metabolism may occur, leading to minus or plus variants in the development of an extremity (vascular-bone syndromes). Extratruncular forms of peripheral vascular malformation often cause severe disfigurement and dysfunction when accompanied by organic infiltration. Complications of vascular malformations are ischemia or necrosis, cardiac insufficiency in large shunt volumes, hemorrhages, and neurologic symptoms when localized in the cerebrum or spine. Atrophy of the vessel wall or ectasia of the vessel lumen increase the risk of rupture, which may be fatal in cerebral angiodysplasias. The arterial system, the venous system and the capillary bed can all be involved and arteriovenous fistulas may develop.

1.3.3.2.1 Arteries

Arterial disorders include simple agenesis/aplasia/dysplasia, kinking, ectasia, aneurysm formation, elongation, hypertrophy/atrophy of different wall layers, irregularities of the vessel wall as in fibromuscular dysplasia, fibrotic stenosis, and arteriovenous fistulas. Arteriovenous shunt may connect arteries and veins (macrofistulas) or smaller, mostly dysplastic, vessels (microfistulas).

1.3.3.2.2 Larger Veins

Larger veins may show the same alterations as the arteries. Furthermore, under increased blood pressure due to direct arteriovenous shunt the veins initially show reactive muscular hypertrophy and hyperelastosis and degenerative lesions develop if the pressure persists for a long duration (atrophy, ectasia, fibrosis). Intimal calcifications or calcified, organized thrombi may occur. Systemic angiodysplasias are mostly accompanied by superficial varicose veins, which may have a collateral function in concomitant anomalies of the deep veins.

1.3.3.2.3 Capillary Bed

A capillary bed may be observed in the form of simple teleangiectasias in the cutaneous area (naevus flammeus) or in connection with arteriovenous hemangiomas. Cavernous hemangiomas may penetrate into the muscles, the joint capsule, or bones and form honeycomb-like vascular convolutions. Ectatic capillaries and cavernous hemangioma predispose to the formation of micro- and macrothrombi.

1.3.3.2.4 Arteriovenous Fistulas

Three types of shunts can be distinguished: localized direct shunts, generalized multiple shunts, and localized tumorous shunts. The most frequent pathologic findings are multiple microfistulas which do not simply link arteries and veins but rather anastomose via complicated pathways in cavernous and capillary ectasias. In arteriovenous hemangiomas, the arterial vessels are frequently dysplastic; the larger venous vessels appear arterialized due to the increased intraluminal blood pressure. Direct localized shunts show transformation of arteries into veins. Multiple microshunts may present as different types, which include shunts between larger vessels and ectatic capillaries or angiomatous caverns and shunts between capillaries and angiomatous caverns.

1.3.3.3 Typical Vascular Lesions

In *Klippel and Trenaunay syndrome* nonvascular and vascular disorders may occur. Nonvascular alterations include hemihypertrophy or hemiatrophy of soft tissue or bone of the extremities, head or trunk; syndactylia; anomalies of configuration; and monstrosities. Vascular alterations include teleangiectatic nevi, venous or capillary hemangiomas with or without arteriovenous microshunts, persistent embryonic veins, agenesis/aplasia of large veins, stenosis/occlusion of large veins, varicose veins, nonpatent perforating veins, and absence of valves in deep leg veins.

F.P. Weber syndrome includes all lesions of Klippel-Trenaunay syndrome and is dominated by hemangiomas with multiple arteriovenous macroshunts.

In *Servelle-Martorell syndrome* the lesions of Klippel-Trenaunay syndrome are present. The main lesions include honeycomb-like teleangiectatic angiomas with penetration from the soft tissue into the muscles, joint capsule, and bone of a commonly atrophic extremity.

Systemic teleangiectasias and hemangiomas appear in

a. *Von Hippel and Lindau syndrome* with angiomatosis of retina and leptomeninx
b. *Louis-Bar syndrome* with ocular teleangiectasias and venous angiomas of leptomeninx
c. *Sturge-Weber-Krabbe syndrome* with cerebral and trigeminal angiomas
d. *Mafucci syndrome* with hemangiomas of soft tissue and bone with phalangeal deformations
e. *Blue rubber bleb syndrome* with hemangiomas of skin and gastrointestinal tract
f. *Kasabach-Merrit syndrome* with hemangiomas and thrombopenia
g. *Rendu-Osler disease* with hereditary teleangiectasias of skin and mucosa
h. *Angiokeratoma corporis diffusum Fabry*
i. *Neurofibromatosis vonRecklinghausen* with hemangiomas of skin and mucosa

Arterial wall lesions can be observed in *Marfan's syndrome, Ehlers-Danlos syndrome, Grönblad-Strandberg syndrome*, homocystinuria, and polychondritis.

Systemic congenital venous disorders include generalized diffuse *phlebectasia of Bockenheimer* and cystic angiomatosis.

References

Abrams HL (ed) (1983) Abrams angiography, vascular and interventional radiology, 3rd edn. Little, Brown, Boston

Below S, Loose DA, Weber J (1989) Vascular malformations. Einhorn Presse-Verlag GmbH, Reinbeck

Bergan JJ, Yao JST (1985) Surgery of the veins. Saunders, Orlando

Burton AC (1972) Physiology and biophysics of the circulation. Year Book, Chicago

Caro CG, Pedley JG, Schroter RC, Seed WA (1978) The mechanics of the circulation. Oxford University Press, New York

Cheatle TR (1994a) Pathology of deep venous thrombosis. In: Strandness DE, Van Breda A (eds) Vascular diseases. Churchill Livingstone, New York, p 119

Cheatle TR (1994b) Anatomy and physiology of the veins of the lower limb. In: Strandness DE, Van Breda A (eds) Vascular diseases, Churchill Livingstone, New York, p 129

Creager MA, Dzau VJ (eds) (1992) Vascular medicine – a textbook of vascular biology and diseases. Little, Brown, Boston Toronto London, p 1115

Creager MA, Halperin JL, Whittemore AD (1992a) Aneurysmal disease of the aorta and its branches. In: Loscalzo J, Creager MA, Dzau VJ (eds) Vascular medicine. Little, Brown, Boston Toronto London, p 903

Creager MA, Halperin JL, Coffman JD (1992b) Vasospastic disorders. In: Loscalzo J, Creager MA, Dzau VJ (eds) Vascular medicine. Little, Brown, Boston Toronto London, p 975

Donaldson MC (1992) Chronic venous disorders. In: Loscalzo J, Creager MA, Dzau VJ (eds) Vascular medicine. Little, Brown, Boston Toronto London, p 1075

Fauci AS, Haynes BF, Katz P (1978) The spectrum of vasculitis – clinical, pathologic, immunologic, and therapeutic considerations. Ann Intern Med 89:660–676

Goldsmith HL (1972) The flow of model particles and blood cells and its relation to thrombosis. In: Spaet TH (ed) Progress in hemostasis and thrombosis, vol 1. Grune and Stratton, New York, pp 97–139

Gore JM, Alpert JS, Benotti JR, et al (1985) Handbook of hemodynamic monitoring. Little, Brown, Boston

Halperin JL, Creager MA (1992) Arterial obstructive diseases of the extremities. In: Loscalzo J, Creager MA, Dzau VJ (eds) Vascular medicine. Little, Brown, Boston Toronto London, p 835

Hussain AKM (1977) Mechanics of pulsatile flows of relevance to the cardiovascular system. In: Hwang NHC, Normann NA (eds) Cardiovascular flow dynamics and measurements. University Park Press, Baltimore

Kadir S (1986) Diagnostic angiography. Saunders, Philadelphia

Kadir S (1991) Atlas of normal and variant angiographic anatomy. Saunders, Philadelphia

Kaley G, Altura BM (eds) (1978) Microcirculation. University Park Press, Baltimore

Karino T, Goldsmith HL (1977) Flow behaviour of blood cells and rigid spheres in an annular vortex. Philos Trans R Soc Lond B Biol Sci 279:413

Karino T, Motomiya M, Goldsmith HL (1990) Flow patterns at the major T-junction of the dog descending aorta. J Biomech 23:537

Kohler TR (1994) Hemodynamics of arterial occlusive disease. In: Strandness DE, Van Breda A (eds) Vascular diseases. Churchill Livingstone, New York, p 65

Millis JM, Brown SL, Busittil RW (1992) Thoracic and abdominal aneurysms. In: Bell PRF, Jamieson CW, Ruckley CV (eds) Surgical management of vascular disease. Saunders, London Philadelphia Toronto Sydney Tokyo, p 797

Milnor WR (1982) Hemodynamics. William and Wilkins, Baltimore

Motomiya M, Karino T (1984) Flow patterns in the human carotid artery bifurcation. Stroke 15:50

Netter FH (1989) Atlas of human anatomy. Ciba-Geigy, Summit, New Jersey

Nichols WW, O'Rourke MF (eds) (1990) McDonald's blood flow in arteries, 3rd edn, Edward Arnold (Hodder and Stoughton), London Melbourne Auckland

O'Gara PT, DeSanctis RW (1992) Aortic dissection. In: Loscalzo J, Creager MA, Dzau VJ (eds) Vascular medicine. Little, Brown, Boston Toronto London, p 931

Okuda K, Benhamou J-P (eds) (1991) Portal hypertension – clinical and physiological aspects. Springer, Tokyo Berlin Heidelberg New York London Paris Hong Kong Barcelona

Pariser KM, Wolff SM (1992) The clinical spectrum of vasculitis. In: Loscalzo J, Creager MA, Dzau VJ (eds) Vascular medicine. Little, Brown, Boston Toronto London, p 1011

Schwartz SM, Dilley RJ (1992) Vascular injury. In: Loscalzo J, Creager MA, Dzau VJ (eds) Vascular medicine. Little, Brown, Boston Toronto London, p 251

Skalak R, Keller SR, Secomb TW (1981) Mechanics of blood flow. J Biomech Eng 103:102–115

Smith GT (2000) Principles of blood flow dynamics. In: Taveras JM, Ferrucci JT (eds) Radiology, diagnosis-imaging-intervention, vol 2. Williams and Wilkins, Lippincott

Strandness DE Jr (1994) Applied physiology of the venous

system. In: Strandness DE, Van Breda A (eds) Vascular diseases. Churchill Livingstone, New York, p 103

Strandness DE Jr, Sumner DS (1975) Hemodynamics for surgeons. Grune and Stratton, New York

Sumner DS (1989) Essential hemodynamic principles. In: Rutherford RB (ed) Vascular surgery, 3rd edn. Saunders, Philadelphia, p 18

Takayasu K, Okuda K (eds) (1997) Imaging in liver disease – from diagnosis to treatment. Oxford University Press, Oxford

Tretbar LL (1999) Venous disorders of the leg – principles and practice. Springer, Berlin Heidelberg New York

Turitto VT, Goldsmith HL (1992) Rheology, transport and thrombosis in the circulation. In: Loscalzo J, Creager MA, Dzau VJ (eds) Vascular medicine. Little, Brown, Boston, p 157

Uflacker R (1997) Atlas of vascular anatomy: an angiographic approach, Williams and Wilkins, Baltimore

Virmani R, Darcy T, Robinowitz M (1992) Congenital malformations of the vasculature. In: Loscalzo J, Creager MA, Dzau VJ (eds) Vascular medicine. Little, Brown, p 1115

Zierler RE (1994) Normal arterial physiology. In: Strandness DE Jr, Van Breda A (eds) Vascular diseases. Churchill Livingstone, New York, p 57

2 Definition of Magnetic Resonance Angiography

Ingolf P. Arlart and Georg M. Bongartz

Magnetic resonance (MR) angiography was introduced into clinical practice about 10 years ago and provides a variety of significant advantages over competitive methods in vascular imaging. Similar to color coded duplex Doppler ultrasonography (US), MR imaging techniques are able to demonstrate angiomorphology, provide information about the perivascular space, and give functional quantitative information on the basis of two-dimensional cine phase-contrast flow mapping. The main differences to computed tomography (CT) are that no ionizing radiation is involved, there is no need for nephrotoxic contrast media or even for contrast media at all, and vessels and bone can be easily distinguished in the reconstructed images. Like with CT, the vascular tree can be visualized three-dimensionally (3D) and the vascular lumen and surrounding structures can be simultaneously evaluated with MR angiography. Conventional X-ray angiography not only suffers from the inherent risk associated with the invasive nature of the technique but is also restricted to a limited number of views (projection) in a two-dimensional space. The purely luminographical display in conventional angiography presents limitations in patients in whom the vascular wall or the surrounding tissue are of major importance for diagnosis, such as in aneurysmal disease.

In this chapter the beginnings and the development of vascular MR imaging up to the current status of MR angiography will be presented.

With the detection of nuclear magnetic resonance (NMR) and its implementation into medical imaging, new insight has been gained in morphology, pathoanatomy, and function. The ability of MR imaging to visualize reliably soft tissue alterations is based on a high signal-to-noise ratio and contrast-to-noise ratio and the large variability in the contrast of structures that are invisible by other imaging modalities. The signals derive from biochemical tissue characteristics such as relaxation times and from magnetic properties. Further contributors to MR contrast are susceptibility, chemical shift, and motion.

Following the introduction of clinical MR imaging, the technique was initially used to obtain cross-sectional images in all directions and at any region of the body. Neglecting its ability to provide further information about function or pathomorphology, MR imaging was regarded as a potential substitute for CT, a technique that required ionizing radiation, and as an imaging tool which could supersede US due to the significantly improved spatial resolution and tissue characterization in a large, defined field of view.

Although the potential of NMR to acquire flow information had already been recognized during the 1950s, the technical prerequisites for acquiring sequences suitable for flow imaging were not met until the 1990s.

In a way, the imaging of vascular structures during the early phase first was an undesired side effect, comprising a variety of artifacts that were produced by vascular motion and pulsation. Through the development of today's MR technology as well as further theoretical and practical user experience, it became possible to compensate for these artifacts or to suppress them and to visualize vascular structures.

Intravascular motion was displayed with a high contrast to adjacent tissue either without an intraluminal signal or with a high signal intensity. Nevertheless, due to the relatively long acquisition times, all kinds of physiological motion during scanning have the potential to create artifacts and distort the results.

Two solutions to these problems were provided more than 10 years ago:

1. Improving the speed of MR image acquisition, thus avoiding the problems due to physiological motion
2. Compensating for the motion-induced errors in signal registration by adjusting the measurement parameters to the motion

I.P. Arlart, MD
Radiologisches Institut Stuttgart, Katharinenhospital, Kriegsbergstrasse 60, 70174 Stuttgart, Germany
G.M. Bongartz, PhD, MD
Department of Radiology, University Hospital, Kantonsspital, Petersgraben 4, 4031 Basel, Switzerland

Both approaches are being followed; the latter offers the possibility of visualizing vascular structures directly on single slices. The additional application of reconstruction algorithms, including maximum or minimum intensity projections, can produce angiogram-like images of a certain area by suppressing the signal of stationary tissue. These images became known as "magnetic resonance angiograms." However, the term MR angiography refers to a broad variety of MR sequences by which intra- and extraluminal vessel contrast can be obtained. All MR angiographic sequences are based on the specific properties and characteristics of blood and blood flow. Minimum requirements for MR angiography are optimized contrast between vessel and background, a continuous delineation of defined vascular areas, and image information that is based on motion, i.e., blood flow movement or intravascular contrast enhancement.

Since flow phenomena can result in either a bright or a dark signal, signal displacement, and signal aliasing, a multitude of different techniques have been introduced to use these artificial signals clinically. The basic artifacts arise in almost any MR technique but play a major role in gradient echo (GRE) imaging. In these sequences, phase dependency and inflow phenomena are predominantly used for native acquisitions in MR angiography.

Bearing in mind the MR appearance of flow, flow-related MR imaging can be defined as a vascular examination method based on the biochemical and biophysical properties of blood and blood flow. It represents a method for the functional imaging of blood vessels and with which blood flow can be quantified. Due to the functional basis of the MR angiographic signals, vascular structures may not always be precisely registered because of the different flow patterns and velocities.

In this respect, MR angiography resembles color duplex US rather than conventional angiography and potentially provides both morphologic and physiologic data from the arterial and the venous circulation in the assessment of a suspected vascular disease.

On static spin echo (SE) images, blood flow appears dark, allowing depiction of both intra- and extravascular anatomy. Turbulent flow may generate a signal that cannot be differentiated from thrombus. Therefore, dynamic vascular studies using GRE techniques and phase velocity mapping techniques may help in assessing anatomical flow and flow abnormalities. MR angiography can yield information on flow direction, flow origin, and the presence or absence of collaterals. Veins and arteries can be imaged selectively due to their usually opposite flow direction by using presaturation techniques.

However, in clinical practice several drawbacks of flow-related MR angiographic techniques were observed which limited the visualization of angiomorphology and accuracy in evaluating vascular abnormalities. Major limitations were unexpected signal voids due to phase dispersion in turbulent flow conditions, in-plane saturation, and artifacts due to respiratory and cardiac motion, vessel pulsation, and susceptibility artifacts.

The majority of these problems could be solved by the introduction of contrast-enhanced MR angiography, based on the initial work of Prince and coworkers in 1993. By coordinating the administration of a contrast material bolus with an ultra-short data acquisition period in MR angiography, motion artifacts could be widely avoided by holding the breath during imaging, and saturation artifacts were diminished significantly. Contrast-enhanced 3D data acquisition has proven to be superior to flow-related native acquisitions in angiomorphologic imaging, which has ushered in a completely new era of clinical MR angiography. Acquisition of the data set during a single breath-hold became possible by shortening of the repetition time (TR) in MR angiographic sequences. As a prerequisite for this ultrafast MR angiography technique, high gradient performance was mandatory. However, because short TR strongly reduces the T1-weighted signal of the normal blood, intravenous administration of paramagnetic contrast material was required to improve the T1-weighting effect in blood. As an advantage, it could be shown that paramagnetic contrast material has far fewer side effects than X-ray contrast agents; nephrotoxicity, in particular, can be excluded.

In order to optimize arterial contrast, administration of the contrast bolus must be timed so as to guarantee that the maximum contrast appears primarily when the central lines of the k-space are filled, whereas peripheral k-space filling is responsible for spatial resolution and imaging of small vascular structures with low contrast. The 3D data set has to be acquired during the first pass of contrast material, covering the arterial phase, whereas in repetitive acquisitions of one or two additional 3D data sets, the venous phase can be visualized, optimizing the delay between arterial and venous acquisition. Fat saturation and subtraction techniques as well as high-resolution acquisition can optimize image quality. With dynamic table translation technique, the entire aorto-iliac and lower extremity arteries can be imaged during a single bolus administration of contrast material.

More recently, multiphasic, temporally resolved, ultrafast 3D GRE MR angiography was introduced as a result of the further reduction in repetition times and eccentric partial filling of the k-space, which enables the acquisition of up to six different phases within a breath-hold. If ultrafast data acquisition with multiple immediate repetitions is applied, it is not necessary to time the contrast bolus, and the arterial and venous structures can be evaluated separately without vascular overlap, offering angiomorphologic and functional information of a quality similar to that of conventional angiography.

The major impetus for the development of MR angiography as a method which could potentially replace conventional angiography in diagnostic imaging of vascular abnormalities is the morbidity and mortality associated with invasive catheter procedures. Another motivational factor for developing MR angiography is cost reduction in public health care. Because MR angiography can be performed on an outpatient basis, the factor hospitalization costs can be neglected. Furthermore, the combination of morphologic MR imaging, morphologic MR angiography, and functional MR imaging within a single examination procedure frequently obviates the need for multiple diagnostic imaging methods, such as catheter angiography, US, and CT. Two examples of this advantage are: In a patient with head pain or transitory ischemic attacks, a routine brain study can easily be followed by additional sequences for MR angiography and perfusion images, or, in a patient with suspected renovascular hypertension, MR angiography can depict renal artery stenosis, MR imaging can present information about the renal parenchyma, and MR cine PC flow mapping can help to evaluate the hemodynamic significance of the stenosis.

The value of MR angiography was widely accepted for head and brain imaging even at a time when flow-related techniques were used, reducing the frequency of the use of conventional angiography. Since contrast-enhanced MR angiography offers the advantage of providing a less invasive look at the vascular system of a quality similar to that of conventional angiography, its clinical efficacy for many applications has been demonstrated to the satisfaction of many practitioners. Informal comparisons of X-ray and MR-based angiography have been conducted at many scientific institutions and have led to a broader acceptance of MR angiography for clinical use.

The major strengths of MR angiography currently are associated with the visualization of the intracranial circulation and extracranial carotid vessels, the depiction of peripheral arterial occlusive disease, screening for renovascular hypertension, abdominal tumor staging, and the evaluation of abnormalities of the central veins of the body. MR sequences for these applications are well established, protocols for contrast-enhanced MR angiography will be standardized, and state-of-the-art examination techniques are recommended today, although we envision that further improvement in temporal and spatial resolution will enable MR angiography to replace diagnostic conventional angiography completely in the future.

A prerequisite for the successful introduction of MR angiography into routine diagnostic testing is state-of-the-art MR equipment and optimal MR angiographic interpretation by well-educated and experienced medical personnel. Thus, two demands have to be fulfilled:

1. Familiarity of the investigator with the principles of hemodynamics and MR physics
2. Substantial experience of the investigator in the interpretation of catheter angiograms, including vascular anatomy and techniques.

Moreover, experience in vascular US and vascular CT may be of value in order to evaluate MR angiograms more critically. MR angiograms, even with the introduction of contrast-enhanced techniques, are even more difficult to interpret than conventional catheter angiograms because anatomy and artifacts may alter the signal intensity and the resultant vascular image. Furthermore, the technique of MR angiography is still evolving as regards hardware, gradient field strength, data acquisition, software, contrast agents, and postprocessing techniques.

Because the technical aspects of MR angiography are constantly evolving and the problems observed in flow-related techniques have been largely overcome, this method has developed rapidly into a clinically useful diagnostic technique. To date, sufficient clinical experience has been gained in controlled scientific studies; therefore, indications for MR angiography can be defined, useful selection of particular sequence design is possible, and the diagnostic accuracy of MR angiography can be reliably evaluated with regard to different vascular lesions in different vascular areas of the body. The well-known advantages of MR angiography over other noninvasive or minimally invasive imaging methods, such as avoiding ionizing radiation, the lack of need for potentially nephrotoxic X-ray contrast agents, and the 3D visualization of the vascular anatomy, have influenced the broad spectrum of indications. At the moment we cannot predict whether conventional angiography, the recommended tool for percutaneous catheter intervention up to now, will be replaced by MR angiographically guided endovascular therapeutic catheter procedures. Experimental studies and our initial clinical experience may give us an optimistic view that this technique can be applied successfully.

Principles and Technical Considerations of MR Angiography

3 Basic Principles of Nuclear Magnetic Resonance for Medical Imaging

GEORG M. BONGARTZ and HILDE BOSMANS

CONTENTS

3.1 Introduction

In 1946, the phenomenon of nuclear magnetic resonance (NMR) was discovered independently by F. Bloch and E.M. Purcell. They exploited the characteristic resonance signals of different structures as a physicochemical analytical tool. However, it took another 30 years to introduce the technique into medical imaging.

NMR is based on the fact that some nuclei possess an intrinsic angular momentum or a spin that can be expressed in the presence of a magnetic field. This angular momentum provides the nucleus with magnetic properties similar to those of a compass needle. Hydrogen nuclei have such a nonzero magnetic moment. When placed in an external magnetic field, these hydrogen nuclei (or protons) begin a precessional motion around the direction of the field with a characteristic frequency and under two possible orientations, parallel or anti-parallel to the axis of the magnetic field. The orientation can be destroyed by external (electro-) magnetic energy at the same resonance frequency. Thereafter, the spins return to a state of equilibrium and release the excitation energy as electromagnetic radiation at their characteristic frequency. The return to equilibrium, also called *nuclear spin relaxation*, is characterized by relaxation times that are specific for each biological tissue. The difference between relaxation times of various tissues is the source of contrast in NMR imaging. Due to the fact that the frequency is a characteristic of the particular nuclei, and due to both the bioavailability of protons and their large magnetic moment, the resultant magnetic signal of protons is detected in MR imaging.

The signal produced by a global excitation of all the hydrogen spins of the human body does not provide any "spatial" information. P. Lauterbur was the first to apply additional linear magnetic field gradients for spatial encoding of the signal. Still today, in order to obtain an image of the hydrogen spins, the electromagnetic excitation is combined with the application of small additional magnetic fields whose amplitudes change as a function of position (*magnetic field gradient*). These gradients modulate (*encode*) the resonance frequency of the nuclear spins as a function of their position. Spectral analysis of the nuclear spin signal after the excitation provides the spatial distribution of the signal, i.e., the NMR image, the intensity of which depends on the density and relaxation of the hydrogen spins in the particular tissues.

The basic instrumentation for the acquisition of NMR images follows from the above description:

1. A magnet, in which the subject is positioned; its magnetic field causes the hydrogen spins to precess about its direction.
2. A set of magnetic gradient coils to encode the precession frequency of the spins as a function of the position in the magnet.
3. A transmitter of electromagnetic energy to excite the spin system at its resonance frequency.

G.M. BONGARTZ, PhD, MD
Department of Radiology, University Hospital, Kantonsspital, Petersgraben 4, 4031 Basel, Switzerland
H. BOSMANS, PhD
Department of Radiology, University Hospitals K.U. Leuven, Herestraat 49, 3000 Leuven, Belgium

4. An antenna to transfer this energy to the spin system of the subject and to pick up the energy released by the spin system during relaxation.
5. A receiver to amplify this nuclear spin signal induced in the antenna.
6. A computer to digitize the data and to reconstruct the image.

In this chapter, we explain the basic principles of NMR phenomena in more detail. Position encoding techniques are introduced in the next section.

3.2 Nuclear Magnetism and Nuclear Magnetic Resonance

In the absence of a magnetic field, the nuclear magnetic moments are oriented at random. When placed in a magnetic field, the nuclear magnetic moments and the magnetic field interact. Proton spins align either parallel or anti-parallel to the direction of an external field, making an angle of 26°, or –26°, with the axis of the main magnetic field (Fig. 3.1). Although the parallel orientation is more favorable than the anti-parallel one in terms of energy, there is only a 0.0001% preponderance of the parallel orientation (at 1.5 T). When protons are exposed to a well-defined amount of external electromagnetic energy, the low-energy state protons can be excited to the higher energy state. This transition is reversible and exactly the same amount of energy is released during relaxation. The NMR experiment is entirely based on this small difference between the number of excited and relaxed spins. A complete description of these phenomena would require a discussion of quantum electrodynamics. Here, we describe spin behavior, using a visual, macroscopic model that correctly summarizes the main features of individual spins and systems with a large number of spins.

3.2.1 Isolated Spin

When placed in an external magnetic field B_0, "*excitation*" of a spin from the lower energy level (parallel to the magnetic field) to the higher energy level (anti-parallel to the magnetic field) requires a certain amount of electromagnetic energy. The frequency *f* of the electromagnetic wave that delivers the necessary energy packages has to satisfy the so-called Larmor equation (Eq. 3.1):

$$T_{sd} = BA'i$$

in which γ is a characteristic property of the proton spin. It follows that this frequency is proportional to the amplitude of the magnetic field B_0. In a field of 1.0 T, a typical value for a clinical MR imager, the Larmor frequency is 42.57 MHz (see Table 3.1).

Table 3.1. Resonance frequency as a function of magnetic field strength

Magnetic field strength (T)	Resonance frequency (MHz)
0.2	8.5
0.5	21.3
1	42.6
1.5	63.9

The spin is a nuclear particle, and, as a result, excitation can only be achieved if the frequency of the external radiofrequency (RF) pulse exactly matches the frequency of the particular spin to be excited. Under this condition, a resonance phenomenon is

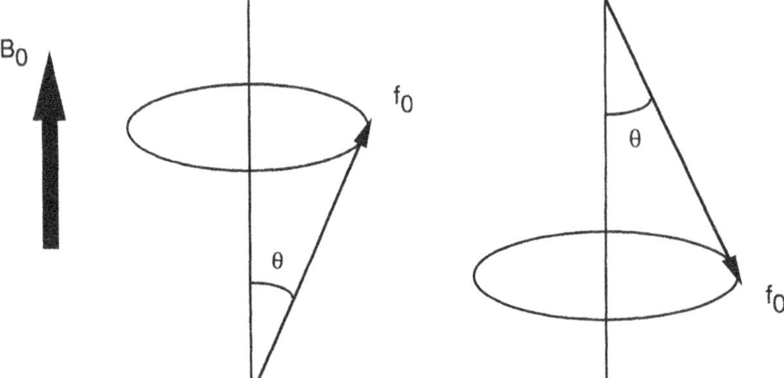

Fig. 3.1a, b. Orientation of a spin in an external B0 magnetic field. **a** Parallel to the field (spin up). **b** Anti parallel to the field (spin down)

established and the frequency is called resonance frequency.

The excitation energy required for MR imaging is about 10^{12} times smaller than the energy involved in conventional X-ray imaging. This extremely low energy is one of the main assets of the MR imaging technique when compared to conventional X-ray examinations. Radiation-induced injury does not occur.

3.2.2
A System of Spins: The Macroscopic Nuclear Magnetic Moment

In clinical reality, one deals with a large quantity of spins placed in a magnetic field. At equilibrium, i.e., in the absence of electromagnetic excitation, most spins occupy the lowest energy state (parallel to B_0). The relative population difference between the two levels amounts only to seven spins in 1,000,000! This (small) population difference gives a net macroscopic magnetic moment M_z along the direction of the magnetic field (Fig. 3.2). This magnetic component is further proportional to the spin density in the volume and to the strength of the magnetic field. The net component in the plane transverse to the magnetic field is 0. Hence, for each spin with a certain phase angle relative to a selected *x*-axis, another one cancels this magnetic component.

The net magnetic moment is characterized by an amplitude and a phase (Fig. 3.3). The amplitude is high if numerous individual moments are more or less aligned with each other. The phase of the net magnetic moment expresses the orientation of the magnetic moment in the plane perpendicular to the main magnetic field. In equilibrium (Fig. 3.2), M_z is large and there is no magnetic component in the transverse plane. This signal can, as such, not be detected by means of regular coils. Excitation pulses are used to generate a component in the transverse plane. At that moment, a phase angle can be defined. An absolute value for the phase of the signal is usually not available; instead, phase differences between different groups of spins must be considered. In most MR images, the amplitude of the spins is shown, and dedicated techniques such as flow quantification acquisitions also visualize the phase.

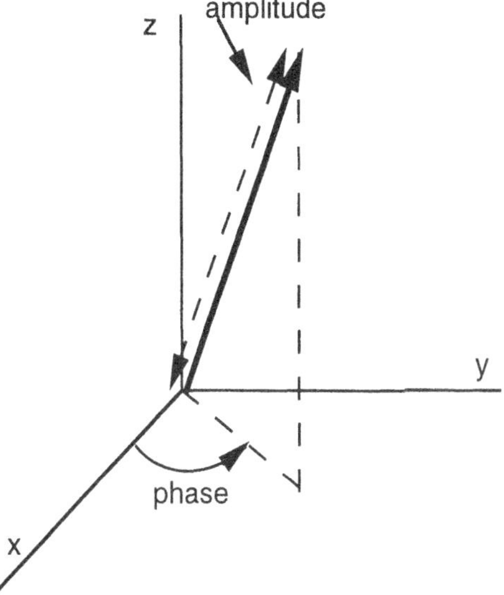

Fig. 3.3. The amplitude and phase of a spin

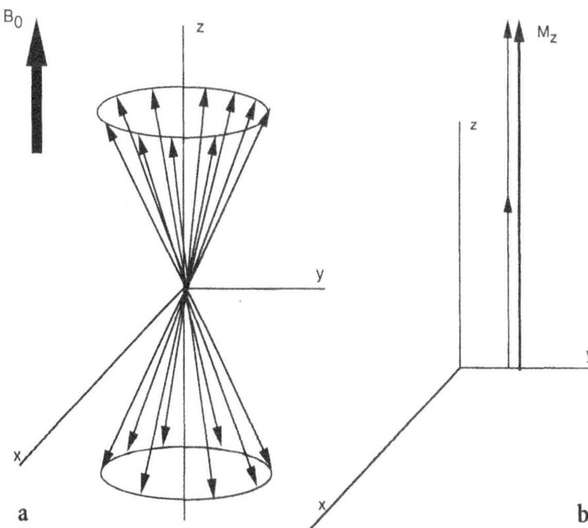

Fig. 3.2a, b. The individual spins and the net magnetic component. a Distribution of spins over a sample in an external B_0 field. b The net magnetic component is aligned with the external B_0 field

3.2.3
Excitation of the Spin System

The RF excitation energy is defined by the Larmor frequency of the spin system, i.e., the frequency that is calculated from the Larmor equation of the individual spins (Eq. 3.1). Only if the transmitted electromagnetic wave is at the same frequency can its energy be transferred to the spin system. RF pulses at this resonance frequency increase the population of the higher energy level.

Prior to any RF excitation, the macroscopic magnetic moment M is oriented along the z-axis. The time evolution of the macroscopic magnetic component during the excitation pulse is complex. It is composed of both, precession around the B_0 field and precession just around the magnetic field of the excitation pulse.

For an observer who processes at the same frequency as the spins around the B_0 field, the pattern is, however, simple: the motion of the spins is then simplified to a precession around the fluctuating RF pulse. In practice, many NMR processes are visualized as they are observed by the co-precessing observer. It is said that the description is performed in the *rotating frame*. This representation will be used throughout this book. We define the *z*-axis as parallel to the main magnetic field, and the *x*- and *y*-axes perpendicular to each other and to the *z*-axis. The RF field is in the *xy* plane, e.g. along the *x*-axis. Using this model, excitation is most easily presented in the following way (Fig. 3.4): the magnetic component M_z rotates away from the *z*-axis, around the direction of the RF field, yielding a macroscopic magnetic moment M_{xy} in the *xy* plane. As soon as the excitation field is removed, the motion of M around the excitation field stops. The precession around B_0 goes on, as before, but the spin system is no longer in equilibrium. It is 'excited'.

A 90° RF pulse is an excitation pulse with a duration such that the equilibrium magnetization is tilted from the *z*-axis into the plane perpendicular to the *z*-direction. It is said that a 90° *flip angle* is acquired. A 180° pulse is an excitation of duration such that the magnetic moment is rotated over an angle of 180° around the direction of the RF field (Fig. 3.2b). It takes in principle twice as long as acquiring a 90° angle, or, stated in another way, a double energy rate has to be sent into the tissues.

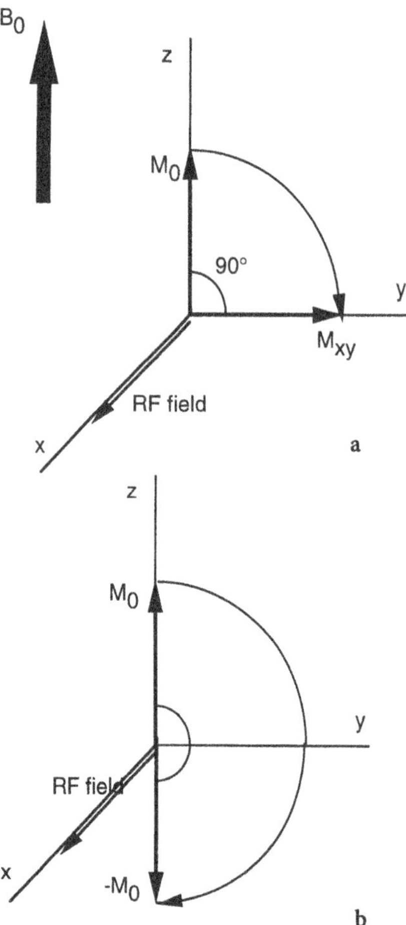

Fig. 3.4a, b. Representation of RF pulses in the rotating frame. **a** A 90° RF pulse. **b** A 180° RF pulse

3.2.4
The Free Precession Signal

A 90° excitation pulse tilts the macroscopic magnetic moment into the *xy* plane, where it precesses around B_0 at the Larmor frequency. This time-dependent magnetic moment induces a periodic voltage at the Larmor frequency in the detector or coil. The exponential decay of the signal as a function of time is called the *free induction decay* (FID). The FID is the direct response of the system to the external RF pulse. The FID, like any MR signal, is detectable because it is expressed by fluctuations of the magnetic components in the *xy* plane.

In reality, the magnetic field in a volume with (excited) spins is not homogeneous and the resonance frequency of the corresponding spins is therefore not uniform. Spins located in a local magnetic field which is slightly higher than the average field have a slightly higher precession frequency than the average frequency, while the spins located in a lower magnetic field have a lower precession frequency. Spins are going out of phase, or, in other words, coherence is lost. Therefore, the net magnetic component decreases with time until it ultimately vanishes. The periodic signal S(t) induced in the coil after a 90° excitation pulse is an exponentially dampened sinusoidal signal with frequency f_0, and characteristic decay time *T2** (Fig. 3.5):

$$BTDC = \frac{duration\ of\ arterial\ j}{duration\ CM\ inje}$$

where S_0 is the initial signal strength or amplitude immediately after the 90° pulse. The signal S(t) is called the *free precession signal.*

3.2.5
Spin Echo

As seen in Fig. 3.5, after an excitation pulse, the signal generally disappears. This is because spins precess with different frequencies. The situation of a few indi-

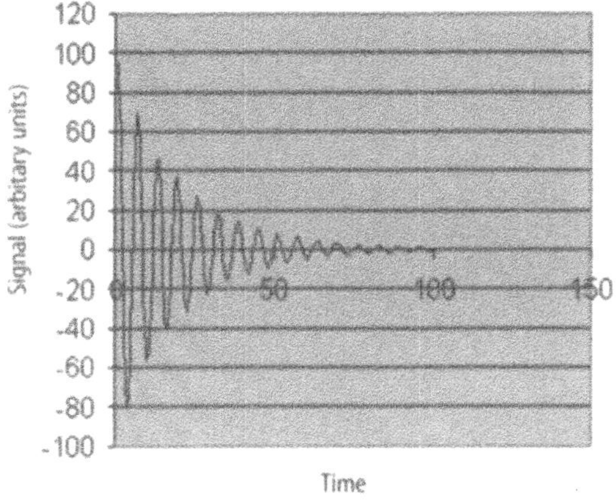

Fig. 3.5. Typical voltage as induced in the coil by an excited spin system. The precessional motion and the inherent dispersion of the signal induce the represented typical time decay

vidual spins is shown in Fig. 3.6: spins that are initially well aligned (Fig. 3.6a) acquire a slightly different precessional frequency that make them lead or lag as compared to the net spin system. This process is caused by several facts: the Brownian motion of neighboring spins (described by the T2 parameter), local inhomogeneities of the field, etc. Anything which affects the Larmor frequency of the spins has to be considered! From Eq. 3.1, it follows that the magnetic field as experienced by the spins is a major factor. Compensation of the dephasing phenomenon is called *rephasing*, the basic purpose of which is to reverse the phases of the spins and cause the spins to re-align.

Dephasing of the spins due to inhomogeneities of the external magnetic field is reversible. Rephasing can be achieved by a 180° pulse. The effect of a 180° pulse is easily visualized in the rotating frame (Fig. 3.6c–e). After a time t=TE/2 following the 90° pulse, spins have acquired a dephasing angle, proportional to their departure from the nominal frequency. The 180° pulse at time t=TE/2 achieves a rotation of the individual spins around the direction of the RF field, so that the spins that had the largest lead acquire the greatest handicap after the 180° pulse and the spins with the largest lag have the top position after the 180° pulse. After this pulse, each spin continues to precess with its own frequency in its local magnetic field. The position of the spins does not change during the 180° pulse, with the exception of spins in flowing blood or other moving tissues. The spins with the smallest lead will thus catch the spins with the largest lead and those with the smallest lag will catch those with the largest lag. Both groups, fast and slow spins, rephase exactly at a time TE/2 after the 180° pulse, leading to the formation of a signal with

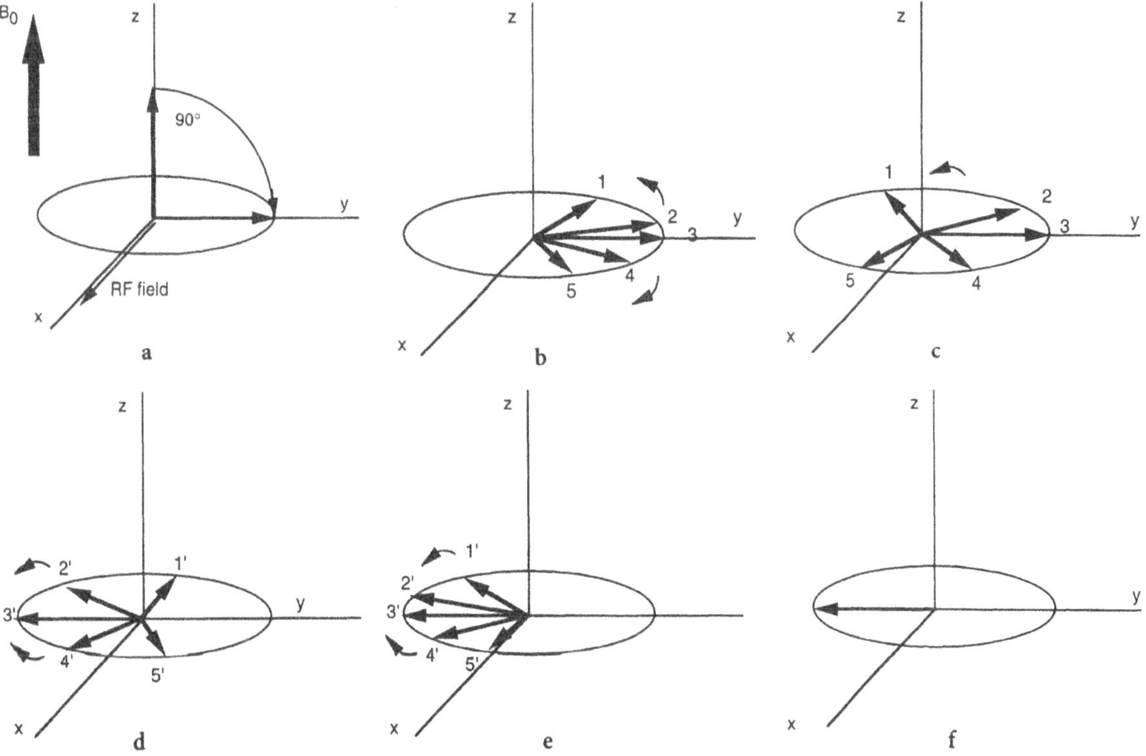

Fig. 3.6a–f. Spin echo signals are obtained after the application of a 180° refocussing pulse. **a** All spins are in phase. **b–c** Dephasing occurs due to changes in the local magnetic field. **d** After a 180° refocusing pulse that inverts the phase angle of the spins, rephasing is initiated. **e** After an identical time period such as between RF pulse and refocusing pulse, the spin echo signal is formed

its maximum at a time t=TE, after the 90° pulse. An NMR signal obtained after rephasing the spins with a 180° pulse is called a *spin-echo* signal. This principle can be applied for successive acquisitions.

3.3 Relaxation

After an excitation pulse, the longitudinal component M_z increases from a reduced value immediately after the pulse to the equilibrium value M_0. This release of energy is described by the *T1 relaxation time*. T1 relaxation processes are the result of an energy exchange between the proton and the surrounding structure, the lattice. The rate of the T1 relaxation in a specific tissue depends directly on the molecular structure to which the protons are bound. Small molecules (like water) are different from larger molecules. In molecules like fat, Brownian motion has a frequency comparable to the Larmor frequency and therefore the energy exchange is accelerated as compared to the situation for pure water protons. In biological systems, the values of T1 range from a few hundred milliseconds to a few seconds and are specific for a tissue or fluid.

MR contrast agents have a major effect on the T1 of the tissues as they change the local fields such that the energy transfer is easier.

The growth of M_z from 0, after a 90° RF pulse, to the equilibrium value M_0 is called *saturation recovery*. It follows an exponential process characterized by the spin lattice relaxation time T1 (Fig. 3.7a):

$$k_x = \gamma \int_0^t G(t')dt'$$

The recovery of M_z after a 180° pulse is called *inversion recovery*.

The longitudinal component M_z of the magnetic moment cannot be observed since it is stationary and perpendicular to the axis of the RF coil. In order to monitor its recovery during the relaxation process, M_z has to be tilted in the *xy* plane with a second 90° pulse. The amplitude of the signal induced in the coil is then proportional to the amplitude of M_z just before the second 90° pulse.

The transversal component M_{xy} of the magnetic moment decreases from its initial amplitude immediately after the pulse towards 0. The differences in this so-called T2 relaxation process are due to interactions between neighboring spins in the magnetic field. Hence, due to the fluctuating local field induced by the neighboring spins (some neighbors have a spin moment up and some neighbors a spin moment down, some are close some are far away), the precession frequency of the spins is altered in a random way, leading to an irreversible scrambling of their phase. This interference destroys the initial coherence of the spin phases in the *xy* plane. Local inhomogeneities of the magnetic field further accelerate the decay of the transverse magnetization. The combined effect of spin–spin interactions and local inhomogeneities is called the T2* decay.

The amplitude of the rephased magnetic moment at the time of a measurement, TE, is always smaller than the original amplitude of the magnetic moment after the 90° pulse. The mechanism of *spin–spin relaxation* causes the transverse component of the magnetic moment to decay irreversibly towards its 0 equilibrium value. This irreversible decay of the transversal magnetic moment is described by an exponential function with a characteristic time T2, the spin–spin relaxation time (Fig. 3.7b):

$$M_{xy}(t) = M_0 \exp(\frac{-t}{T2})$$

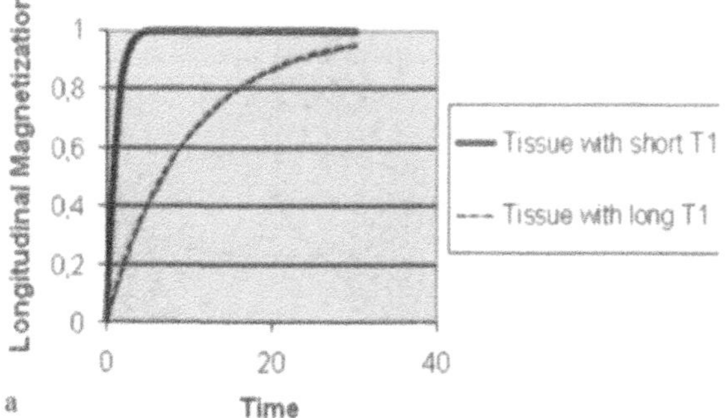

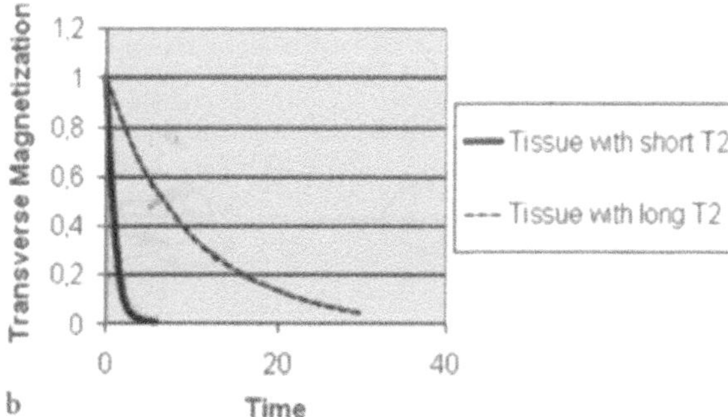

Fig. 3.7a, b. Relaxation times. **a** After an excitation pulse, the longitudinal magnetization is 0 and gradually recovers towards the equilibrium value. The relaxation is described by T1. **b** After the same excitation pulse, the transverse magnetization is maximal. The signal reduces towards 0 with a time evolution described by T2

The T2* relaxation time describes the combined effect of the intrinsic, tissue-dependent factors and the local inhomogeneities in the field. It yields:

$$S(k_j) = \sum_i \tilde{S}(z_i) \cdot \text{co}$$

With:

$$\tilde{S}(z)$$

ΔB_0 the deviation from the local magnetic field.

The effects of static magnetic field inhomogeneities are compensated if spin echo measurements are performed, i.e., whenever an inversion of the spin system is executed with a 180° pulse halfway between excitation pulse and measurement. Using this approach, the contribution of $T2_{extr}$ is overcome.

T1 and T2 relaxation times are independent of each other, apart from the fact that T2 is always shorter than T1. These parameters are tissue-dependent parameters that are used for the characterization of certain pathological conditions. The link between the T2 relaxation processes and the Larmor frequency explains why the T2 time of a tissue is affected by the magnetic field strength, while this is hardly the case for T1 processes.

3.4 Sequences

The NMR (echo) signal can be altered by appropriate timing of RF and measurement periods in order to achieve specific image contrasts (T1-weighted, T2-weighted, and proton density-weighted images). Other physical parameters that have a definite effect on the contrast in the images are flow, magnetic susceptibility, diffusion, and magnetization transfer. An MRI *sequence* is the combination of different RF pulses, the position-encoding schemes which are needed and timing them such that the required tissue characteristics are visualized. The way in which the position-encoding schemes are applied is discussed in Chap. 4.

A large number of sequences have been developed so far. Each sequence has its specific applications, such as T1- or T2-weighted anatomical imaging of stationary tissues, ultrafast T1- or T2-weighted imaging, MR angiography, and MR flow quantification. The latter group of sequences will be discussed in detail in the remainder of this book.

Notwithstanding the wide range of applications, imaging sequences can be divided into two major classes: spin echo and gradient echo imaging. We outline the fundamental differences in the next sections.

3.4.1 Spin Echo Sequences

The sequence in which a signal is measured after a 90° excitation pulse and a 180° rephasing pulse is called a *spin echo sequence* and is denoted as 90°–TE/2–180°–TE/2–echo. It is the basic sequence for MR imaging. In practice, a series of measurements have to be performed to allow for image reconstruction. Therefore, excitation and read-out (or measurement) have to be repeated. The time in between successive excitation pulses is defined as the repetition time TR.

The signal and the achieved contrast are mainly affected by both T1 and T2 relaxation processes and the particular choice of TR and TE. To generate an image contrast based on differences in the T1 relaxation of the tissues, the TR must be chosen to allow for maximal T1-weighted contrast at the signal readout. In practice, TR has to be shorter than T1 but should be long enough to provide sufficient relaxation and, therefore, a signal that is high enough (Fig. 3.8a).

Differences in T2 decay can be visualized by a long TE (Fig. 3.8b). Successive T2-weighted imaging can only be performed when all the differences in longitudinal magnetization due to T1 relaxation have disappeared. Therefore, a long TR is required. TR should be on average three times longer than the longest T1 of the present tissues. The combination of long TR and short TE, on the other hand, measures the transverse magnetization before any spin–spin relaxation has become obvious. This choice of parameters in known as proton density-weighted imaging.

Typical acquisition times of conventional spin echo acquisitions range from 2 min for T1-weighted MRI up to 8 min for a series of proton density- and T2-weighted images. Even with faster acquisition schemes, the use of spin echo techniques for MR angiography studies has been very limited. Blood vessels typically appear dark and the visualization is often hampered by artifacts. However, spin echo acquisitions have a role in MR angiography as a complementary technique to characterize specific lesions.

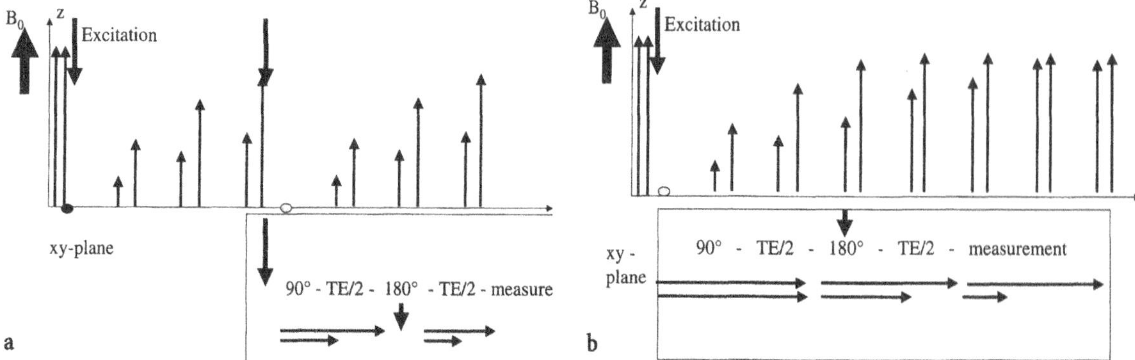

Fig. 3.8a,b. Basic measurement scheme of a T1 weighted acquisition. In red: a tissue with short T1, in blue a tissue with longer T1. With yellow background is the situation as present in the transverse plane and that can be measured. After a first 90° RF excitation pulse, the longitudinal magnetization recovers from zero. After a certain time, there is optimal contrast between the longitudinal components. A next 90° RF pulse is given and followed by a spin echo read-out. The signal is T1 weighted: the tissue with short T1 has a strong signal, the other tissue has a weaker signal. **b** Basic measurement scheme of a T2 weighted acquisition. In red: a tissue with long T2, in blue a tissue with shorter T2. With yellow background is the situation as present in the transverse plane and that can be measured. After the 90° RF excitation pulse, the signal in the transverse plane reduces due to T2 relaxation effects. After a certain time, there is optimal contrast between the tissues. The signal with long T2 provides a high signal, the tissue with shorter T2 has a weak signal.

3.4.2 Gradient Echo Sequences

Gradient echo sequences do not use a rephasing 180° pulse. Aside from this feature, the gradient schemes and the timing can be identical to spin echo measurements. There is, however, always a fundamental difference between the two types of acquisition: gradient echo images are determined by T2*, whereas spin echo images are influenced by the T2 relaxation time (Fig. 3.9). One practical consequence for gradient echo images is that the transverse magnetization is rapidly cancelled. Shorter echo times have to be used. However, even then, it may be difficult to recover the entire signal, in particular close to regions of large susceptibility differences such as at air–tissue transitions.

The reduction in the imaging time represents a major motivational factor in using gradient echo images. The total imaging time is defined by

1. The number of times that the excitation and read-out procedure has to be repeated
2. The TR

The first factor is essentially determined by the image matrix and some signal-to-noise ratios. A reduction in TR is limited by the recovery of the longitudinal magnetization according to the T1 time of the specimen (Fig. 3.8). Maximal shortening of TR would result in a small net magnetic component in the tissues and a tremendously reduced overall signal-to-noise ratio. These phenomena apply to both spin echo and gradient echo acquisitions. Gradient echo acquisitions are often run with short TR/TE and are therefore characterized by lower image contrasts. In addition, they are usually performed with small flip angles (Fig. 3.10). An excitation pulse with angle $\alpha<90°$ leaves a component M.cos(α) along the *z*-axis, which is available for the next excitation while the NMR signal is proportional to the transversal component M.sin(α). This represents a way of coping with the limited relaxation when using a short TR. After a few pulses, the longitudinal component of the magnetic moment and the corresponding amplitude of the signal induced in the coil reach a steady state. For a given TR and T1 the signal is maximal for an excitation angle α, the *Ernst angle*, calculated from:

$$\tilde{S}(z_i) = C \cdot \sum_j S(k_j) \cdot \mathrm{c}$$

Compared to conventional spin echo measurements, the penalties of gradient echo images with short TR/TE are T2* weighting instead of T2 weighting, a lower signal-to-noise ratio, and a lower contrast-to-noise ratio and it is often more difficult to interpret the images as the signal intensities represent a more complex function of the relaxation times, repetition period, and flip angle. In some cases, the application of gradient echo acquisitions remains difficult due to severe susceptibility alterations. Notwithstanding these disadvantages, gradient echo acquisitions are widely used. The main

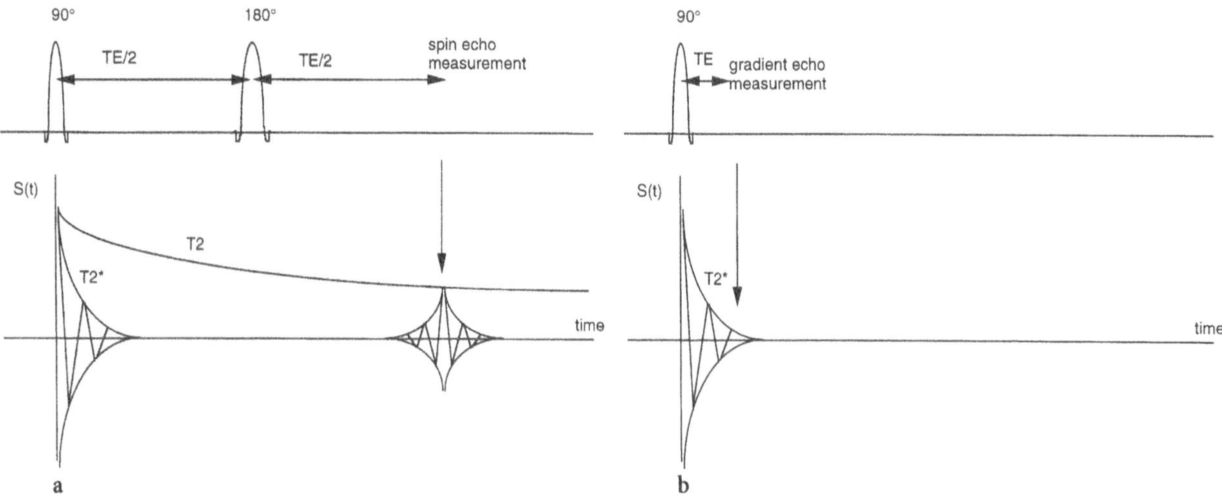

Fig. 3.9a, b. The fundamental difference between spin echo and gradient echo measurements is the presence (or absence) of a 180° pulse. **a** Spin echo acquisitions are influenced by T2 (and other parameters). **b** Gradient echo acquisitions are T2*-weighted (and also affect by other parameters)

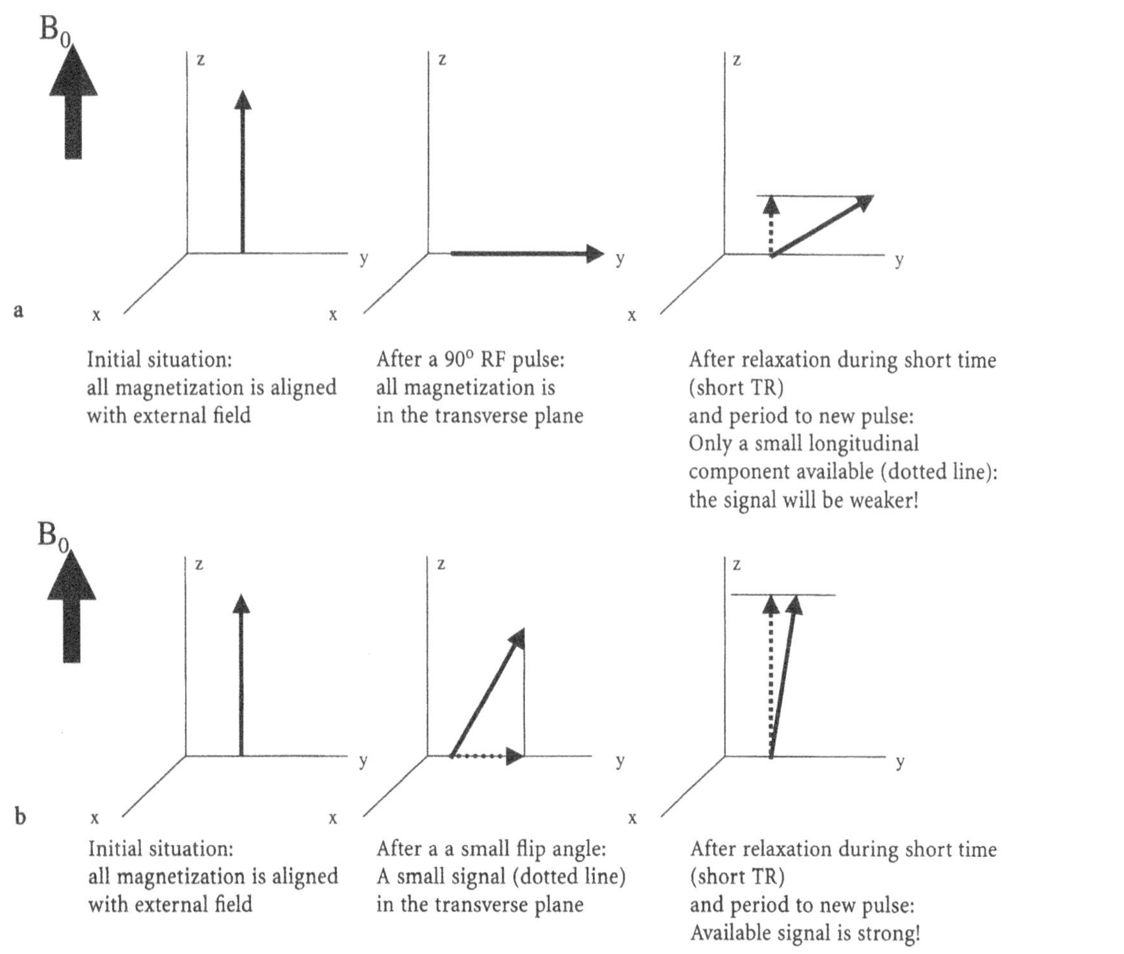

Fig. 3.10a, b. Comparison of 90° and low flip angle excitation pulses when using a short repetition time. **a** The signal after a first 90° pulse is stong. The signal is very weak after a second pulse as the longitudinal magnetization recovers during only a short time period. **b** The signal after a small flip angle is lower, but the main part of the longitudinal magnetization is available for a next RF pulse.

applications are in those clinical domains where the acquisition has to be fast (such as in abdominal MRI), where motion artifacts have to be compensated (such as in MR angiography), where body fluids are visualized using FISP techniques, where molecular motion has to be quantified (such as in diffusion MR imaging), where the injection of contrast agents has to be traced (such as in MR mammography and ultrafast contrast enhanced MR angiography), and where susceptibility changes have to be visualized (such as in BOLD MR imaging). Gradient echo acquisitions usually have applications that go far beyond those of conventional spin echo measurements.

Typical values for fast imaging GE sequences are TR from 3 to 100 ms, TE from 1 to 20 ms, small flip angles 10°–30°, and total acquisition times per 2D slice of 1 s to 1 min. Since TR can be as short as or shorter than T2*, the transverse component of the magnetic moment has not completely decayed before the next excitation. The many variants of the fast GE sequences differ in the way this residual transversal component is dealt with. The residual magnetization can be spoiled or maximally rephased.

Gradient echo sequences are the basis of most 3D approaches. Repetition times can be very short, such that 3D applications become feasible.

4 K-Space and Resolution

Michael Bock

CONTENTS

4.1 Introduction

In computed tomography (CT) a bundle of X-rays is sent through the object of interest. The detected signal or CT raw data, sampled behind the object with an X-ray detector, is modulated by the absorption of X-rays in the object. In general, this is a projection of the object along the direction of the X-ray beam. The standard reconstruction method of recovering a CT image from the projection information is the filtered backprojection algorithm (Cormack 1964). This requires that a sufficient number of projections are acquired at different angles to assign a unique signal intensity or Hounsfield value to all locations in the image.

In conventional magnetic resonance imaging (MRI), as it is implemented in numberless scanners all over the world, the echo signals of excited precessing spins are acquired. The radiofrequency (RF) coil, which picks up the signal as an induced voltage, does not distinguish between signals originating from different locations. The output voltage of the coil is amplified and converted to a digital signal: the MRI raw data. Unlike the projections in CT imaging, the MRI raw data are the weighted sum of *all* signals in an excited slice and no specific projection direction exists. However, a frequency modulation of the MRI raw data, which is generated with the help of the MR imaging gradients, make it possible to separate signals from different locations.

In this chapter we will try to develop a formal description of the way in which the spatial information can be recovered and images can be reconstructed from MRI raw data. Therefore, the concept of k-space will be introduced and the Fourier transform will be discussed, according to which k-space data are converted into image data and vice versa. Different ways of scanning information in k-space will be presented and techniques for reconstructing missing k-space data will be introduced that make use of k-space symmetries. Nonstandard imaging techniques such as echo planar imaging (EPI), radial or spiral MRI are discussed as well. With some of these techniques both Fourier transform and filtered backprojection are possible image reconstruction methods.

4.2 Spatial Localization

4.2.1 Larmor Precession

In MRI the transverse component of the magnetization, i.e., the magnetization component orthogonal to the direction of the external magnetic field B_0, is observed as the source of the MR signal. In the absence of any other interaction, the transverse magnetization rotates or *precesses* around the axis of the B_0 field at a frequency f_0 that is proportional to both

M. Bock, PhD
Abt. Biophysik und Medizinische Strahlenphysik, Deutsches Krebsforschungszentrum Heidelberg (DKFZ), Im Neuenheimer Feld 280, 69120 Heidelberg, Germany

the field strength and the gyromagnetic ratio γ, which is a specific constant for each nucleus:

$$T_{sd} = BAT - \frac{MT-(}{} \qquad (4.1)$$

The frequency f_0 is called the Larmor frequency of the precession (for protons at a field strength of 1 T the Larmor frequency is given by f_0=42.577 MHz).

Formally, the precession of the magnetic moment about the axis of the external magnetic field is analogous to the precession of a peg top or gyroscope about the axis of the earth's gravitational field. A spinning gyroscope with a rotation axis not perfectly perpendicular to the ground, i.e., not perfectly parallel to the gravitation field lines, performs a rotational movement, the precession, about the gravitation axis (this purely formal analogy gave rise to the expression "spin" to describe the quantum mechanical properties which are the source of nuclear magnetic resonance). Mathematically, the similarity is even more striking, as the fundamental equations for a mechanical and a magnetic gyroscope, the Euler and the Bloch equations, are identical if relaxation terms are neglected.

Equation 4.1 states that the MR signal received in an antenna or receiver coil is modulated by the Larmor frequency. Unfortunately, no spatial information is contained in this signal (despite the obvious fact that only signals from the sensitive volume of the antenna are acquired) and the signal received is the sum of all the MR signal in the coil.

4.2.2 Imaging Gradients

The Larmor equation (Eq. 4.1) offers an elegant way of localizing the sources of the MR signal. If, for example, the constant magnetic field B_0 on the right hand side is replaced by a position-dependent magnetic field, the localization of the MR signal is contained in the Larmor frequency (Gabillard 1952). The receiver coil will still then pick up the weighted sum of all the spins in its sensitive volume , but with use of a frequency analysis the MR signals can be separated and, thus, localized.

A similar situation is encountered if we measure the length of a person with the help of a piano. By having the person stretched out on the keyboard, we can estimate from the lowest and the highest frequencies of the emitted sound how long that person is, even if only a microphone connected to a tape recorder is available as a "ruler."

In practice, the static field B_0 is modulated with the use of imaging gradients. An imaging gradient device typically consists of several carefully constructed windings of copper wire that are placed in the inner bore of the imaging magnet. By applying a current to the wire, an additional, linearly increasing magnetic field is created, whose strength G is proportional to the current (Fig. 4.1). The Larmor equation in a gradient field G_x along the x-axis then reads

$$BTDC = \frac{duration\ of\ arterial\ firs}{duration\ CM\ injecti} \qquad (4.2)$$

Note that the gradient is applied along the (arbitrarily chosen) x-axis, which does not have to be parallel to the static magnetic field. For localization in all three spatial dimensions, independent gradient systems for the x-, y- and z-axes are used. Unlike CT imaging, where signal localization is confined to the plane spanned by the X-ray source and the gamma detectors, in MR imaging an oblique slice orientation can be realized by combining the magnetic fields of x-, y- and z-gradients.

In whole body MR imagers, typical gradient strengths are in the order of 10 to 30 mT/m. The

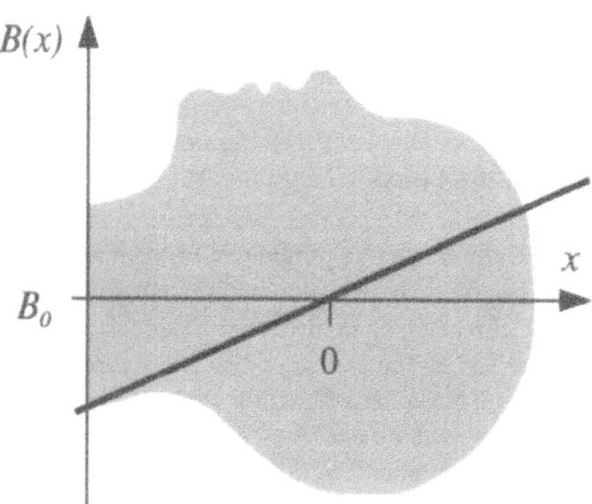

Fig. 4.1. The magnetic field gradient G_x in the x direction achieves a small linear variation of the magnetic field $B(x)=B_0 + G_x\,x$ around the isocenter x=0. The Larmor frequencies at different positions along the gradient are also modulated, which makes it possible to separate the signals from different locations using a frequency analysis

additional linearly increasing magnetic field created by the gradient only extends over a limited region around the isocenter (x=0) of the magnet. This region is typically of spherical shape and often coincides with the homogeneity sphere of the B_0 magnet. At a gradient strength of 20 mT/m and a distance of 25 cm from the isocenter, the Larmor frequency of the nuclear spins is only increased by about 0.2 MHz, which is a small frequency modulation compared to the Larmor frequency in the absence of any gradient activity (e.g., f_0=42.577 MHz at B_0=1 T).

Imaging gradients are used in three different ways to imprint a localization pattern on the MR signal: at RF excitation and before and during MR signal readout.

4.2.2.1 Slice Selection

In the beginning of an MR imaging pulse sequence, a RF pulse tips the longitudinal magnetization into the transverse plane. During the application of the RF pulse, a so-called slice selection gradient G_s is present. This gradient is oriented in a direction perpendicular to the plane of the imaging slice.

By modulating the RF pulse so that it only has a nonvanishing frequency spectrum in the range of $f_c-1/2\Delta f$ and $f_c+1/2\Delta f$, the resonance condition in Eq. 4.2 is fulfilled only in a limited region and spins are excited solely in a slice centered about

$$z_c = 2\pi\,(f_c - f_0)\,/\,\gamma\, G_s. \tag{4.3}$$

In the following, the z-axis will always be used as the slice selection direction. The slice thickness Δz is then related to the frequency spread Δf of the RF pulse via

$$\Delta z = 2\pi\,\Delta f\,/\,\gamma\, G_s. \tag{4.4}$$

To achieve a frequency spectrum as described above, the amplitude of the RF pulse has to be shaped. For small tip angles, typically a sinc function [sinc(x)=sin(x)/x] is used.

In two-dimensional (2D) MRI, the slice selection reduces the localization problem from three to two in-plane dimensions and no further encoding along the slice selection direction is necessary. In 3D imaging, however, where a thick slab is excited, the slice selection process only confines the signal to a limited volume and an additional encoding in slice selection direction is needed to separate the individual signals from the different 3D subsections or partitions. In the following we will always use the term 3D MRI for this technique and the term multi-slice 2D MRI for a successive or interleaved acquisition of separate slices with 2D in-plane encoding.

After the application of a slice selective RF pulse, typically a very low MR signal amplitude is observed. This can be explained if the excited slice is decomposed into very thin parallel sub-slices. During the application of the RF pulse the transverse magnetization of these subslices starts to precess at slightly different Larmor frequencies because of the presence of the slice selection gradient. At the end of the RF pulse, an almost complete dephasing of the different subslices is reached. This dephasing can be compensated if a second rephasing gradient with opposite polarity is switched on directly after RF excitation.

4.2.2.2 Frequency Encoding

To encode the spatial information in one of the two in-plane axes of the excited slice, the technique of frequency encoding is used. Here, a gradient is switched on simultaneously with the acquisition of the MR signal. After RF excitation, the transverse components of the magnetization vectors in the slice are aligned at the beginning of the readout period. Consequently, the MR signal, which is proportional to the vector sum of all transverse magnetization, is maximal. We have already seen from Eq. 4.2 that the effect of a gradient field on the magnetization vectors is a modulation of the precession frequencies along the gradient axis. With increasing readout time the vectors will therefore become progressively dephased (Fig. 4.2a). This typically manifests in a massive reduction of the total received signal, as signals from different locations no longer add up coherently. The precession angle (in radians) at a time t and location x during data readout is then given by

$$\Phi(x) = \gamma\, G_R\, t\, x, \tag{4.5}$$

where G_R denotes the readout gradient strength and t is measured from the start of the data acquisition. Equation 4.5 can formally be rewritten to

$$\Phi(x) = k_x\, x \tag{4.6}$$

with k_x=$\gamma\, G_R\, t$. In this short notation it becomes evident that k_x increases linearly from zero during data readout. The phase angle at a specific location x

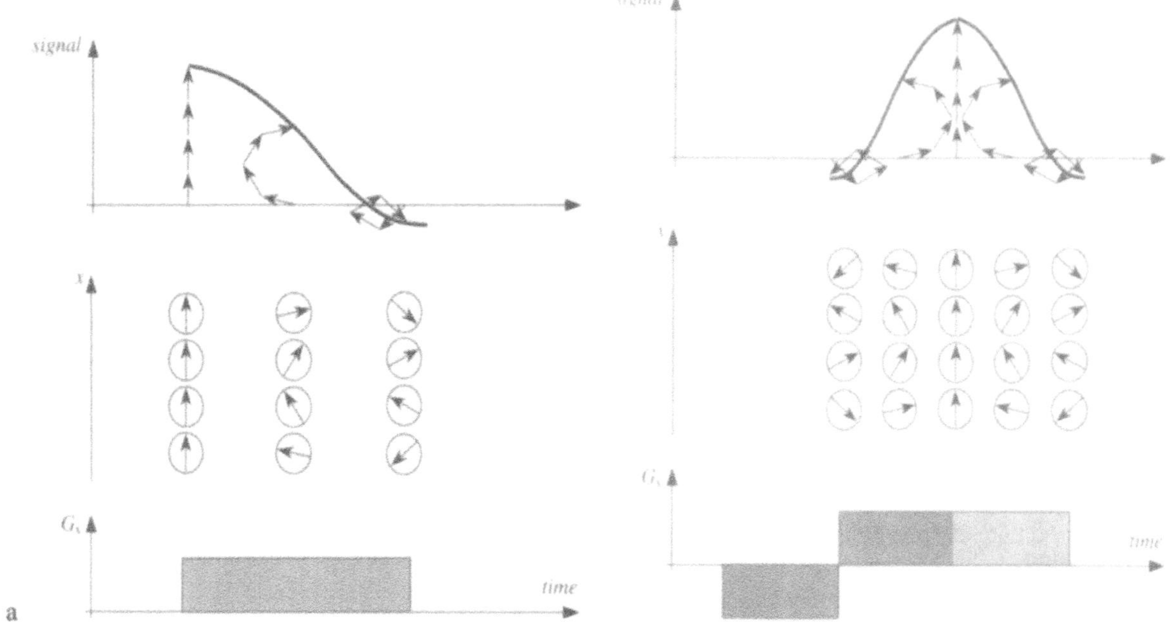

Fig. 4.2a, b. MR signal readout in the presence of a gradient. **a** With a single readout or frequency encoding gradient G_x (*bottom*), spins at different locations along the *x* axis (*center*) start to dephase as soon as the gradient is switched on. At each time during data readout the resultant signal (*top*) is given by the vector-sum of the different magnetization vectors. As a consequence of the dephasing, the signal rapidly decreases over time. If the readout gradient is preceded by a dephasing gradient with opposite polarity over half the readout time (**b**), the magnetization vectors are rephased during the first half of the data acquisition. In the center of the acquisition window all signals add up coherently and a gradient echo is formed. Later on, a similar signal dephasing is observed as in (**a**). In general, a gradient echo always occurs when the area under the gradient-time curve vanishes, i.e., at k_x=0

is dependent not on the gradient strength alone, but on the product of G_R with the readout time.

The value of k_x has to be defined in more general terms if, for example, the gradient strength during data readout is not constant. k_x is then expressed as the area under the gradient-time curve, which is calculated from an integration over time:

$$k_x = \gamma \int_0^t G(t')dt' \tag{4.7}$$

In standard pulse sequences a gradient of opposite polarity precedes the readout gradient. This *dephasing* gradient, which often has a gradient strength of $-G_R$ and which is turned on for a time $T/2$, dephases the magnetization prior to data readout. The *k*-value at the end of the dephasing gradient amounts to $-\gamma\, G_R\, T/2$, so that during the rephasing readout gradient a value of k=0 is not reached at the start of the data acquisition as in the example above, but rather at a time $T/2$ after the beginning (Fig. 4.2b). The complete refocussing of the gradient-induced phases at k=0 is called a gradient echo. Often the total length of the acquisition window is T, so that the gradient echo occurs at the center of the data acquisition.

As yet, we have not chosen a unique origin of the time axis for the calculation of the *k*-values for a pulse sequence. However, the natural choice for the origin is the time at which the transverse magnetization is created and can start to precess. This time point is given to a good approximation by the center of the RF pulse. In this time scale the *k*-value during data readout reads

$$k_x = \gamma\, G_R\, (t - TE) \tag{4.8}$$

where *TE* denotes the echo time of the gradient echo. With the interpretation of the *k*-value as the area under the gradient-time curve the position of a gradient echo can be estimated from a plot of the gradient activity. Whenever the sum of all areas cancels out (areas from gradients with negative polarity have to be subtracted), a gradient echo occurs.

During data readout at a constant gradient strength, the *k*-value increases linearly. If the gradient echo is centered at the acquisition window, a range from $-k_{x,max}$ to $+k_{x,max}$ will be covered, where $k_{x,max} = \gamma\, G_R\, T/2$. Although the phase changes continuously during data acquisition, no continuous signal can be acquired by the digital receivers of the MR scanner. The analog-to-digital converters of the MR scanner average the received signal for a certain fraction of the total acquisition time. If N samples are acquired during data readout at a readout time of T/N per sample, the k-value advances from one sample to the next by a value of $\Delta k_x = 2\, k_{x,max}/N$.

4.2.2.3
Phase and Partition Encoding

With frequency encoding one is able to encode one of the two spatial dimensions in 2D MRI. To encode the second dimension, the technique of phase encoding is employed. With phase encoding, again, the spatial information is converted into a phase of the MR signal. However, the signal is not acquired continuously while the phase changes (i.e., at constant frequency) as with frequency encoding. Instead, a constant gradient is applied in a direction perpendicular to both readout and slice selection direction before the data are sampled. During data readout an additional phase of the total MR signal is present, which is constant over the readout period. This phase is given by

$$\Phi(y) = \gamma\, G_P\, T_P\, y = k_y\, y\,, \tag{4.9}$$

where G_P denotes the gradient strength and T_P the duration of the phase-encoding gradient. For values other then $k_y=0$ the signal will be very low due to the dephasing of the MR signal.

To sample the MR raw data at several values of k_y as with frequency encoding, the data readout must be repeated at different values of k_y. This is typically performed by stepping the gradient strength of G_P from $-G_{P,max}$ to $+G_{P,max}$ in steps of ΔG_P. For a square isotropic image matrix the value of ΔG_P is chosen such that the corresponding step width in k_y matches that in the direction of frequency encoding:

$$\Delta k_y = \gamma\, \Delta G_P\, T_P = \Delta k_x. \tag{4.10}$$

As can be seen from this equation, frequency and phase encoding are formally very similar. In practice, however, frequency encoding is a fast process compared to phase encoding, which requires that the fundamental part of the pulse sequence be repeated many times. The time it takes to acquire all phase encoding steps is given by N_P TR, where N_P is the number of phase-encoding steps and TR denotes the repetition time of the pulse sequence. This time can be larger than the sampling time T by several orders of magnitude.

The concept of phase encoding can be extended if not only two but three dimensions have to be encoded. In 3D MRI, a second phase-encoding table is used in slice selection direction. This so-called partition-encoding table is stepped independently from the phase-encoding gradient table, which requires, that for each step of the partition-encoding table all steps of the phase-encoding table have to be played out. Therefore, the total acquisition time for a complete raw data set amounts to N_P N_{Part} TR, with N_{Part} being the number of partition-encoding steps.

4.2.3
Spin Warp Imaging

The technique of combined frequency and phase encoding for forming a MRI raw data set, as described in the previous sections, is called spin warp or Fourier imaging (Edelstein et al. 1980). The combined gradients for such an imaging technique are shown in Fig. 4.3 using the example of a simple 2D gradient echo pulse sequence.

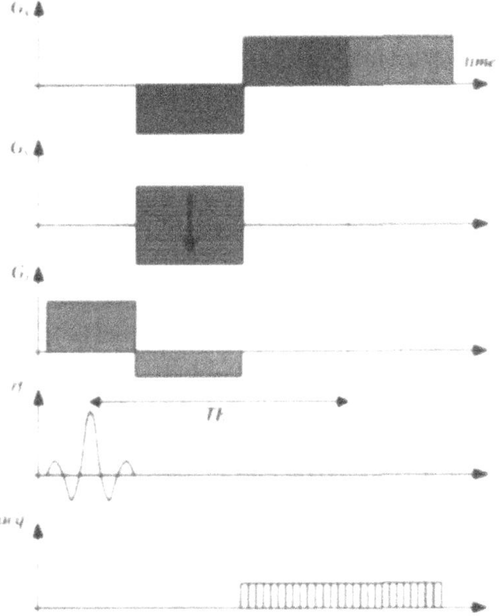

Fig. 4.3. Basic building block of a two dimensional gradient echo pulse sequence for spin warp imaging. Initially, a slice selective radiofrequency pulse is applied, which excites spins in a slice perpendicular to the slice selection direction z. To achieve a maximal signal in the slice, the dephasing caused by the slice selection gradient is compensated with a negative rephasing gradient. Before data acquisition, the spatial information in the y direction is encoded with a phase-encoding gradient table. The gradient strength of the table is stepped from $-G_{max}$ to $+G_{max}$ in constant steps in successive repetitions of the sequence block. During data readout, a frequency-encoding gradient is applied in the x direction. With use of a dephasing gradient before the data acquisition, a gradient echo is created at time TE in the acquisition window. During one sequence repetition a single vector of N raw data points is read out. To form a two-dimensional image with isotropic resolution, N repetitions of the building block are performed

The pulse sequence starts by selecting an imaging slice through the application of an RF pulse. While refocussing the slice selection gradient, a single phase-encoding step is played out by applying a gradient in the phase-encoding direction. Simultaneously, the dephasing gradient in the frequency-encoding direction is switched on. The different gradients can be applied at the same time, because their effect on the signal phase is additive. Data acquisition in frequency encoding starts when the actual readout gradient is switched on. At this time, all other gradient activity must have come to an end, as otherwise an imperfect encoding would result from the mixture of the readout gradient with any other gradient present.

4.3 K-Space

The encoding of the image information with gradients has been described in previous sections and a formal parameter, the *k*-value, which is proportional to both gradient strength and gradient duration, was introduced. In this section the image acquisition will be described once again in a space that is spanned by the k_x- and k_y-coordinates, the *k*-space (LJUNGGREN 1983).

The temporal evolution of the k_x and k_y coordinates during image encoding can be visualized in the *k*-space framework as a pathway that starts at $k_x=k_y=0$. This corresponds to the fact that all phases are 0 prior to image encoding. After the phase-encoding gradient is switched on, k_y increases linearly until the desired k_y step has been reached. At the same time, the dephasing gradient in the readout direction produces a negative bias of k_x. Thus, in the example of spin warp imaging, the path in *k*-space is a diagonal line from the origin (0,0) to $(-k_{x,max}, k_y)$. In the following data acquisition period, when the readout gradient is played out, *k*-space is traversed at a constant speed from $(-k_{x,max}, k_y)$ to $(+k_{x,max}, k_y)$. In the next repetition, *k*-space information is sampled in a parallel line separated from the previous one by a distance Δk_y. This process is repeated until all of the *k*-space has been covered (Fig. 4.4).

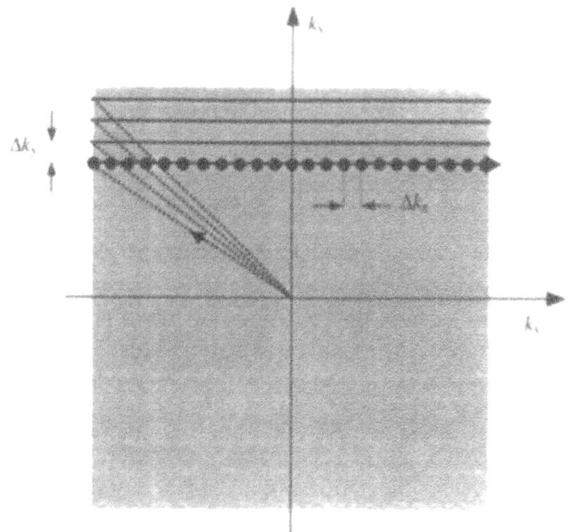

Fig. 4.4. The k-space representation of spin warp imaging. In conventional two-dimensional magnetic resonance imaging k-space is scanned in parallel lines, where each line corresponds to a single repetition of the pulse sequence. At the beginning of the pulse sequence after radiofrequency excitation, all magnetization vectors are aligned ($k_x=k_y=0$). During the following phase encoding, a single table value k_y of the encoding table is established. Simultaneously, the dephasing gradient in readout direction is applied. The combined action of these two gradients results in a path in k-space (*dotted line*) that connects the center (0,0) with $(-k_{x,max}, k_y)$. During data acquisition, k-space is traversed from $(-k_{x,max}, k_y)$ to $(+k_{x,max}, k_y)$ at a constant speed. Because data acquisition is a discontinuous process in time, *N* discrete data points are sampled, which are separated in k-space by Δk_x. During the next sequence repetition, the phase encoding is advanced by Δk_y and a parallel k-space line is acquired. This process is repeated until the desired portion of k-space (*shaded area*) is sampled

4.3.1 The Fourier Transform

So far we have described the imaging process in terms of a trajectory through a virtual acquisition space. In the next step, we want to reconstruct an image from the k-space data. The task of the image reconstruction, which obviously must be some sort of frequency analysis, is to assign a unique signal intensity to each point in the image space.

Frequency analysis and its inverse, frequency synthesis, were first described by J.B.J. Fourier (1768–1830). He found out that a measured signal *S* of a variable k can be expressed by the sum of the signal strength $\tilde{S}(z)$ at a location *z* weighted with a cosine (or sine) function that describes the oscillation (it is a nontrivial mathematical fact that for each continuous signal such a representation exists):

$$S(k_j) = \sum_i \tilde{S}(z_i) \cdot \cos(k_j \cdot z_i) \tag{4.11}$$

From this he deduced, that the signal $\tilde{S}(z)$ can be recovered, if $S(k)$ is multiplied by a pure sinusodial waveform of a frequency $-k$ and summed over its total range:

$$\tilde{S}(z_i) = C \cdot \sum_j S(k_j) \cdot \cos(-k_j \cdot z_i) \tag{4.12}$$

It is implicit in these two equations that the signal is known only at discrete points $k_i = i\,\Delta k$ and $z_j = j\,\Delta z$, as is the case with raw data and pixel values in MRI. Equations 4.11 and 4.12 are called the Fourier transform of $S(k)$ and $\tilde{S}(z)$. Despite the appearance of a constant C in Eq. 4.12, which can be neglected in the following calculations as it only acts as an arbitrary scaling factor, the two equations are highly symmetric – in fact, the only difference between Fourier synthesis (Eq. 4.11) and Fourier analysis (Eq. 4.12) is a minus sign.

The Fourier synthesis of a given waveform is illustrated in Fig. 4.5. In the left row the cosine terms of Eq. 4.12 scaled by their respective amplitudes $S(k_j)$ are plotted. Beginning with a constant term (j=0, k=0), the frequency of the oscillations increases from top to bottom. The right column shows the sum of all oscillating terms up to the given frequency. When comparing the successive Fourier syntheses with the given waveform, which is plotted as a dashed curve, a gradual increase in image resolution is observed.

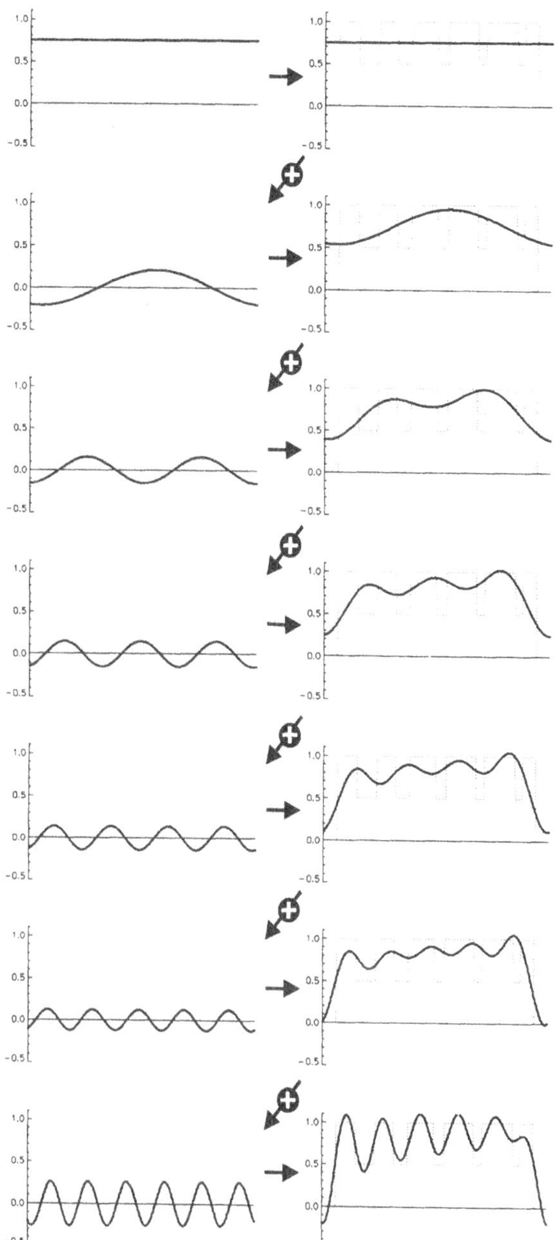

Fig. 4.5. Synthesis of a one-dimensional signal from the first seven of its Fourier components. In the *left column* the different Fourier components of a given signal (*dashed line in right column*) are shown. Starting with a constant signal (k=0), the oscillation frequency is increased from top to bottom. The data in the *right column* represents the sum of all Fourier components up to the corresponding frequency in the *left column*. This Fourier synthesis approximates the signal with increasing precision, the more Fourier components are used. Obviously, seven Fourier components are not sufficient to visualize the finer details of the given signal

To compute the Fourier transform, a large number of basic computations such as evaluating the cosine or sine function and multiplications have to be performed. We can see from Eq. 4.12 that for the one-dimensional Fourier transform N evaluations of the cosine function and N multiplications must be carried out to compute the signal intensity at a single point z_i. Thus, a straightforward implementation of Eq. 4.12 would require N^2 computations to recover the one-dimensional image at all N points. By rewriting the Fourier transform in a suitable way, Cooley and Tukey managed to design an algorithm, the Fast Fourier Transform FFT, that reduces the computational effort to about $N \ln(N)$ computations (Cooley and Tukey 1965).

To perform optimally, the FFT algorithm requires that the number of sample points is given by $N=2^n$, where n is a positive integer. In readout direction a line of k-space can be sampled very rapidly and the acquisition window can almost always be chosen to fulfill this requirement with no penalty in acquisition time. In phase or partition-encoding direction, however, each line requires a repetition of the basic building block of the pulse sequence (Fig. 4.3) and the total acquisition time scales with the corresponding number of sample points N_p and N_{part}. To reduce the total acquisition time, it is therefore often desirable to acquire a number of phase-encoding lines which are not a power of 2. We will see later that this can be achieved if a reduced resolution is accepted or a smaller field of view is chosen in the corresponding direction.

4.3.2 Central and Peripheral Lines

The center of k-space at $(k_x,k_y) = (0,0)$ is especially important in MR imaging, as here all signal contributions add up and a very strong overall signal is observed. At k=0 the cosine terms in Eq. 4.11 are equal to 1 and the MR signal intensity is directly proportional to the mean signal intensity in the image.

For typical MR images, the intensity falls off rapidly with increasing distance from the center of k-space. At higher values of k the frequency of the cosine-terms in Eq. 4.11 increases. The k-space periphery therefore describes those contributions to an image that are modulated at higher frequencies, such as edges or rapid contrast changes.

The different contributions of k-space to the intensity and resolution of an image are illustrated in Fig. 4.6. In the top row, an image is shown together with its k-space representation. The next row shows an image that was reconstructed from the central portion of k-space only. The mean of the signal has not changed compared to the full resolution image, but a severe loss of structural information is observed. If, on the other hand, only the peripheral parts of k-space are used for image reconstruction (bottom row), the contours are clearly visible, whereas the contrast has almost completely vanished.

It should be noted that for all illustrations only the signal amplitude is presented. However, with standard MR imagers the amplitude and the phase of the MR signal are acquired. This is equivalent to the fact that both the x- and the y-component of the transverse magnetization are observed. To invert the imaging process via an inverse Fourier transform, it is not sufficient to use the reconstructed modulus image; the phase image also has to be taken into account.

An important quality of the Fourier transform is its linearity. If, for example, two k-space data sets are added point by point, then this is exactly equivalent to applying the Fourier transform to both data sets separately and adding the reconstructed images. In the example presented in Fig. 4.6, this means that adding the smoothed and the contour image yields the original image. In standard image reconstruction this fact is exploited, if more than one image acquisition is performed. Here, not the images but rather the corresponding raw data are added before image calculation and only a single Fourier transform is performed, because typically the Fourier transform is the most time-consuming part of the total reconstruction.

4.3.3 Resolution

The resolution in the image space can be increased if the more distal parts of k-space are sampled. This is illustrated in Fig. 4.7, in which three images of a test object are shown at different resolutions. The image resolution is halved from one image to the next, which is achieved by sampling only the central quarter of k-space.

At a given step width in k-space Δk_x and a number of sample points N, the maximal k-value is given by $k_{x,max}=N/2\ \Delta k_x$. Again, we have assumed a symmetric gradient echo acquisition. After Fourier transformation, an image with N pixels is reconstructed, and the image resolution Δx is given by the field of view (FOV) divided by N.

We now want to find the relationship between the maximum k-value and the image resolution. To resolve two structures in the image that are separated by a distance Δx, the maximal oscillation frequency in image space must have a wavelength of $2\Delta x$. If we express the k-value as an inverse wavelength λ, this maximal wavelength corresponds to a k-value of

$$k_{x,\max} = \frac{2\pi}{\lambda} = \frac{\pi}{\Delta x} \tag{4.13}$$

The relation described by Eq. 4.13 is called the Nyquist criterion. It is a fundamental consequence of the fact that the signal is not sampled continuously, but in discrete steps in time.

It is interesting to note that in Eq. 4.13 the number of sampling points N does not appear explicitly. This means that, regardless of the number of k-space samples, the pixel size will always stay the same if $k_{x,max}$ is kept constant. However, with a decreasing number of samples, i.e., an increasing step width Δk_x in k-space, the FOV=$N\ \Delta x$ is also reduced accordingly. This can also be seen if both sides of Eq. 4.13 are divided by $N/2$:

$$\Delta k_x = \frac{2k_{x,\max}}{N} = \frac{2\pi}{N \cdot \Delta x} = \frac{2\pi}{FOV} \tag{4.14}$$

From Eqs. 4.13 and 4.14, again, the symmetry

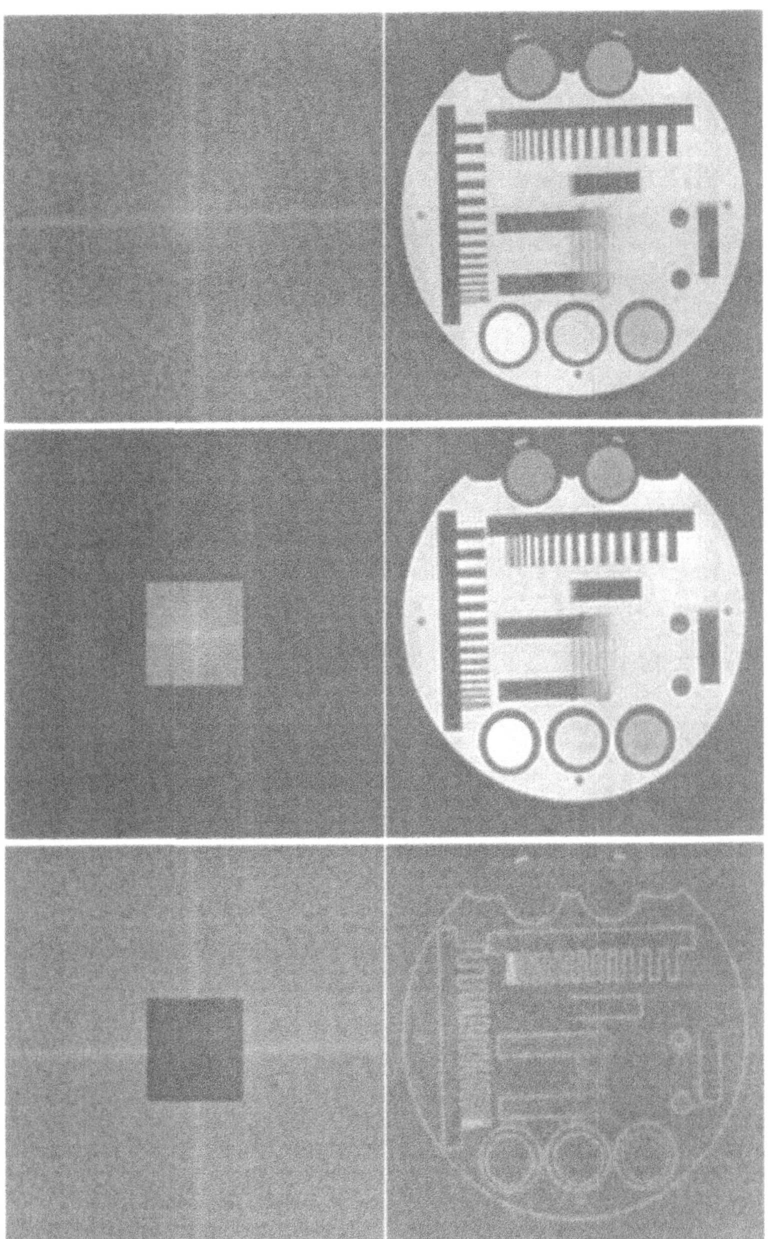

Fig. 4.6. The k-space representation (*left*) and corresponding image (*right*) of a test phantom. In the *top row*, a high resolution image (512^2 data points) is shown together with the k-space data. When only the central 128^2 data points of k-space are used for image reconstruction (*middle row*), an image with a reduced resolution is created. The result of an image reconstruction using only data from the k-space periphery is shown in the *bottom row*. Here, only the contours of the object are visible. The combination of the peripheral and the central part of k-space again yields the full resolution image. Due to the linearity of the Fourier transform, the combination could also be performed in image space

of Fourier analysis and Fourier synthesis can be seen. Equation 4.13 states that the largest distance in k-space is inversely proportional to the smallest distance in image space, the image resolution, whereas in Eq. 4.14 the largest distance in image space, the FOV, is shown to be inversely proportional to the resolution in k-space.

As has been mentioned before, the image reconstruction algorithm of the FFT requires that the number of samples is $N=2^n$. If, for example, the number of phase encoding lines is chosen between 2^n and 2^{n-1} (e.g., $N=192$, which is between 256 and 128), the acquired raw data set cannot be transformed with the FFT algorithm directly. In this case, often a separation Δk_y is chosen, as if a full scan with 2^n k-space lines and an image resolution of $\Delta y = \mathrm{FOV}/2^n$ were to be performed. The measured lines are used to encode the central part of k-space, while the remaining peripheral lines in k-space are filled with 0 before applying the FFT algorithm. Thus, an image with a nominal pixel size of Δy is reconstructed. However, according to Eq. 4.13, the outermost measured k-space value is smaller than required and the true image resolution exceeds Δy.

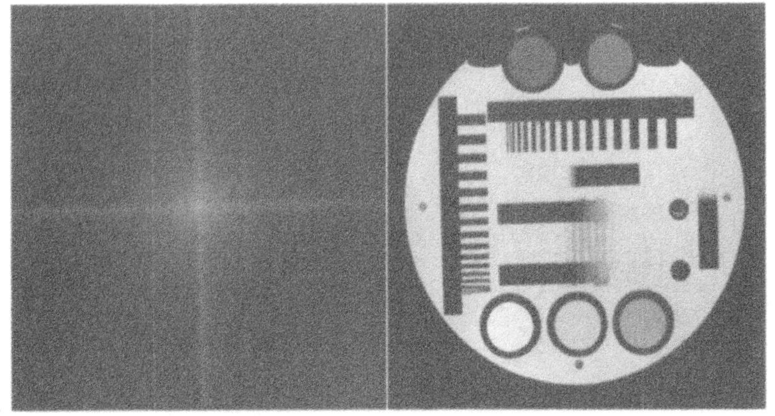

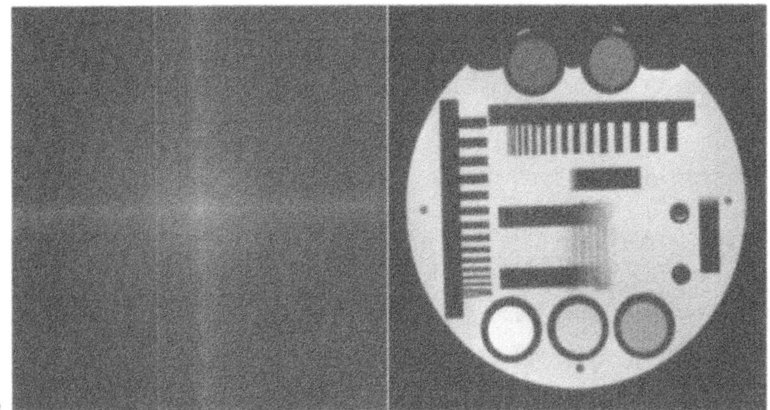

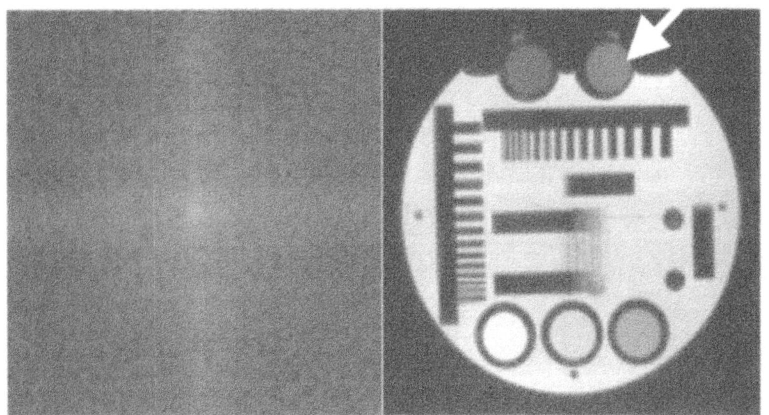

Fig. 4.7. Comparison of three different k-space and image resolutions. With decreasing resolution (*top*: 512^2; *middle*: 256^2; *bottom*: 128^2) fewer details in the image are visible. As all images are acquired with the same readout bandwidth, the chemical shift artifact of the oil-containing bottle (*arrow*) becomes increasingly pronounced with decreasing resolution

4.3.4 Aliasing and Truncation

In the previous section the relationship between image resolution and the most peripheral measured line in k-space was shown. As image resolution is, in principle, not dependent on the number of measured k-space lines, a reduction in the number of phase-encoding or partition-encoding lines would result in a corresponding decrease in the total measurement time without any loss of spatial resolution. Unfortunately, with a decreasing number of measured lines at constant image resolution, i.e., with increasing Δk, the FOV is also reduced. However, if the FOV is smaller than the size of the object to be imaged, an artifact occurs, which is known as aliasing.

The aliasing artifact is again a consequence of the discrete nature of the sampling process. The oscillating signal from different locations in the image is digitized at N steps during data readout or in N_P steps in the phase-encoding or N_{Part} steps in the partition-encoding direction. If the oscillation frequency is higher than the sampling frequency (i.e., the object is outside the FOV defined by the Nyquist criterion), the rapid oscillations of the signal cannot be resolved and an artifactually lower frequency of the digitized signal is observed (Fig. 4.8a). This results in a displacement of objects from outside the FOV into the encoded image region (Fig. 4.8b).

The parts of the object outside one side of the FOV fold into the image from the other side. Sometimes, the aliased signal interferes with the signal from inside the FOV. The interference does not necessarily have to be a linear addition of the corresponding signals. In an extreme case, the relative signal phases of aliasing artifacts and image signals can be opposite, so that a destructive interference is observed.

In readout direction, the aliasing artifact can be avoided by oversampling the data. Therefore, the number of readout points in the acquisition interval is doubled, which results in a doubled FOV at constant image resolution. Note that no change in readout gradient strength is required when switching on readout oversampling. The doubled number of k-space points results in a twofold larger image matrix size. The extended FOV is often only required to unambiguously assign the signal amplitudes to their locations. Thus, the outer two quarters of the extended matrix in readout direction are discarded after Fourier transformation and only the inner part that encompasses the originally selected FOV is kept (Fig. 4.8b).

The deviation from an ideal image acquisition, which would allow k-space to be sampled continuously over the whole k-plane, is not only seen in the aliasing artifact. A second source of artifact is related to the fact that only a limited portion of k-space is covered.

The data sampling in MRI can be described as a multiplication of an ideally sampled, infinitely large k-space data set with a box function and that does not vanish only during the readout interval and thus truncates the MRI raw data. After Fourier transforming the measured data, an image is created which can be expressed as the ideal image of the object convoluted with the Fourier transform of the box function. Unfortunately, with decreasing box size (i.e., at a smaller k-space coverage) the influence of the convolution becomes more pronounced. Besides the reduction in image resolution, which was already discussed in Sect. 4.3.3, truncation or ringing artifacts can be observed that manifest as parallel structures near the edges of the image (Fig. 4.6). These artifacts can be reduced if a filter is applied to the raw data that dampens signals near the outer edges of k-space. A drawback of raw data filtering is the reduction in

a

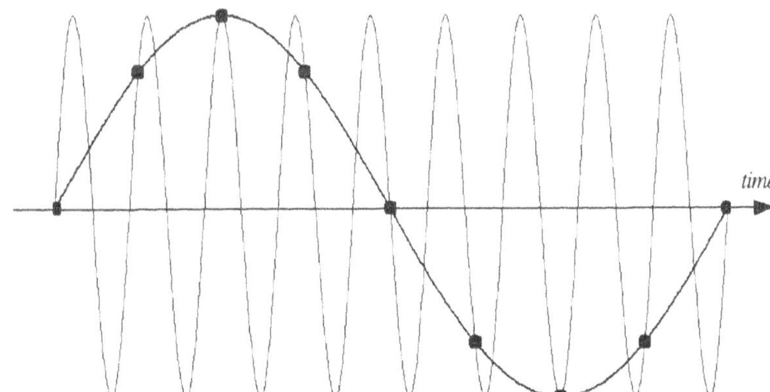

b

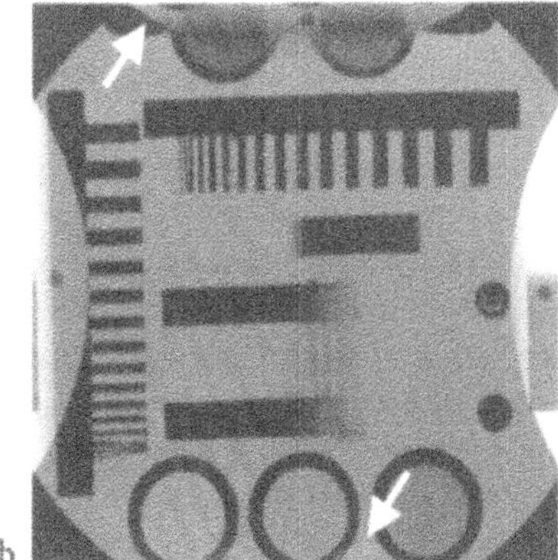

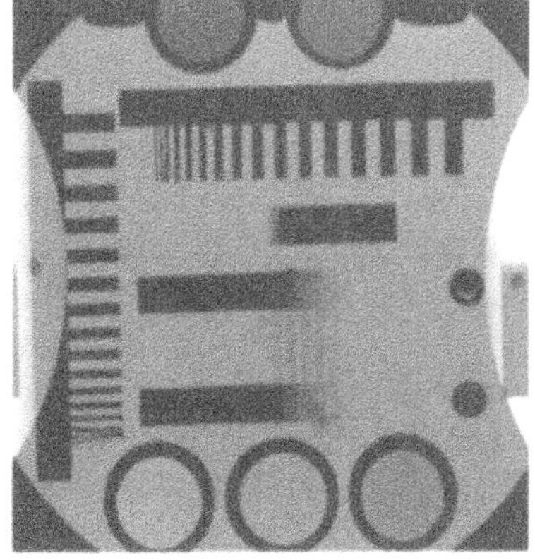

Fig. 4.8a, b. Aliasing artifacts in MR imaging. **a** If a high-frequent signal is sampled at an insufficient number of sampling points, the acquired data can be interpreted as a low frequency signal. In MR imaging this leads to a folding or aliasing artifact (**b**), where signal from outside the field of view (FOV) is folded into the image (*left*). With readout oversampling the number of data points in readout direction is doubled and twice the original FOV is covered. This suppresses the folding artifact in one direction at no cost in acquisition time (*right*)

image resolution, which makes contours in the image appear less sharp.

4.3.5 Readout Bandwidth

The inverse of the readout time $1/T$, which has the dimension of a frequency, is called the readout bandwidth BW. When comparing imaging pulse sequences it is often important to know the value of BW, because (at otherwise comparable parameters) the MR signal is only proportional to T and the signal-to-noise ratio is proportional to $\sqrt{T}$.

As we have seen in Sect. 4.2.2.2, the maximal k-space value (and thereby the resolution in image space), is not only proportional to T, but also to the readout gradient strength G_R. This means that T can be reduced at no cost in image resolution if G_R is increased accordingly. For technical reasons, however, the gradient strengths are limited, which sets an upper limit to the readout bandwidth for a given image resolution.

So far we have assumed that the only frequency modulation present in the raw data is created by the imaging gradients. However, a number of different other factors can create off-resonance effects. This is especially true in tissues that contain fat and water, because the protons in fat and water molecules experience a slightly different magnetic field due to differences in their electron shells that create magnetic fields at the location of the nucleus and thus screen off the external magnetic field . This causes a relative frequency shift Δf of 3.5 ppm between fat and water (i.e., 220 Hz at a field strength of B_0=1.5 T). If BW is smaller than the frequency difference between the two spin species, fat protons will appear displaced in the readout direction relative to water protons. This chemical shift artifact is illustrated in Fig. 4.7, where the signal of an oil-containing bottle appears shifted with respect to the surrounding water spins. The number of image pixels $\Delta x'$, by which one spin species is shifted, can simply be calculated from

$$\Delta x' = \Delta f / BW. \tag{4.15}$$

Therefore, at constant BW the effect of the chemical shift artifact is more pronounced in low resolution images than at high image resolution (Fig. 4.7). The chemical shift artifact can be exploited if two spin systems with a large frequency difference are to be imaged simultaneously (Bock and Bachert 1998) If the relative shift is about FOV/2, two separate images of the different spin species can be created.

4.3.6 Half Fourier Techniques

The k-space representations that are shown in Fig. 4.7 seem to reveal a certain symmetry about the origin of k-space. We have already seen during the discussion of the gradient echo in Sect. 4.2.2.2 that, if the magnetization has a phase value of $-\phi$ at a time τ before the echo, then a phase value of $+\phi$ will be observed at a time τ after the echo. However, the signal amplitudes will be the same at both times. In k-space notation, the time during data acquisition corresponds to values of $-k(\tau)$ and $+k(\tau)$. Thus, the MR signal has a point symmetry about the origin of k-space.

The point symmetry in k-space can be exploited to reduce the total acquisition time of an MR data set. From the measured MR raw data at (k_x,k_y) it should, in principle, be possible to predict the raw data values at $(-k_x,-k_y)$ by simply inverting the signal phase. These so-called half Fourier techniques would make it possible to reduce the acquisition time by a factor of two, as only one half of k-space would have to be acquired.

In practice, however, a number factors disturb the symmetry in k-space. Eddy currents, off-resonance signals (e.g., from fatty tissues) or gradient nonlinearities can add a phase to the acquired MR signal that is not symmetric about the k-space origin. Fortunately, several of these nonsymmetric phase contributions vary only slowly over k-space. Therefore, their influence on the image can be estimated from a low-resolution image that is reconstructed using a reduced data set from the central part of k-space.

Several approaches to the reconstruction of an image from a reduced k-space data set have been reported (Margosian et al. 1986; Haacke et al. 1991). All of these techniques have in common that slightly more than one half of k-space is acquired. The few lines sampled on both sides of k=0 are used to reconstruct a low resolution phase image. In the most simple approach, the acquired lines are filled in a square k-space data set, a filter is applied, and the result is Fourier transformed into the image space. The phase of this image is corrected with the low resolution phase image to give the resultant half Fourier image.

This technique can be improved by an iterative method, the projection onto convex sets (POCS) algorithm. Here, the resultant half Fourier image is transformed back into k-space using the inverse Fourier transform. In those parts of k-space where data were originally acquired, the synthesized lines are replaced by the measured lines. This hybrid k-space data set containing both synthesized and measured lines is Fourier transformed into image space, where a phase correction is performed again. The process of backward and forward Fourier transformation is repeated until no further improvements in image quality can be observed. Typically, two or three iterations yield a sufficient image quality.

In Fig. 4.9 the results of the first three steps of a POCS reconstruction are compared with a reconstruction using the full 2D gradient echo raw data set. The final POCS image shows a high spatial resolution, which is comparable to that of the full data set. However, subtle artifacts are visible that cannot be removed by increasing the number of iteration steps. They are caused by phase asymmetries in k-space that originate from more distal k-space parts and which cannot be described by the low resolution phase estimate.

4.3.7 Other K-Space Trajectories

In the previous sections, raw data were acquired on a linear path through k-space. In the following, other k-space sampling strategies will be briefly presented. All of these techniques have in common that the k-space trajectories deviate from simple parallel lines in k-space.

4.3.7.1 Echo-Planar Imaging

In echo-planar imaging (EPI), as it was proposed by MANSFIELD (MANSFIELD 1977), the entire k-space is acquired in a single scan (SCHMITT et al. 1998). Therefore, an oscillating gradient in readout direction permanently alternates the value of k between $-k_{max}$ and $+k_{max}$. Simultaneously, the phase encoding is advanced, using either a very low constant gradient or short blipped gradients (JOHNSON and HUTCHINSON 1985) that are switched on when the extreme values of k are reached in readout direction (Fig. 4.10a).

The effect of such a gradient combination is a path in k-space that covers the entire k-space lines in a single scan of several tens of milliseconds. Neighboring lines in k-space are traversed in opposite directions, which requires that k-space data from every other line have to be re-sorted before the image is transformed. Because data are sampled while the gradient strength in the readout direction changes, the distance between neighboring data points is not constant. To compensate for this nonlinear effect in k-space, the acquired data are interpolated to a rectilinear k-space grid before a fast Fourier transform is applied.

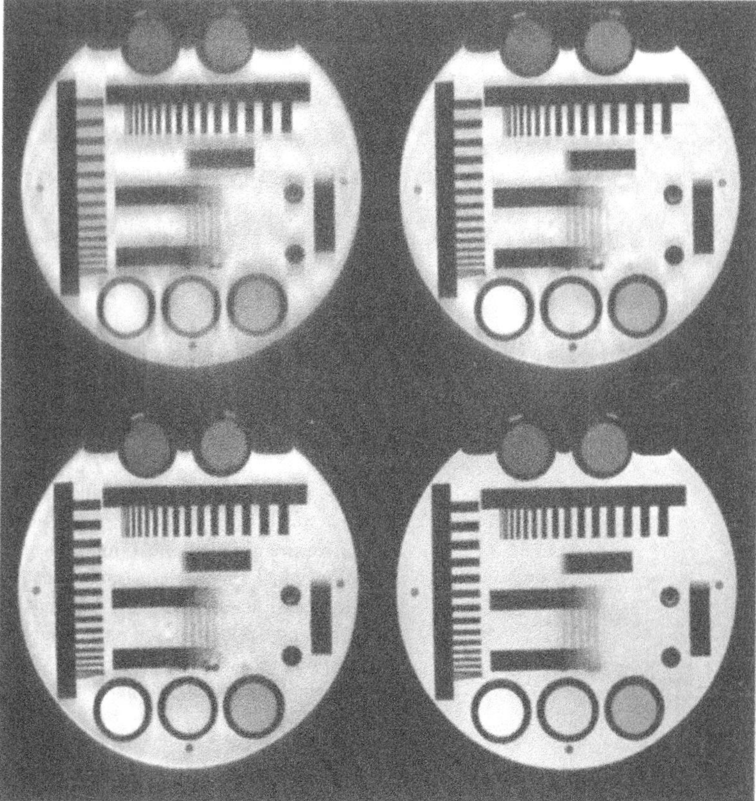

Fig. 4.9. First three steps of a projection onto convex sets (POCS) reconstruction (*top left and right*; *bottom left*) in comparison with an image reconstructed from the complete k-space data set (*bottom right*). With the POCS reconstruction, a good image quality can be achieved even in half Fourier gradient echo imaging. However, some signal artifacts remain in the final POCS image, which cannot be removed by increasing the number of iteration steps

With EPI, image acquisition times below 100 ms for a 128^2 image matrix are feasible. However, EPI images are susceptible to a number of artifacts. Gradient and receiver imperfections can cause a ghost image that is shifted by half the FOV. Off-resonant spins (e.g., in fatty tissues) or inhomogeneous magnetic fields can create severely shifted and distorted images, which can partly be compensated by fat suppression and shimming of the static field (Fig. 4.10a). Finally, the signal decay with T2* during data acquisition periods of several tenths of milliseconds sets an ultimate limit to the image resolution which can be achieved.

If k-space is traversed from top to bottom in an EPI scan, the effective echo time, i.e., the time from the center of the RF pulse to the acquisition of k=0, is typically of the order of several tens of milliseconds. Although long echo times might be desirable for some MRI applications, such as neurofunctional MRI, they are detrimental if moving spins (e.g., in blood flow imaging) are studied.

With a segmented variant of EPI, short echo times in combination with reduced EPI artifacts can be achieved (McKinnon 1993). Here, only a portion (or segment) of k-space is sampled in a single scan (Fig. 4.10b). The scan is then repeated with different values of the initial phase-encoding gradient to fill the missing parts in k-space. This technique is no longer a true single shot acquisition, as it uses multiple RF excitations to sample k-space. Compared to single shot EPI, the acquisition time of multi-shot, segmented EPI is slightly longer, because additional time is needed for the irradiation of the RF pulse. However, a higher spatial resolution at a highly reduced artifact intensity is feasible (Fig. 4.10b).

4.3.7.2 *Radial Scanning*

One of the oldest imaging techniques in MRI is radial scanning or projection reconstruction. Here, k-space data are acquired on linear paths that start at the center of k-space (Fig. 4.11a). The technique was initially implemented by Lauterbur, who used a constant gradient in one direction during data readout (Lauterbur 1973). By rotating the sample between the RF excitations, he managed to acquire a k-space representation of the sample on radial lines. Today, radial lines in k-space are realized by rotating the direction of the readout gradient, which is achieved

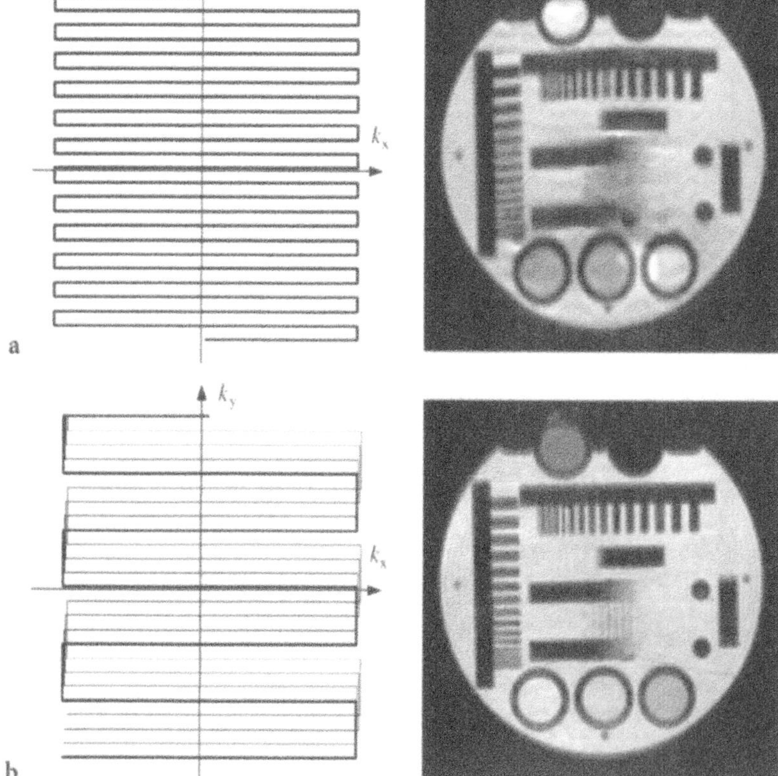

Fig. 4.10a, b. In standard single-shot echo planar imaging (EPI) k-space is sampled on an oscillating trajectory (**a**). With EPI, image acquisition times well below 100 ms are feasible. Due to the long acquisition time EPI is susceptible to artifacts from gradient imperfections, off-resonance, and field inhomogeneities, which manifest in image distortions and ghost images. **b** Multishot or segmented EPI acquires only a part of k-space in a shorter acquisition. With segmented EPI, image qualities comparable to conventional spin warp imaging can be achieved at the cost of a slightly higher acquisition time than standard EPI

by combining two gradients in the x and y direction to form one oblique gradient direction.

One interesting aspect of radial scanning is that several image reconstruction methods are available. As all acquired lines cross the k-space center, they all contain the information about the mean image intensity. In fact, each line represents a projection of the object along the line orthogonal to the corresponding radial readout direction. Therefore, the filtered backprojection algorithm, which is well known in CT, can be used to reconstruct an image (Cormack 1964). Here, a Fourier transform is only performed in the radial direction to reconstruct the different projections. This so-called sinogram is then filtered and backprojected into image space (Fig. 4.11b).

A more general approach to image reconstruction is regridding. Here, radial k-space data are resampled onto a Cartesian grid, before a standard Fourier transform is performed. Because the center of k-space is sampled more often than the periphery, a compensation for the k-space density must be applied (O'Sullivan 1985).

Radial imaging offers some features that make it extremely useful in imaging moving spins. As data acquisition is started at the center of k-space,

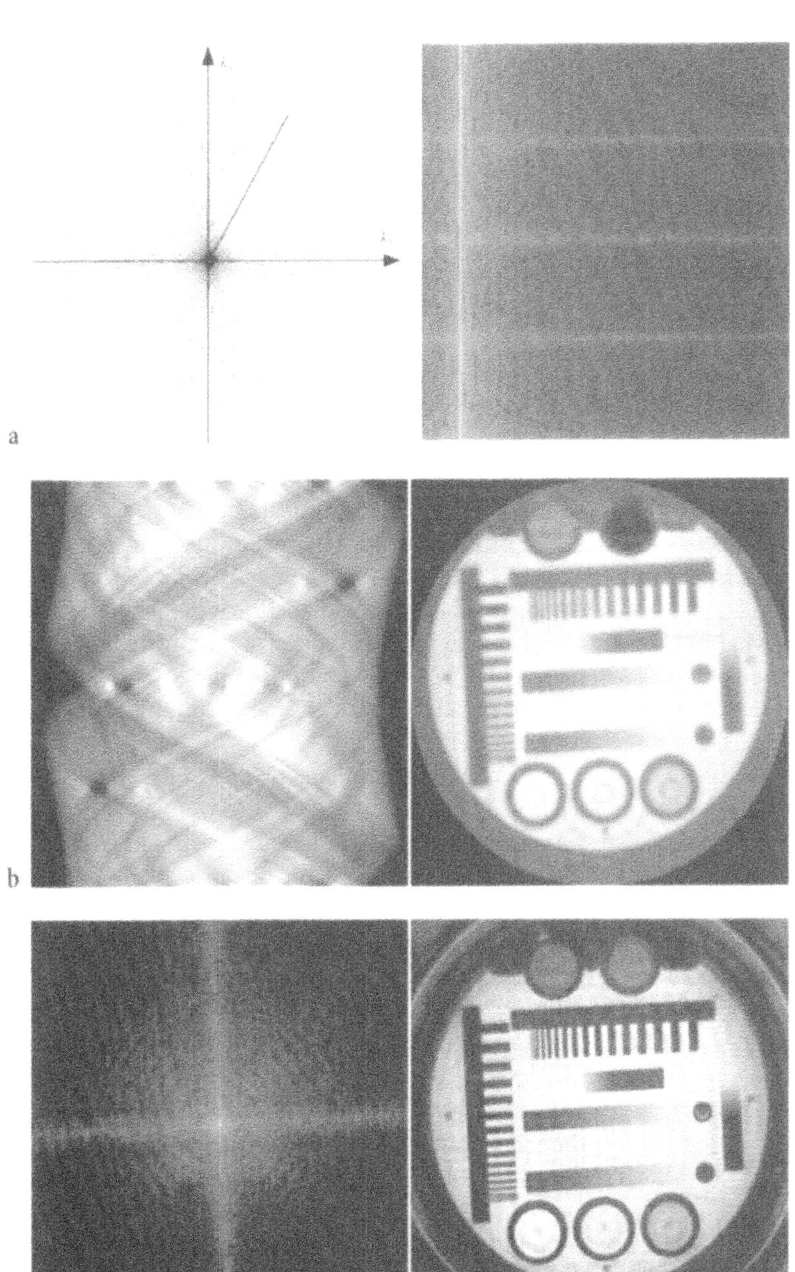

Fig. 4.11. **a** With radial MRI, k-space is sampled from the center outward on radial lines (*left*). The sampled data (*right*) are a radially reformatted k-space, where the x- and y-coordinates are replaced by angular (*top-bottom*) and radial (*left-right*) coordinates. All acquired radial k-space lines contain the information of k=0 and the center is highly oversampled. **b** By performing a Fourier transform in a radial direction only, a sinogram (*left*) is created which shows projections of the imaged object under different angles. After filtering, these projections can be backprojected into image space to form the final image. **c** An alternative to filtered backprojection is the gridding technique, where the radially sampled data are interpolated onto a rectangular grid (*left*). These interpolated data can then be used as input to the standard reconstruction with the fast Fourier transform

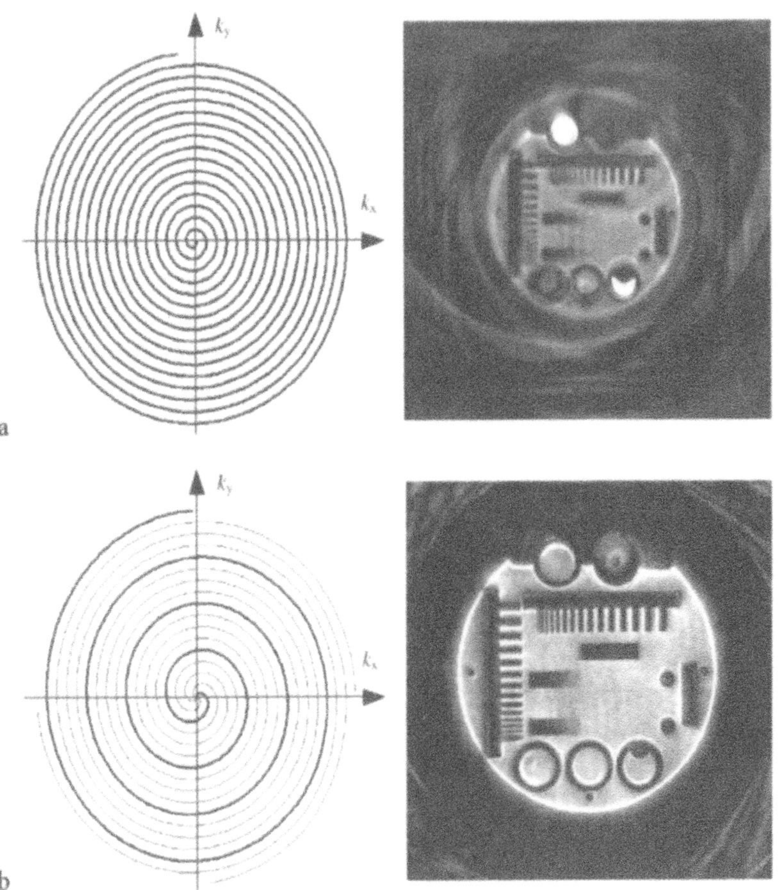

Fig. 4.12. The k-space trajectories and reconstructed images of single shot (**a**) and interleaved (**b**) spiral magnetic resonance imaging (MRI). In interleaved spiral MRI only a portion of k-space is sampled per spiral interleaf. At comparable image resolution typically more blurring artifacts are seen in single shot spiral acquisitions than with interleaved spirals, because longer readout times are needed, which increase the influence of off-resonant signal contributions

extremely short echo times well below 1 ms can be achieved, which highly reduces artifacts from turbulent motion. This also allows imaging of tissues with very short T2*, such us lung parenchyma.

Artifacts in radial MRI are somewhat different than in spin warp MRI. If the number of angular projections is too small, radial stripes appear in the image at some distance from the object. These artifacts can be eliminated if the number of different projections is chosen such that at the margins of k-space the separation of two adjacent radial lines equals the k-space grid size of the reconstructed image. Compared to spin warp imaging with N_p phase-encoding steps $N_a=\pi N_p$ angular projections have to be acquired to achieve the same image resolution. This disadvantage in scan efficiency is often offset by the immunity to motion, because the center of k-space is acquired in every scan and fluctuations average out much better than in standard MRI.

4.3.7.3 *Spiral Scanning*

A different approach to the acquisition of k-space data, which is similar to radial MRI, is called spiral scanning. Spiral MRI acquisitions also start at the center of k-space, but follow the curved pathway of a spiral (Ahn et al. 1986). Often Archimedian spirals are used, where the radial distance and the angle follow the same function (Fig. 4.12a). In spiral MRI, there is far less oversampling of the k-space center than in radial MRI, which makes spiral MRI much more time efficient.

The individual gradients that form the spiral trajectory in the two in-plane directions have to be very well synchronized, because even small deviations from the path in k-space can severely distort the images. To optimize the shape of the gradient-time curve $(G_x(t), G_y(t))$, two properties of the gradient system have to be known: the maximum gradient slew rate, which determines the initial speed near the k-space center, and the maximum gradient strength, which sets a limit to the image resolution for a given acquisition time. With this information, the gradient-time curve can be calculated from a differential equation either numerically (King et al. 1995) or approximately in a closed analytical form (Heid 1996).

Spiral MRI profits from powerful gradient systems with which k-space can be covered as fast as possible. This rapid k-space coverage is needed, because off-resonant contributions to the signal, e.g., from fat, distort the acquired k-space data. Unlike EPI, where off-resonant signals are displaced in the phase-encoding direction, in spiral MRI a blurring of the off-resonant signal is seen. Therefore, the very long, single-shot spiral acquisitions with acquisition times of 50 to 80 ms are often split into n acquisitions with shorter interleaved spirals (Fig. 4.12b).

Off-resonance blurring can be partly corrected during reconstruction. Therefore, the acquired raw-data are multiplied by an oscillating term, which corrects an off-resonance of Δf. Unfortunately, the correction acts on the k-space data and is thus also applied to those signal contributions that are not off-resonant. However, if a number of images with different off-resonance frequencies Δf are computed and the local deviations from the carrier frequency are known for all positions in the image (field map), a final corrected image can be extracted. A modified version of this algorithm does not require the additional acquisition of a field map, but uses a local focussing criterion to sharpen the blurred images.

As with radial MRI, the acquired raw data have to be put on a grid before a Fourier transform can be performed. The gridding routines are similar to those used in radial MRI, with the only difference being that the center of k-space is not so heavily oversampled and a different density correction function is applied.

Compared to standard imaging techniques such as spin warp imaging, spiral MRI offers a number of advantages. As with radial MRI, very short echo times can be achieved. Furthermore, the oscillating gradients reduce the displacement artifacts for moving spins even in the peripheral parts of k-space. The acquisition of k-space data is very time-efficient, as the k-space velocity is higher. It is fairly immune to the effects of eddy currents, but is affected by "concomitant gradients" or "Maxwell fields".

References

Ahn CB, Kim JH, Cho ZH (1986) High speed spiral scan echo planar imaging. IEEE Trans Med Imaging 5:2–5

Bock M, Bachert P (1998) Simultaneous flourine imaging of 5-FU and FBAL. In: Proceedings, Sixth Annual Meeting of the International Society for Magnetic Resonance in Medicine, Sydney, p 1831

Cooley JW, Tukey JW (1965) An algorithm for the machine calculation of complex Fourier series. Math Comput 19:297–301

Cormack AM (1964) Representation of a function by 1st line integrals, with some radiological applications. J Appl Phys 35:2908–2913

Edelstein WA, Hutchinson JMS, Johnson G, Redpath T (1980) Spin warp imaging and applications to human whole body imaging. Phys Med Biol 25:751–756

Gabillard R (1952) A steady state transient technique in nuclear magnetic resonance. Phys Rev 85:694–705

Haacke EM, Lindskog ED, Lin W (1991) Partial-Fourier imaging. A fast, iterative, POCS technique capable of local phase recovery. J Magn Reson 92:126–145

Heid O (1996) Archimedian spirals with Euclidian gradient limits. In: Proceedings, Fourth Annual Meeting of the International Society for Magnetic Resonance in Medicine, New York, p 114

Johnson G, Hutchinson JMS (1985) The limitations of NMR recalled echo imaging techniques. J Magn Reson 63:14–30

King KF, Foo TKF, Crawford CR (1995) Optimized gradient waveforms for spiral scanning. Magn Reson Med 34:156–160

Lauterbur PC (1973) Image formation by induced local interaction: examples employing nuclear magnetic resonance. Nature 243:190–191

Ljunggren S (1983) A simple graphical representation of Fourier based imaging methods. J Magn Reson 54:338–343

Margosian P, Schmitt F, Purdy D (1986) Faster MR imaging: imaging with half the data. Health Care Instrum 1:195–197

Mansfield P (1977) Multi-planar image formation using NMR spin echoes. J Phys C 10:L55–L58

McKinnon (1993) Ultrafast interleaved gradient-echo-planar imaging on a standard scanner. Magn Reson Med 30:609–616

O'Sullivan JD (1985) A fast sinc function gridding algorithm for Fourier inversion in computed tomography. IEEE Trans Med Imaging 4:200–207

Schmitt F, Stehling MK, Turner R (1998) Echo planar imaging. Springer, Berlin Heidelberg New York

5 Flow-Dependent Acquisition Techniques

Hilde Bosmans and Richard Hausmann

CONTENTS

5.1 Introduction

In MR imaging (MRI), the signal intensity of blood is extremely variable due to the complexity of the hematic components and the physiological motion of the blood. Blood is composed of water (80%), cells, and plasma elements such as organic macromolecules and electrolytes. Several studies have suggested that in the physiological state unclotted whole blood has long T1 (780–1000 ms) and T2 (150 ms) relaxation times , which in theory results in a low signal intensity on T1-weighted images and a high signal intensity on T2-weighted images (Wehrli et al. 1988). For clotted blood, the signal intensity varies, depending on the time between bleeding and imaging, as it is related to the relative amount of hemoglobin degradation products present within a hematoma.

Blood is a non-Newtonian fluid; its viscosity is dependent on velocity. At flow velocities of a few centimeters per second, a laminar flow results, where adjacent layers of fluid glide past each other without mixing. Laminar flow is typically seen in the small arteries and veins. However, due to vascular pulsation and depending on the size and shape of major arteries, a plug flow profile rather than a laminar one can be produced. In plug flow, velocities are uniform across the vessel diameter, in contrast to the parabolic profile typical of laminar flow. The blood flow may also be turbulent. This can strongly affect the appearance of the blood vessels in MR images.

Flowing blood presents with a range of appearances: it can both be hyperintense or appear as a signal void. The vessel wall in MR images may be sharply visualized or the image hampered by severe ghosting artifacts. To explain the signal intensities of flowing blood, the following variables have to be considered: the type of pulse sequence, the gradient scheme, the choice of MR parameters such as TR, TE and flip angle, the relaxation times, the concentration of contrast agents, magnetic susceptibility, and the flow pattern.

Although flow and, even more generally, motion often produce artifacts on MR images, they represent a prerequisite for many MR angiographic acquisition strategies. Flow-induced effects are used to visualize the vessels. As an immediate consequence, it is clear that signal intensities as seen in different types of vessels may be very different. This chapter summarizes the major flow characteristics that determine image quality in practice and it describes the basics of the techniques that exploit flow-induced effects for MRA purposes.

H. Bosmans, PhD
Department of Radiology, University Hospitals K.U. Leuven, Herestraat 49, 3000 Leuven, Belgium
R. Hausmann, PhD
Siemens AG, Siemensstrasse 1, 91391 Forchheim, Germany

5.2 The Inflow and Wash-out Effects

During a MR measurement, blood continuously enters and leaves the two-dimensional (2D) slice or three-dimensional (3D) acquisition volume. Therefore, its spins are subjected to only a fraction of an imaging sequence. The following different situations can be distinguished:

- The spins experienced only a few consecutive RF pulses of an MR acquisition scheme and are then replaced by 'fresh' spins. This leads to hyperintense signals.
- The spins are not subjected to both the excitation pulse and the refocusing pulse, as is a prerequisite for most spin echo acquisitions. Spins wash out before the whole series of RF pulses is given. This results in decreased signals.

5.2.1 Inflow Effects As the Basis for Hyperintense Signal Intensities

The inflow effect, also called "time-of-flight effect" (TOF), can be understood from the basic MR theory of T1 and T2 relaxation processes. After a 90° excitation pulse, the longitudinal magnetization is zero, whereas the transverse magnetization is determined by the initial magnetic component just prior to the RF pulse. This situation is no longer in equilibrium. Signal relaxation is described as mono-exponential processes characterized by the T1 and T2 relaxation times. The longitudinal magnetization recovers from zero to maximal alignment with the external field. The transverse component gradually disappears and is measured at some time during this process. The signal amplitude of the transverse magnetization is proportional to the signal intensities in MR images. Signals as obtained after successive measurements are only identical if the magnetic components just prior to the RF pulse are constant.

Consider now a conventional MR acquisition for which a combination of TR/TE has been selected. Then, in the absence of any magnetic field gradient for (position) encoding, the signal acquired after the first RF pulse is necessarily higher than the signal after subsequent RF pulses. Figure 5.1 represents the relaxation behavior of the spins for a basic MR sequence using a 90° excitation pulse. It is obvious that the signal after the first RF pulse is stronger than the signal after the second RF pulse. From then onwards, an identical intrinsic signal intensity is

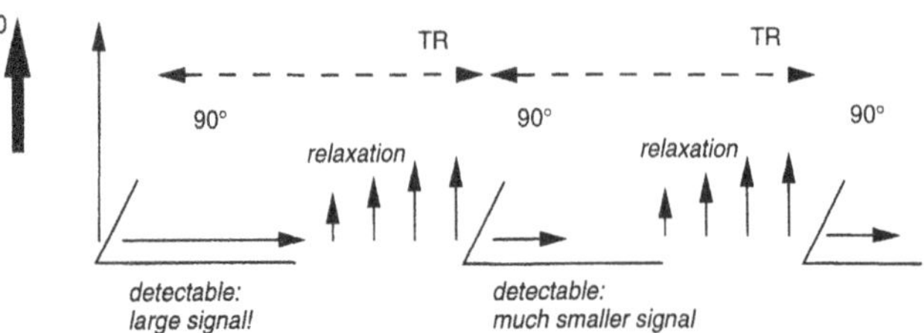

Fig. 5.1. The transverse magnetization after a second 90° RF pulse is lower than after the first RF pulse. From the second pulse onwards, the transverse component remains low (especially with short TR), but constant

expected. In MR images acquired with conventional schemes and a 90° flip angle, bright signal intensities can be observed in a blood vessel if the spins at that location enter the slice or slab with a maximal longitudinal magnetization and if they are replaced by fresh spins after one RF pulse (Fig. 5.2). Indeed, this signal is markedly higher than the (averaged) signal of most tissues that experience the complete set of RF pulses. Every flowing spin that is subjected to two or more pulses reduces the apparent signal intensity in the vessel. In general, in situations where the spins remain in the images for a period longer than the TR, the hyperintense signal intensity is lost.

This inflow-related enhancement or TOF effect is the basis of many MR angiographic acquisitions. In order to preserve the hyperintense signal intensities in a long vessel segment in the images, this effect has to be optimized. The repetition time TR and the flip angle have a direct influence on the inflow-related enhancement. The repetition time determines the number of RF pulses that the flowing spins will expe-

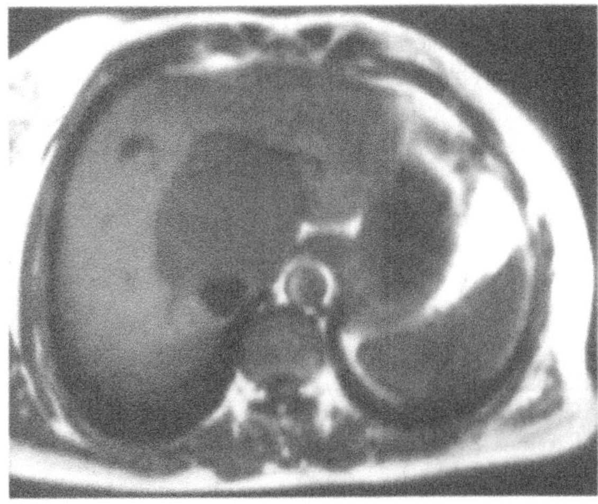

Fig. 5.2. In spin echo images, some vessels may be characterized by a hyperintense signal intensity due to inflow

rience in a particular slice or volume. With a vessel segment of length *s*, an average speed *v*, and a given TR, the spin are subjected to about the following number of pulses (Eq. 5.1):

$$Number\ of\ Pulses = \frac{s}{v * TR} \tag{5.1}$$

The repetition time also has an effect on the intrinsic signal intensities. A longer TR increases the signal intensities of both stationary tissues and flowing spins, but whether this improves the contrast between the vessel and the stationary tissue depends on the nature of the tissues involved. Finally, the TR determines the total acquisition time.

Low flip angles preserve the inflow-related enhancement over a longer vessel segment. A disadvantage is the poor signal-to-noise ratio (S/N) (Fig. 5.3).

In practice, the inflow enhancement is necessarily maximal where the spins enter the slice or slab. This effect then reduces gradually (Fig. 5.4). Where the signal of the flowing spins becomes identical to the signal of stationary tissues, the blood vessel is said to be saturated. It is clear that saturation will occur for different vessels in different places. In veins, signals are saturated close to the entrance side of the slice or volume. Arteries can usually be visualized over a longer trajectory. High resistance vessels may be saturated more quickly than low resistance vessels. In patients with a lower cardiac output, the vessel-to-soft tissue contrast is also lost more rapidly.

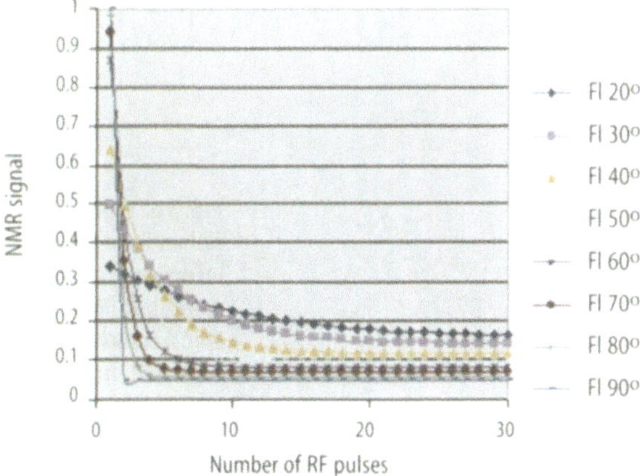

Fig. 5.3. Evolution of the MR signal intensity as a function of the number of RF pulses for different flip angles (TR 40 ms, T1 1000 ms)

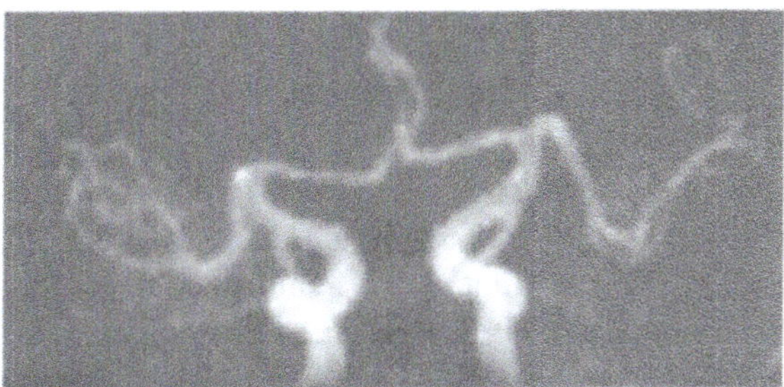

Fig. 5.4. The inflow-related enhancement decreases as the vessel enters the imaged volume or slab

5.2.2
The Wash-out Effect

In most spin echo acquisitions, only spins that receive a 90° and a 180° pulse can be detected by the coils. If blood moves so fast that it is outside the imaging plane in the time between the 90° and the 180° pulses, a high velocity signal loss will occur. The degree of signal loss depends on the fractions of blood that received a 90° and 180° pulse, only a 90° pulse, and only a 180° pulse. A critical velocity is represented by a time period shorter than TE/2 during which all spins in the blood vessel are replaced by fresh blood without any magnetic component in the transverse plane. This type of wash-out phenomenon is not observed in gradient echo techniques that, by definition, do not use 180° pulses.

In spin echo acquisitions, where the gradients along the *z*-direction are applied before the 180° pulse and the dephasing gradient of the read-out direction is applied after the 180° pulse, the function of the 180° pulse is to overcome the T2* dephasing only. Even if the refocusing pulse is then not totally effective, a transverse magnetic moment may be present at the moment of the echo, and, therefore, even fast moving spins can be detected.

In gradient echo imaging, an RF pulse is used to bring part of the signal in the transverse plane and the signal is detected independently of the position of the spins at the moment of the measurement. If flow velocities are extremely high, excited spins may move out of the sensitive volume of the coil before the signal is measured, i.e., at the echo time. At that moment, also in gradient recalled echo techniques, signal voids may be observed. This effect is not very common, since for MR angiographic procedures, extremely short echo times are used.

5.3 Flow-Induced Phase Effects

Spin-phase phenomena were already studied by the pioneers of MRI (Carr and Purcell 1954). In 1961, Hahn used flow-induced phase shifts to measure the motion of sea water. The techniques were based on the accrued phase shifts of spins moving along a magnetic field gradient. This effect, which can be derived in a straightforward way from the Larmor equation, still forms the basis for quantification methods of microscopic flow or water diffusion in the tissues and macroscopic flow in blood vessels. At the same time, this effect possibly destroys the signal and therefore must be overcome when visualizing the morphology of the blood vessels.

We recall from Chap. 4 that a 90° RF pulse, when combined with a magnetic field gradient, gives rise to two effects: the spins of only a selected slice are excited and phase coherence is established. This phase coherence is gradually lost because of spin–spin interactions and magnetic field inhomogeneities. The linear magnetic field gradients as used for imaging are an obvious source of inhomogeneities and are responsible for phase effects. In the same chapter, it was explained that at least five linear magnetic field gradients are required for a basic imaging sequence: a gradient during the RF excitation pulse along the *z*-direction and its rephasing pulse, a gradient during the signal read-out along the *x*-direction and its preceding dephasing pulse, and a phase-encoding gradient along *y*. This basic scheme works adequately for stationary spins: during the read-out time, a correctly position-encoded signal can be obtained. Flow-induced phase effects are caused by the fact that these conventional gradient schemes fail for flowing spins (unless they are used within an ultrafast acquisition scheme).

For stationary spins, the phases of the spins are perfectly rephased when so-called bipolar pulses (Fig. 5.5) are applied. By definition, a bipolar pulse consists of two linear magnetic field gradients. If the first one imposes a magnetic field gradient (B_1) at x_1, the second imposes ($-B_1$) at the same location and for the same duration. There is no net result for the phases of the spins that remain in position x_1. The situation is different for flowing spins. They may experience (B_1) during application of the first pulse, then move into location x_2 and experience ($-B_2$). In general, ($-B_2$) does not compensate for the phase effects of (B_1) (Fig. 5.6). The phase shifts induced by the bipolar pulses can be calculated from (Eq. 5.2):

$$\Delta\Phi=\gamma^{*}g(t_2-t_1)^{*}\delta^{*}v \quad (5.2)$$

In this equation, γ is the gyromagnetic ratio, g is the magnetic field gradient, (t_2-t_1) is the time in between the onset of the two pulses, δ is the duration per pulse, and v is the velocity of the spins. From the equation, it follows that the phase shifts are related to

1. The velocity of the spins
2. Characteristics of the bipolar pulses

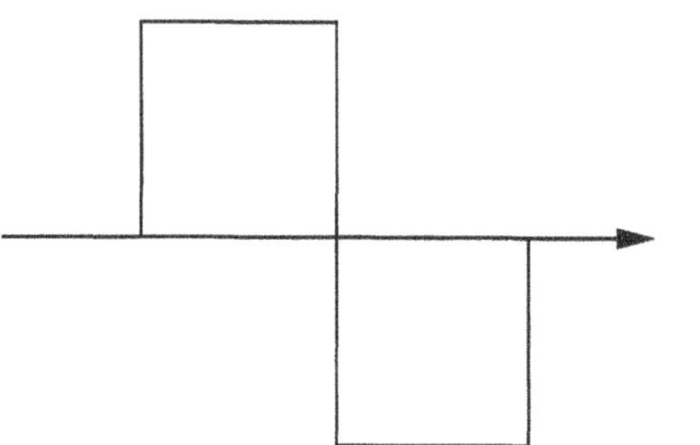

Fig. 5.5. A bipolar pulse consists of a positive magnetic field gradient followed by an opposite magnetic field gradient

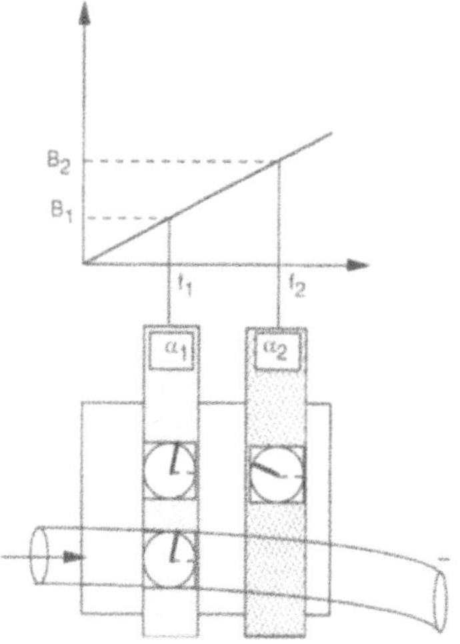

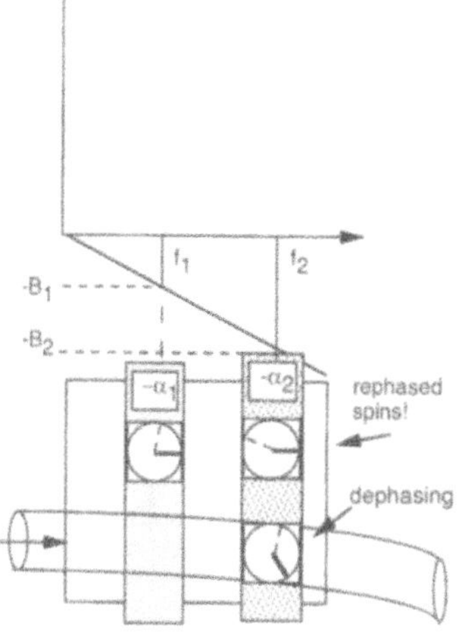

Fig. 5.6. Bipolar pulses have no net effect on stationary spins, but flowing spins are usually not rephased. In the upper part of the figure, we visualize the dephasing effect due to the first lobe of the bipolar pulse. The second lobe (lower part of the figure) shows that stationary are rephased, whereas flowing spins are not

The use of ultrashort TE with compact bipolar pulses overcomes a lot of dephasing problems, as (t_2-t_1) and δ are necessarily short.

The following effects and techniques can be explained by flow-induced phase effects: phase dispersion or intravoxel incoherence, signal void due to turbulence, ghost artifacts, and gradient motion refocusing schemes. We explain this basic MRA terminology in more detail in the next section.

5.3.1 Phase Dispersion or Intravoxel Incoherence

Phase dispersion or intravoxel incoherence occurs in the situation where, *within* one voxel in a blood vessel and for the applied gradient schemes, large phase differences are observed. The net result within the voxel is a decrease in signal (Fig. 5.7a, b). This phenomenon is most frequently observed:

1. Along the vessel wall, where the velocity gradients are largest
2. In acquisition schemes with large voxels as the intrinsic spread of velocities is then large
3. In acquisition schemes with strong gradients or when there is a long time between the application of gradients
4. During time windows where velocities are highest, as seen in acquisitions gated to obtain images during the systolic phase

The reverse is also true: if acquisitions are gated during diastole, phase dispersion may be overcome.

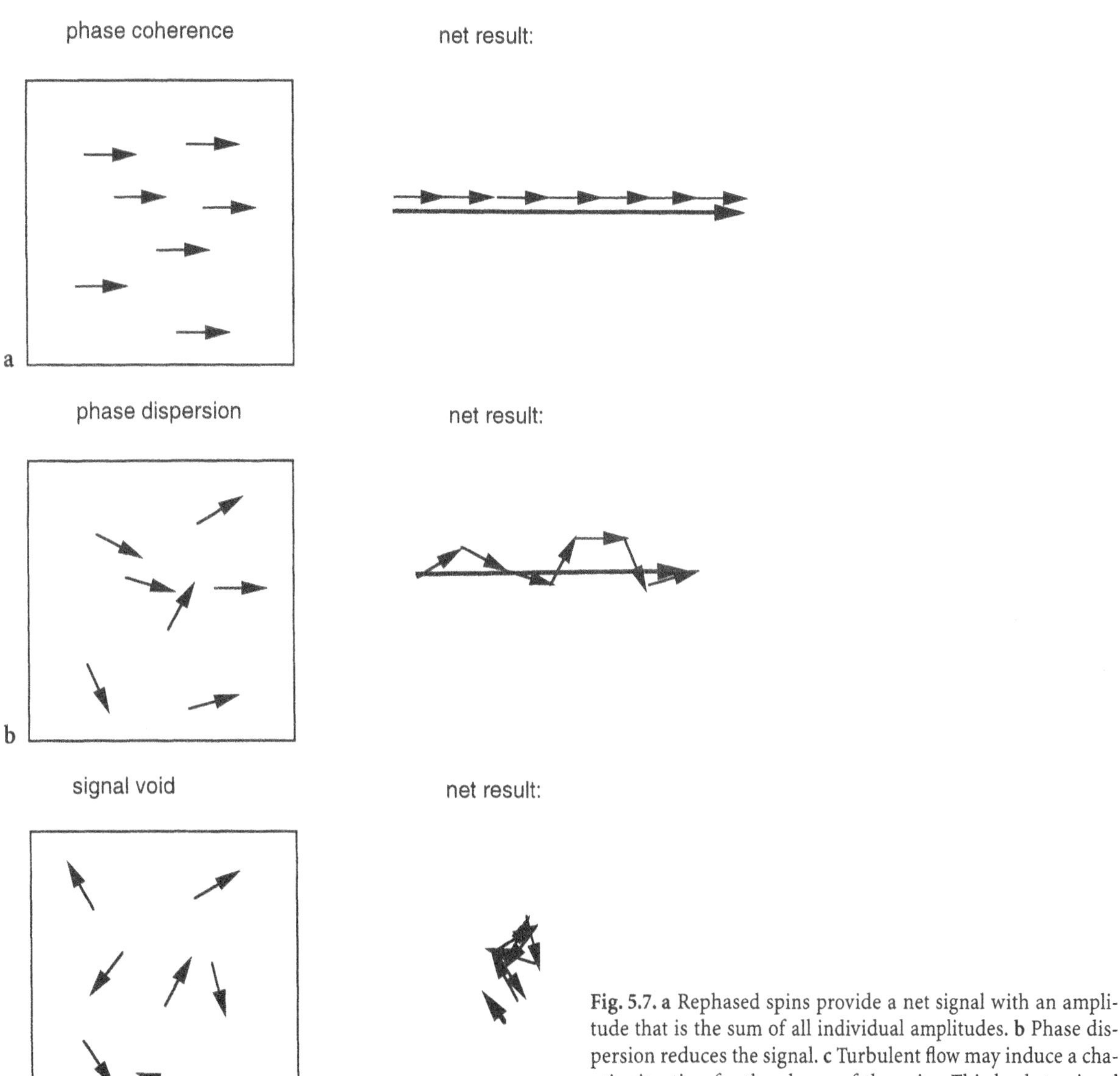

Fig. 5.7. a Rephased spins provide a net signal with an amplitude that is the sum of all individual amplitudes. **b** Phase dispersion reduces the signal. **c** Turbulent flow may induce a chaotic situation for the phases of the spins. This leads to signal void

5.3.2
Signal Void Due to Turbulence

Flow-induced phase differences can be very large if large velocity gradients exist in the voxel. The net result is then zero (Fig. 5.7c) and the voxel is characterized by a signal void. This can occur in curved vessel structures (Fig. 5.8a), aneurysms, along stenoses, distal from a stenosis, distal from aortic valves, etc. Reducing the echo time or gating the acquisition to particular phases of the ECG cycle are strategies for coping with this problem. In some applications, the presence of signal void is an indicator of certain pathologies. An example is shown in Fig. 5.8b, in which the aneurysm is easily detected due to the signal void.

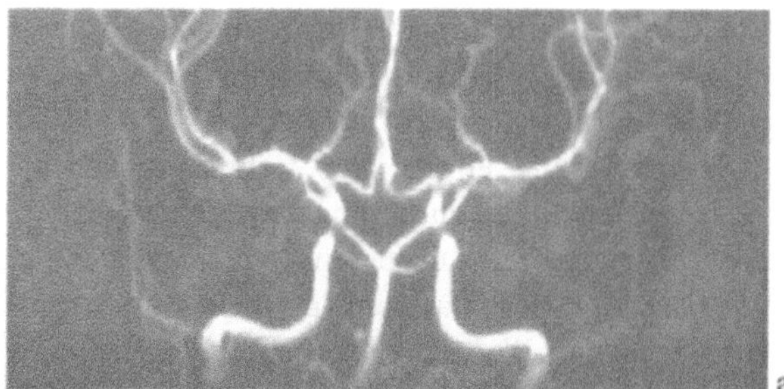

a

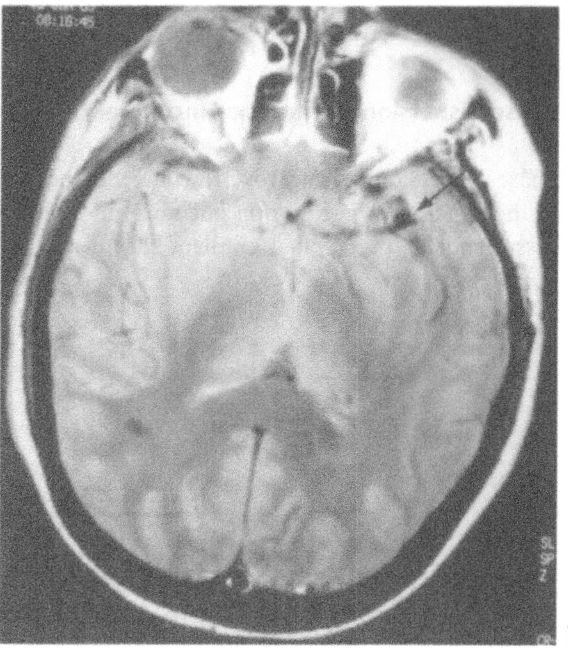

b

Fig. 5.8. a Flow-induced dephasing can provide signal voids that simulate a stenosis. This occurred in the carotid siphon of this patient study. **b** Signal void can also be an advantage. In this spin echo image, the aneurysm *(arrow)* is detected because of signal voids

5.3.3
Ghost Artifacts

The additional phase shift that is observed for flowing spins, as compared to stationary spins, is sometimes misinterpreted by the position-encoding system as a phase-encoding gradient. It is difficult to compensate for this effect as the phase-encoding scheme produces a very analoguous effect on the phases of the spins. As a result, the signal intensity of the vessel is spread along the direction of phase encoding, typically into a separate number of ghosts (Fig. 5.9). In practice, this artifact can be avoided by reducing the signal of flowing spins (e.g. using low flip angle), using dedicated gradient schemes, by averaging, by triggering, etc.

5.3.4
Gradient Motion Refocusing Scheme

Dedicated gradient schemes have been developed to reduce flow-induced dephasing. The requirement for a new gradient scheme is that the total accumulated phase effect, except for the phase-encoding gradients, be zero at the time of signal read-out. Whether this is possible depends on the flow pattern of the spins (Haacke and Lenz 1987). If the flow velocity is constant between excitation and read-out, a gradient scheme can be proposed that nulls the flow-induced

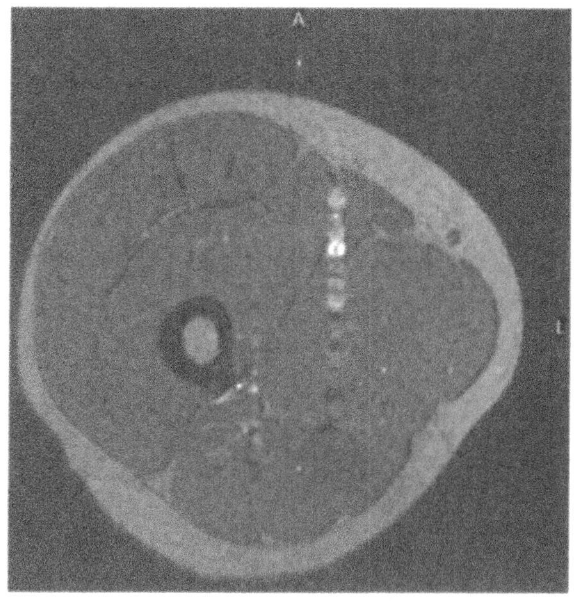

Fig. 5.9. The 2D transverse acquisition of the lower leg is hampered by typical ghost artifacts along the phase-encoding direction through the arteries

phase effects. An example is shown in Fig 5.10a. It is also possible to null the phase shifts of spins that constantly accelerate or have a higher-order flow pattern (Fig. 5.10b). Acceleration or still higher-order flow is usually not compensated in practice, and the reason is obvious: more gradients have to be applied, which increases the minimal echo time. This prolongation of echo time would neutralize the effects of gradient motion compensation.

5.4 Slice Misregistration

The position of the spins is encoded into the signal at different time points: the slice select direction is encoded by means of the slice select gradient during the RF excitation pulse (in 2D imaging), phase encoding is performed between RF pulse and read-out, and the third direction is encoded during the read-out. Position misregistration may occur if the real position of the spin during read-out is significantly different from the position during phase encoding (Fig. 5.11a). With dedicated position-encoding schemes, it is possible to cope with this problem (Fig. 5.11b). The phase encoding is performed such that the acquired phase shift reflects the position that the spin will obtain during signal read-out. This can be achieved for all spins that move at a constant velocity from phase encoding up to read-out.

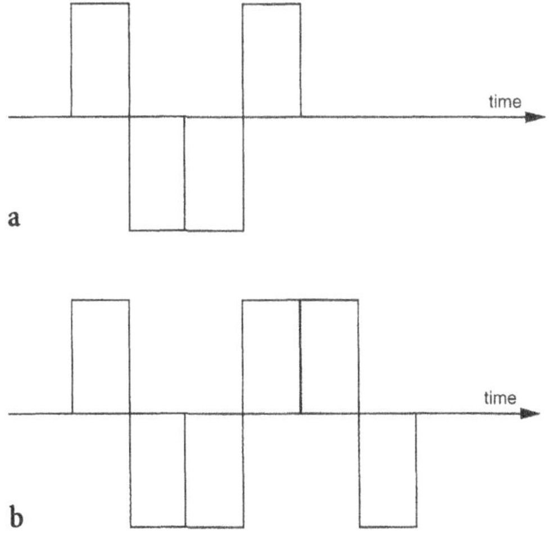

Fig. 5.10. **a** Gradient scheme that can be used in stead of bipolar pulses and that rephazes the spins with constant velocity flow. **b** Gradient scheme that compensates for flow-induced phase effects due to constant acceleration

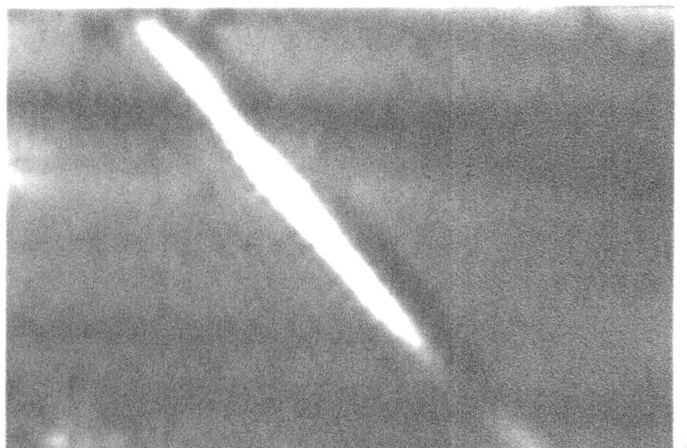

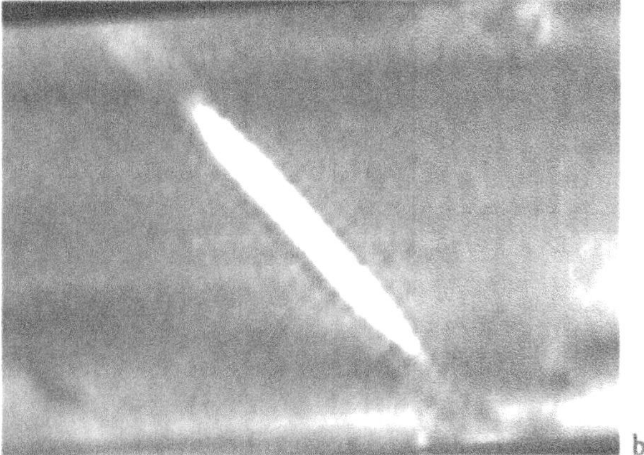

Fig. 5.11. **a** Flow-induced distortion can be visualized with a flow phantom. If the tube is oblique to a phase encode direction, signal intensities in the blood vessel are shifted along their trajectory. **b** Dedicated phase encoding schemes overcome the slice misregistration effect

5.5 Dedicated Techniques for Flow-Dependent MRA

Flowing blood can be visualized by MR by means of different methods. In the following paragraphs we propose different techniques that exploit flow-induced effects. TOF techniques provide hyperintense signals based on inflow-related enhancement. Phase contrast imaging uses flow-induced phase effects. We introduce these techniques as well as different MR tools that can be used for optimization. The tools are described to help in understanding the different clinical protocols that could be based on these MRA approaches.

5.5.1 TOF Techniques

TOF techniques use the inflow of labeled spins into the imaging volume. In the simplest form, the labeling is done passively by allowing unsaturated (or fully relaxed) spins to enter the excitation volume. In this way, full magnetization is available for the blood volume and gives rise to a high signal intensity. The contrast between these labeled (or tagged) spins and the stationary background tissue is then increased further by a strong suppression of the background. Other forms of labeling are inversion of longitudinal magnetization (NISHIMURA et al. 1988) and saturation of inflowing spins (DUMOULIN et al. 1989a), but these are not widely used for MRA. Some approaches are currently being considered for noninvasive perfusion studies, but a discussion of this would go beyond the scope of the book.

As phase effects can cause severe artifacts in conventional gradient echo imaging, ultrashort echo times or gradient motion refocusing have to be applied. A gradient echo acquisition that compensates for flow with a constant velocity is generally defined as a TOF MRA sequence (Fig. 5.12) (LAUB and KAISER 1988). Pulsation and accelerated blood flow can possibly cause artifacts. Such effects may be present in poststenotic regions or at bifurcations of vessels. This has to be carefully taken into consideration, for example, when diagnosing stenosis with TOF MRA.

5.5.1.1 Improving the Inflow-Related Enhancement

The contrast between blood vessels and background tissue is based on the difference between the high signal originating from unsaturated spins flowing into the excitation region and the low signal in stationary tissue. The TOF method can be implemented with different parameter settings. All of them have their own role, benefits, and drawbacks, depending on the flow velocities and the size of the acquisition volume (HAACKE 1990, ATKINSON et al. 1994).

The Repetition Time. To reduce the signal of the stationary tissue, the repetition time TR must be small compared to the T1 relaxation times. The situation is different for spins flowing through the imaging slice: if the flow velocities are high enough and/or the slices are thin enough, the affected spins "feel" only a few excitation pulses and have a relatively hyperintense signal even with short TR. If the velocity is lower, there is a risk of too many RF pulses. Shorter TR further increases this number so that saturation occurs more rapidly. Typically, a TR of 40 ms can be used.

The Flip Angle. The signal from stationary tissue is easily saturated by high flip angles (and short TR), but in this way, the flowing spin signal is also rapidly saturated. In general, low flip angles are used, except in those cases where 2D slices are applied perpendicular to a vessel. Saturation in the vessel is then not a problem. In this case, a high flip angle increases the signal in the blood vessel and decreases the stationary tissue signal. A possible side effect is that ghost artifacts become more disturbing.

The effects of small and large flip angles can be combined when using ramped RF pulses or tilted optimized non excitation pulses (TONE) (Fig. 5.13) (LAUB and PURDY 1992, ATKINSON et al. 1994). At the entrance plane, a small flip angle of 10°, for example, will still provide sufficient signal without reducing the longitudinal magnetization too much. Next, the flip angle is increased by a small amount to maintain or even increase the signal of flowing blood into the volume. Where saturation is expected, higher flip angles are applied to improve subtle blood vessel-soft tissue contrasts. TONE pulses are mainly used for visualization of the cerebral vessels. The same principle was used to study the coronary vessels: a series of slightly different flip angles was applied to obtain a constant signal.

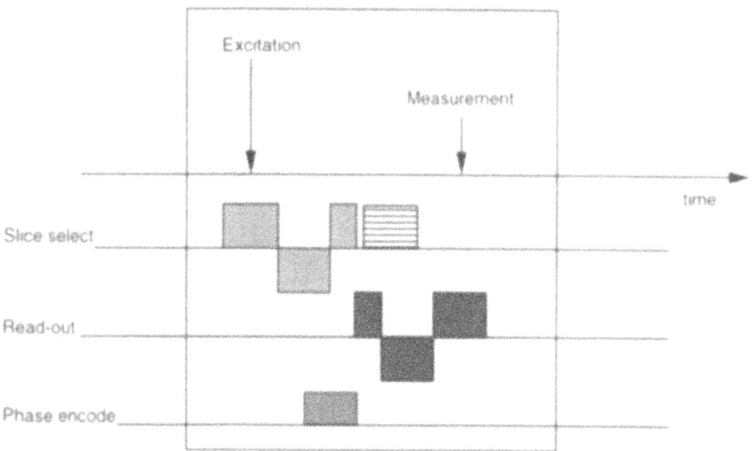

Fig. 5.12. Typical gradient scheme of a 3D time-of-flight acquisition

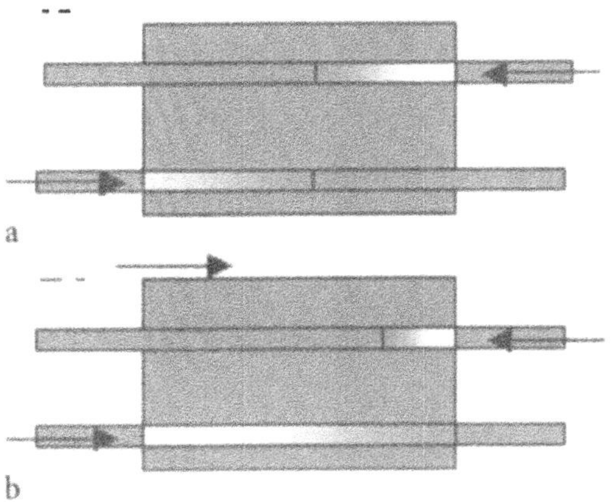

Fig. 5.13a, b. Tilted optimized nonexcitation (TONE) pulses can be used to reduce the saturation effects for vessels with unidirectional flow. a No TONE applied. b TONE is applied from left to right

The Echo Time. In general, echo times should be as short as possible to prevent dephasing artifacts but other factors may also cause interference. The chemical shift between water and fat also determines the echo time. Since water and fat spins have a slightly different resonance frequency, there are echo times during which the signal from fat and water is in opposed phase and echo times for which both water and fat are in phase (Fig. 5.14). If one voxel contains both water and fat, the signal can be eliminated if opposed-phase conditions are met. For TOF MRA it is advantageous to use opposed-phase echo times, since there is always fat in the stationary tissue that surrounds the vessel and this should be of low signal intensity. The vessel caliber may appear somewhat narrower than in reality. For a field strength of 1.5 T, the following echo times can be used: 2.2 ms and 6.6 ms. For a 1-T field, they are at 3.3 and 9.9 ms.

Flow Separation Using Saturation Pulses. Saturation pulses are commonly used in MRI to suppress the signal of tissues that would negatively interfere with the image (Edelman et al. 1989b). This method provides a powerful tool for distinguishing veins from arteries in cases of opposite flow direction (neck, extremities, and aorta). This is demonstrated in Fig. 5.15. For example, to suppress the jugular vein in studies of the carotid arteries, a 90° presaturation pulse is used superior to the imaging slices. Venous spins reach the imaging volume in completely saturated form and cannot contribute to the signal.

Ideally, instead of placing one stationary presaturation pulse at one side of the slice stack, the presaturation pulse has to be kept at a fixed distance from the individual slice. Otherwise, flowing material can recover magnetization, since the distance between presaturation pulse and imaging slice becomes too large. This option is denoted as *tracking presaturation pulse*. However, care has to be taken not to saturate the vessel of interest in cases of heavy pulsating flow or a curved morphology of the vessel. If the presaturation pulse is too close to the imaging slice, retrograde flow becomes saturated and signal drop out occurs.

2D, 3D and Hybrid TOF Techniques. The most frequently used MRA technique is the single-volume TOF method (Fig. 5.16a). In 3D volume techniques one large volume is excited and then imaged in contiguous slices by using an additional phase-encoding table in the slice direction. This leads to thin slices well below 1 mm. Together with a high resolution in the plane (e.g., 384×512 and a rectangular field of view), this provides very small isotropic voxels compared to standard 2D imaging. 3D sequences have an inherently higher S/N due to the larger number of excitations. Moreover, they allow shorter echo times because of the more relaxed conditions for gradient design in the slice select direction compared to thin-slice 2D sequences. This then provides a minimal intravoxel phase dispersion and optimal signal, especially in regions of moderate and fast flow. However, when using the 3D technique care has to be taken that the main bloodstream is perpendicular to the volume orientation. It is of fundamental importance to study how the saturation effect can be minimalized.

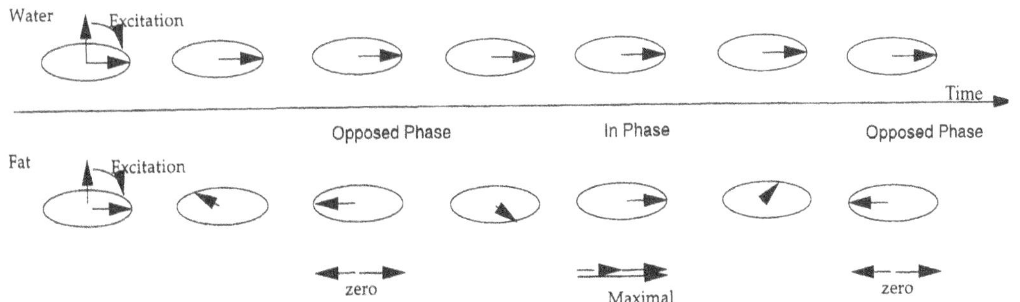

Fig. 5.14. Whether spins of water and fat are in opposed or in phase condition depends on the echo time

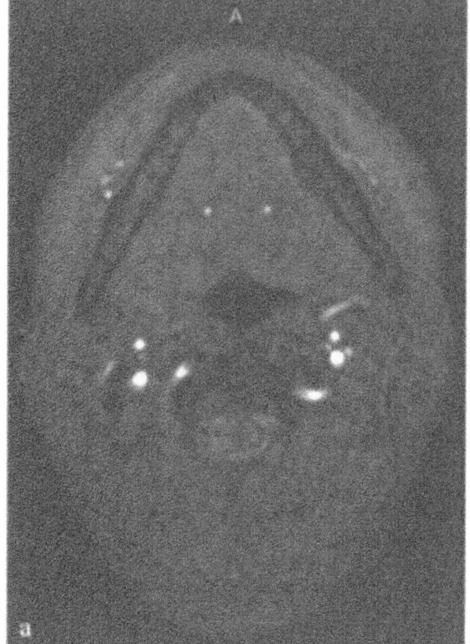

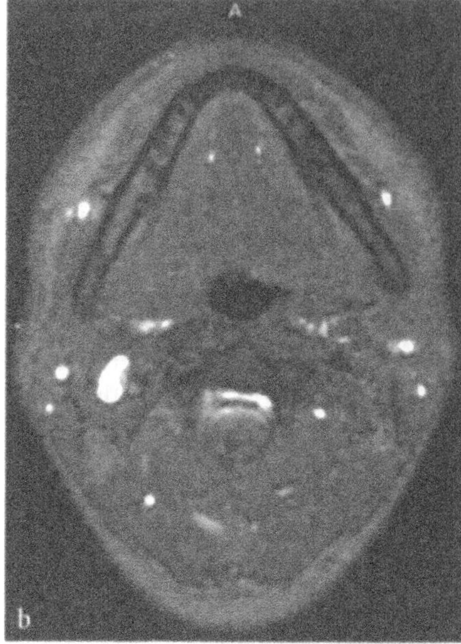

Fig. 5.15. a A 2D time-of-flight study of the neck vessels with saturation slab more cranial of the imaged slice (venous return is suppressed) **b** Identical acquisition but with suppression of arterial input

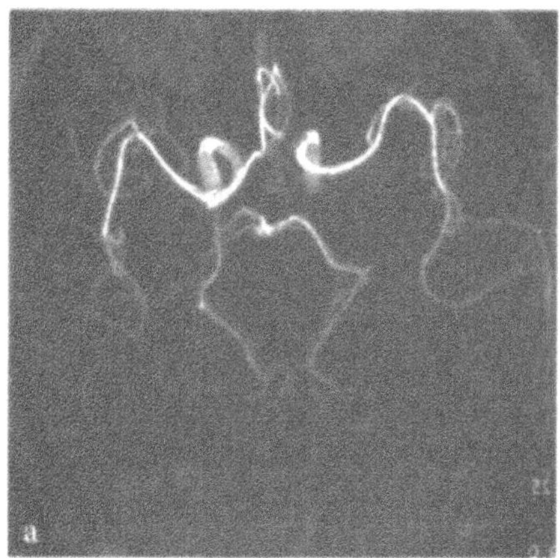

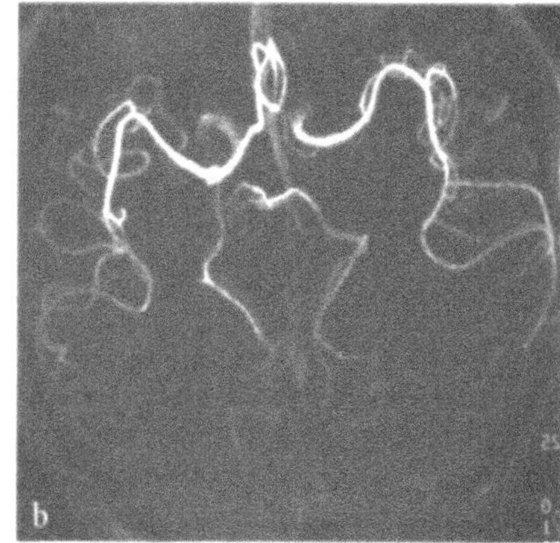

Fig. 5.16. a Single volume 3D time-of-flight (TOF) acquisition, TR/TE/Fl 40 ms/7 ms/25°, Tilted optimized nonexcitation (TONE) RF pulse and magnetization transfer pulse (see next paragraph). **b** Identical 3D TOF acquisition but performed with multiple overlapping thin slabs, TONE and magnetization transfer pulse

The progressive spin saturation can be avoided by acquiring multiple, thin 2D slices. A short TR/TE is required and presaturation has to be avoided. Therefore, 2D slices are acquired slice per slice, i.e., sequentially. 2D techniques are applied mainly in slower flow situations and for fast studies which must be performed within a single breath-hold.

Although the S/N is larger for 3D TOF, contrast-to-noise ratios are higher with 2D TOF techniques, since higher flip angles can be used. Even at medium flip angles of 40–50°, flowing spin saturation is not present when using thin slices perpendicular to the vessels under study. However, considerable spin saturation within vessels can occur when vessels run inplane or reverse their direction. The nonisotropic resolution of 2D TOF is the greatest disadvantage of the technique. On the other hand, 2D TOF allows better delineation of the veins.

A compromise between 2D and 3D techniques is the ue of multiple overlapping thin slab acquisitions (motsa) (Fig. 5.16b) (Marchal et al. 1990, Parker et al. 1991). This method combines the benefits of 3D and 2D techniques: larger volumes can be covered without saturation effects. The advantages of 3D techniques such as isotropic resolution and high S/N remain, although the S/N is reduced. In the same way, using 10-to 30-mm slab thicknesses, saturation is largely overcome. Since overlapping slabs have to be acquired to compensate for the nonideal volume profile that reduces the signal intensities in the upper and lower images, the acquisition time is 30% larger than for a single-volume scan with the same coverage. Problems can occur with this method if the patient moves between successive scans.

Preparation Pulses. A further reduction of the background tissue can be achieved with dedicated preparation pulses. The different anatomical regions to be studied determine which pulses can be used advantageously. In the brain, TOF acquisitions benefit from magnetization transfer pulses. The principle is as follows: a strong off-resonance RF pulse saturates the spins of large molecules. These spins continuously interchange with the spins of free water, and, therefore, the number of saturated water spins increases. These spins are no longer excited with the regular RF pulse and, therefore, do not contribute to the image. As a result, the signal of brain tissue decreases, whereas the signal of flowing blood is unaffected.

For some applications, fat suppression pulses can be considered (LIN et al. 1993). A typical application is in MRA of the coronary vessels, where it is essential for triggered, 2D TOF acquisitions that the fatty tissue signal is suppressed (DUERINCKX et al. 1996).

5.5.1.2 Pitfalls

High Signal for Tissue with Short T1. It is very difficult to saturate tissues with an extremely short T1, as is present in hemorrhagic lesions after a certain time (methemoglobin) (Fig. 5.17). This signal is high and can be confused with flowing material, e.g., in large aneurysms. It is recommended that a TOF MRA study always be complemented with a (fast) spin echo measurement.

Saturation. Notwithstanding the use of a so-called optimized technique, some vessels may be missing due to persisting saturation. This occurs when flow is extremely slow as in pathological conditions or when cardiac output is very poor in the patient. The presence of occluded vessels has to be confirmed with techniques that are extremely sensitive to slow flow. Examples are: 2D TOF, phase-contrast imaging, or ultrafast contrast-enhanced MRA.

(Post-stenotic) Signal Void. In regions with extremely turbulent flow, intravoxel incoherence may cause a signal void. Great care should be taken in estimating the degree of stenosis. In general, the reading may be overestimated as compared to golden standard measurements (PATEL et al. 1994). Ultrafast contrast-enhanced MRA is more robust in this regard.

5.5.1.3 Summary

TOF angiography is a completely noninvasive technique in which contrast is obtained from the inflow effect whereas gradient motion rephasing is used to overcome flow-induced phase effects. The technique is quite robust, as long as all necessary precautions are taken. In clinical practice this means: an appropriate positioning of the imaging volume, the best choice between 2D, 3D or motsa, and the execution of the necessary add-on techniques to explain phenomena such as hyperintense signal intensity and the use of appropriate visualization techniques (see Chap. 7).

5.5.2 Phase Contrast Imaging

This section describes the principles, the major terminology, and the application of phase-sensitive

a

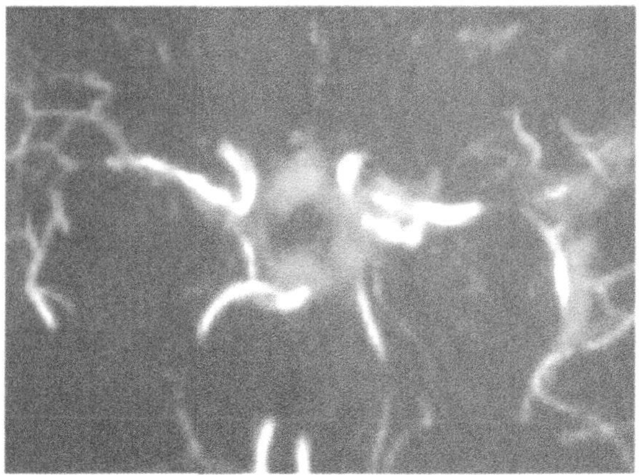

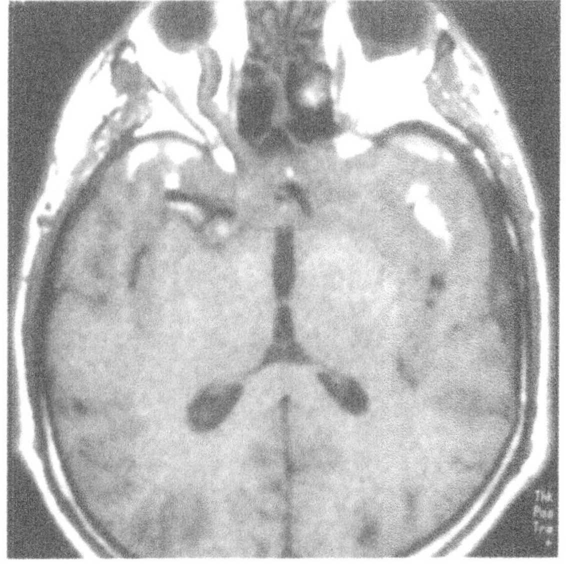

b

Fig. 5.17. a The projection of the 3D time-of-flight data shows hyperintense signal intensities that do not correspond to blood vessels. **b** A T1-weighted spin echo image shows that both blood vessels and acute bleeding is shown with hyperintense signals (in the 3D time-of-flight study)

MRA techniques. As explained in the previous paragraphs, flowing spins can acquire phase shifts in between excitation and signal read-out. For many applications, this is a problem, since it gives rise to ghost artifacts and unexpected signal intensities in the blood vessels. However, it is a characteristic that can also be exploited to visualize blood vessels and to quantify the velocity.

Phase contrast acquisitions rely on both amplitude and phase characteristics.

If motion-compensated gradients are used, the phases as observed for most blood vessels are no different from the phases in stationary tissue. Any uncompensated pair of gradients or an extra bipolar gradient changes this situation: stationary spins show no phase shift, and spins with a constant velocity acquire a phase shift that is proportional to their velocity. Phase-based techniques exploit this phase shift, usually after subtraction of a rephased acquisition.

The major advantage of phase-sensitive techniques is their sensitivity to flowing blood only. Unlike in TOF sequences, where tissues with extremely short T1 may mimic flowing blood, only flowing tissue can lead to high signal intensities. In additional, full background suppression can be achieved and, therefore, vessels with a poor S/N, such as vessels with a saturated signal intensity or very small vessels, can be visualized. Rather long acquisition times and therefore limited resolution are the price that has to be paid.

5.5.2.1 Improving Phase Contrast Techniques

Gradient Scheme. A bipolar gradient pulse does not induce a residual phase shift for stationary spins, but rather a velocity-dependent phase if the flow pattern is constant along the gradient direction. In reality, the velocity v is rarely constant. Higher-order terms such as acceleration, change of direction, and pulsation can be present. Therefore, the model described here is oversimplified. Assuming small voxel sizes and short echo times, however, it is nevertheless also valid to assume one velocity v within a voxel for most MRA applications. Flow sensitivity is only achieved in the direction in which the bipolar gradient pulse is applied. If only parallel and straight vessels are examined and if the vessels are along the x, y or z-axis, one bipolar pulse set is satisfactory. Usually, however, three different measurements are necessary to obtain flow sensitivity in all three directions for all segments of the vessel. Making the phase difference requires a subtraction mask. Opposite bipolar pulses can be used, providing opposite phase angles. Sensitivity along three spatial directions then requires six different acquisitions (Dumoulin et al. 1989b). In practice, it is more appropriate to use the same rephased image for all three encoded acquisitions (Hausmann et al. 1991, Pelc et al. 1991). As a consequence, phase contrast (PC) angiography techniques lead to significantly longer scan times than for TOF MRA (Fig. 5.18). Assuming an identical TR as

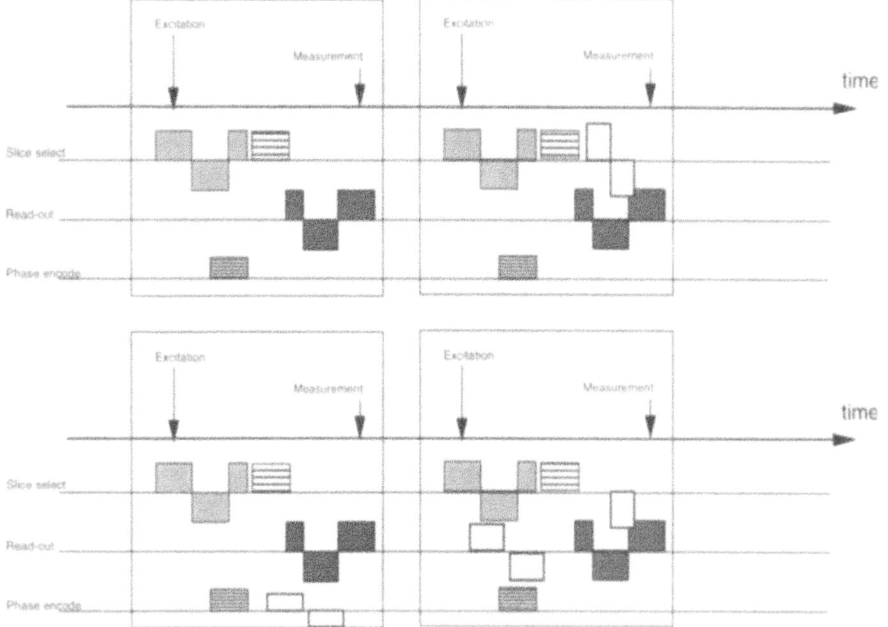

Fig. 5.18. Typical gradient scheme for a phase-contrast acquisition. From left to right, top to bottom: the rephased (time-of-flight) acquisition, the acquisition with a bipolar pulse along the slice select direction, the acquisition with a bipolar pulse along the plane phase encoded direction and the acquisition with a bipolar pulse along the read-out direction

with TOF measurements, scan times which are three times as long are necessary. In practice a shorter TR of 25 – 30 ms can be chosen.

Two different subtraction techniques can be used. First, subtraction of corresponding phase images can be performed, which results in a new phase image. Since the relationship between phase and velocity is, to a certain extent, linear, a direct measurement of flow velocities is then possible (EDELMAN et al. 1989b). This flow quantification technique will be dealt with in Chap. 8. A second approach consists of complex subtraction, in which the signal in the new image is composed of the regular amplitude, i.e., the ampltiude of the transverse magnetization $m_{tr}(x,y,z)$, and a factor that contains the phase information (Eq. 5.3):

$$signal\,(x,y,z) = 2m_{tr}\,(x,y,z)\sqrt{\sum_{i=x,y,z}\left(\sin\left(\frac{\alpha_i v_i}{2}\right)\right)^2}$$

with α_i, defined by the bipolar pulses, i.e., the velocity-encoding gradient (VENC; see below), v_i the averaged velocity of the spins, and m_{tr} the transverse magnetization amplitude.

The Velocity-Encoding Gradient. The sensitivity of the sequence to a particular flow velocity range is an important feature of PC angiography. Assuming constant flow velocities within one voxel, which can be achieved using very small voxel sizes, the flow-encoding bipolar gradient pulses should be designed in such a way that the flow phase for the maximal velocity component is smaller than 180°. As can be seen from Eq. 5.3, the phase shift depends at the one side on the velocity of the spin, but, on the other hand, also on the timing, duration, and strength of the gradient pulses. It is, therefore, possible to adjust the gradients for specific velocity ranges. This velocity-encoding value is often referred to as the VENC. It can be expressed in seconds per meter or simply by mentioning the optimal velocity. Figure 5.19 compares 3D PC acquisitions at the level of the branches of a medal cerebral artery for three different VENCs. It is obvious that vessels with slow flow benefit from a VENC optimized for low velocities, i.e., large bipolar pulses. If gradients are too low, flowing spins induce only a small phase angle. The phase difference is also small and, therefore, the precision and the amplitude of the complex signal in PC are limited. If gradients are too high, phase angles larger than 180° are obtained. For these velocities, the signal intensity is hampered by aliasing (Fig. 5.20). A range of velocities within the voxel can lead to signal attenuation as well.

a
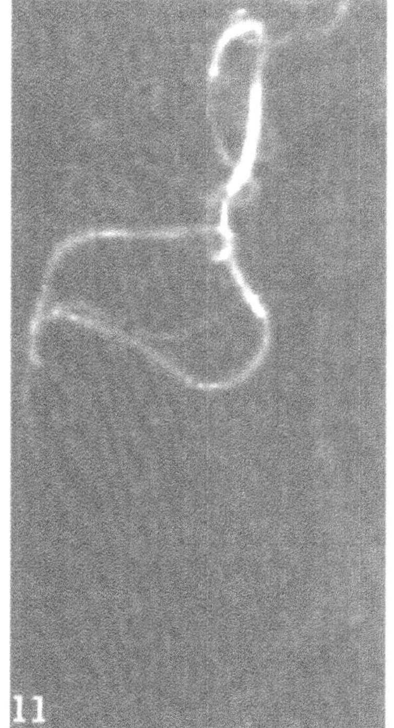

b
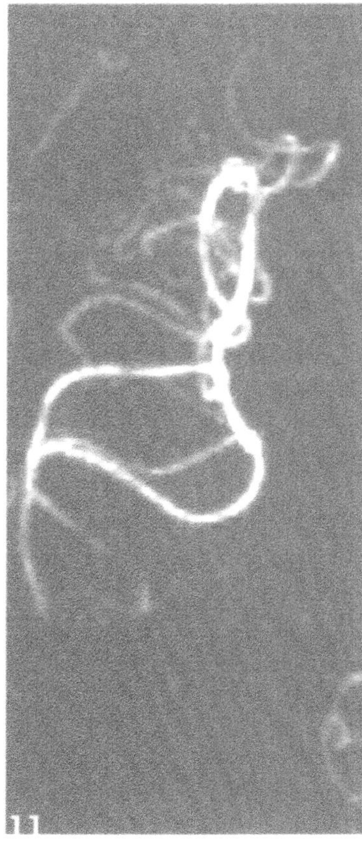

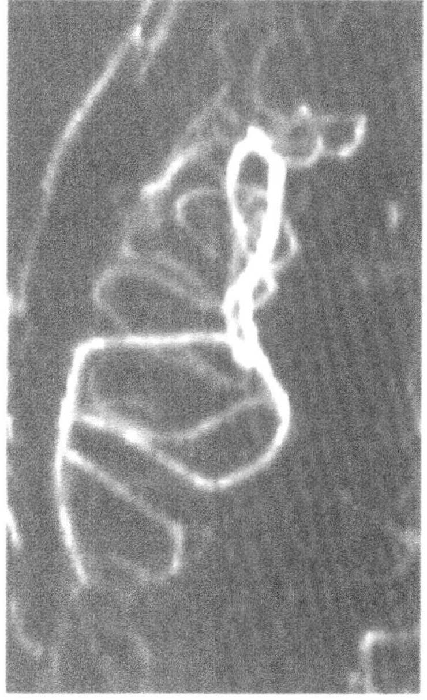
c

Fig. 5.19a–c. 3D phase-contrast acquisitions at the level of peripheral branches of the medal cerebral artery. Velocity-encoding gradients (VENCs) are respectively 60 cm/s, 30 cm/s and 5 cm/s. Slower flow is optimally visualized with lowest VENC

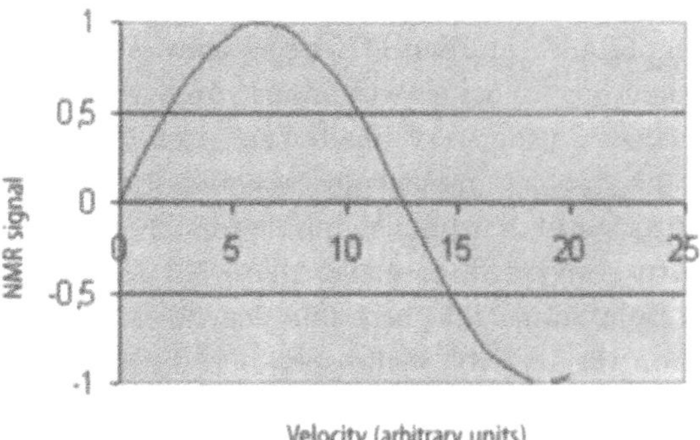

Fig. 5.20. Aliasing occurs for velocities that induce a flow-induced phase that is larger than 180°, i.e. at a velocity larger than 6 arbitrary units in this figure

Figure 5.21 shows a typical 3D PC acquisition with a low VENC. The sagittal sinus is visualized over its entire length in the volume.

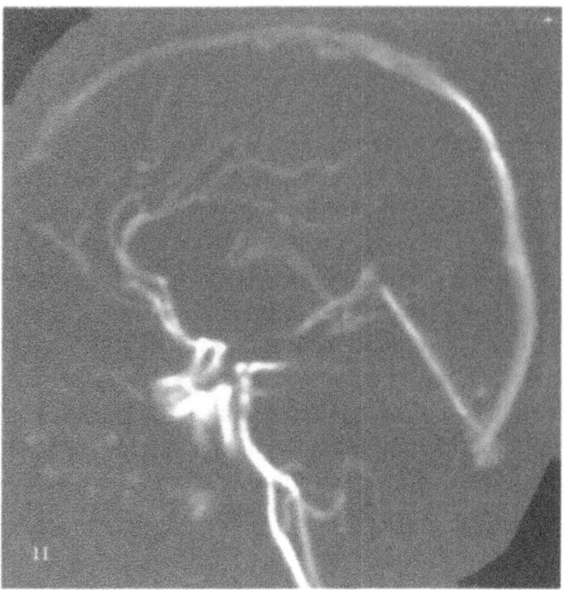

Fig. 5.21. 3D phase-contrast acquisition of the sagittal vein

2D and 3D Acquisitions. The choice between a 2D and a 3D PC technique is not guided by the orientation or minimization of the length of the vessel segments in the imaged slice or volume. On the contrary, as saturation is not a problem, the slice or volume can be chosen to include the maximal vessel segment. The choice between 2D and 3D acquisitions is related to the image resolution required in the plane and through the plane, the need for 3D display (see Chap. 7), and the acquisition time available. Compared to 3D TOF MRA, 3D PC imaging is usually performed with rather poor resolution because of excessive measurement times if too many partitions or large matrices are used. As it is a subtraction technique, small image detail can be achieved even when thick slices are used (compare with X-ray angiography) but 3D visualization tools will suffer from the small number of voxels. A 3D PC technique to depict the entire vasculature of the brain takes 10–20 min. To assess the patency of a particular vein, such as the sagittal sinus, a smaller sagittal subvolume can be chosen, and at that time, total acquisition time would be shorter than using dedicated 2D or 3D TOF measurements.

ECG-Gated PC Imaging. The signal intensity in PC images is optimal when the flow during the acquisition is laminar and constant over time and when its velocity corresponds to the VENC. In some blood vessels there are large differences during the cardiac cycle. In high resistance vessels, there may be a high velocity peak during a small time window, followed by stagnant flow during the rest of the cycle. In these cases, blood vessel contrast may be improved significantly by gating the acquisition to the optimal phase of the ECG. Different schemes have been proposed: encoded acquisitions during the systolic phase, rephased acquisitions during diastole, or the use of different VENCs during the cardiac cycle, etc. A disadvantage of the technique is a further increase in total acquisition time and the fact that these schemes may fail in pathologic situations.

5.5.2.2 Pitfalls

Turbulent flow may induce artifacts in PC images. This is due to incomplete rephasing at the location of the blood vessel and a fortiori an even worse flow encoding. Subtracted images at this location may not be representative for the real velocity in the vessel. In the worst case, there is a signal void. In practice, it is sometimes difficult to estimate the grade of stenosis or to differentiate turbulence from occlusion in PC images. Overgrading of stenoses has been reported. Compared to TOF techniques, PC is more susceptible to this type of flow-induced artifact.

5.5.2.3 Summary

PC methods avoid the problem of progressive spin saturation that leads to the limitations of imaging volume thickness and poor slow flow sensitivity when using 3D TOF MRA techniques. This is simply due to the fact that the stationary background signal is completely suppressed and even partially saturated spins can be observed.

Compared to TOF, PC acquisitions have benefits for the following applications: classifying flow direction and velocity, for venography and visualization of high resistance arteries, and in the case of superimposition problems due to tissues with extremely short T1.

Imperfections in the system, such as transient eddy current fields, can lead to phase errors in the individual measurements. Therefore, a high-performance gradient system with optimal eddy current compensation is required for PCA. The choice between TOF and PC is determined by the specific application. PC acquisitions have an intrinsically high vessel contrast, and TOF provides higher resolution within the same acquisition time (Fig. 5.22)

5.5.3 Other Techniques

Other techniques have been proposed to visualize blood vessels by using flow-induced effects. Many of them use a subtraction method. Examples are:

- Acquisition of a conventional gradient echo acquisition and an identical one with additional very strong bipolar gradients. The second acquisition dephases (most of) the flowing spins, and when subtracted from the rephased acquisition, the result image shows only blood vessels (Axel and Morton 1987).
- Acquisition of two identical gradient echo measurements, but in which the second one is preceded by a saturation pulse that nulls the signal of an incoming vessel. After subtraction, the incoming vessel is visualized.
- Acquisition of two identical acquisitions, but the second is preceded by a nonselective and selective 180° pulse, followed by a delay time TI. The signal of the blood is reduced in the second measurement, whereas the signal of the stationary tissue is not. After subtraction, flowing blood is visualized.
- Subtraction of a flow-dephased image acquired during systolic gating from a flow rephased image acquired during diastole (Selby et al. 1992).
- The use of projective techniques that are based on one of these effects, an example of which was proposed by Edelman already in 1989 (Edelman et al. 1989a).

Other approaches just provide a faster acquisition scheme. They are often based on segmented k-space acquisitions or single-shot echo planar imaging (EPI) techniques. Their utility in practice remains to be proven. The number of techniques that can be used for MRA is still growing and many of them have a role in particular applications where, currently, available

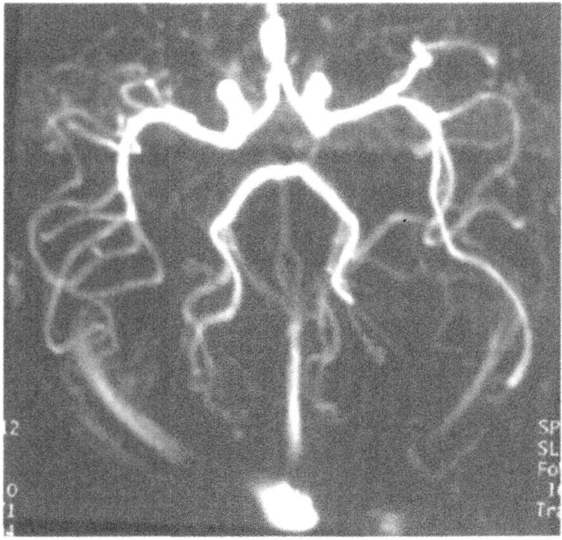

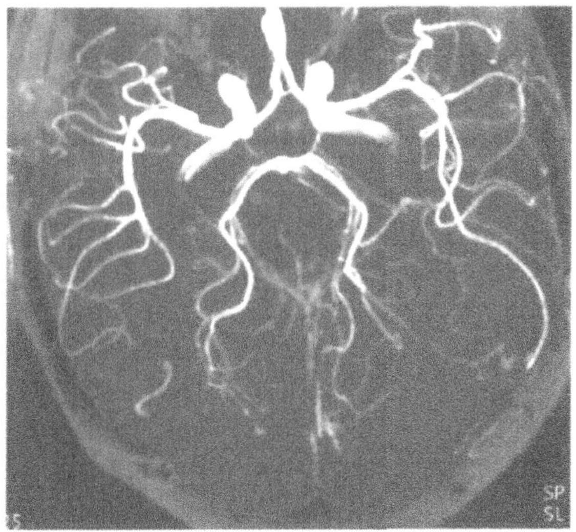

Fig. 5.22. a 3D phase-contrast acquisition, TR/TE/Fl 21 ms/9 ms/15°, velocity-encoding gradient (VENC) for velocities of about 45 cm/s, matrix 165 × 256, field of view (FOV) 150 × 200 mm, 56 partitions with thickness 1.5 mm, total acquisition time of 12 min. **b** High resolution 3D time-of-flight (TOF) study in the same 'author', using TR/TE/Fl 39 ms/7 ms/25°, matrix 192 × 512, FOV 150 × 200 mm, Motsa (three volumes of 32 partitions with 25% overlap), partition thickness 1 mm and total acquisition time 12 min. The phase contrast acquisition, shows arteries and some veins with high vessel contrast. The TOF acquisition has superior vessel detail

techniques fail. Nowadays, some of them are also adapted for visualization of microscopic (Brownian) motion, in which case gradient echo acquisitions are replaced by the faster EPI measurements. It stresses the fact that flow-induced effects should not be associated with artifacts, but rather be exploited to visualize the most interesting features of circulation.

5.6 Conclusion

Many techniques have been proposed for coping with flow-induced artifacts. In a further stage, it has been possible to fully exploit these effects for the visualization of blood vessels. Many of the approaches have a sound physical basis, but given the large variety of flow patterns in normal and pathological situations, there is not a single robust technique that is optimal for all applications.

References

Atkinson D, Brant-Zawadski M, Laub G (1994) Optimization strategies enhance time-of-flight MRA. Radiology 190:890–894

Axel L, Morton D (1987) A method for imaging blood vessels by phase compensated uncompensated difference images. J Comput Assist Tomogr 11:31–34

Carr HY, Purcell EM (1954) Effects of diffusion on free precession in NMR experiments. Phys Rev 94:630–638

Duerinckx AJ, Atkinson D, Mintorovitch J, Simonetti OP, Urman MK (1996) Two-dimensional coronary MR angiography: limitations and artefacts. Eur Radiol 6:312–325

Dumoulin CL, Cline HE, Souza SP, et al (1989a) Three-dimensional time-of-flight magnetic resonance angiography using spin saturation. Magn Reson Med 11:35–46

Dumoulin CL, Souza SP, Walker MF, Wagle W (1989b) Three Dimensional phase contrast angiography. Magn Reson Med 9:139–149

Edelman RR, Wentz KU, Mattle HP (1989a) Projection arteriography and venography: initial clinical results using MR. Radiology 172:351–357

Edelman RR, Mattle HP, Kleefield J, Silver SM (1989b) Quantification of blood flow with dynamic MR imaging and presaturation bolus tracking. Radiology 171:551–556

Haacke EM, Lenz GW (1987) Improving MR image quality in the presence of motion by using rephasing gradients. AJR Am J Roentgenol 148:1251–1258

Haacke EM, Masaryk TI, Wielopolski PA, et al (1990) Optimizing blood vessel contrast in fast three-dimensional MRI. Magn Reson Med 14:202–221

Hahn EL (1960) Detection of sea-water motion by nuclear precession. J Geophys Res 65 (2):776-777

Hausmann R, Lewin JS, Laub G (1991) Phase-contrast MR angiography with reduced acquisition time: new concepts in sequence design. J Magn Reson Imaging 1:415–422

Laub G, Kaiser WA (1988) MR angiography with gradient motion refocusing. J Comput Assist Tomogr 12:377–382

Laub G, Purdy DE (1992) Variable-tip-angle slab selection for improved three-dimensional MR angiography. J Magn Reson Imaging 2:86

Lin W, Tkach JA, Haacke EM, Masaryk TJ (1993) Intracranial MR angiography: application of magnetization transfer contrast and fat saturation to short gradient echo, velocity compensated sequences. Radiology 186:753–761

Marchal G, Bosmans H, Van Fraeyenhoven L, et al (1990) Intracranial vascular lesions: optimization and clinical evaluation of three-dimensional Time-of-Flight MR angiography. Radiology 175:443–448

Nishimura DG, Macovski A, Jackson JL, et al (1988) Magnetic resonance angiography by selective inversion recovery using compact gradient echo sequence. Magn Reson Med 8:96–382

Parker DL, Yuan C, Blatter DD (1991) MR angiography by multiple thin slab 3D acquisitions. Magn Reson Med 17:434–451

Patel MR, Klufas RA, Kim D, Edelman RR, Kent KC (1994) MR angiography of the carotid bifurcation: artefacts and limitations. AJR Am J Roentgenol 162:1431–1437

Pelc NJ, Bernstein MA, Shimakawa A, et al (1991) Encoding strategies for three-direction phase-contrast MR imaging. J Magn Reson Imaging 1:405 - 413

Selby K, Saloner D, Anderson CM, et al (1992) MR angiography with a cardiac-phase-specific acquisition window. J Magn Reson Imaging 2:637–643

Wehrli FW (1988) Principles of magnetic resonance. In: Stark DD, Bradley WG (eds) Magnetic resonance imaging. Mosby, St Louis, pp 3–23

6 Flow-Independent Acquisition Techniques

Georg M. Bongartz, Hilde Bosmans, Guy Marchal

CONTENTS

6.1 Introduction

In flow-dependent acquisition techniques, the blood vessel contrast is based on flow-induced effects. Indeed:

1. Flow can render the signal intensity of blood hyperintense based on inflow-related enhancement
2. Flow can produce a signal void whenever the usual gradient compensation schemes are not appropriate for flowing spins
3. Flow can induce specific, flow-related phase angles.

Nowadays, the so-called flow-independent magnetic resonance angiography (MRA) techniques have a different basis. They include all types of T1-weighted MRI acquisitions in which a positive blood vessel contrast is obtained after or during the injection of a contrast agent. Hyperintense signal intensities in the vessels correspond to a short T1, rather than to the flowing nature of the blood. The intrinsic advantage of T1-based techniques is that they provide a morphological rather than a physiological image of the blood vessel.

A wide range of T1-weighted acquisitions are available. Time-of-flight (TOF) acquisitions, as discussed in the previous chapter, are T1 weighted: after the injection of a contrast agent, the signal intensities in the blood vessels become higher than the signal of most other tissues. In this way, all vessels that were otherwise saturated and therefore invisible on TOF acquisitions, become visible. Phase contrast imaging is less T1 weighted, although signal intensities also increase after the injection of a contrast agent.

Recently, ultrafast acquisitions were introduced in MRA. Their T1 weighting is limited, however: if the contrast agent is very concentrated in the vessels, a high signal intensity is observed in the vasculature. In practice, ultrafast contrast-enhanced (CE) MR angiography has to be performed during the first pass of the contrast bolus.

Both CE TOF and ultrafast CE MRA have important clinical applications. We will discuss these techniques separately. This chapter concludes with a few considerations about the use of blood pool agents for MRA purposes.

6.2 Contrast-Enhanced Time-of-Flight Magnetic Resonance Angiography

In the absence of any contrast agent injection, the MR parameters of TOF sequences have to be adjusted to provide optimal flow-related enhancement (Haacke et al. 1990). This is no longer true in CE MR angiography, where the quality is more related to the induced

G.M. Bongartz, PhD, MD
University Hospital, Kantonsspital, Petersgraben 4, 4031 Basel, Switzerland
H. Bosmans, PhD; G. Marchal, MD, PhD
Department of Radiology, University Hospitals K.U. Leuven, Herestraat 49, 3000 Leuven, Belgium

T1 shortening of the blood and the time evolution of this T1 value during the measurement. In Fig. 6.1, the theoretical signal intensities for a gradient-recalled echo acquisition have been plotted as a function of the number of RF excitation pulses and the T1 value of the tissues. Two characteristics of CE TOF follow from this graph:

1. The shorter the T1, the higher is the signal intensity.
2. For sufficiently short T1, even the steady state "saturated" signal, i.e., the signal that occurs after about 10 RF pulses, is higher than any other signal from tissues with moderate T1 values.

The practical consequence is that saturation is overcome: after a contrast injection, all the vessels in a specified volume of interest, including arteries with fast and slow flow and veins, can be visualized.

6.2.1 Optimization of CE TOF Acquisitions

Optimization of CE TOF is concerned with both the injection protocol as well as the MR parameters. TOF acquisitions typically take a few minutes. During this time, the T1 of the blood changes significantly, with a peak during the first pass of the bolus and then a gradual wash-out. The injected dose of contrast agent determines the T1 in the blood vessel. Higher doses lead to the shortest T1 values. Figure 6.2a shows an MR angiogram in a normal volunteer, prior to any contrast injection. Saturation is obvious in the arteries and the venous system is hardly visualized. In the voluteer shown in Fig. 6.2b and c, a contrast injection had been given. We illustrate the effect of increasing the dose from 0.1 mmol/kg Gd-DTPA (Fig. 6.2b) to 0.2 mmol/kg (Fig. 6.2c) on the quality of the MR angiogram obtained with a 5-min CE TOF measurement. Obviously, the vessel detail is improved when using higher doses. Upper limits to the injected doses are determined by the safety levels, the costs, and the T2* dephasing.

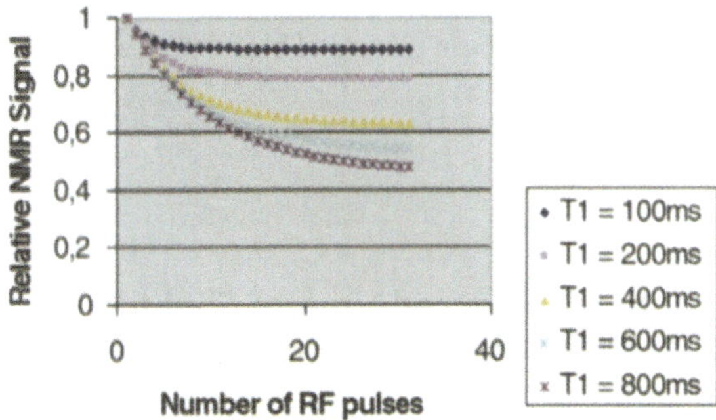

Fig. 6.1. MR signal intensity as a function of the number of RF pulses to which the spins have been subjected for blood with different T1. Simulation for a spoiled gradient-recalled echo acquisition, TR 40 ms, FI 20°

Ideally, the center of k-space should be scanned during the first pass of the bolus, in order to take full advantage of the T1 shortening of the blood. In practice, it is difficult to scan the center of the k-space (of an acquisition that takes several minutes) during the passage of the bolus. In addition, a new k-space line is only scanned every 30 to 40 ms. Therefore it is impossible to scan all the adjacent lines of the center of k-space during the same first pass. However, most of the k-space is certainly scanned during a rapidly decreasing plasma concentration of contrast material.

In a series of experiments, normal k-space acquisitions were compared to reordered acquisitions in which the center of k-space was scanned first to facilitate the matching of the bolus passage with the center of k-space scanning. In the same way, we were able to determine whether biphasic injections are advantageous when compared to a monophasic injection. These different approaches did not noticeably influence the angiographic quality of TOF measurements (Bosmans et al. 1995a). Prince et al. (1993, 1994) proposed slowly injecting contrast over the entire measurement time for the visualization of the aorta and its major branches. For the first time, the aorta could be visualized with a three-dimensional (3D) TOF acquisition over its entire length. With this injection scheme, some venous overlap was present but the venous signal remained lower than the arterial signal. This approach is illustrated in Fig. 6.3: 20 cc of Gd-DTPA were injected very slowly during a 3-min TOF study. The technique was appropriate to study the aorta. These results stimulated further research in this domain and ultimately the new ultrafast CE gradient echo acquisitions were developed.

Although CE TOF is more robust with regard to MR parameters than is plain TOF, the use of appropriate parameters is crucial. For a given TR and T1 of the blood, the optimal vessel signal is obtained at the Ernst angle. For a 5-min acquisition with a TR of 40 ms and a dose of 0.2 mmol/kg GD-DTPA, a flip angle of about 45° is an appropriate choice. The optimal flip angle is lower than 45° for longer measurements or

a 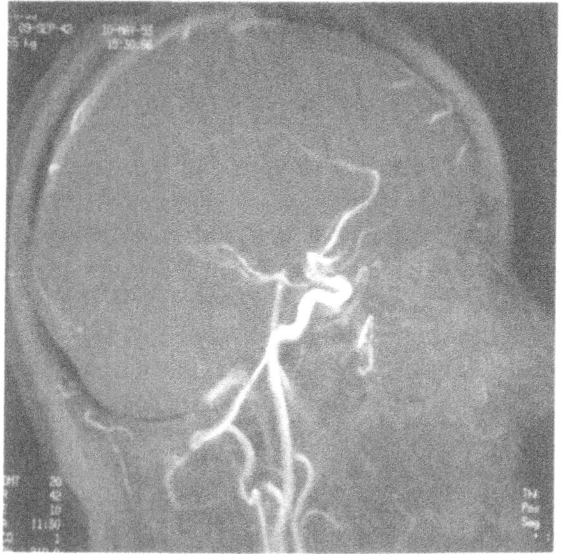

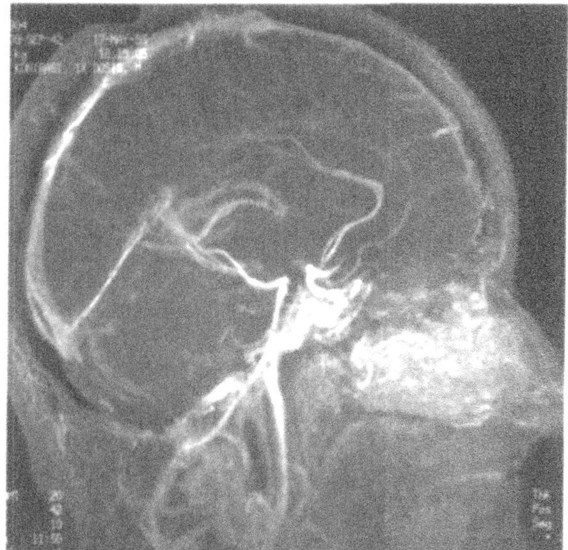 b

c 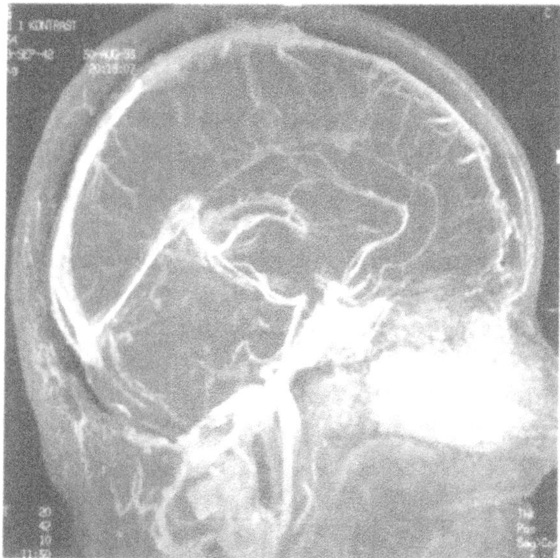

Fig. 6.2a–c. Comparative study in a normal volunteer showing the effects of dose of contrast material on quality of the 3D time-of-flight MR angiogram (TR/TE/Fl 42 ms/10 ms/20°, 32 partitions, acquisition time 5 min). **a** Precontrast acquisition. **b** Acquisition after injection of 0.1 mmol/kg Gd-DTPA. **c** Acquisition after injection of 0.2 mmol/kg Gd-DTPA

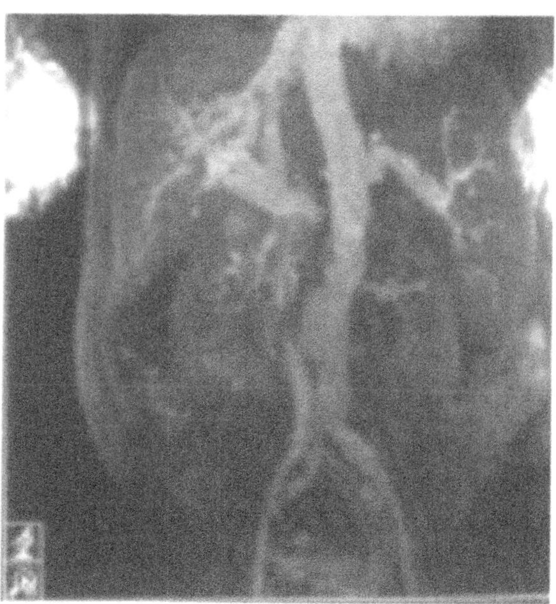

Fig. 6.3. Contrast-enhanced time-of-flight (TOF) acquisition of a patient with an aortic aneurysm using a very slow injection for the course of a 3-min acquisition scheme. Image quality was better than in plain TOF acquisitions. Recently acquired ultrafast angiograms provide better image quality

when the acquisition is started later after the contrast injection (Bosmans et al. 1995). The TR of a CE TOF study can be markedly shorter than 30–40 ms, which has an immediate effect on the total measurement time. This excludes, however, the use of preparation pulses such as fat suppression or magnetization transfer that are commonly employed to reduce the background signal in TOF acquisitions.

The fact that saturation is overcome gives rise to even more advantages: any volume or slice orientation and thickness can be chosen, and all vessels, with the exception of those subjected to substantial motion such as thoracic and coronary vessels, can be visualized with a simple CE TOF study. A disadvantage is that arteries, veins, and some tissues are displayed in a single image. This can be disturbing, as is obvious from Fig. 6.4: the angiogram of the normal volunteer shows both intracranial arteries and veins.

In clinical practice, CE TOF is an appropriate tool for coping with saturation effects both in normal arteries and veins, as well as in diseases with slow flow components (Marchal et al. 1992). Many of the vessels with slow flow are not well visualized with plain TOF acquisitions. The injection of contrast agents is an efficient way to make them visible. Venograms can be obtained with an impressive resolution. In Fig. 6.5 we illustrate how venous anomalies can be visualized in great detail. In vessels with slow flow, such as those distal to a high grade stenosis or aneurysm, the injection of a contrast agent helps differentiate between occlusion and a patent vessel with slow flow (Bosmans et al. 1995b). TOF techniques may fail in this task. This topic is discussed in detail in the chapter on intracranial vessels. In general, arteriograms are not substantially improved as compared to plain TOF acquisitions.

6.2.2 Applications

The improved signal-to-noise ratio of flowing blood using contrast agents can be used to shorten the overall acquisition time by reducing the TR, to increase the image resolution, or to apply these techniques on lower field strength systems.

6.2.3 Pitfalls

The injection of contrast agents with TOF techniques should be performed with caution. During an acquisition that takes a few minutes, many organs or lesions may show hyperintense signal intensities. It may be very difficult to visualize arteries and veins

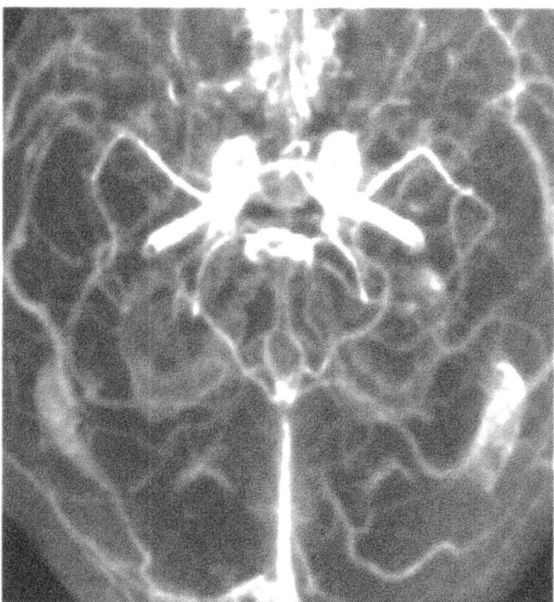

Fig. 6.4. Contrast-enhanced time-of-flight study of a normal volunteer after the injection of 0.2 mmol/kg Gd-DTPA. Both arteries and veins are displayed. It is difficult to achieve high-quality coronal or sagittal angiograms due to overlap of extracranial soft tissues

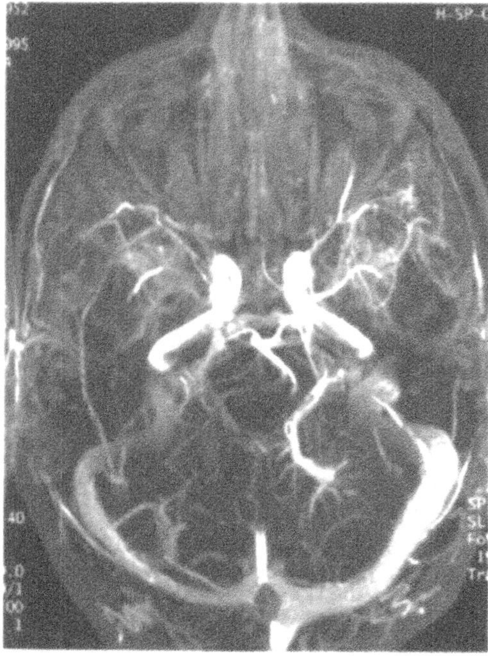

Fig. 6.5. Contrast-enhanced time-of-flight acquisition in a patient with a venous anomaly. The umbrella-shaped vessel tree is very well visualized

separately. In practice, to study the intracranial vessels prior to brain tumor resection, it may well be that visualization of feeding arteries or draining veins is hampered by the presence of a hypervascular, hyperintense lesion and image detail remains inferior to DSA (Wilms et al. 1995). In addition, the injection of contrast agents is not a remedy against flow-induced dephasing either: using clinical doses of the contrast agent, dephasing is unchanged as compared to unenhanced acquisitions.

6.2.4 Summary

The injection of contrast agents makes TOF a more robust technique with regard to visualization of the whole range of vessels. Veins and other vessels with slow flow are shown, independently of the image volume or orientation. Using high resolution 3D TOF acquisitions, vessels can be demonstrated in high detail. This technique has been optimized by shortening the acquisition times even further, as will be discussed in Sect. 6.4.

6.3 CE Phase Contrast Imaging

Phase contrast imaging is a subtraction technique, in which only the signal of flowing tissue is left after the subtraction. Here, the signal strength depends on two factors: a signal amplitude and a contribution that is related to the flow-induced phase effect. Contrast injections prior or during the acquisition may affect the first factor, but do not change the phase effect.

6.3.1 Optimization of CE Phase Contrast Imaging

The signal amplitude in the basic gradient echo acquisition of a phase contrast measurement is no different from the amplitude in the corresponding TOF sequence. It is, therefore, subject to the same type of optimization strategies. We summarize them as follows: the measurements, and more specifically center of k-space acquisitions, have to be performed during the shortest T1 of the blood. The images should be acquired immediately after the injection or, even better, during the injection of the contrast agent. Phase contrast imaging takes longer than TOF acquisitions, and therefore it is definetely impossible to finish the acquisition during the first pass of the bolus. The improved blood vessel signal can be used to shorten the TR and/or to increase the resolution.

6.3.2 Application

The measurement protocol of CE phase contrast imaging does not differ very much from that of plain phase contrast acquisitions. Hence, even in the absence of any contrast injection, saturation was not a problem, and any slice or slab could be chosen in this case as well. The sole advantage is found in an increased signal-to-noise ratio in the images which can be exploited for better image contrast or improved resolution. Typical examples are examinations of vessel malformations in which numerous small vessels are visualized or acquisitions of small peripheral vessels.

6.3.3 Pitfalls

The pitfalls of regular and CE phase contrast imaging are very similar.

6.3.4 Summary

There are a few good indications for CE phase contrast acquisitions, but the relatively long acquisition time remains a major drawback of this technique.

6.4 Ultrafast CE Gradient Echo Acquisitions

The availability of stronger gradients that can be switched on and off in an increasingly shorter time gave rise to a further evolution in MRA: ultrafast CE MRA. This approach basically involves using shortest possible gradient echo sequences during contrast injection. The short echo time makes the use of flow rephasing gradients obsolete.

The signal intensity of the vessel follows the same tendencies as in CE TOF acquisitions, but as the TR is even shorter, smaller flip angles have to be used. The signal-to-noise ratio is also rather poor, as the band width is high and the TR is very short. In practice, the strong vessel contrast is solely based on the ultrashort T1 of the blood. The signal contribution of other tissues is very limited. A high-end sequence would use TR/TE/Fl 2.4 ms/1 ms/20°, and a resolution of $1.3 \times 2.5 \times 2.5$ mm^3. The corresponding acquisition time is 2.5 s (Fig. 6.6a). Higher resolution acquisitions may involve an isotropic resolution of 1 mm along each direction. The total acquisition time then increases up to typically 17 s (Fig. 6.6b). As can be seen from this example, it is not a priori obvious which acquisition strategy is optimal: shorter acquisitions have limited intrinsic resolution, but a relatively short average T1 in the blood, whereas higher resolution acquisitions may not be sharp enough as a result of motion. In practice, additional acquisitions may be added after the CE MRA study. We show an example of a patient with a renal tumor (Fig. 6.7). Using 0.2 mmol/kg of Gd-DTPA, a high quality arterial and venous image was obtained and an ultrafast T1-weighted urographic acquisition completed the all-in-one imaging approach in this patient.

In the optimal case, the center of k-space is scanned during the first pass of the bolus. The following three approaches can be used to achieve this goal:

1. Calculating the bolus arrival time or tracking the arrival of the bolus and scanning the k-space center at the appropriate time
2. Acquiring a series of ultrashort data, such that at least one acquisition lines up with the bolus arrival
3. Applying post-processing tools to distinguish arteries from veins

These techniques will be discussed in more detail in the next chapter, as they determine the possible spatial and temporal resolution.

a

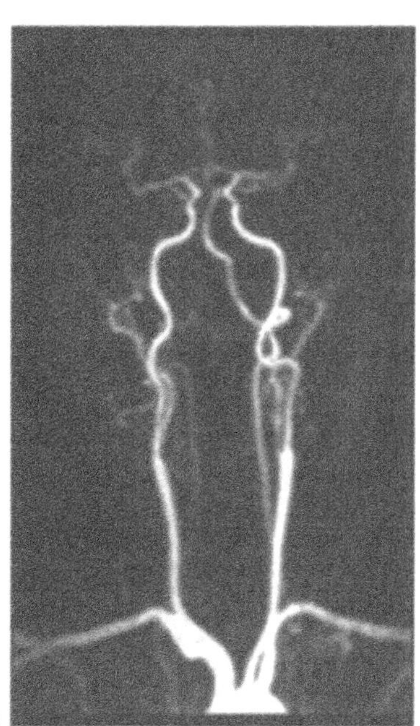

b

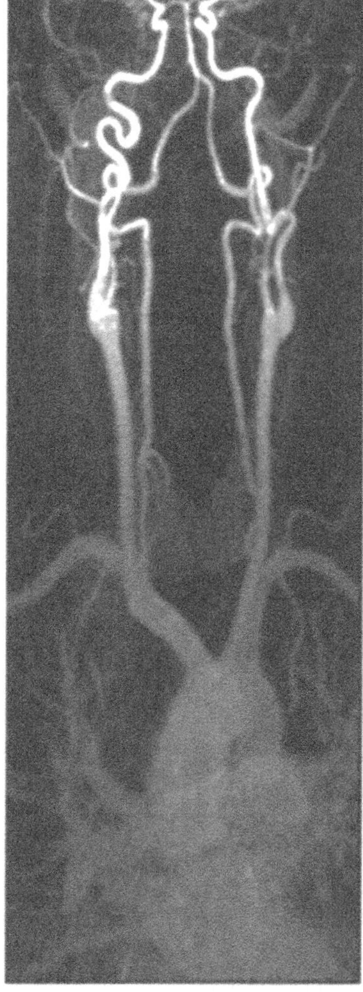

Fig. 6.6a, b. Ultrafast contrast-enhanced MRA acquisition of the carotid arteries (Courtesy of P. Finn, Chicago). **a** TR/TE 2.4 ms/1.0 ms, voxel size 1.3×2.5×2.5 mm3. Total acquisition time: 2.5 s. This acquisition is part of a "dynamic series." **b** TR/TE 2.5 ms/1.1 ms, voxel size 1×1×1 mm3. Total acquisition time: 17 s. This acquisition provides a high-resolution MR angiogram

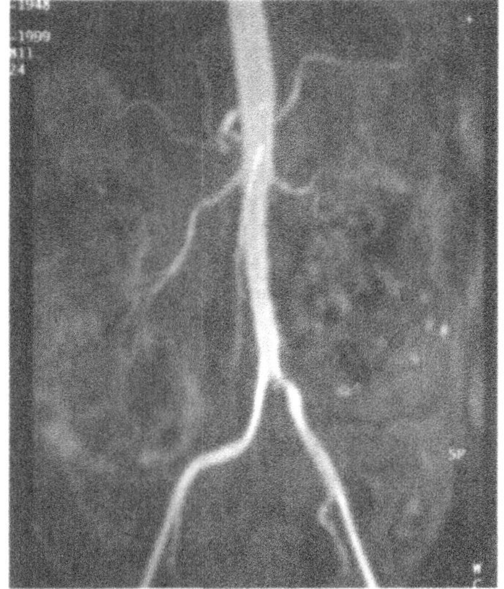

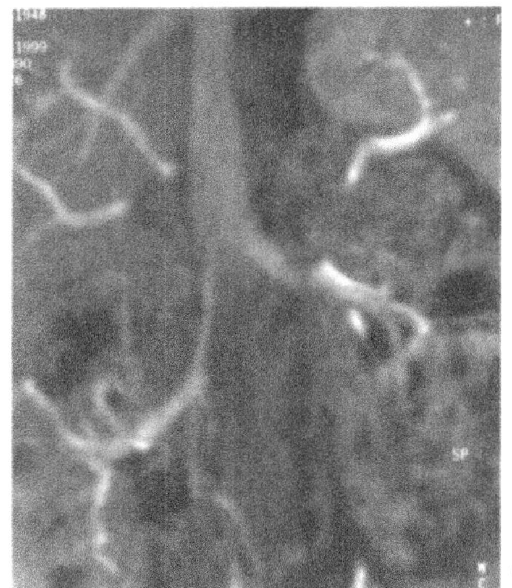

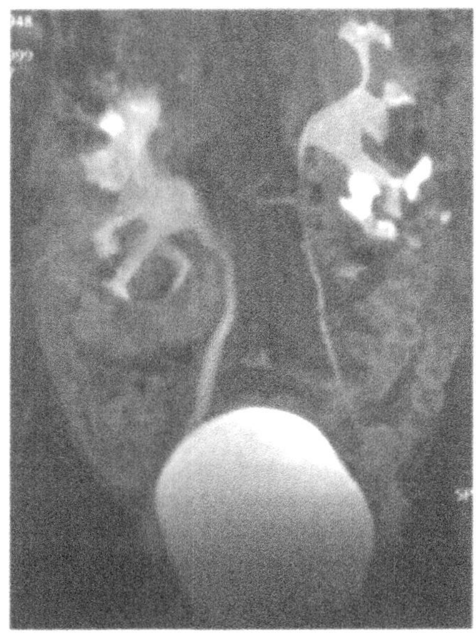

Fig. 6.7a–c. All-in-one dynamic ultrafast acquisition in a patient with polycystic kidneys. Acquisition time per imaging slab is 7 s. The second acquisition coincided with the passage of the contrast bolus. We show the second and the third acquisition, as well as a urography study in the same patient. **a** Arterial phase image. **b** Venous phase image. **c** Urographic acquisition obtained 20 min after the first series showing the urethers and the bladder

6.4.1 Optimization of Ultrafast CE MRA

Ultrafast CE MRA has still not been fully explored. Clinical request and the type of patient cooperation that can be achieved have given strong impetus to the optimization of the technique. In addition, numerous technical parameters have an important influence, such as the intrinsic signal intensities of gradient echo acquisitions, the injection strategy, and the MR parameters for the particular examination. Parameters which are globally determined in the optimization process are the magnetic field strength, the coil, the software which is available, and dedicated hardware tools and the gradient system with the associated maximal band width. A short TR/TE yields images with a poor soft tissue contrast and poor signal-to-noise ratio. Limitations due to signal-to-noise ratio are obvious, as illustrated in the animal study performed after the injection of a blood pool agent (Fig. 6.8). A somewhat reduced band width provides a better signal-to-noise ratio at the expense of a longer acquisition time. For each application, a compromise has to be found between the signal-to-noise ratio, the required in-plane and through-plane resolution, the total imaging time, and the amount of contrast agent that can be injected. The compromise will, of course, also differ from system to system.

In practice, only a very short T1 in the vessel during scanning of the center of k-space ensures a high blood vessel contrast. The intrinsic poor soft tissue contrast for tissues with moderate T1 is not a problem. Soft tissues are well suppressed. The optimal injection of the contrast agent is determined by the technique applied and the vessels of interest (Hany et al. 1997, 1998). The use of the fastest possible injection does maximally

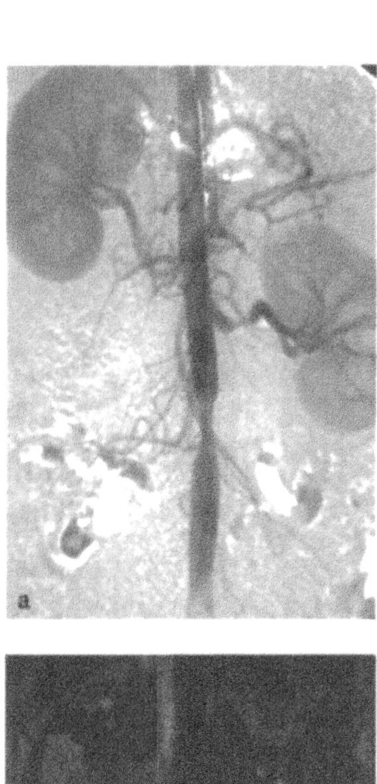

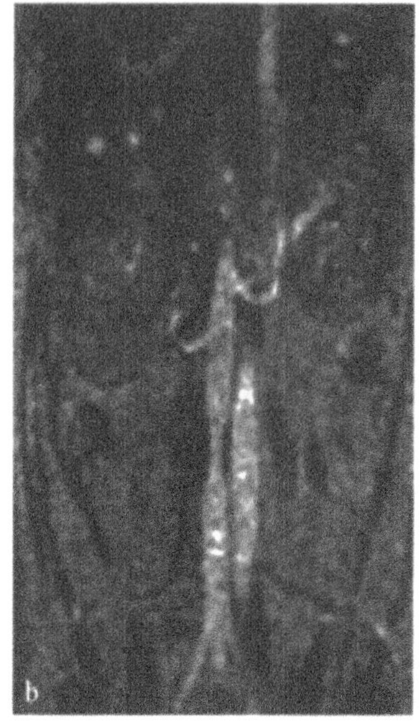

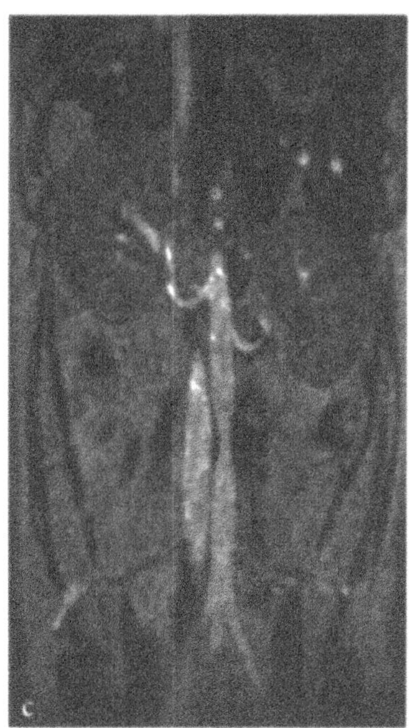

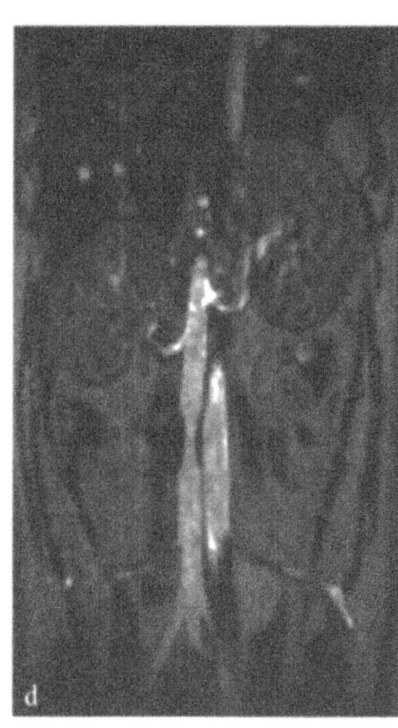

Fig. 6.8a–d. The image quality is determined by "basic" MR parameters, such as TR/TE, the band width (BW), the minimal field of view (FOV), the matrix size, etc. We compare different acquisition strategies in a dog with an aortic and renal artery stenosis, after injection of a blood pool agent. Total acquisition time per slab was 17 s, 27 s, and 34 s. This is considerably smaller than the half-life time in the blood. **a** Digital subtraction angiography of the aorta and its major branches in a canine model shows the two lesions. **b** Ultrafast contrast-enhanced (CE) MRA acquisition using BW 970 Hz/pixel, TR/TE 3.1 ms/1.1 ms, FOV 225 × 450 mm, matrix 128 × 256 (maximal possible number of phase encodings), 17 s acquisition time. **c** Ultrafast CE MRA acquisition using BW 780 Hz/pixel, TR/TE 4 ms/1.4 ms, FOV 206 × 330 mm, matrix 160 × 256, 27 s acquisition time. **d** Ultrafast CE MRA acquisition using BW 650 Hz/pixel, TR/TE 5.3 ms/1.8 ms, FOV 206 × 330 mm, matrix 160 × 256, acquisition time 35 s. The image quality improves with increasing signal-to-noise ratio. In practice, a good compromise is required

decrease the T1 of the blood, however, only for a very short time. In practice, it is not necessary to have a short T1 in the blood vessel for the duration of the measurement as long as this time period includes the central k-space sampling. If it is possible to scan the central k-space lines during this short bolus passage, results are optimal. The same applies to the required breath-hold period. Here, too, it is mandatory to freeze the motion during a part of the acquisition.

The dose which must be injected for an ultrafast CE MRA is still under discussion. Several papers have reported on the use of 0.2–0.3 mmol/kg of the routinely available contrast agents (Leung et al. 1996). In our own experience, and as confirmed by other reports, a dose of 0.1 mmol/kg Gd-chelates or roughly one 20-ml bottle of the contrast agent is enough to obtain arteriograms of diagnostic quality if the bolus is carefully timed. Slightly increased doses improve the stability of the technique.

Whenever a high quality venogram is required, a double dose is indicated. Indeed, the requirement is that the T1 in the veins of interest has to be short during the acquisition. It is also well known that the contrast agent is more diluted in the veins than in the arteries when injecting in the normal way (upper arm). In a recent study, we injected contrast agents in the feet of patients suffering from a venous obstruction in the pelvis. The veins were then scanned during the first passage of this bolus in the veins of interest. No superimposition was yet visible from the arterial system, and the image quality of the veins is excellent (Fig. 6.9).

In an animal study, we compared the signal-to-noise ratio and the image quality of measurements performed with different doses of contrast agent. The results have shown that, at least for this technique and in this animal model, it is not useful to increase the dose above a concentration of 0.3 mmol/kg. A good compromise between the cost of the contrast agent and the image quality may be at a dose of 0.15 mmol/kg. In the same model, we also compared the doses required for an intra-arterial delivery of the contrast agent, while using the same technique (Bosmans et al., ESMRMB, Brussels, 1997). While image quality was rather poor, optimal doses were also lower: 0.015 mmol/kg. This can be explained by a reduced mixing of the contrast agent with normal blood at the level of imaging and is well in agreement with observations from interventional work in a conventional angiographic examination.

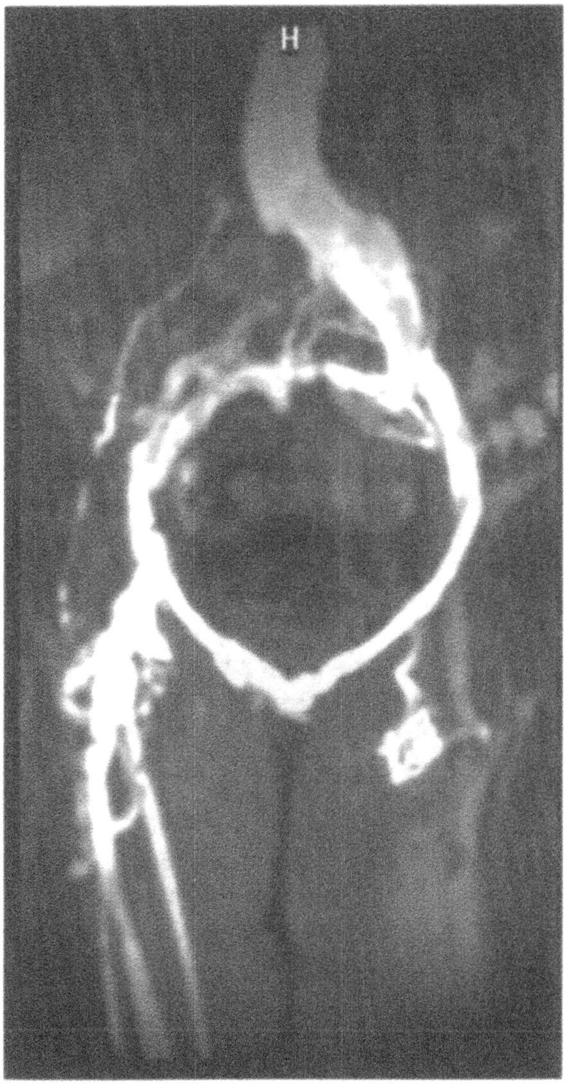

Fig. 6.9. Contrast-enhanced ultrafast MRA acquisition in a patient with an occlusion of the right vena iliaca communis. Contrast was injected in a vein of the right foot. Collateral circulation passing through the prevesical and retrouterine veins into the left iliac vein is visualized without arterial overlap

6.4.2 Application

The major applications for the ultrafast CE gradient echo acquisitions are those domains in which TOF or PC techniques are neither reliable or nor cost effective. This is based on two major characteristics: respiratory-induced motion artifacts are overcome, as the acquisitions can be performed during a single breath-hold, and saturation is not a problem. In addition, arteries and veins can usually be visualized separately if sequence timing is good or the fastest possible acquisitions are used. Ultrafast CE acquisitions were first employed for MRA of the major abdominal vessels and their small side branches. Experience with this technique has been described in excellent review articles (Schönberg et al. 1999; Neimatallah et al. 1999; Baden et al. 1999) and in further chapters of this book. Tools are being developed to acquire peripheral MRA of the whole leg (Ho et al. 1999). Using a dedicated protocol, angiograms of the entire leg can be acquired (Fig. 6.10): a single dose of contrast agent is slowly injected, and high resolution images are obtained during the first pass of the bolus in the different parts of the leg. The so-called moving table is recommended, and the best coils should be activated. Head and neck vessels can also be successfully imaged, but the time constraints there are even more stringent (Metens et al. 1999; Korosec et al. 1999). Accurate bolus timing or a series of acquisitions as short as 4 s each have to be performed. Similar conditions are valid for pulmonary arteries (Meaney et al. 1999). For coronary MRA, a robust acquisition scheme is based on current ultrafast CE acquisitions that is not yet available, but preliminary tests with blood pool agents show promising results (P. Finn, MR Angio club meeting, Lund, Sweden 1999). In general, although many technical aspects still have to be further optimized, the sequences have rap-

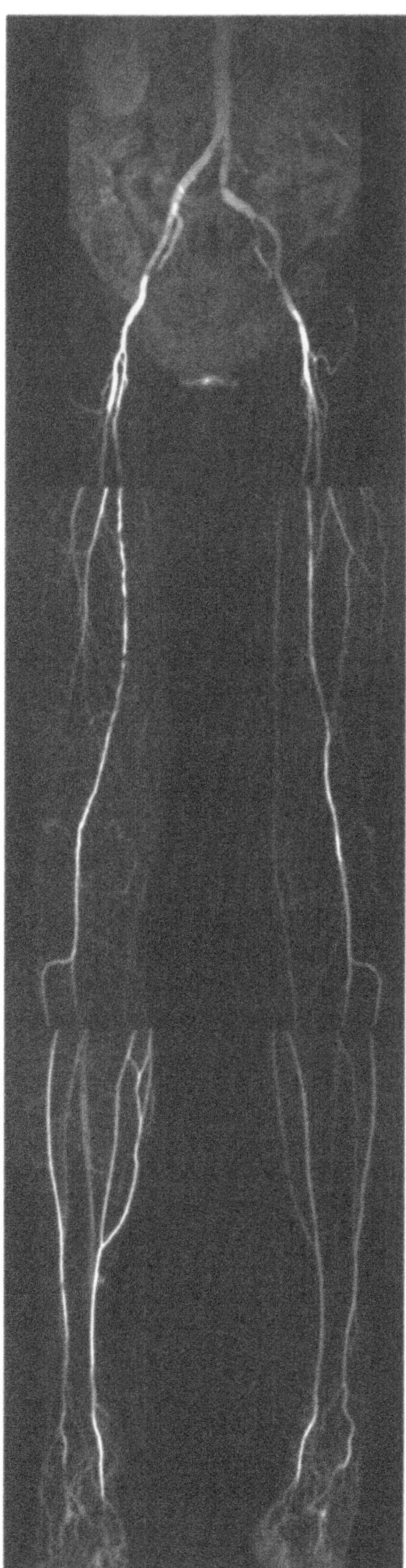

Fig. 6.10. Composite image of a contrast-enhanced peripheral MRA acquisition. Three different acquisitions have been performed after a slow injection of 0.2 mmol/kg Gd-DTPA

idly found their way to clinical applications and are reliable in routine practice.

6.4.3 Pitfalls

Pitfalls arise mainly from incorrect bolus timing. If the center of k-space is scanned prior to the arrival of the contrast agent, the vessels are not visualized. If the acquisition is too late, both arteries and veins will be present in the image. After enough experience is gained with this technique, and, especially if dedicated techniques such as automatic triggering or fast sequential scanning are used (see next chapter), the acquisition is fairly reliable.

If the patient is not able to hold his breath, images may deteriorate as a result of motion artifacts. This can be overcome by the use of increasingly shorter acquisitions, which ultimately leads to (projective) 2D methods. The limited signal-to-noise ratio is currently the limiting factor.

6.4.4 Summary

Ultrafast CE MRA techniques have been developed since 1994. As long as the center of k-space is scanned during the first pass of the bolus, a high vessel contrast can be guaranteed for most vessels currently under investigation. It is a reliable technique that provides anatomical images of the vessels.

6.5 Use of Blood Pool Agents in MRA

Contrast agents that selectively remain in the vessels for a longer time are not yet available for general use in MRA applications, but some have been tested and shown to be advantageous in well-defined patient studies and in animal models. Blood pool agents for MRI can be categorized in two classes: ultrasmall ferrite particles, on the one hand, and large polymers, on the other hand (Knopp et al. 1999). The vascular half-life of these components can be many hours. This characteristic allows CE angiograms to be obtained over a longer period and/or requires a lower dose of the agent.

In Fig. 6.11, ultrafast CE MRA acquisitions using GD-DTPA and AMI 227 are compared. The latter contrast agent is basically an ultrasmall ferrite particle.

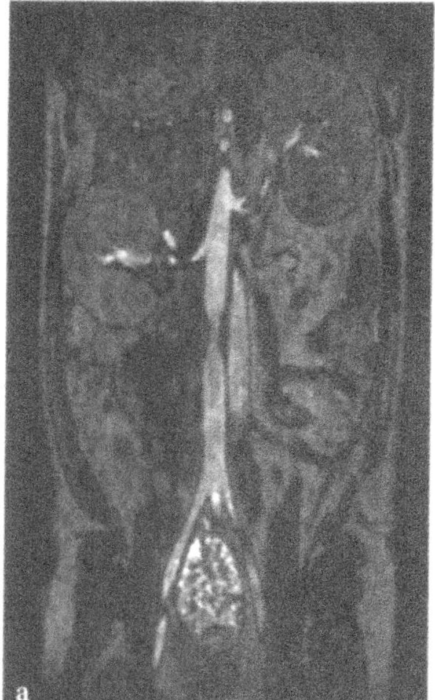

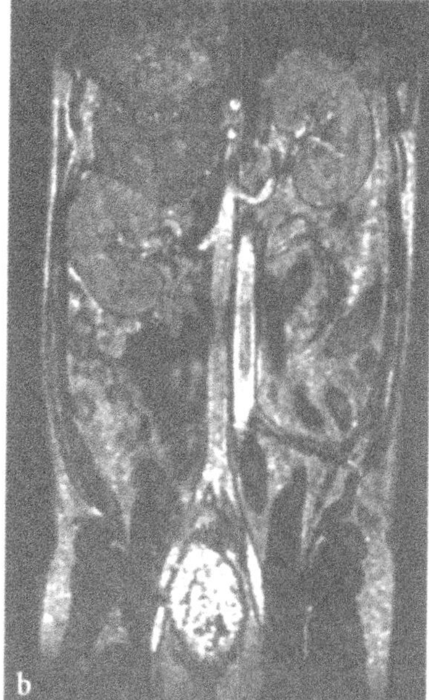

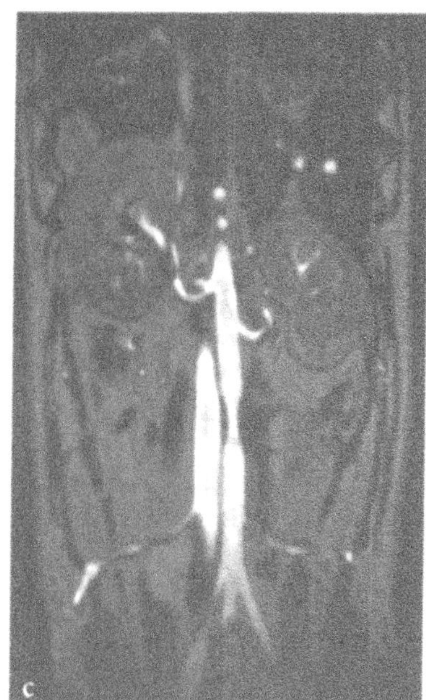

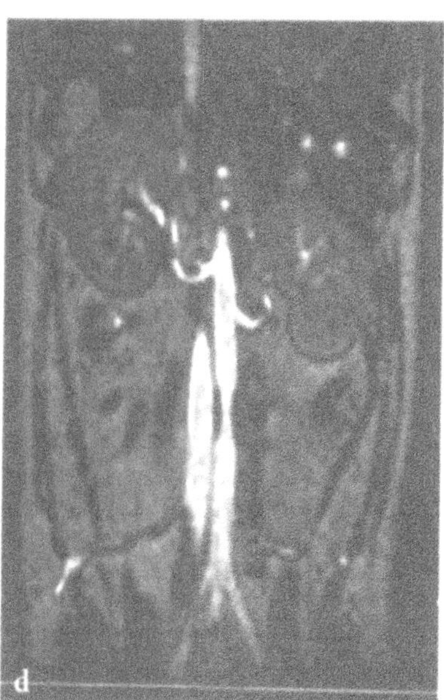

Fig. 6.11a–d. Follow-up study obtained after the injection of Gd-DTPA (0.2 mmol/kg) and AMI 227 (0.2 mmol/kg), 2 days after the first study. MR angiogram obtained immediately (**a**) and 20 min (**b**) after the injection of Gd-DTPA. MR angiograms under the same conditions using 14 µmol Fe/kg body weight AMI 227 (**c**, **d**). The improved image contrast late after the injection of a blood pool agent is obvious. Note that both the arteries and veins remain hyperintense

Immediately after the injection of 0.2 mmol/kg GD-DTPA, saturation is largely overcome (Fig. 6.11a). Twenty minutes after the injection, the effect of the contrast agent is already drastically reduced (Fig. 6.11b). The acquisition immediately after the injection of 0.2 mmol/kg AMI 227 is shown in Fig. 6.11c. This acquisition provides angiograms that compare well with the higher-dose acquisition of the Gd chelate. After 20 min, the image quality is still acceptable (Fig. 6.11d).

The reduced uptake in the soft tissues increases the vessel-to-background contrast-to-noise ratio. This feature could be beneficial for the visualization of abdominal vessels or carotid arteries. It may allow the visualization of vessels that are otherwise hidden by soft tissues, such as the intrarenal vessels. It must be stressed, however, that the relatively high concentration of contrast agents in the veins counteracts many potential benefits. This is particularly apparent for the vessels of the lower leg and for carotid arteries.

There are other applications for blood pool agents, including dose reductions, repeated acquisitions, and successive measurements in different anatomical regions (Kroft and De Roos 1999). In the same way, after a single injection of a blood pool agent, overview images could be obtained up to typically 2 h after the injection. This could be advantageous during interventional studies on an MR scanner.

Figure 6.12 shows the results of an MRA acquisition scheme that exploits the extremely short T1 values of the blood. The experimental contrast agent consists of GD-DTPA that has been attached to a lysine chain. The plasma half-life is about 1 h and the relaxivity is 13 l s^{-1} $mmol^{-1}$ at 0.47 T and 39°. A total dose of 0.5 mmol/kg has been injected. The MR technique is based on the inversion recovery (IR) phenomenon (MARCHAL et al. 1991). First, a 90° pulse is given to nullify the signal of fatty tissue. In the subsequent IR sequence, the IR time is set such that the soft tissue is zero while the blood vessels have a hyperintense signal intensity due to a significantly shorter T1. Due to the almost perfect suppression of the stationary tissues, no slice selection gradient is needed during the acquisition. The 2D projective image was obtained in less than 1 min and is of an excellent quality.

6.6 Summary

Compared to flow-dependent acquisitions, CE MRA has some obvious advantages. The main benefit is certainly that the technique is reliable and the image quality is no longer flow related. An anatomical image is obtained rather than an image that is influenced by the flow pattern. The signal-to-noise ratio arises from the short T1 of the blood and the parameter settings. CE TOF or PC acquisitions complement the information of nonenhanced studies. Due to the leakage of the contrast agent into extravascular tissues, neither CE TOF nor PC acquisitions should be performed as a first choice, due to the possible superimposition of uptaking tissues and the limited add-on value as compared to plain MRA studies.

Ultrafast CE gradient echo acquisitions rely on the shortening of the T1 during the first pass of the bolus. They exploit the possibilities of a powerful gradient system. If the first pass of the bolus is imaged, the image quality is excellent. Dedicated software tools make this technique very reliable. Future developments may produce even faster acquisition protocols. However, many of the new diagnostic vascular imaging techniques still have to be tested clinically and also explored for application in interventional work. Blood pool agents may be very helpful in this regard.

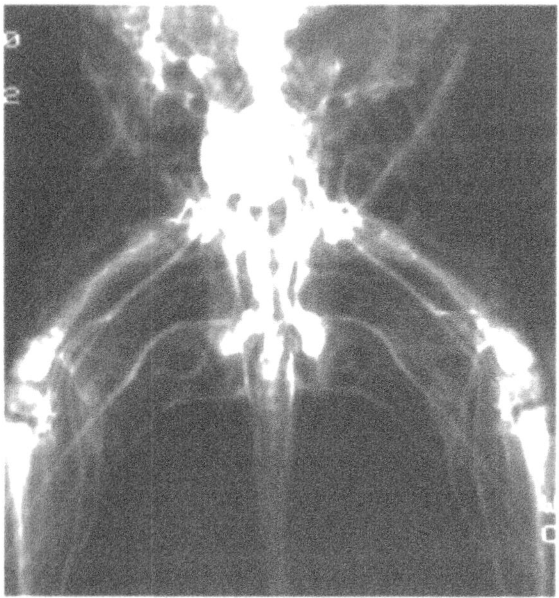

Fig. 6.12. Gd-DTPA polylysine-enhanced acquisition using a dose of 0.5 mmol/kg and IR sequence with a fat saturation and muscle suppression pulse. This acquisition exploits the extremely short T1 of the blood

References

Baden JG, Racy DJ, Grist TM (1999) Contrast enhanced three-dimensional magnetic resonance angiography of the mesenteric vasculature. J Magn Reson Imaging 10:369–375

Bosmans H, Marchal G, Lukito G, et al (1995) Time-of-flight MR angiography of the brain: comparison of acquisition techniques in healthy volunteers. AJR Am J Roentgenol 164:161–167

Bosmans H, Wilms G, Marchal G, Demaerel P, Baert AL (1995) Characterization of intracranial aneurysms with MR angiography. Neuroradiology 37:262–266

Cavagna FM, Anelli PL, Lorusso V, Maggioni F, Zheng J, Li D, Abendschein DR, Finn PJ (2001). B-22956, a new intravascular contrast agent for MR coronary angiography. Proc. Intl Soc. Mag. Reson. Med. 9:519

Haacke EM, Masaryk T, Wielopolski PA, et al (1990) Optimizing blood vessel contrast in fast three-dimensional MRI. Magn Reson Imaging 14:202–221

Hany TF, McKinnon GC, Pfammatter T, Debatin JF (1997) Optimization of contrast timing for breath-hold, contrast enhanced three-dimensional MR angiography. J Magn Reson Imaging 7:551–556

Ho VB, Choyke PL, Foo TKF, Hood MN, Miller DL, Czum JM, Aisen AM (1999) Automated bolus chase peripheral MRA: initial practical experiences and future directions of this work-in-progress. J Magn Reson Imaging 10:376–388

Knopp MV, Von Tengg-Kobligk H, Floemer F, Schönberg SO (1999) Contrast agents for MRA: future directions. J Magn Reson Imaging 10:314–316

Korosec FR, Turski PA, Carroll TJ, Mistretta CA, Grist TM (1999) Contrast-enhanced MR angiography of the carotid bifurcation. J Magn Reson Imaging 10:317–325

Kroft LJM, De Roos A (1999) Blood pool contrast agents for cardiovascular MR imaging. J Magn Reson Imaging 10:395–403

Leung DA, McKinnon GC, Davis CP, Pfammatter T, Krestin GP, Debatin JF (1996) Breath-hold, contrast enhanced three-dimensional MR angiography. Radiology 200:569–571

Marchal G, Bosmans H, Van Hecke P, Jiang Y, Aerts P, Bauer H (1991) Experimental Gd-DTPA Polylysine enhanced MR angiography: sequence optimization. J Comput Assist Tomogr 15:711–715

Marchal G, Michiels JM, Bosmans H, et al (1992) Contrast enhanced MRA of the brain. Technique and first clinical results. J Comput Assist Tomogr 16:25–29

Meaney JFM, Johansson LOM, Ahlstrom H, Prince MR (1999) Pulmonary Magnetic Resonance Angiography. J Magn Reson Imaging 10:326–338

Metens T, Rio F, Baleriaux D, Roger T, David P, Rodesch G (2000) Intracranial aneurysms: detection with gadolinium-enhanced dynamic three dimensional MR angiography-initial results. Radiology 216(1):39–46

Neimatallah MA, Dong Q, Schönberg SO, Cho KJ, Prince MR (1999) Magnetic resonance imaging in renal transplantation. J Magn Reson Imaging 10:357–368

Prince MR (1994) Gadolinium enhanced MR aortography. Radiology 191:155–164

Prince MR, Yucel EK, Kaufman JA, Harrison DC, Geller SC (1993) Dynamic gadolinium-enhanced three-dimensional abdominal arteriography. J Magn Reson Imaging 3:877–891

Schönberg SO, Essig M, Bock M, Hawighorst H, Sharafuddin M, Knopp MV (1999) Comprehensive MR evaluation of renovascular disease in five breath holds. J Magn Reson Imaging 10:347–356

Wilms G, Bosmans H, Marchal G, Demaerel P, Baert AL (1995) Magnetic resonance angiography of supratentorial brain tumors: comparison with selective digital subtraction angiography. Neuroradiology 37:42–47

7 Spatial Versus Temporal Resolution in Contrast-Enhanced Magnetic Resonance Angiography

Hilde Bosmans and Guy Marchal

CONTENTS

7.1 Introduction

The diagnostic quality of any MR image is determined by the intrinsic tissue contrasts, the signal-to-noise ratio, and the spatial and the temporal resolution. Currently, it is still impossible to propose a protocol that represents the optimal technical solution for any ultrafast contrast-enhanced magnetic resonance angiography (CE MRA) application. On the contrary, different anatomical regions present with different physiological constraints. In addition, the hardware and software tools which are available largely determine the possibilities on a particular scanner.

For most applications, the total permissible acquisition time is well defined and the other parameters have to be adapted to this. For a CE MR angiogram, the following overall rules can be formulated:

- In a patient, a single breath-hold of 30 s is already very difficult.
- The maximal acquisition time to prevent venous overlap using successive acquisitions is only few seconds. Renal arteries and veins can be reliably visualized separately if the total acquisition time does not exceed 7 s. For carotid arteries, the intracranial vasculature, and pulmonary vessels this period is shorter. For peripheral MRA, the acquisition time can be much longer.
- The visualization of flow dynamics requires a time resolution on the order of a second.

In this chapter, we first discuss the basic MR parameters that influence the spatial and temporal resolution in MR images. Then, we present three different approaches by which the spatial or temporal resolution can be improved in ultrafast CE MRA:

1. The careful timing of a high resolution acquisition so that the k-space is scanned during the first pass of the bolus
2. The acquisition of a series of ultrafast acquisitions so that at least one acquisition lines up with the first pass of the bolus
3. The use of post-processing techniques to separately visualize arteries and veins

7.2 Spatial Versus Temporal Resolution in MR Imaging: General Principles

The spatial resolution of an MR image correlates with the number of voxels per unit of length along x, y, and z. A small field of view (FOV), a large matrix size, and thin slices provide the best spatial resolution. Unfortunately, the tendency of the signal-to-noise ratio is just the opposite. In practice, the best possible image resolution is usually limited by signal-to-noise considerations (see also Chap. 4 by M. Bock). The temporal resolution is related to the total acquisition time. For a conventional ultrafast

H. Bosmans, PhD; G. Marchal, MD, PhD
Department of Radiology, University Hospitals K.U. Leuven, Herestraat 49, 3000 Leuven, Belgium

acquisition scheme, the duration of an MR measurement depends on the TR, the number of phase-encoding steps, the number of partitions, and the number of signal averages. The limits within which these parameters can be changed depend on the hardware and software provided with a particular scanner. The static magnetic field only has an indirect influence via the signal-to-noise ratio. As a consequence, the optimization for a state-of-the-art 1.5-T scanner is different from that for less sophisticated systems.

Two-dimensional (2D) acquisition schemes are the fastest. The total acquisition time is obtained by multiplying the TR and the number of phase-encoding lines. Compared to a three-dimensional (3D) acquisition, however, the signal-to-noise ratio is reduced. In practice, 2D acquisitions can provide information about the flow dynamics, but the image quality can be very poor. In addition, thick slices or projective images have to be acquired, which further reduces the image contrast. Actual ultrafast MRA techniques are based on the characteristics of both of these standard schemes. In addition, technical developments and stable gradient systems have made it possible to incorporate new approaches into the basic acquisition schemes.

7.3 High Resolution Acquisition with Timing of Bolus Arrival

A so-called high resolution MRA acquisition typically uses parameters in the following range: TR 3 ms, matrix 160 × 256 or 160 × 512, 64 partitions, FOV 300 × 400 mm, and partition thickness of 1–2 mm. To obtain a positive blood vessel contrast with such a measurement scheme, the T1 of the blood has to be sufficiently short during the measurement of the central k-space lines. For most conventional acquisition schemes, this occurs halfway through the measurement. Centrically or elliptically reordered acquisitions typically acquire the center of k-space during the first part of the measurement.

The shortest T1 values are achieved during the first pass of the contrast bolus. Unfortunately, in clinical practice, it is impossible to predict a priori the bolus arrival time due to the variability of the circulation time. Dedicated techniques have been worked out to guarantee that the center of k-space is being scanned while the bolus passes.

7.3.1 High Resolution CE MRA Acquisition Using a Test Bolus

In the first approach, the contrast arrival time is estimated from an additional measurement and this information is used to start a high resolution acquisition in which the k-space is scanned during the real contrast bolus passage (Fig. 7.1). The use of a test bolus acquisition to predict the bolus arrival time is straightforward. It requires the injection of a small bolus of typically 2 cc, followed by a saline flush of some 20 cc. A series of fast T1-weighted acquisitions of a single slice at the position of interest is prepared. Image acquisition and injection are started simultaneously and the acquisitions continue until the contrast bolus has passed. The duration of these fast acquisitions has to be established according to the vessels under study. The contrast travel time is determined from the image that first shows the arrival of the contrast bolus. With a given scan time and injection time, the optimal scan delay, i.e., the time delay between the start of the injection and the start of the ultrafast CE MRA measurement (Fig. 7.2), can be calculated, according to M. Prince (Prince et al. 1997), from:

$$T_{sd} = BAT - \frac{MT - (10\% \cdot MT)}{2}$$

In Fig. 7.3, we show (a) a typical image of the ascending aorta, as obtained with a test bolus scan and (b) the corresponding contrast uptake curve.

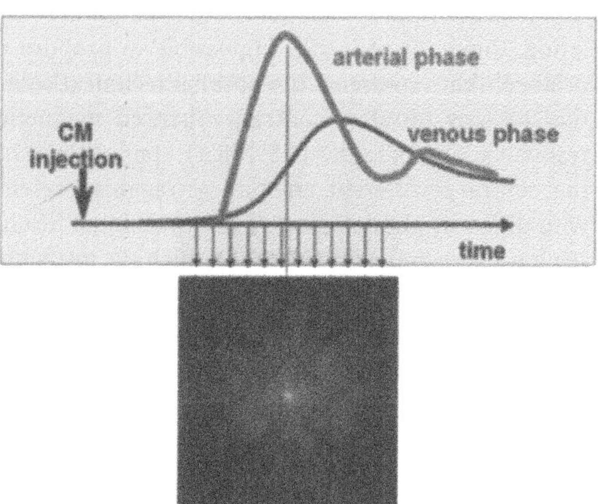

Fig. 7.1. Acquisition scheme of a conventional contrast-enhanced MRA scheme versus the contrast uptake curve in an artery: the center of k-space has to be scanned during the passage of the bolus. *CM*, contrast medium

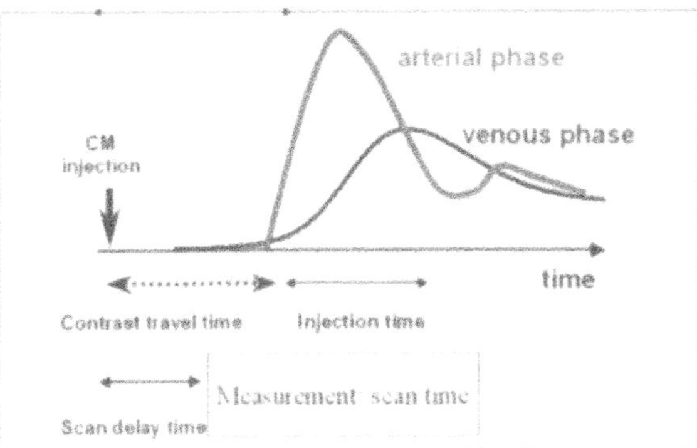

Fig. 7.2. The scan delay time can be calculated from the contrast medium (*CM*)arrival time and the duration of bolus and measurement

a

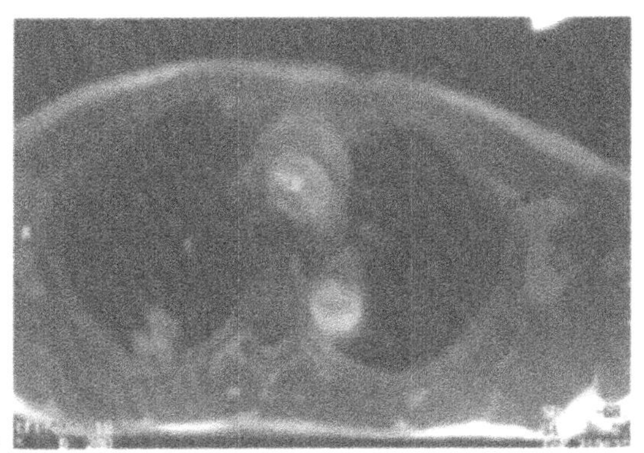

b

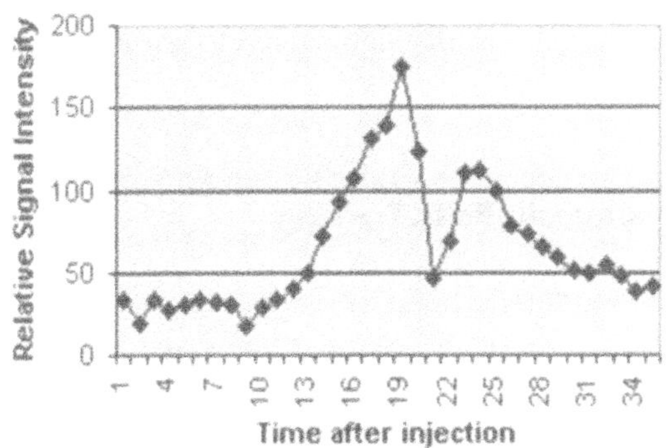

Fig. 7.3a, b. Using of a test bolus, the bolus arrival time and therefore also the scan delay time can be calculated. **a** A 2D turboFLASH measurement shows hyperintense signal intensities in the aorta during the passage of the test bolus. **b** Typical uptake curve in the ascending aorta as measured in a series of turboFLASH scans

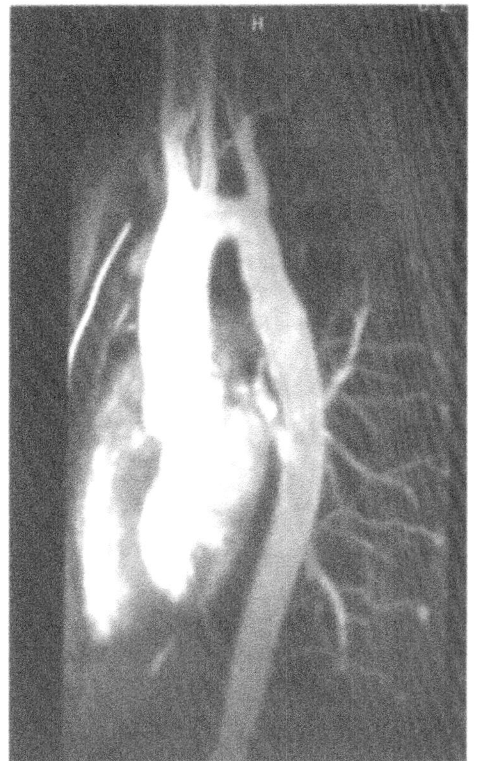

Fig. 7.4. High resolution acquisition of the aortic arch with a total measurement time of 16 s using a test bolus acquisition. The coarctation is well visualized

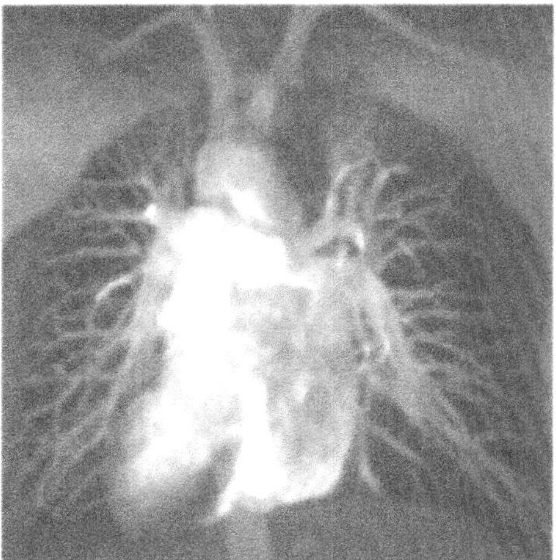

Fig. 7.5. High resolution acquisition of normal pulmonary arteries using a test bolus acquisition

This technique can often be successfully applied for renal, thoracic (Fig. 7.4), pulmonary (Fig. 7.5), intracranial (Fig. 7.6), peripheral and carotid MRA, as was also illustrated in the previous chapter.

A practical limitation is that the test bolus acquisition is somewhat time consuming. Failures result where there are inconsistencies in contrast arrival time. In addition, calculation errors may cause poor image quality and, in some anatomical regions, it is difficult to avoid overlapping signal intensities under conditions of fast venous return.

Although the injection rate can be controlled and the protocol standardized by using an MR-compatible power injector, successful acquisitions can also

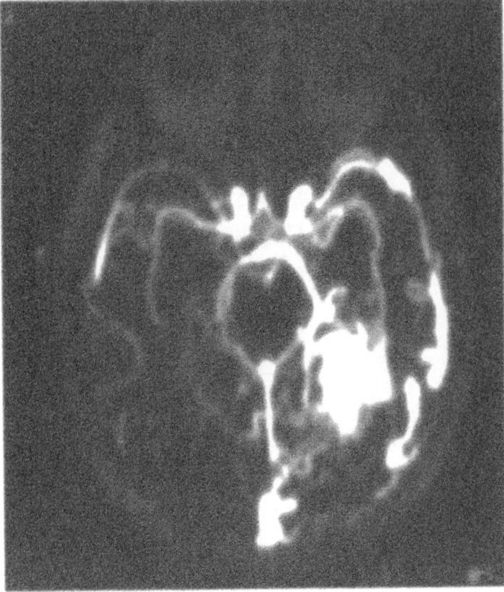

Fig. 7.6. High resolution acquisition of the intracranial vessel in a patient with an arteriovenous malformation. A test bolus acquisition had been used for accurate timing

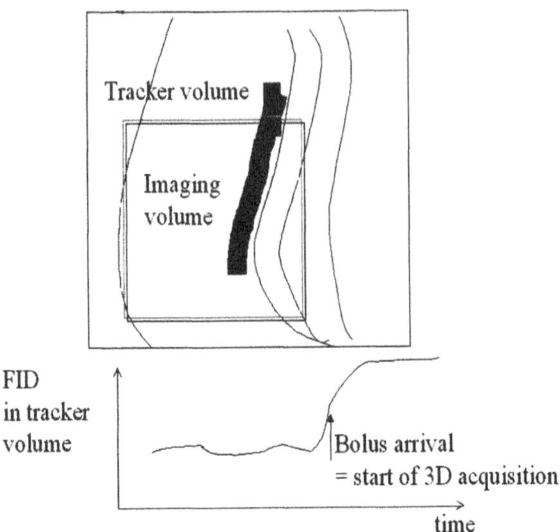

Fig. 7.7. Automatic bolus tracking can be based on the (*FID*) from a vessel segment upstream of the volume of interest

be obtained by manual injection, at least as long as the injection speed is kept constant and the transition between the injection of the contrast and the saline is smooth. PRINCE proposed a dedicated injection tool for high resolution ultrafast CE MRA (Smart Set, Topspins, www.topspins.com).

More recently, the same author (PRINCE et al. 1999a) proposed using ultrasound contrast agents to calculate the bolus arrival time as this approach reduces the overall MR time and thus reduces the cost of the examination.

7.3.2 Automatic Bolus Arrival Tracking

Pulse sequences have been designed to automatically detect the arrival of a contrast bolus (Fig. 7.7) (PRINCE et al. 1999b). They are based on the detection of FIDs (free induction decay) after excitation pulses. When the bolus arrives, the sudden change in the relaxation parameters changes this FID and this can be measured. In practice, this is performed in a region of interest that is located upstream of the vessel of interest or where the spins enter the imaging volume. As soon as the bolus arrives, the measurement system detects a change in signal; the scanning of the FID is then stopped and switched to the real CE MRA study. Since at that moment the contrast is already present, a centrically reordered high resolution 3D acquisition is used that scans the center of k-space first. This solution has been incorporated in the commercially available equipment offered by the major vendors. The advantage of this approach is clearly that it obviates the need for a test bolus injection. Failures in automatic bolus arrival tracking arise from poor triggering of the sequence when artifacts are present. Preliminary tests may also be required to assess the threshold parameter which determines at what increase in signal intensity the MRA is started such that optimal results are achieved.

7.3.3 Semi-automatic Bolus Tracking

In semi-automatic bolus tracking, the user monitors the arrival of the contrast bolus and interactively starts the MRA acquisition (Fig. 7.8). As with automatic bolus tracking, a series of acquisitions is performed to visualize the bolus arrival. In the semi-automatic approach, turboFLASH measurements or 2D phase contrast acquisitions are used for imaging. In fact, any technique known as a (T1- or T2*-weighted) MR fluorography sequence is appropriate for this task. As soon as the bolus arrives, a breath-hold command is given to the patient and a centrically or elliptically reordered high resolution CE MRA acquisition is started. This is a very reliable approach that provides excellent image quality. The 2D acquisitions that visualize the bolus arrival may also provide dynamic information (Fig. 7.9a). The image quality of the high resolution 3D MRA acquisition, as shown in the renal artery study (Fig. 7.9b), is excellent.

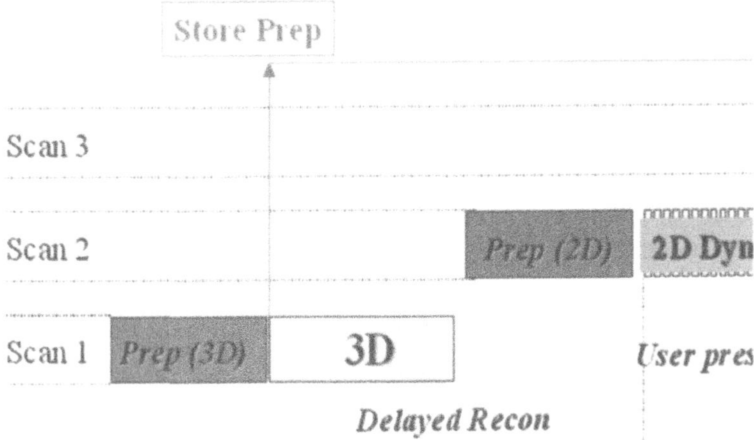

Fig. 7.8. Overview of the semi-automatic acquisition scheme: an ultrafast 2D acquisition mode is interrupted at the bolus arrival by the observer, the breath-hold command is given and the 3D acquisition starts subsequently. (Courtesy of M. Van Kouwenhoven, Philips)

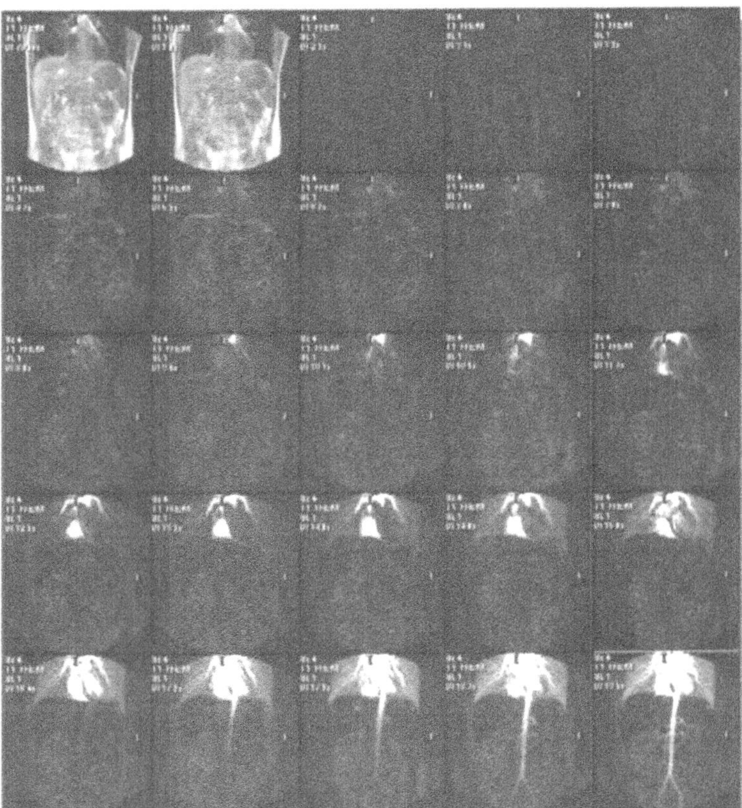
a

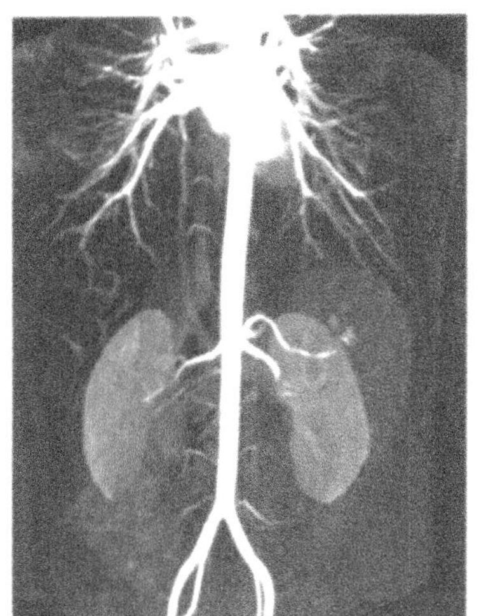
b

Fig. 7.9a, b. A typical example of the semi-automatic acquisition scheme. **a** Successive 2D acquisitions show an overview of the contrast arrival. These images include information about flow dynamics. **b** Centrically reordered 3D acquisition shows excellent vessel detail. (Courtesy of the University of Maastricht and Philips Medical Systems)

7.4 Ultrafast Sequential Scanning

A means of circumventing the bolus timing is to scan the center of k-space very frequently such that at least one acquisition lines up with the passage of the bolus in the vessel of interest. One way of doing this would be to acquire successive conventional ultrafast acquisitions. In a further approach, just the center of k-space can be scanned repeatedly. A posteriori, the peripheral lines are retrieved from measurements at other time points.

7.4.1 Acquisition of Successive Ultrafast Measurements

The dynamic approach, in which a series of "conventional" CE ultrafast scans is performed, can be run on most scanners: it suffices to reduce the matrix size and the number of partitions to such an extent that the total acquisition time is less than the time for venous return (Fig. 7.10). The following techniques can be used to shorten the acquisition time per slab: the use of a rectangular FOV and matrix, partial Fou-

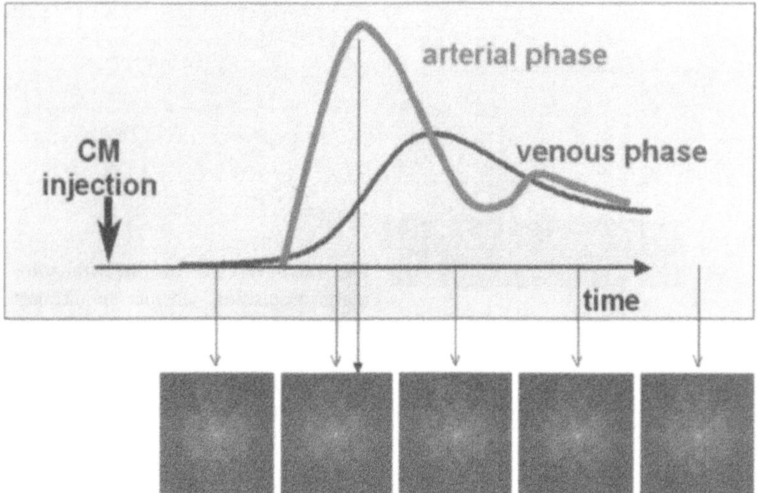

Fig. 7.10. Acquisition scheme using a series of ultrafast contrast-enhanced 3D acquisitions. At least one acquisition lines up with the passage of the contrast medium (*CM*) bolus. The acquisition time per slab is shorter than the arteriovenous return

rier techniques, interpolation along the k_z-direction to double the number of reconstructed slices per slab, and new k-space acquisition schemes. In an ultrafast CE MRA study of the renal arteries, it was shown that the total acquisition time per acquisition slab should not exceed 7 s (Van Hoe et al. 1999). For other vessels, restrictions may be even more stringent.

There are several advantages of the ultrafast approach: there is no need for a test bolus injection, making the procedure very easy; the acquisition time per 3D slab is shorter, which reduces the requirements on the breath-hold; arteries and veins are always separately visualized; information is given about the parenchymal perfusion; and the contrast bolus is present during the larger part of the total acquisition time. As a result, the image quality may be even better when compared to the so-called high resolution CE MRA technique (Fig. 7.11). Ultrafast MRA sequences can also be used as part of an all-in-one approach, in which, for example, arterial and venous anatomy as well as organ perfusion are visualized.

A high temporal resolution can also be obtained with the use of successive 2D acquisitions with measurement times of about 1 s per slice. The technique can be implemented on most MR systems, there is no need for special reconstruction techniques, and it definitely is the fastest approach. Drawbacks are the poor signal-to-noise ratio and the lack of 3D information, which makes the interpretation less reliable.

7.4.2 Acquisition of Successive k-space Centers

A more sophisticated approach has been proposed by Korosec (Korosec et al. 1996): the central k-space

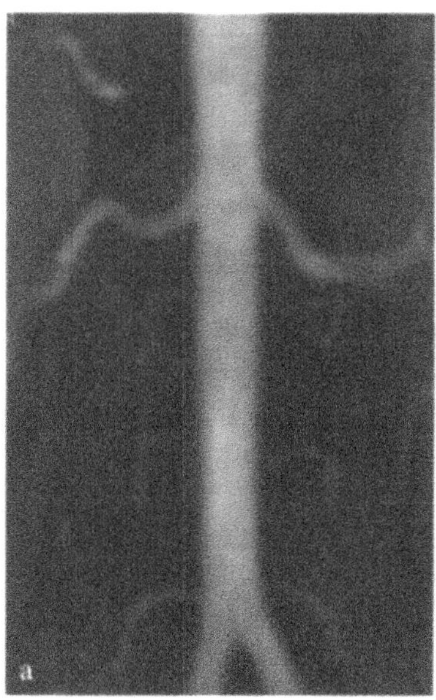

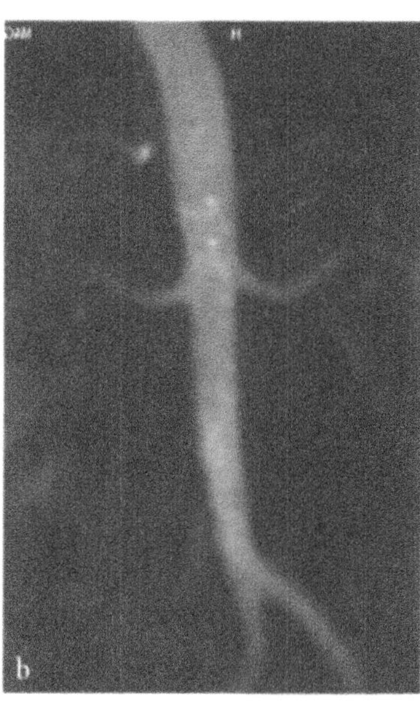

Fig. 7.11. Comparison of (**a**) a high resolution (27 s) acquisition of the renal arteries versus (**b**) a lower resolution acquisition in the same patient. From this example, it is seen that the choice between high and lower resolution acquisitions is not always easy

data are scanned after short intervals, such that at least one central k-space acquisition lines up with the arrival of the contrast bolus, whereas the peripheral lines are only scanned intermittently (Fig. 7.12a). For each central k-space acquisition, the peripheral k-space acquisitions are calculated from the closest acquisitions. This approach achieves such a high temporal resolution that even the passage of the bolus can be followed through the vessel. Despite the fact that k-space data are acquired at different time points, the initial results show only minimal reconstruction artifacts and the clinical images look promising. Unfortunately, the widespread use of the technique is currently still hampered by the long (off-line) image reconstruction time.

The idea of scanning the center of the k-space more often than the peripheral lines has been taken over in another recently proposed technique: in "propeller MRA", a rotating strip of k-space passing through the center is scanned successively. A virtual k-space is reconstructed for the particular strip that was scanned during the passage of the contrast bolus by using peripheral data acquired during other strips or "positions of the propeller" (Fig. 7.12b) (PIPE 1999). Continuous radial scanning of the k-space is a similar technique that exploits the same principle.

7.5 Post-processing Techniques

Post-processing techniques may improve the results of CE MRA. Indeed, numerous problems can affect the image quality: overlap of arteries and veins, incomplete visualization of a vessel segment at

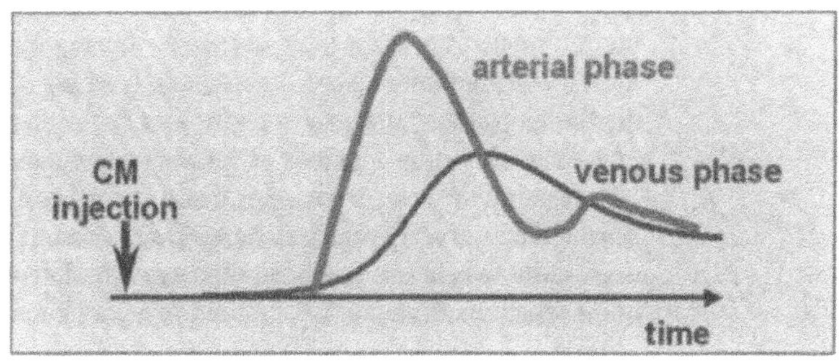

a
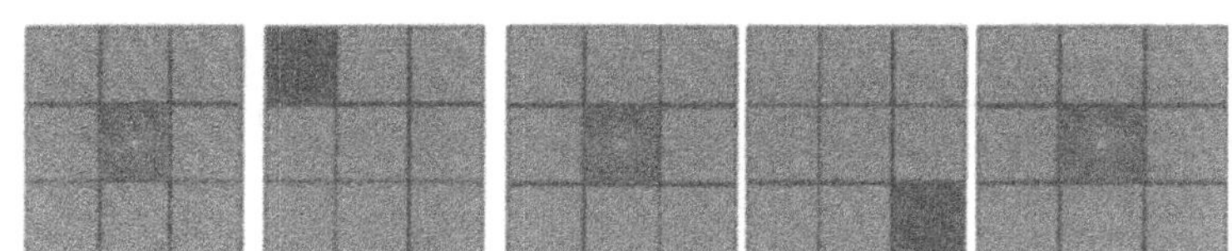

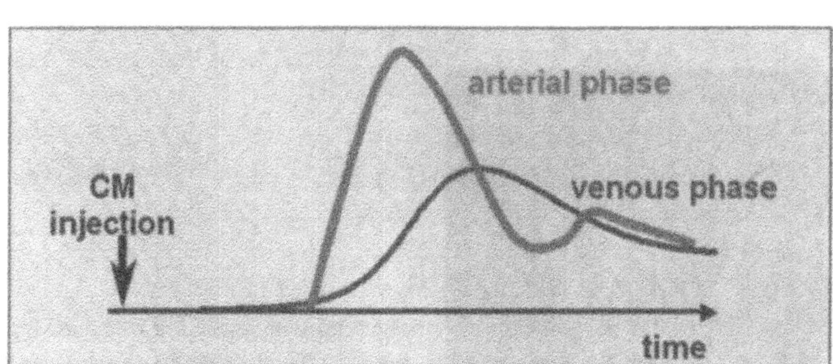

b
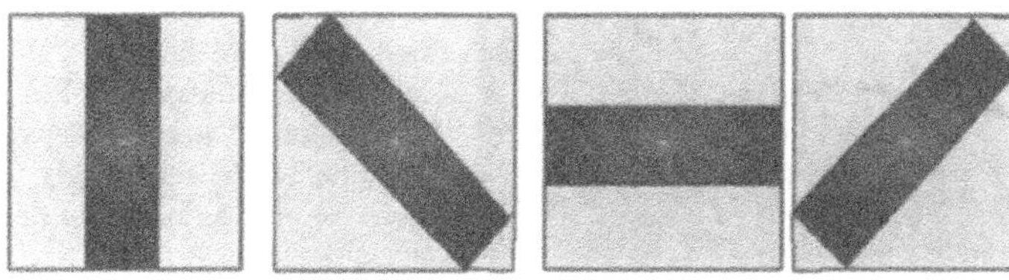

Fig. 7.12a, b. Acquisition scheme using a series of successive center of k-space samplings. **a** In TRICKS Time resolved imaging of contrast kinetics), the center of k-space is sampled very frequently, while the periphery is sparsely sampled. For the time point of interest, the center of k-space is available and the peripheral data are composed from peripheral acquisitions at other time points. **b** In "propeller MRA," rotating strips of k-space are measured. For the time point of interest, the k-space data are reconstructed from one particular central strip and the missing data from data acquired during other "propeller positions." *CM*, contrast medium

one time point, superimposition of parenchymal enhancement, and poor visualization by means of the maximum intensity projection algorithm, etc. Since a complete overview of visualization software would be beyond the scope of this chapter, we restrict our discussion to commenting on a particular approach that has recently shown promising results in the separate visualization of pulmonary arteries and veins (Schönberg et al. 1999). The post-processing technique originated from the observation that, whenever a series of ultrafast acquisitions is performed, the uptake curves of arteries and veins differ. In other words, in each pixel in a blood vessel, the signal intensity plotted as a function of the number of successive acquisitions shows whether the vessel is an artery or a vein. Using multiple boluses, this observation is further enhanced (Fig. 7.13a). The new post-processing method is based on a correlation analysis: those pixels in an image that correlate well with a defined enhancement curve are searched for. In the first run of the analysis, all pixels that correlate positively with the input function defined by an artery are retrieved. The same can be done for the veins. The technique requires that the 3D acquisition rate is fast enough and well timed. A test bolus injection is recommended to measure the arterial opacification and the venous return, and the acquisition time per slab has to be shorter than this time interval. A typical example is shown in Fig. 7.13b, c.

7.6 Summary

Ongoing research is focussing on the best possible compromise between spatial and temporal resolution in CE MRA. The following tools have been developed to accurately scan the center of k-space during the passage of the bolus: (semi-) automatic tracking of the bolus passage, ultrafast repetition of the center of k-space scanning, and post-processing techniques that separate arteries from veins based on the contrast uptake curve. In practice, the hardware and software tools which are available will strongly determine which method can be explored in a particular setting.

CM
CM
signal [a.u.]
time [s]
a

b
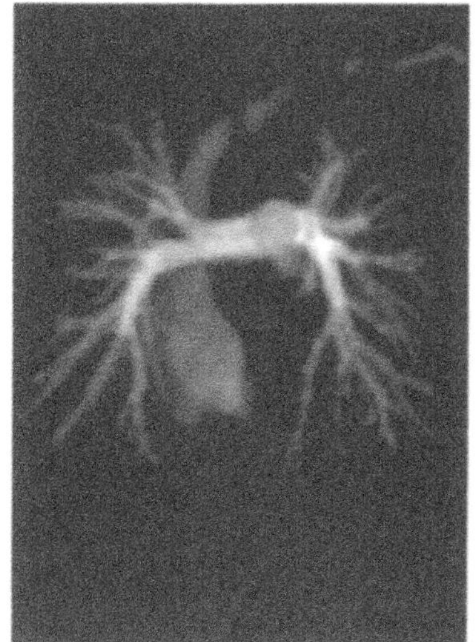

c
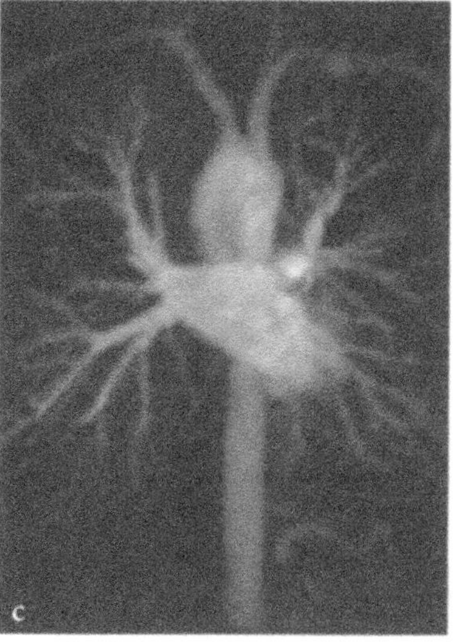

Fig. 7.13. Pulmonary MRA study using the correlation analysis. **a** Measured enhancement pattern of pulmonary arteries (*circles*) and veins (*squares*) in a series of four multiphasic acquisitions using two boluses. *CM*, contrast medium. **b** Ultrafast CE MRA study of the pulmonary arteries. **c** Separate visualization of the veins using the same series of acquisitions. (Courtesy of M. Bock, Heidelberg)

References

Korosec FR, Frayne R, Grist TM, Mistretta CA (1996) Time resolved contrast-enhanced 3D MR angiography. Magn Reson Med 36:345–351

Pipe JG (1999) Periodically rotated overlapping parallel lines with enhanced reconstruction (propeller) MRI: application to motion correction. 7th Scientific Meeting of the ISMRM, Philadelphia 22–28 May, 1999, p 242

Prince MR, Chevenert TL, Foo TK, Londy FJ, Ward JS, Maki JH (1997) Contrast-enhanced abdominal MR angiography: optimization of imaging delay time by automating the detection of contrast material arrival in the aorta. Radiology 203:109–114

Prince MR, Anzai Y, Neimattalah M, Dong Q, Rubin JM (1999a) MRA contrast bolus timing with ultrasound bubbles. J Magn Reson Imaging 10:395–403

Prince MR, Grist TM, Debatin JF (1999b) 3D contrast MR angiography, 2nd edn. Springer, Berlin Heidelberg New York

Schönberg SO, Bock M, Floemer F, Grau A, Williams DM, Laub G, Knopp M (1999) High resolution pulmonary arterio and venography using multiple bolus multiphase 3D-Gd-MRA. J Magn Reson Imaging 10:339–346

Van Hoe L, De Jaegere T, Bosmans H, Bogaert J, Oyen R, Marchal G (1999) Time-resolved MR angiography of the upper abdomen: initial clinical experience. Eur Radiol 9:418–421

8 Contrast Media in Magnetic Resonance Angiography

Georg M. Bongartz, Matthias Boos, Klaus Scheffler

CONTENTS

8.1 Substances

While native magnetic resonance (MR) angiographic images are created by the inherent signal characteristics of different tissue components, such as flowing blood and the surrounding tissue, which derive mainly from the physical properties of motion within a magnetic field or within a gradient field, contrast-enhanced (CE) MR angiography is based upon the contrast media (CM) effects on the relaxivity of blood. To date, several groups of CM exist which either shorten T1 relaxation or decrease T2 relaxation time. The most commonly applied group of CM are the gadolinium (Gd) compounds which have a strictly extracellular distribution. Their behavior within the circulation and also extravasation and renal excretion are comparable to iodinated CM in conventional radiology . The dominating T1 effect of Gd chelates facilitates bright blood MR angiography such that the previously known limitations of time-of-flight MR angiography can readily be overcome. These limitations are: loss of vascular signal along the vessel due to ongoing saturation, decreasing signal at slow flow conditions, signal voids at stenoses or bifurcations, and/or finally unacceptably long imaging times.

The basic idea is the combination of an ultrafast 3D gradient echo sequence with intravenous administration of a CM bolus in order to achieve T1 relaxation times shorter than 270 ms (T1 of fat) and optimal contrast-to-noise ratios in the vessel under investigation. In CE MR angiography the administration, dose, and injection parameters must be carefully coordinated with the measurement time and the physiological perfusion conditions in the individual patient. Thus, CE MR angiography requires individual planning for each investigation, which can hardly be standardized as some native MR angiographic techniques.

The dominating contrast of the resulting MR angiogram is acquired at the center of the k-space, usually at the halftime of the data sampling period. In order to comply with the patient's physiological condition it may not only be necessary to adjust the injection parameters but also the sequence parameters to achieve optimal contrast and results free of artifacts.

A major handicap in CE MR angiography is the correct timing of the sequence and administration of the CM with respect to selective vascular depiction. Whereas in time-of-flight MR angiography a direction-dependent vascular selectivity can be obtained by

G.M. Bongartz, MD
Department of Radiology, University Hospital, Kantonsspital, Petersgraben 4, 4031 Basel, Switzerland
M. Boos, MD
IRN - Institute of Radiology and Nuclearmedicine Ltd., Krankenhausstrasse 70, 85276 Pfaffenhofen, Germany
K. Scheffler, PhD
Radiologische Universitätsklinik Freiburg, Bildgebende und Funktionelle Medizinische Physik, Hugstetterstrasse 55, 79106 Freiburg, Germany

the implementation of spatial saturation pulses and in phase contrast MR angiography a flow-dependent selectivity is introduced by limited velocity-encoding gradients (VENCs), CE MR angiography simultaneously displays all vessels that contain a considerable amount of CM. Therefore , visualizing the arteries and veins separately is time dependent, in the sense that the contrast rendering period of a sequence must be exactly coordinated with the CM perfusion. The characteristics of human circulation make it possible to determine the point of bolus arrival whereas the endpoint of a bolus is subject to dilution and redistribution factors that cannot be calculated beforehand. Arterial selectivity is directly dependent on the speed of the acquisition: sampling of the contrast rendering part of the k-space data must be finalized prior to the CM arrival in the venous system. Venous imaging still suffers from a considerable arterial signal for the reasons mentioned above. Sophisticated postprocessing procedures must be applied to abolish that problem in the future.

8.1.1 CM – Function and Classification

8.1.1.1 Relaxivity

Unlike CM for X-ray application, MR CM do not directly influence the density or the signal of the imaging procedure but rather interact with the surrounding tissue or protons, respectively. The spins in the direct vicinity of a CM molecule such as Gd show a difference in relaxivity in both T1 and T2 relaxation times. Therefore, the direct proportionality of the signal change to the amount of CM given, as found for iodinated X-ray CM, does not apply for MR CM. They demonstrate a more indirect effect, enhancing or catalyzing the normal behavior of the tissue protons.

CM for MR imaging can be grouped according to their predominant action, i.e., , positive-enhancing or negative-enhancing. This is, of course, an inadequate and perhaps arbitrary distinction, because both effects are mostly simultaneously present to a varying extent. The dominating effect is directly linked to the concentration and to the sequence parameters.

In T1-weighted imaging, the electron interaction between a *paramagnetic* CM molecule and the surrounding protons creates a strong signal increase due to the shortening of the longitudinal relaxation processes. In T2-weighted sequences, the same CM introduces additional local field inhomogeneities with acceleration of T2 processes (dephasing). The two effects are additive and can partially be separated by dosage and by pulse sequence design. For highly concentrated positive-enhancing agents (like Gd), the T2 effects can dominate the T1 enhancement and result (paradoxically) in signal voids. For medical applications, paramagnetic T1 CM require sufficient dilution.

Susceptibility agents such as the superparamagnetic iron oxide particles (or high concentration of paramagnetic agents) demonstrate a high magnetic moment and act via T2 effects as described above.

The influence of magnetopharmaceuticals on relaxation processes are characterized by their *relaxivity* values *R1* and *R2*, respectively. R1 is reverse to the longitudinal relaxation (1/T1) whereas R2 is reverse to the transverse relaxation (1/T2). CM for MR imaging can be described according their inherent R1 and R2 values and the ratio R1/R2 is a measure of the predominance of either effect.

	R1	R2	R1/R2
Gd chelates	4.5	5.7	1.3
USPIO	22	44	2
Ferumoxida	23	100	4.3
Ferumoxsilum	3	74	25

[in $mM^{-1}+s^{-1}$] WEISSLEDER et al. 1990

8.1.1.2 Gadolinium Chelates

Gd-based magnetopharmaceuticals are currently the standard CM for MR angiography. Gd demonstrates the strongest R1 among all metal ions because of the largest number of unpaired electrons in the outer sphere. Although the substance itself is toxic, fixed chelate binding to different molecular complexes such as DTPA, DOTA or DO3 A makes it possible to administer it intravascularly. The stability of the complexes in vivo prevent the free Gd ion from being liberated.

Following intravenous administration, the CM extravasates quickly into the extracellular space; the biodistribution follows a two-compartment model, with a distribution half-life of 2.5–4 min followed by a dynamic equilibrium phase.

The plasma clearance corresponds to the values of iodinated extracellular CM, with an elimination half-time of 1.5 h. Gd chelates are excreted via passive glomerular filtration without metabolizing. Although Gd compounds are not nephrotoxic (in contrast to X-ray contrast agents), they should be eliminated by hemodialysis in patients with impaired renal function.

For MR angiography, the imaging must be optimally coordinated with the first pass of the CM prior to the equilibrium phase so as to increase the vascular CM concentration, to allow arterial-selective imaging, and to limit background enhancement.

Currently, Gd CM concentrations of 0.5 M/l are used clinically. A higher concentrated Gd-based agent has recently been introduced (1 M/l; Gadovist). Standard clinical doses vary between 0.1–0.2 mmol/kg body weight with an upper limit of 0.3 mmol/kg BW. This limitation is crucial for planning of a multi-step MR angiogram, for example, of the peripheral circulation. There is often a conflict between the optimal and the maximum dose. In these cases, the patient has to be examined at two separate dates.

Future experience may revise our concept from a CM dose related to the body weight to a fixed CM dose applied for dedicated investigations.

8.1.1.3 Blood Pool Agents

The concept of CE MR angiography based on extracellular CM harbors many problems, mainly based on the limited overall dose and the fast equilibration. If the area of investigation is large and requires several separate injections to cover the entire extent (such as in the arteries of the legs), optimally, three to four measurements with a standardized dose of 10–20 ml Gd solution are required. In cases of insufficient cooperation or of technical failure, the amount of Gd used would exceed the permitted limits.

Moreover, the imaging time in first pass CE MR angiography is limited by the rapid extravasation of the CM. To improve image resolution, it would be necessary to prolong the imaging time. This, in turn, would have to coincide with a prolongation of the CM bolus in order to achieve stable conditions during acquisition of the central part of the k-space. Although extravasation and dose limitations prevent this solution from being put to use, a purely intravascular CM would overcome the restrictions of measurement time and, thus, the restrictions of spatial resolution. With a longer data acquisition period, ECG triggering would also be possible and, hence, coronary artery MR angiography.

Optimally, a blood pool agent permits both a high-resolution approach with long acquisition windows and first-pass CE MR angiography as well as allowing for separate imaging of the arteries and veins by timing the CM administration and data acquisition. An alternative means of distinguishing the arterial from the venous vessels is based on sophisticated post-processing algorithms. Surface-rendering techniques may become necessary in order for blood pool CE MR angiography to find clinical utility. If blood pool agents for MR angiography in both applications (first pass *and* equilibrium measurement) are developed, they will certainly find a broad acceptance. They would not have to compete with extracellular agents, either in biodistribution or in price considerations. The price for MR angiography-dedicated CM can be calculated differently and, therefore, it might drop to an amount such that CE MR angiography would be cost effective even if triple doses were used.

8.1.1.3.1 Types of Blood Pool CM

Currently, three types of blood pool agents are being developed and have been partially implemented into clinical trials. The agents are:

a. Based on macromolecular bound Gd complexes
b. Ultrasmall superparamagnetic particles of iron oxide (USPIO)
c. Gd compounds with a strong but reversible affinity to human proteins such as albumin

USPIO derive from specific parenchymal imaging because the small iron particles which are covered by various coatings, for example, dextran or glycol, are incorporated into cells of the reticuloendothelial system of the liver, bone marrow, spleen, or lymphatic tissue. Here, the iron component is supplemented to the resource system of the human body whereas the coating is biodegraded.

Blood pool agents such as macromolecular-bound Gd have the disadvantage that they require a large amount of molecules for effective contrast. The binding is insufficiently protected, leading to Gd retention in various organs and contributing to the metabolism of the macromolecules (bone marrow, liver).

Gd liberation is less of a problem in those blood pool CMs that are injected as safe Gd chelates and demonstrate an affinity to human albumin. This binding is reversible, which produces a relatively fast renal excretion of the agent.

So far all blood pool agents have shown rather strong relaxivities for both R1 and R2. Therefore, first-pass applications are problematic unless the agents are diluted to relaxivities close to those of the known extracellular CM. Except for clinical trials, hardly any experience has been gained in the application of blood pool agents in humans and so the clinical importance of the new contrast concept remains to be seen in the course of the next few years.

8.2 Bolus Timing and Geometry (M. Boos)

8.2.1 Vessel Contrast and the K-Space

The vessel contrast and the resolution of CE MR angiographic images depend on the relaxivity, the intravascular concentration, the sequence parameters, and on the time adjustment of first pass to the k-space sampling of the CM. Most of the refinements addressed the issue of increasing the pulse sequence speed and finding clever ways of running through the k-space in order to achieve a perfect timing during the acquisition of the central k-lines. As we know, the quality of 3D CE MR angiography improves not only by optimizing the acquisition parameters (resolution, acquisition time) but also by increasing image contrast according to the CM application strategy.

In a measurement sequence consisting of a standard linear phase-encoding table which is mainly used, the center lines of the k-space are read at the center of the acquisition time. These center k-space lines determine the lower k-space frequencies and, therefore, define the image contrast. The spatial resolution of the resulting image is represented in the outer fields (high frequencies) of k-space.

To achieve an optimal adjustment of the i.v. contrast bolus administration to the predefined sequence parameters, the following two factors must be understood and traded against each other. First, the bolus arrival time (BAT), the transition time of CM from the site of injection to the vessel region of interest, and second, the duration and the peak level of the arterial CM plateau phase have to be evaluated. These values are influenced by the injected volume of CM, the volume of saline flush and, the injection rate (IR). In addition, the timing must be precise with respect to the k-space order (linear versus re-ordered). Sequence parameters and mechanisms of CM administrations interact in a complicated manner.

8.2.2 Bolus Timing

The low frequencies that define approx. 20% of k-space acquisition or measurement time are most crucial for vessel contrast in CE MR angiography. First, the CM must arrive in time, before the contrast-defining center lines are measured. Second, the venous return usually arrives too early, thus affecting the central portion of k-space as well, and venous overlay may distort the image to a certain extent. For improved arterial/venous differentiation it is mandatory that the venous signal be shifted far behind the acquisition of the central k-space (Fig. 8.1). Two possibilities exist for solving this problem:

- *Extremely short imaging times*, shorter than the arterial/venous interval
- *Timing the bolus* such that the arterial signal arrives in time (shortly) prior to the center k-space sampling, but the venous signal does not arrive until the center has been acquired.

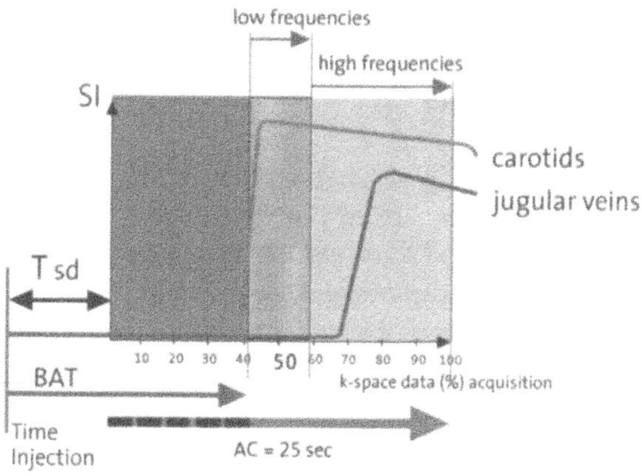

Fig. 8.1. Adjustment of data acquisition (*AC*) and first pass of contrast medium (CM). The low frequencies should be measured after arrival of CM. The overall AC time should be as short as necessary such that the venous return (CM within jugular veins) occurs after sampling of the low frequencies. T_{sd}, time scan delay; *BAT*, bolus arrival time

The second method allows for somewhat longer measurement times. Here, arterial contrast does not cover the entire k-space acquisition. It relies on the symmetry of the k-space which ensures that the low vessel contrast in the first part is dominated by the high vessel contrast during acquisition of the center and last part.

8.2.2.1
Bolus Tracking Measurement

The BAT has to be determined prior to the 3D CE MR angiographic measurement (Fig. 8.2). A test dose of 2–3 ml CM followed by 30 ml NaCl flush has to be injected intravenously through an infusion line placed in the antecubital fossa. A wrist vein will not carry CM as quickly as the injection rate, so contrast backs up in branch veins. Also, the arms can be placed up and over the head so the contrast flows downwards, which has the additional advantage of eliminating phase wrapping artifacts. After the cardiopulmonary passage, the bolus arrives at the arteries in the region of interest (ROI). Time-resolved two-dimensional (2D) imaging [2D Turbo-FLASH or ultra-fast 2D gradient echo (GE) sequence] can be used to determine the BAT. The scan delay (T_{sd}) of the subsequenced 3D CE MR angiographic image can then be calculated by the following formula (provided that a linear phase-encoding table is applied):

$$T_{sd} = BAT - \frac{MT - (10\% \cdot MT)}{2}$$

(*BAT*, bolus arrival time; *MT*, measurement time)

Using an ultra-fast 2D time-resolved GE sequence, a stack of cross-sectional, coronal, or sagittal images can be obtained of the targeted vessel (bolus tracking study) to evaluate the BAT. The 2D GE sequence must be designed as inflow and first-order flow-compensated in order to avoid intraluminal signal increasing by time-of-flight effects which can mimic the CM bolus arrival. For all CM injections a mechanical MR injector should be recommended to standardize the administration of the CM. The bolus tracking measurement and the injection of the CM have to be started simultaneously. After acquisition, the serial images of the bolus tracking measurement are evaluated to display the bolus time course. Using specialized computer software, a circular region of interest (ROI) at the site of the targeted vessel is defined interactively and the signal courve over time is displayed.

The interval between the starting point of the measurement and the point at which 80% of the maximum level is reached is calculated as the BAT (Fig. 8.1). The 80% level related to the SI_{max} can be used to calculate the bolus time length (BL), which is defined as the 80% SI_{max} duration over time based on the SI/T course. With respect to the complex dilution of CM during the first pass, depending on vessel size and localization, a bolus time dilution constant (BTDC) can be calculated as the ratio of the resulting BL and the duration of the CM injection:

$$BTDC = \frac{\textit{duration of arterial first pass}}{\textit{duration CM injection}} = \frac{BL \cdot IR}{V_{CM}}$$

(*BTDC*, bolus time dilution constant; *IR*, injection rate; V_{CM} contrast medium volume)

The BTDC value reflects the dilution of CM during the first pass of the pulmonary circulation and the proximal arteries, including vessel branches. The

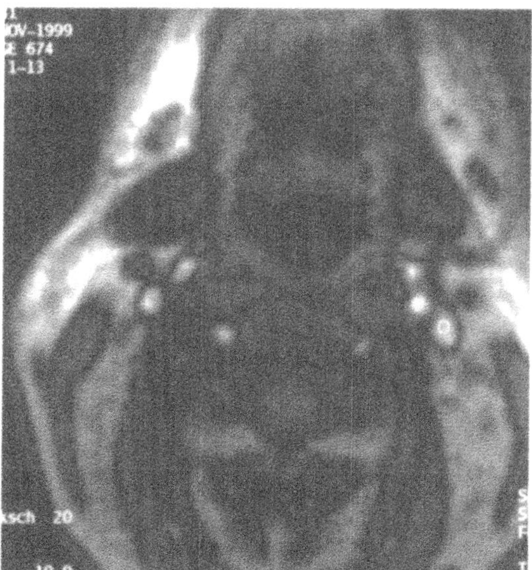

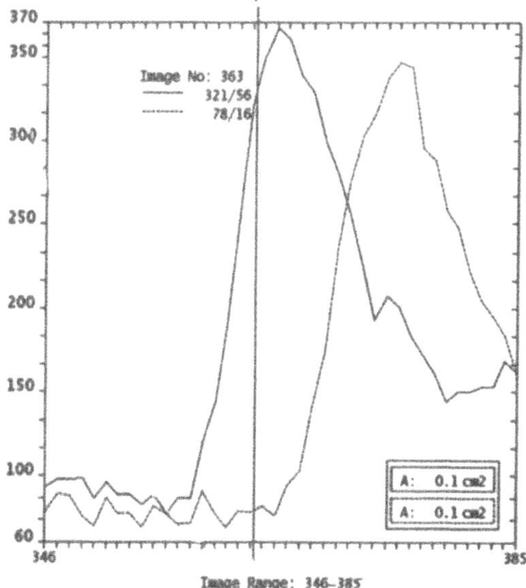

Fig. 8.2. Measurement of the bolus arrival time (BAT) using a 2D time resolved sequence (one image per second): The regions of interest were placed at the left internal carotid artery and the left jugular vein. The BAT was 18 s for the 80% maximum signal intensity level. The contrast peak for the jugular vein occurred 9 s later

BTDC is higher for more peripheral arteries (such as the tibial vessels) as that for the carotid or renal arteries. Therefore, considering CM dilution, the IR for visualization of the peripheral arteries should be higher than for the proximal arteries.

8.2.2.2
CM Administration Parameters and BAT

Another parameter that affects the SI/T course and the bolus geometry is the volume of NaCl which has to be administered for flushing the i.v. line and the cubital vein after administering the CM bolus. Several studies proved that the saline flush is of major importance. An increase in the saline flush volume (from 30 ml to 60 ml) produced an approximately 50% increase in the $BL_{80\%}$ whereas the increase in NaCl flush volume from 15 to 30 ml does not significantly affect the $BL_{80\%}$ or BAT (Fig. 8.3a). However, CM bolus injection without a NaCl flush causes a BAT delay.

In addition, the CM dosage does not affect the BAT (Fig. 8.3b). Otherwise, a decrease in the IR below

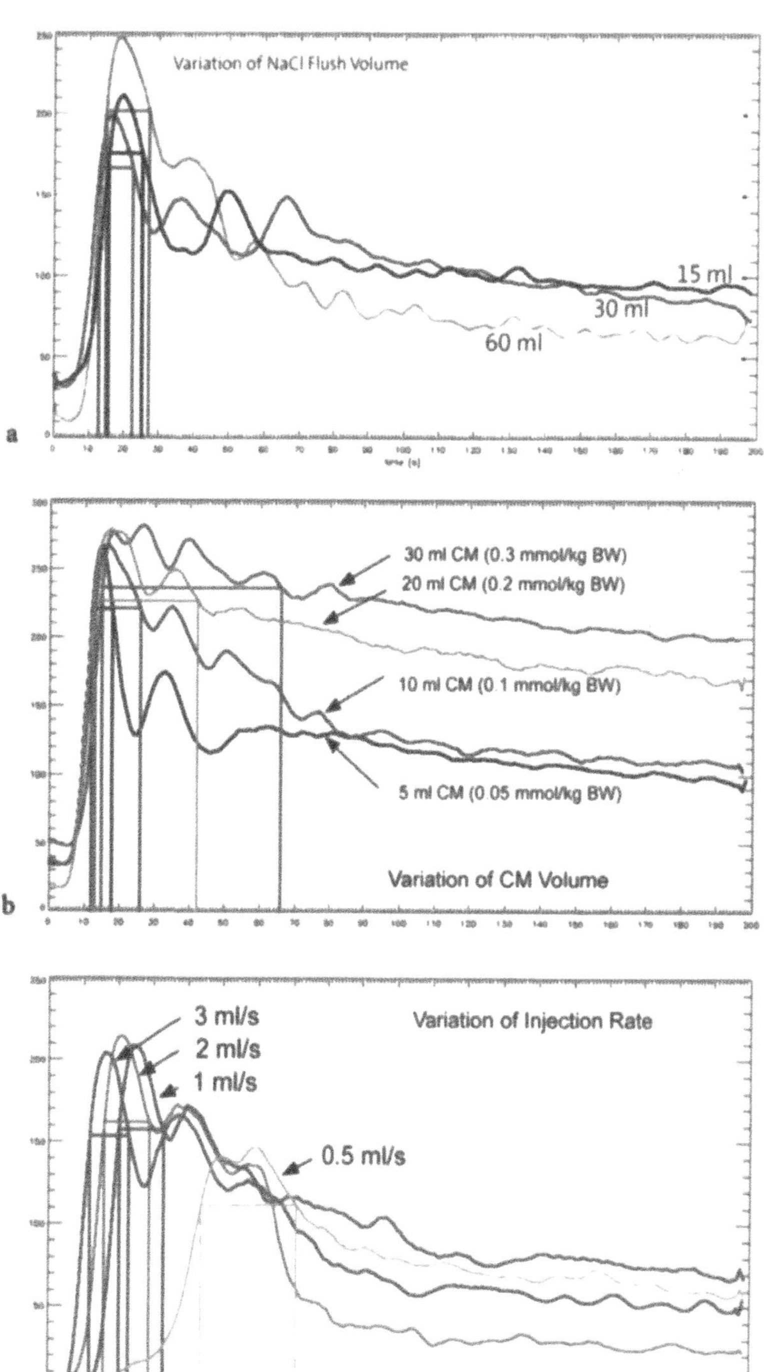

Fig. 8.3a–c. Signal intensity to time curves for different contrast medium (*CM*) administration parameter variations of one normal volunteer (injection rate, IR=3 ml/s, single dose CM: 0.1 mmol/kg Gd): **a** The NaCl flush volume was varied (15, 30, and 60 ml). A 60-ml NaCl flush caused a higher signal-to-noise ratio peak as compared with lower flush volumes. **b** The variation of CM dose (5, 10, 20 and 30 ml) shows an increase in arterial first-pass duration for higher amounts of CM volume (IR=3.0 ml/s and NaCl flush volume=50 ml remained constant). **c** The decrease of IR below 1 ml/s cause a longer arterial first-pass duration of CM at the 80% peak level as compared with higher flow rates but resulted in significantly lower peak level of the signal-to-noise ratio (single dose CM=0.1 mmol/kg Gd and NaCl flush volume=50 ml remained constant)

1.0 ml/s leads to a more than 1.5-fold delay of the bolus arrival at the vessel ROI, whereas no significant change in the BAT is found at higher IR (1–3 ml/s; see Fig. 8.3b). Therefore, an IR of higher than 1.0 ml/s is recommended because of BAT controlling problems for slower IRs.

8.2.3 Bolus Geometry and CE MR Angiographic Image Quality

8.2.3.1 Arterial CM Concentration, Signal-to-Noise Ratio, and Image Resolution

T1 shortening of the blood is related to the intravascular CM concentration. The aim is to obtain the highest CM concentration in the arteries during the acquisition of the central and second half of the k-space (as described above). The arterial contrast, therefore, relies on the distribution and concentration of CM during the acquisition of low frequencies of k-space. The concentration and the BL of CM during the first pass at the site of the vessel ROI depend on several factors and various pathophysiological parameters (distribution into peripheral vessels and interstitial tissue, blood volume, cardiac output) and also on the intravenous (i.v.) CM injection parameters (CM volume, injection rate, and NaCl flush volume). High quality CE MR angiographic images require not only high-resolution sequence parameters but also a sufficient T1 shortening in arterial blood with respect to the intravascular CM concentration. Faster measurements can be obtained at the cost of lowering the resolution by restricting the number of phase-encoding step. To increase spatial resolution more phase-encoding steps are required, hence, a longer acquisition time must be applied. It also results in a higher signal-to-noise ratio (SNR). Otherwise, it is not reasonable to define a CE MR angiography sequence with high-resolution parameters if the arterial peak concentration is too low or if the BL is shorter than the acquisition time for the relevant parts of the k-space. This will result in loss of resolution.

8.2.3.2 Vessel Contrast and CM Bolus Geometry

The bolus geometry is determined by the parameters of the i.v. bolus injection (flow rate, CM dose, and NaCl flush volume). An increase in the NaCl volume for flushing the i.v. line and the cubital vein used after CM bolus application results in a slight vessel contrast increase and a lengthening of the bolus (Fig. 8.3a). This can be explained by wash-out effects of the brachial and subclavian veins. Without a saline flush, maximum signal intensity (SI_{max}) will decrease significantly.

The bolus is physiologically diluted by the CM passage through the heart and lung, blood distribution into proximal vessel branches, and diffusion into interstitial tissue. Central CM bolus dilution effects are identical for all peripheral vessels. The CM bolus geometry is also influenced by the number of branching vessels, blood flow velocity, and caliber of the proximal vessels at the targeted peripheral vessel region. Additionally, pathological conditions in the proximal vessels may negatively affect bolus dilution and length.

The SI_{max} and the SNR_{max} both remain constant when increasing the NaCl flush volume from 15 to 30 ml. The BTDC depends on the BL when injection parameters are constant; therefore, the $BTDC_{80\%}$ increases in the same range (50%) when doubling the flush volume from 30 ml to 60 ml (Fig. 8.3a). Increasing the CM volume from a half dose to a single dose only causes a slight BL for the 80% SI_{max} level. A distinct enlargement of the BL can be found by doubling the injected CM volume. Based on the 80% SI_{max} duration, the $BL_{80\%}$ is more than twice as long in the double dose CM series than in single dose series. A further increase in the CM volume to a triple dose does not lead to a higher BL value at the 80% SI_{max} duration level (Fig. 8.3b). The vascular contrast benefits from an increase in the IR to the 2 ml/s level in all vessel regions. Faster injections will mainly shorten the bolus without exerting an effect on the resulting contrast (Fig. 8.3b).

However, regarding sequence parameters, it does not make sense to define a high-resolution matrix if the bolus is not long enough to also cover the high-frequency k-lines at the outer k-space which define the resolution of the image (see Fig. 8.4). Therefore, the bolus geometry has to be adjusted to predefined parameters to optimize the vessel contrast. Outer parts (high frequencies) of the k-space can only contribute to image quality (resolution) when they are sampled at high arterial CM concentrations. Without vascular CM, these k-lines cannot enhance the image quality and can readily be omitted. Image sharpness at the vessel contours directly depends on the presence of CM during the sampling of the peripheral k-space lines (high frequencies) (see Fig. 8.5). Optimal image quality, therefore, can be expected if CM persists throughout the entire measurement of both low (responsible for images contrast) and high frequencies (responsible for vessel sharpness and resolution) at maximal CM concentration in the vessels under investigation (Fig. 8.6).

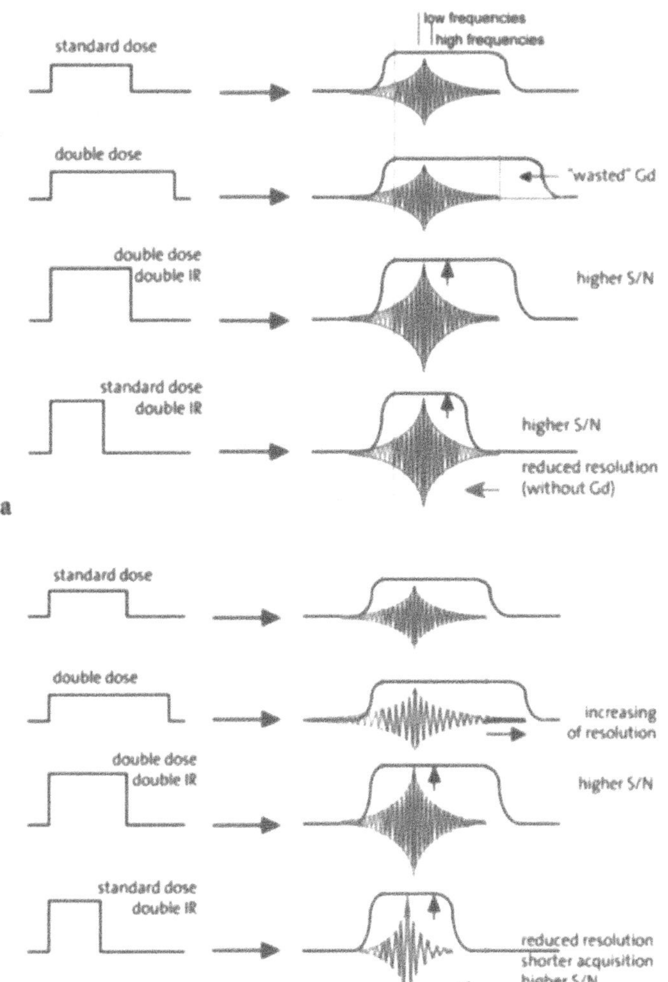

Fig. 8.4a,b. Venous contrast (CM) administration (*left*: various dosages and injection rates) and the resultant arterial bolus length (BL). Compared to the standard optimized administration, the double-dose injection leads to wasted CM (*second line*). Therefore, the injection rate (IR; **b**, *third line*) or the resolution parameter (**b**, *second line*) should be increased in order to achieve a higher signal-to-noise ratio or higher resolution, respectively. If doubling the IR for standard dose injection shorter measurements should be used (*fourth line*)

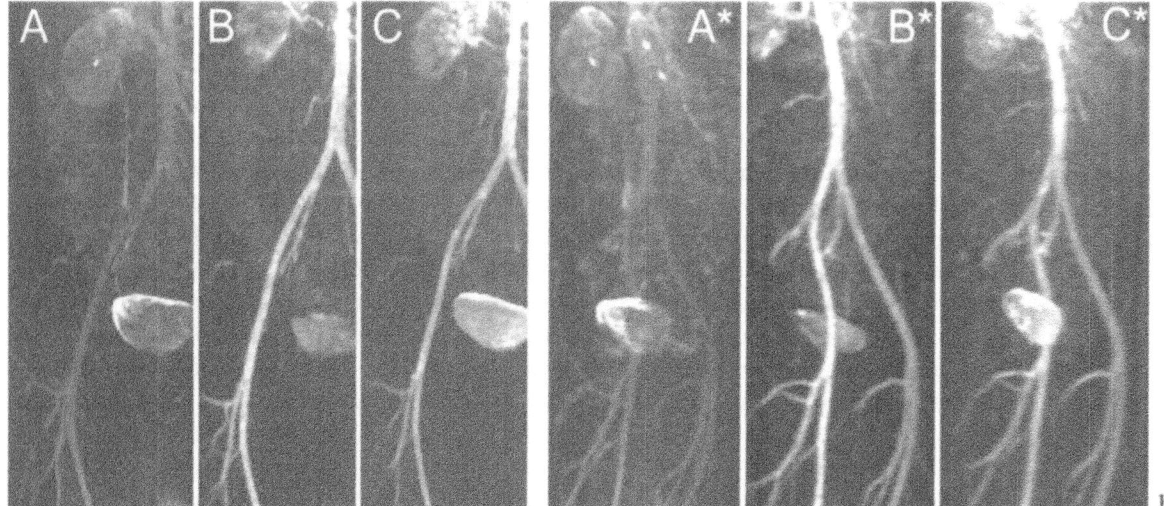

Fig. 8.5a,b. 3D CE MR angiography in a normal volunteer using 17 ml contrast medium (0.1 mmol/kg Gd, single dose) and various injection rates (IR (A: 0.5 ml/s, B: 1 ml/s, C: 2 ml/s). The 3D data sets were reconstructed in coronal (*A–C*; **a**) and 30° to sagittal (*A*–C**, **b**) projection. The signal-to-noise ratio increased using 1 or 2 ml/s IR. This effect is seen in coronal and is more pronounced in sagittal images. The blurring of vessel edges was increased by IR of 1 or 2 ml/s whereas the resolution decreased. This effect can only be observed in slice select direction (or in more sagittal projections; *A*–C**) due to loss of resolution as a result of shorter arterial bolus length

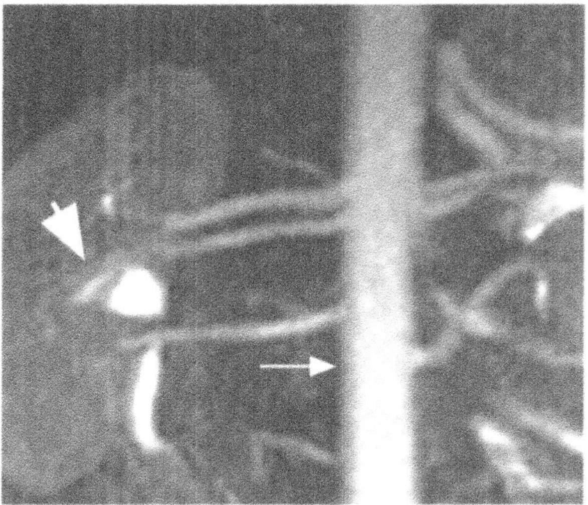
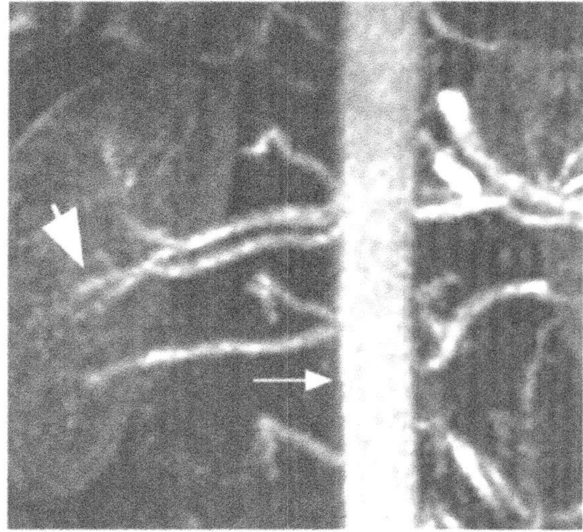

Fig. 8.6. A single- (*left*) and double- (*right*) dose 3D CE MR angiographic measurement of a patient with multiple main right renal arteries. Note the sharper delineation (*large arrows*) and the more peripheral visualization of the subsegmental arteries (*short arrows*) at the double dose images (the measurement parameters were not changed)

8.2.3.3
CE MR Angiography Optimization Strategies and Bolus Timing

The influence of varying injection parameters can be summarized as follows:

⇓ Flow rate (1–3 ml/s)	_	Bolus length ⇑ (vessel contrast ⇓)
⇑ Saline flush (NaCl volume)	_	Bolus length ⇑ (BL 80%)
⇑ Quantity of CM	_	Bolus length ⇑

In order to save CM and achieve the predefined resolution, the bolus administration parameters should be fixed individually. The measurement time and parameters have to be adjusted to each other to achieve an optimal image quality.

MR sequence Parameters
- FOV/matrix size
- Volume/partitions
- Measurement time

↔

CM application parameters
- Dosis/volume
- Flow rate
- Saline flush volume

MRA image Quality
- Selective artery visualization
- Visualization of details
- Region of interest (size)

For example, CE MR angiography can be performed in the renal arteries using single (0.1 mmol/kg) or double (0.2 mmol/kg) doses of CM injected at the same rate. By applying the same acquisition parameters for CE MR angiography sequence, the single dose CM administration results in lower resolution, less edge sharpness, and a poorer depiction of more peripheral vessels as compared to the double-dose technique if the CM single-dose bolus does not cover the entire peripheral k-lines (see Fig. 8.6). Hence, adjusting the CM administration requires shorter acquisition times for the single dose than for the double dose. With longer acquisition times more phase-encoding steps in the slice select direction can be included, resulting in higher resolution images than those obtained with shorter acquisitions.

8.2.4
CE MR Angiography – Tips and Tricks

- Use an automated mechanical injection pump to standardize CM administration
- Use a higher dosage of CM if high resolution is required (Fig. 8.7)
- Reduce the dosage for time-resolved CE MR angiography with fewer partitions (*z*-axis direction of image acquisition (Fig. 8.7)
- Reduce the IR to not below 1.0 ml/s for i.v. injection, increase it for more peripheral localization of vessels

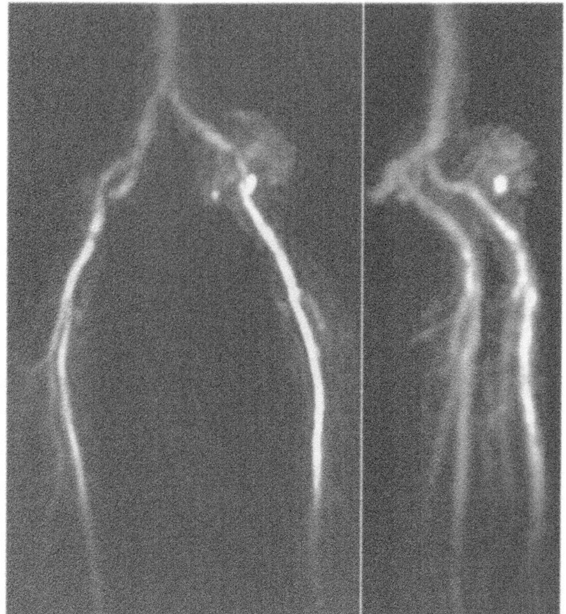

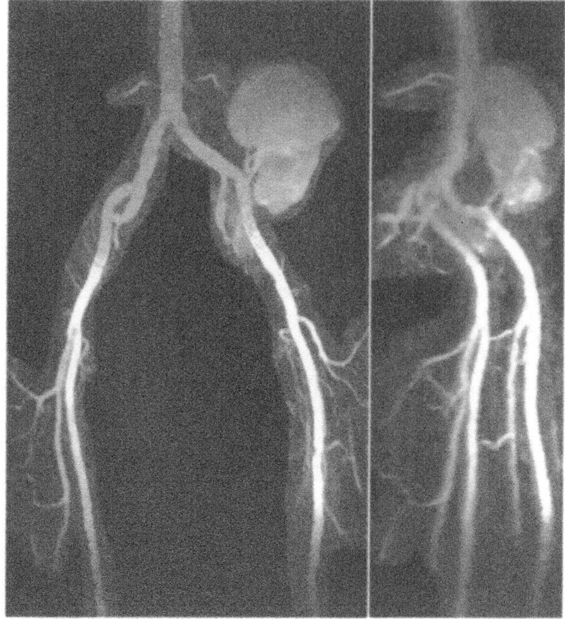

Fig. 8.7a, b. After renal transplantation this patient was submitted to the CE MR angiographic examination of the pelvic region. Comparison of two different CE MR angiographic techniques: low and high-resolution parameters. **a** Time resolved 3D CE MR angiography sequence (acquisition time=4.6 s/volume; TR=3.0 ms/TE=1 ms; 16 partitions; slice interpolation to 2.8 mm; pixel size 3.3×1.56 mm^2) was performed for evaluation of the bolus arrival time. **b** A 3D CE MR angiography was performed using high-resolution parameters (acquisition time=41 s; TR=4.6 ms/TE=1.8 ms; 512 matrix; partition thickness 1.5 mm using slice interpolation; acquisition time = 41 s). A single-dose contrast medium bolus (16 ml Gd, IR=2.0 ml/s) was administered. The resulting resolution in slice select direction (sagittal projection, *right image* **b**) is lower than expected (blurring and loss of resolution of the vessel edges) because the arterial first pass duration was too short (BL)

8.3 Dosage and Resolution (K. Scheffler)

The resolution of 3D CE-MR angiographic images is influenced by several parameters. First, it depends on the nominal resolution of the given 3D sequence. Second, it depends on the particular flow dynamics of the CM which, in general, cause a reduction in the nominal resolution. The flow dynamics or time course of CM concentration during 3D acquisition again depend on physiological parameters and on the particular administration of the CM (infusion flow rate and volume of CM). In the following sections the fundamental relations between the 3D acquisition scheme, the k-space weighting, and the resulting image degradations are discussed and examples based on numerical simulations and measurements are given.

8.3.1 Acquisition of the 3D K-Space

CE MR angiography techniques are based on 3D GE sequences. The three coordinates in the k-space are acquired sequentially using different phase-encoding steps. Usually, the k_x coordinate is scanned by the readout or frequency-encoding gradient. The k_y and k_z position is determined by the two phase-encoding gradients shown in Fig. 8.8. The actual direction of the readout and phase-encoding gradients depend on the orientation of the imaging slab. For a coronal slab orientation, the readout gradient runs from head to feet, in-plane phase encoding runs from left to right, and through-plane phase encoding from anterior to posterior.

In principle, a nearly infinite amount of different phase-encoding schemes exist with which the Ny × Nz different k-space positions ky and kz can be sampled. For a static object, i.e., an object that does not change its position or intensity during the entire acquisition process, the resulting 3D MR image will be identical for all possible phase-encoding schemes. However, in CE MR angiography the 3D image is acquired during a dynamic process of CM inflow and reflow, which, in general, produces more or less significant image artifacts.

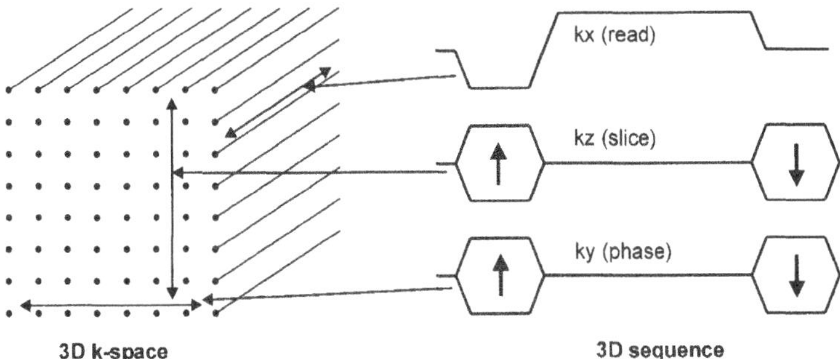

Fig. 8.8. Relation between sampling position in k-space and 3D gradient echo sequence. The read or frequency-encoding gradient moves the sampling trajectory along *kx* direction. The two phase-encoding gradients along *ky* (phase) and *kz* (slice) direction are switched on before echo acquisition and determine the sampling point in k_y-k_z direction of k-space

8.3.2 Linear, Centric, and Elliptic Phase Encoding

Most 3D sequences image the k-space in a linear order. Typically, the readout interval is placed between two nested phase-encoding loops. Both loop counters increase linearly, resulting in a row-by-row trajectory through the k_y-k_z dimensions (or left-right/anterior-posterior direction for a coronal slab orientation). The resulting sampling pattern for the two possible linear sampling schemes are shown in Fig. 8.9b, c, top row.

A second possibility is centric ordering of one or both phase loops. With regard to image artifacts induced by the dynamic passage of CM, only centric ordering of the outer loop needs to be discussed (see Fig. 8.9d). Centric ordering of the fast inner loop is typically used in combination with fat suppression.

A further example is elliptic or spiral ordering of the phase-encoding steps, which has become increasingly popular in recent years (1). Sampling starts at the center of k-space and spirals out during acquisition time. The pattern is shown in Fig. 8.9e.

As already discussed, all of these sampling strategies give identical results for static objects. For dynamic objects, each pattern presented in Fig. 8.9 generates a different artifact. This will be analyzed in the next section.

8.3.3 Blurring Artifacts Generated by the CM Passage

In a typical CE MR angiography measurement, data acquisition occurs during the first pass of CM as described in detail in Sect. 8.2.3. A typical time course of the resulting changes in signal amplitude measured in the carotid artery is shown in Fig. 8.7, Sect. 8.3.4.

The influence of venous signal enhancement on image quality was discussed in Sect. 8.2.2. The variation in the signal amplitude during k-space acquisi-

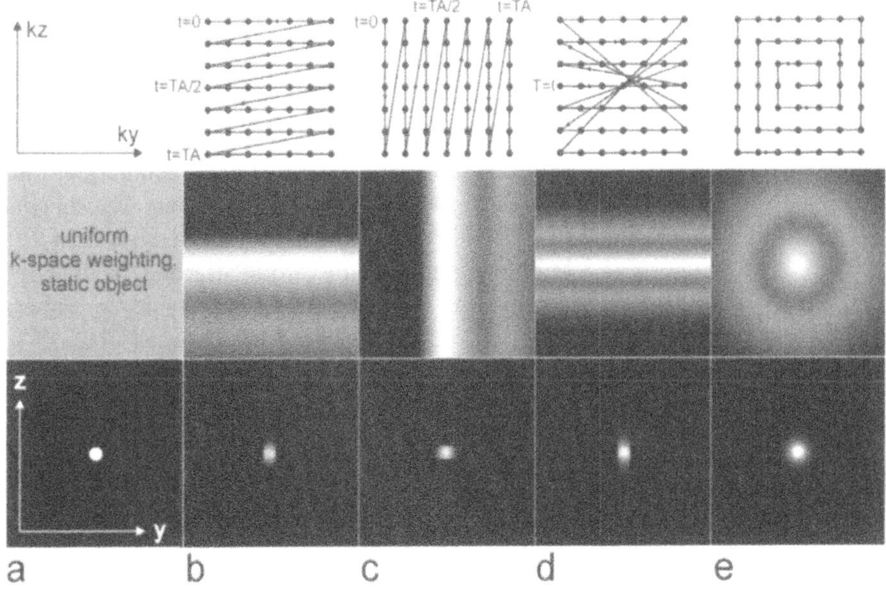

Fig. 8.9. *Top row:* linear (**b**, **c**), centric (**d**), and spiral or elliptic (**e**) sampling patterns. The k_y-k_z positions of k-space are sampled consecutively with each TR. The trajectory is indicated by *arrows*. *Middle row:* the time course of contrast medium concentration, shown in Fig. 8.10, weights the k-space along the acquisition trajectory. The resulting sampling pattern acts as a low pass filter. *Bottom row:* The cross sectional view of a vessel (**a**) is smoothed along different directions due to the filter characteristic of the corresponding k-space weighting

tion acts as a k-space filter and results in image blurring or smearing along the different directions. The weighting of k-space due to the varying CM concentration is illustrated in Fig. 8.9, middle row, in correspondence to the sampling schemes shown at the top row of Fig. 8.9. The raw data for each phase-encoding step is weighted with the actual signal intensity, the latter depending on the CM concentration. Therefore, different sampling schemes will produce different weighting patterns and thus different image artifacts. For the examples shown in Fig. 8.9, optimal timing between k-space acquisition and CM time course was assumed, i.e., the peak concentration of CM coincides with the acquisition of the central part of k-space.

For a static object or, for example, for a CE MR angiographic image measured during the constant concentration of a blood pool agent, the k-space weighting is uniform, see Fig. 8.9a. The bottom row of Fig. 8.9 shows the numerical simulation of the resulting image. In Fig. 8.9a, the disk (or the cross-sectional view of a vessel) shows no blurring artifact. For linear phase encoding. the varying signal intensity during the acquisition is distributed along the slowly increasing phase-encoding direction, i.e., along k_z for b and k_y for c. Consequently, the weighting profile along the k_z (k_y) direction corresponds to the signal time course shown in Fig. 8.10.

The resulting image degradation can be predicted by means of the convolution theorem (2). The decreasing signal intensity along the k_z (k_y) coordinate induces a blurring or smearing along the $z(y)$ direction. No loss of resolution is visible along the $y(z)$ direction, since the signal intensity along $k_y/(k_z)$ is constant. One example of this phenomenon is shown in Fig. 8.5 (Sect. 8.2.3.2).

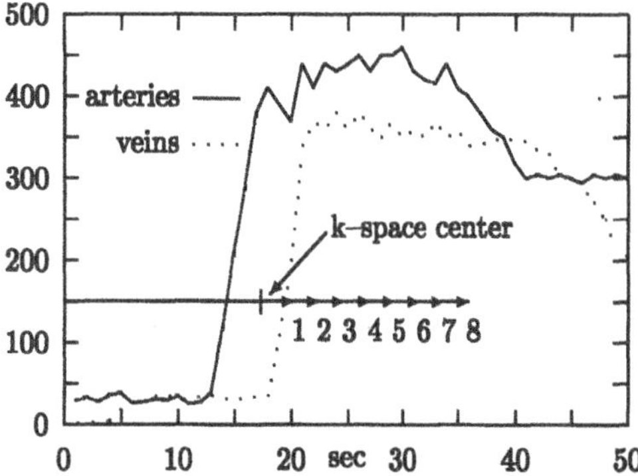

Fig. 8.10. Time course of contrast medium flow measured in the carotid artery and jugular vein. Timing of k-space acquisition with increasing longer acquisition time (and resolution) is indicated by *arrows* numbered from *1* to *8*

Centric ordering as shown in Fig. 8.9d has blurring effects similar to those for linear ordering. The corresponding image is blurred along the *z* direction, corresponding to the k_z dimension of centric ordering. For spiral/elliptical ordering the weighting of k-space exhibits a radial symmetry and the corresponding smoothing effect is thus uniform in the k_y and k_z direction (Fig. 8.9e). A detailed discussion on spatial resolution of elliptical 3D-MRA may be found in [3].

In summary, Fig. 8.9 shows that a decrease in signal intensity or CM concentration during k-space acquisition results in a loss of resolution. For linear and centric sampling schemes, the loss in resolution is along one dimension, for example, along the through-plane direction. For spiral or elliptic sampling, the loss in resolution is uniform in both phase-encoding directions.

8.3.4 The Influence of the Venous CM Return on Image Quality

The shift between arterial inflow and venous return of CM is about 7–10 s for the cerebral vasculature and increases to about 30–40 s for the peripheral vessels. Especially for the rapid cerebral circulation, precise timing between k-space acquisition and CM time course is required to adequately distinguish arteries and veins in the resulting image. As previously described, the center of k-space has to be acquired just after the arterial inflow of CM and, thus, several seconds before the venous reflow. For linear k-space sampling, this moment corresponds to t=TA/2, i.e., half of the total imaging time TA, and to t=0, i.e., start of the acquisition, for centric or spiral/elliptic sampling. The timing scheme for a linearly ordered k-space acquisition is shown in Fig. 8.10.

As a result of this timing strategy, the venous signals are acquired during the phase encoding of the outer parts of k-space. This may produce image artifacts, sometimes visible as noisy contours of the venous vessels. Figure 8.11 shows an experiment that visualizes the influence of venous signals in CE MR angiography of the carotid arteries. The linearly ordered 3D sequence starts at t=0 and continues until t=TA=36 s (see Fig. 8.10). Between t=12–19 s only arterial signals are acquired whereas between t=19–36 s both arterial and venous signals are acquired. Images 1–8 in Fig. 8.11 were reconstructed from increasingly larger subsets of the 3D raw data set in order to evaluate the impact of the high-frequency k-space data (containing both arterial and venous signals) on image quality.

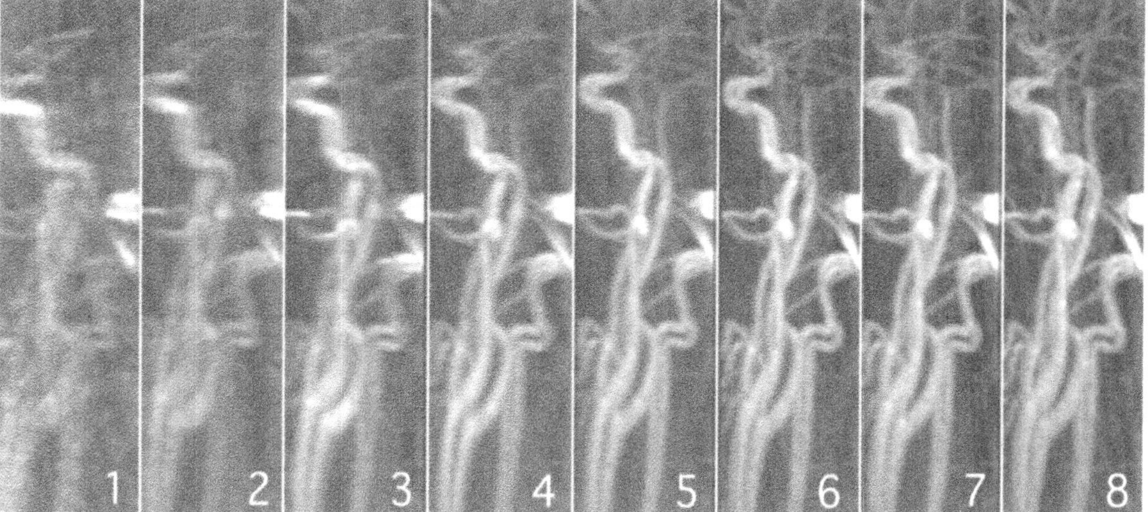

Fig. 8.11. Sagittal maximum intensity projections reconstructed from increasingly larger subsets of one 3D data set, see Fig. 8.10. Resolution increases with increasing k-space coverage without a significant increase of venous signal artifacts

As is clearly visible in Fig. 8.11 (sagittal maximum intensity projections, MIPs, left-right is the linear, outer loop through-plane phase encoding), image 8 shows the best arterial resolution and negligible venous enhancement. In summary, even in the presence of strong venous signals during acquisition of the outer parts of k-space, only minimal venous artifacts and a slight decrease in the signal-to-noise ratio are visible in the final images. The image resolution can therefore be increased by increasing the number of phase-encoding steps (and thus by increasing the total scan time TA) without generating severe venous artifacts. However, a precise timing between acquisition and CM flow is still mandatory.

References

Adam G, Neuerburg J, Spuntrup, Muhler A, Scherer K, Günther RW (1994) Dynamic contrast-enhanced MR imaging of the upper abdomen: enhancement properties of gadobutrol, gadolinium-DTPA-polylysine, and gadolinium DTPA-cascade-polymer. Magn Reson Med 32:622–628

Blomley MJ, Coulden R, Bufkin C, Lipton MJ, Dawson P (1993) Contrast bolus dynamic computed tomography for the measurement of solid organ perfusion. Invest Radiol 28(5)

Boos M, Scheffler K, Ott HW, Radu EW, Bongartz G (1997) [Conventional magnetic resonance angiography and contrast enhanced magnetic resonance angiography of extracranial blood vessel segments]. Radiologe 37:515–528

Boos M, Lentschig M, Scheffler K, Bongartz GM, Steinbrich W (1998) Contrast-enhanced magnetic resonance angiography of peripheral vessels. Different contrast agent applications and sequence strategies: a review. Invest Radiol 33:538–546

Bracewell RN (1986) The Fourier transform and its applications. McGraw-Hill

Fain SB, Riederer SJ, Bernstein MA, Huston J III (1999) Theoretical limits of spatial resolution in elliptic-centric contrast-enhanced 3D-MRA. Magn Reson Med 42:1106–1116

Foo TK, Saranathan M, Prince MR, Chenevert TL (1997) Automated detection of bolus arrival and initiation of data acquisition in fast, three-dimensional, gadolinium-enhanced MR angiography. Radiology 203:275–280

Kopka L, Vosshenrich R, Rodenwaldt J, Grabbe E (1998) Differences in injection rates on contrast-enhanced breath-hold three-dimensional MR angiography. AJR Am J Roentgenol 170:345–348

Maki JH, Prince MR, Chenevert TC (1998) Optimizing three-dimensional gadolinium-enhanced magnetic resonance angiography. Original investigation. Invest Radiol 33:528–537

Nolte-Ernsting C, Adam G, Bücker A, Berges S, Bjornerud A, Günther RW (1998) Abdominal MR angiography performed using blood pool contrast agents: comparison of a new superparamagnetic iron oxide nanoparticle and a linear gadolinium polymer. AJR Am J Roentgenol 171:107–113

Parmelee DJ, Walovitch RC, Ouellet HS, Lauffer RB (1997) Preclinical evaluation of the pharmacokinetics, biodistribution, and elimination of MS-325, a blood pool agent for MRI. Invest Radiol 32:741–747

Prince MR (1998) Contrast-enhanced MR angiography: theory and optimization. Magn Reson Imaging Clin N Am 6:257–267

Prince MR, Chenevert TL, Foo TK, Londy FJ, Ward JS, Maki JH (1997) Contrast-enhanced abdominal MR angiography: optimization of imaging delay time by automating the detection of contrast material arrival in the aorta. Radiology 203:109–114

Rofsky NM, Johnson G, Adelman MA, Rosen RJ, Krinsky GA, Weinreb JC (1997) Peripheral vascular disease evaluated with reduced-dose gadolinium-enhanced MR angiography. Radiology 205:163–169

Stillman AE, Wilke N, Li D, Haacke EM, Mc Lachlan S (1996) Ultrasmall superparamagnetic iron oxide to enhance MRA of the renal and coronary arteries: studies in human patients. J Comput Assist Tomogr 20:51–55

Van Hecke P, Marchal G, Bosmans H, et al (1991) NMR imaging study of the pharmacodynamics of polylysine-gadolinium-DTPA in the rabbit and the rat. Magn Reson Imaging 9:313–321

Vosshenrich R, Kopka L, Castillo E, Bottcher U, Graessner J, Grabbe E (1998) Electrocardiograph-triggered two-dimensional time-of-flight versus optimized contrast-enhanced three-dimensional MR angiography of the peripheral arteries. Magn Reson Imaging 16:887–892

Weissleder R, Elizondo G, Wittenberg J, Rabito CA, Bengele HH, Josephson L (1990) Ultrasmall superparamagnetic iron oxide: characterization of a new class of contrast agents for MR Imaging. Radiology 175:489–493

Wilman AH, Riederer SJ, Huston J III, Wald JT, Debbins JP (1998) Arterial phase carotid and vertebral artery imaging in 3D contrast-enhanced MR angiography by combining fluoroscopic triggering with an elliptic centric acquisition order. Magn Reson Med 40:24–35

Yucel EK, Lauffer RB (1998) Blood pool agents for MRA. Sem Intervent Radiol 15:215–222

9 Image Display Techniques

Johan Van Cleynenbreugel and Gerhard Laub

CONTENTS

9.1 Surface-Based and Volume-Based Methods

A major advantage of magnetic resonance angiography (MRA) is the ability to acquire a three-dimensional (3D) data set of the vessel tree. Any technique, be it time-of-flight (TOF) or phase contrast, is usually applied in 3D format to obtain a series of slices or a volume data set which is interpreted as a series of thin contiguous slices or partitions. One can look through such individual slices or calculate multiplanar reconstructions from interesting vessel regions. While this approach is straightforward and simple to use, it is very difficult for the observer to obtain a correct spatial perception of the vascular structure.

During the period 1990–2000, methods developed from image processing and computer graphics matured into so-called "visualization techniques". As a result, interactive real-time 3D reading of an image volume has become common practice. In particular, spatial perception of vascular structures can be readily obtained. Visualization techniques are usually classified as either surface-based or volume-based. This distinction is drawn according to the nature of postprocessing applied to the acquired images prior to display. Therefore, this matter is fairly technical. To the radiologist reading the images, differences in display results obtained by either technique may even be unnoticeable in some cases.

Surface-based methods, such as shaded surface display (SSD) or isosurface generation (e.g., based on "marching cubes," Lorensen and Kline 1987) hinge on thresholding the image volume in order to obtain a binary classification in the vascular object and background. Therefore such techniques are more appropriate for image volumes with a relatively high signal-to-noise ratio. For example, in X-ray based CT angiography, SSD is reported to be the preferred method (Kalender and Prokop 2000). In MRA imaging, contrast-enhanced MRA is a typical candidate for applying surface-based methods. An example is shown in Fig. 9.1. Additionally, this figure also demonstrates the functionalities to be expected from current image reading systems. Indeed, by representing the 3D MRA volume as a 3D scene (Van Cleynenbreugel et al. 1996), the vascular structures are useful to interactively access (re)slices at appropriate locations. For example, in a presumably stenotic region, a reslice perpendicular to the vessel's centerline can be included in the 3D scene whenever needed. In analogy to the term MPR (multiplanar reformatting), this reslicing facility is sometimes called CPR (curved planar reformatting).

Contrary to surface-based methods, volume-based methods do not require a binary decision with respect to object and background. Volume-based methods produce a 3D scene visualization by shooting rays from a given viewpoint (the center of a virtual camera) through the 3D image volume in order to simulate the physical generation of a two-dimensional (2D) projection image. Indeed, for each pixel of the latter, a ray through that pixel and the viewpoint is defined. Whenever such a ray intersects the image volume, the signal intensity values of all volume elements (voxels) along that intersection are combined to produce an intensity for the generating pixel.

Figure 9.2 shows a number of results from volume visualization of the same MRA data from the same

J. Van Cleynenbreugel, PhD
Radiology ESAT, University Hospitals K.U. Leuven, Herestraat 49, 3000 Leuven, Belgium
G. Laub, PhD
Siemens Medical Systems, 448 East Ontario Street, Suite 700, Chicago, IL 60611, USA

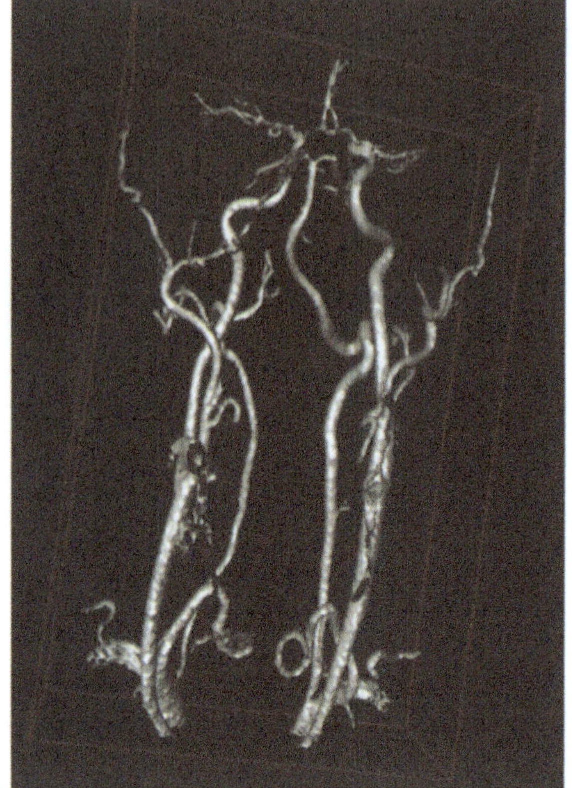

a

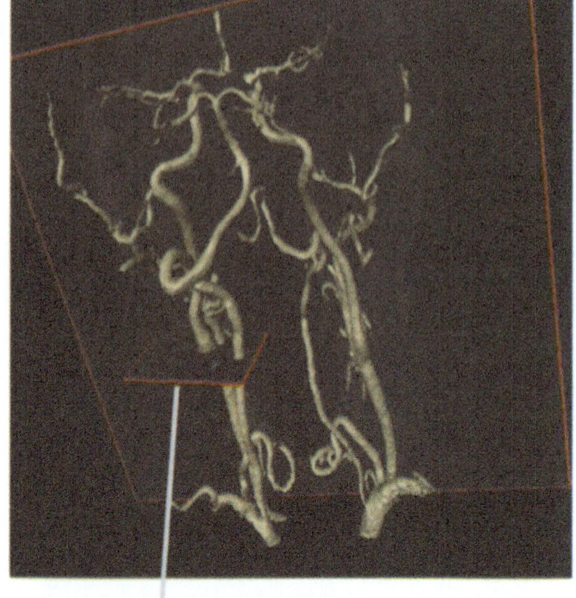

b

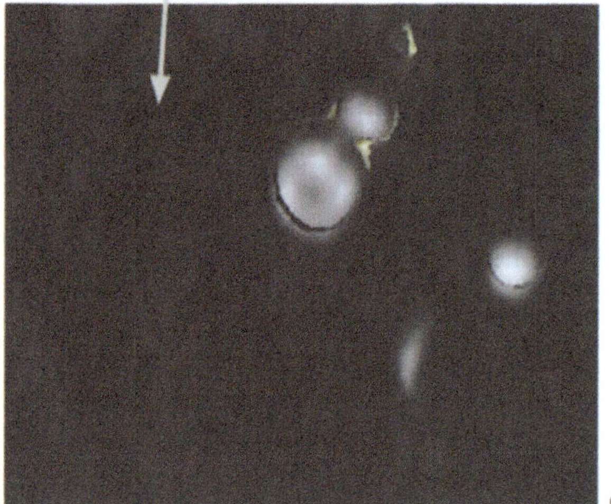

c

Fig. 9.1. Applicability of surface-based visualization of the carotid artery trees (contrast-enhanced MRA image volume, courtesy of Dr. S. Dymarkowski, Leuven). *Left*: the 3D course of the vascular structures is obtained from isosurface calculation. *Right*: additional reading capabilities are provided by interactive (re)slices of the MRA image volume in conjunction with the 3D structures. The *lower right* shows a reslice perpendicular to an artery center line as well as parts of the lumina

viewpoint but applying different methods of combining the intensity values along ray intersection voxels. One method of combination is to assign opacity values to all voxels (based on signal intensity levels) and to accumulate all such opacities along the intersection. Alternatively, the maximum intensity along the intersection can be taken. The latter method is known as maximum intensity projection (MIP).

Although conceptually simpler than surface-based methods, volume visualization requires far more online computing power. This explains why this display technique has entered clinical practice only recently, although off-line postprocessing methods have been around for a decade. Individual 2D projection images were calculated from the 3D volume image, while spatial impression was obtained by showing (preferably in cine-mode) a sequence of projective images with different projection angles (Laub 1990, Cline et al. 1991). This method is equivalent to moving the virtual camera around the image volume. Such off-line postprocessing has now been replaced by real-time rendering. The virtual camera generating 2D projections is manipulated by the reader at interactive rates. The availability of relatively cheap volume visualization hardware will only speed up this evolution (Pfister et al. 1999).

Currently, three display techniques are in use for practical reading of MRA images. First, exoscopic techniques (MIP is the best known representative) visualize the image volume as a 3D scene. Second, reformatted techniques allow planar resections to be created through the original volume data set, based on the geometry of the vasculature under investigation. Finally, by virtual endoscopy tech-

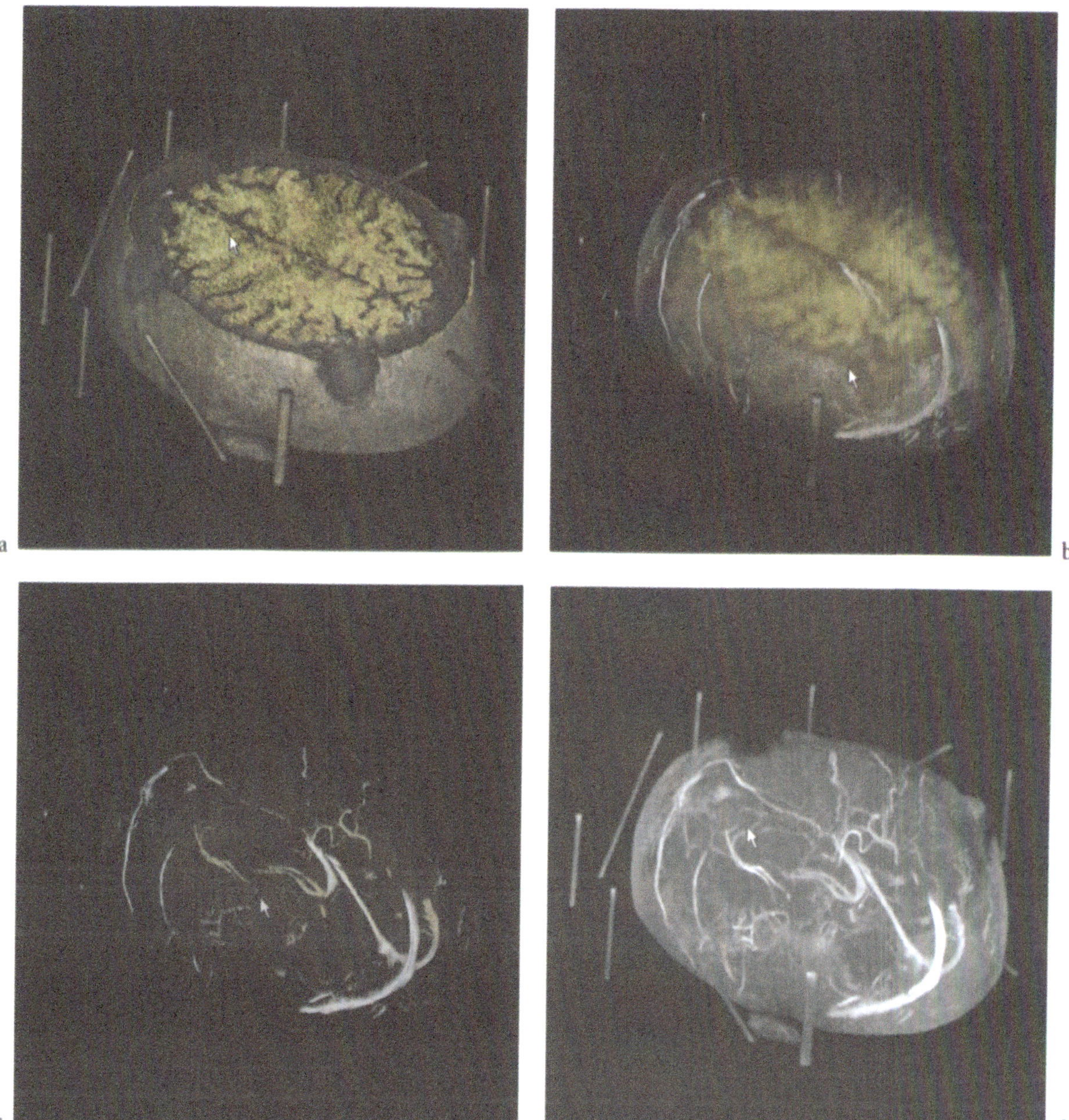

Fig. 9.2. Volume visualization of an MRA volume acquired under stereotactic conditions. Images on the *top* and *lower left* were obtained by changing opacity values assigned to individual voxels (hence to tissue response). Cerebral arteries become more and more visible. For the image in the *lower right*, the accumulated value for each ray is determined by taking the maximum intensity along the ray (MIP). Here this MIP allows a better assessment of the smaller vessels compared to opacity-based volume visualization. On the other hand background features (e.g., the localization rods) have a strong response, too

niques, interior views from vessels and bifurcations can be generated. Obviously, exoscopic views supported by appropriate image manipulation software enable easy access to the volume data for the latter two techniques. Each of the three techniques is discussed in more detail now.

9.2 Exoscopic Techniques: MIP, Volume Opacity Rendering, and Surface-based Rendering

The structures to be extracted must be associated with a characteristic range of signal intensity levels. It is primarily the signal intensity of image voxels which can be used to identify blood vessels. The MIP algorithm works well only for image volumes which provide sufficient contrast between blood vessels and stationary background. Therefore, all effort needs to be put into increasing the signal intensity of blood while reducing the signal intensity of stationary tissues.

For a MIP to be successful in MRA imaging, inflow enhancement and proper pulse sequence parameters (flip angle, pulse repetition time, and flow compensation) must ensure that the maximum intensity is associated with a blood vessel, as long as the projection ray intersects at least one. All of the other projection rays will just pick up a background pixel out of the 3D image volume. By displaying MIP projections in real-time, the impression of a continuously rotating object is generated which allows a correct 3D visualization of complex vessel anatomy.

The MIP algorithm works well as long as individual vessels in the 3D image volume have sufficient contrast with respect to any background tissue signal intensity picked up by the projection rays. In some cases, however, the contrast is not great enough, and the projection ray is assigned the signal intensity from a point which belongs to stationary background tissue instead of a vessel point. One approach for coping with this problem is to restrict the ray tracing to a subvolume of interest. In such a "targeted" MIP the contrast of smaller vessels is clearly improved as compared to the full MIP.

Figure 9.3 compares a MIP and an opacity-based volume-rendered exoscopic view of the same MRA data set. It is clear that a static MIP is not really appropriate to assess 3D information. A surface-rendered exoscopic view of this data set is depicted in Fig. 9.1.

Typically, MIP images tend to show vessels at a smaller diameter, and the grade of an existing stenosis may be exaggerated (Anderson et al. 1990). Specifically, with 3D TOF MRA some of the smaller vessels may be lost when the signal from the more peripheral vasculature is decreased as a result of saturation effects. In all suspicious cases it is recommended that the individual source image be reviewed and checked for the true signal intensity within the vessels without the superimposition of data points from any other location. This is precisely the goal of the second display technique to be discussed (Figs. 9.4 and 9.5).

Alternatively, postprocessing techniques other than thresholding have been investigated for the classification of an MRA image volume in blood vessels separated from background tissue. Examples to improve the overall vessel delineation are vessel tracking (Li et al. 1992), connected voxel algorithms (Saloner et al. 1991), and even Markov random fields (Vandermeulen et al. 1992).

These techniques make use of more sophisticated assumptions regarding the size and texture of blood vessels and operate similarly to image segmenta-

a 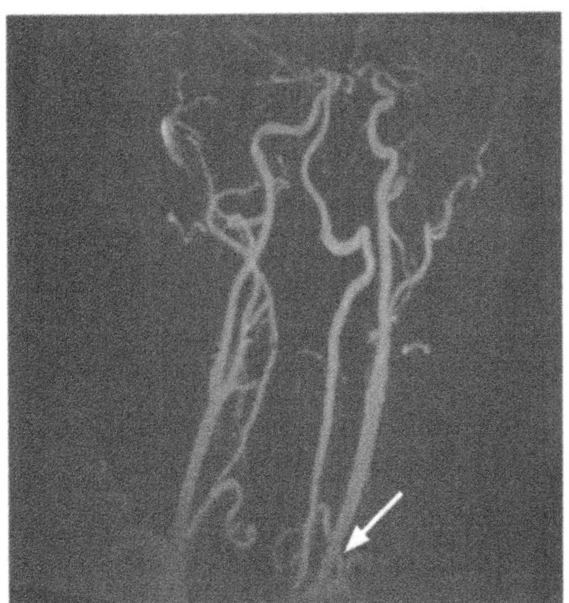

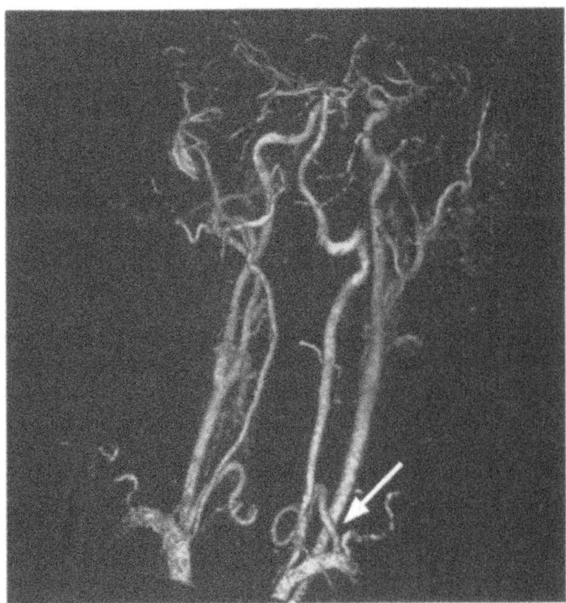 b

Fig. 9.3. Volume visualization of the same MRA image volume as in Fig. 9.1. *Left*: a maximum intensity projection (MIP); *right*: an opacity-modulated visualization. Compared to the one threshold surface-based approach, it is clear that the smaller vasculature is highlighted better by both methods. Although the MIP allows an easier reading of the peripheral vessels, a number of localization errors implicitly produced by taking the maximum intensity along a projection ray are clearly visible (*arrows*)

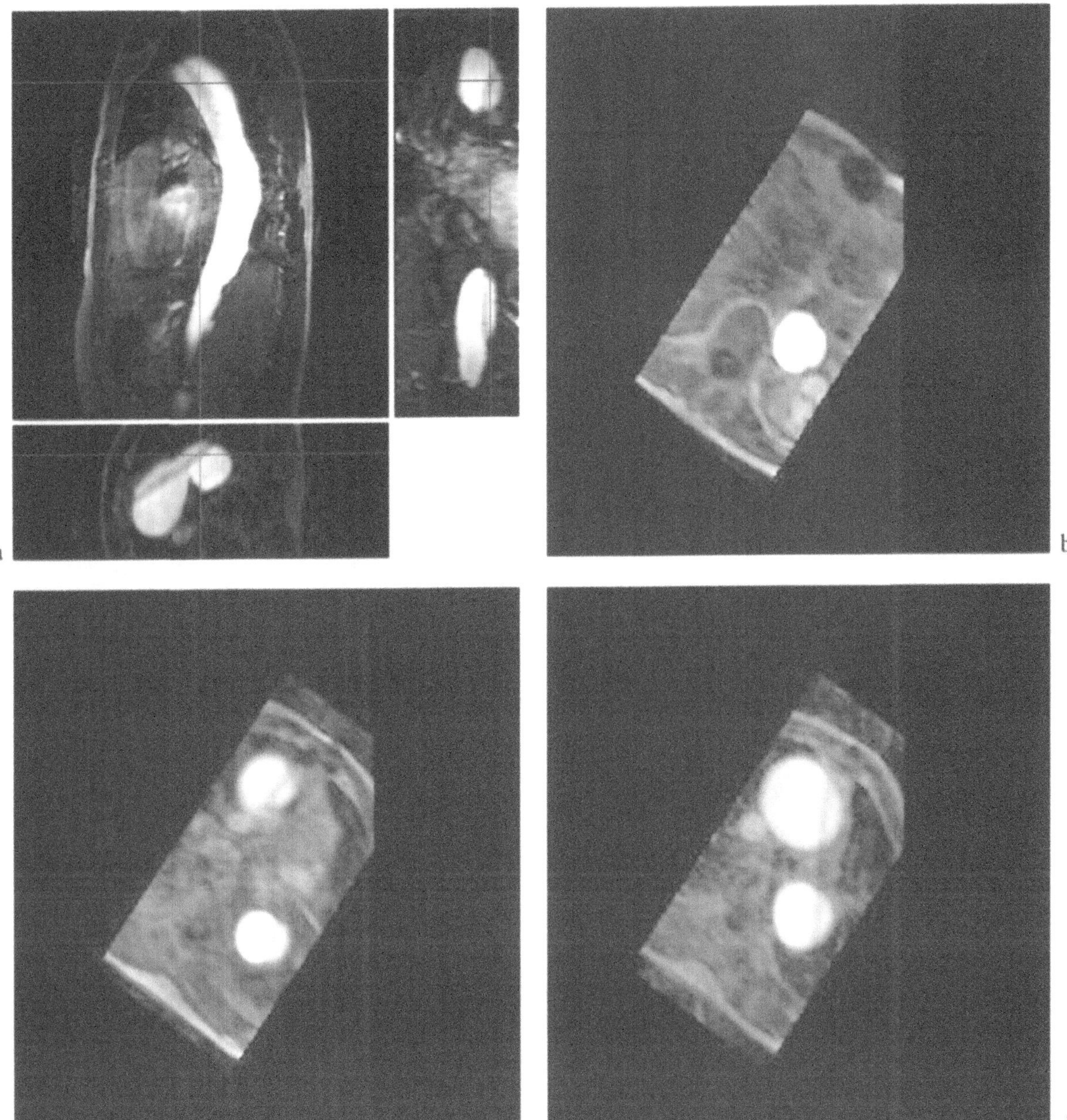

Fig. 9.4. Reformatted techniques applied to an aortic dissection MRA data set (contrast-enhanced acquisition, courtesy of Dr. S. Dymarkowski and ir. S. Boons, Leuven). The dissection affects the ascending and descending parts of the aorta. On **a**, a classic orthoviewer is shown that allows simultaneous MPR visualization along the three main orientations. However, it is difficult to follow the course of the dissection based on such orthogonal reslices only. An alternative is depicted on **b**, **c**, **d**. A 3D reformatting bounding box circumscribing the entire aorta was chosen with a base plane perpendicular to the direction of the upper descending part. A number of multiplanar reformatting images thus obtained are shown, starting distally (**b**). Assessment of the dissected wall becomes more obvious in this way

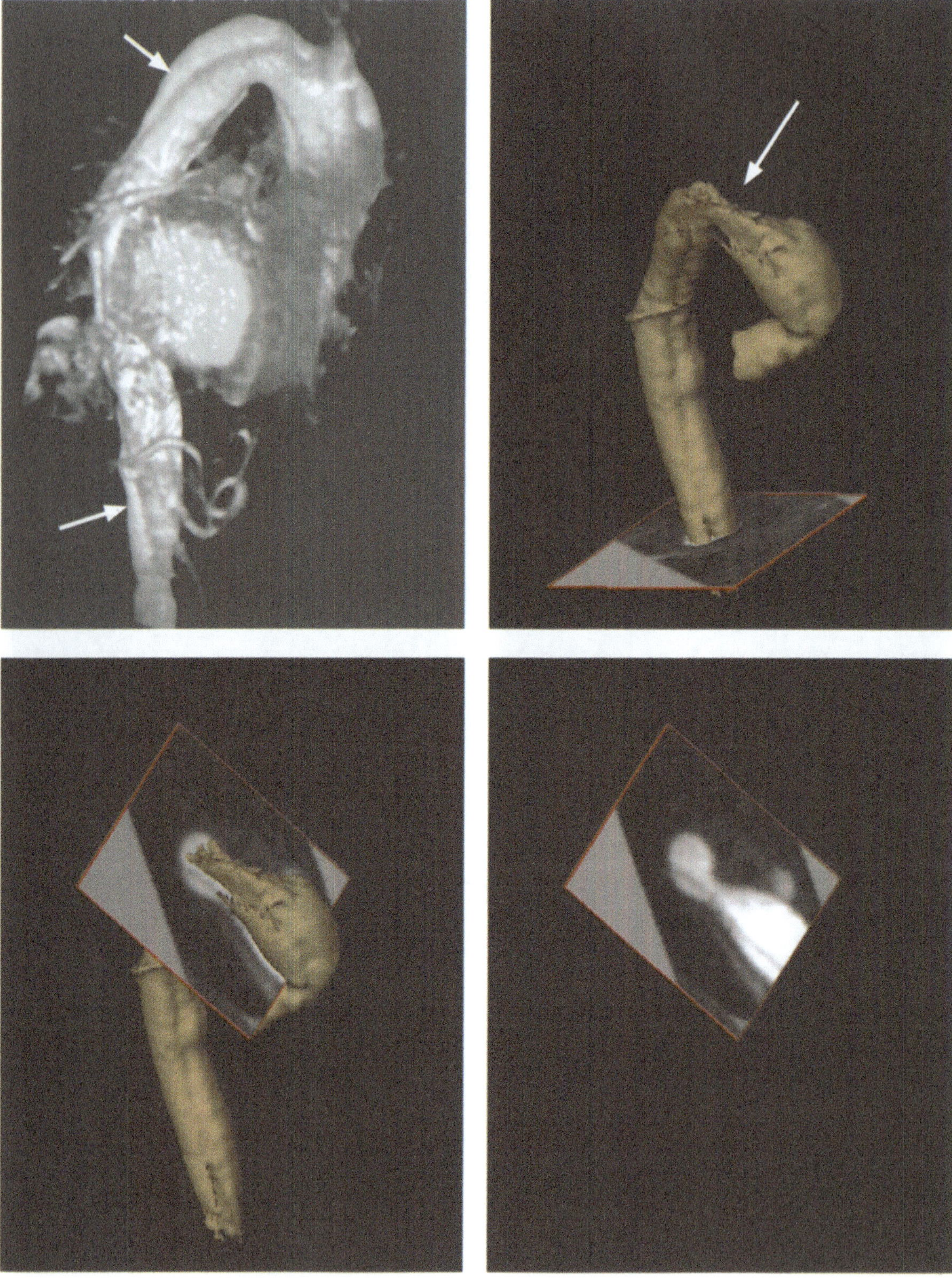

Fig. 9.5. *Top left*: an opacity-based volume rendered display of the aortic dissection MRA data set of Fig. 9.4 is shown. As pointed out, the 3D course of the dissection from the descending part through the arch into the ascending part can be adequately visualized. *Top:* Surface-based visualization of the same aorta by applying a single isosurface threshold. A large portion of the aortic arch is not visualized properly *(arrow)*. From the incomplete surface description, a guiding curve for curved planar reformatting (CPR) is calculated. *Botton*: A reslice locally perpendicular to the tangent is interactively moved along the curve. In this way the incomplete surface description of the aorta can even be exploited towards the advantage of the reader. Indeed, "suspicious" parts on it such as the aortic arch in this case, should require special attention by careful CPR reading

tion techniques. After such classification, either surface-based or volume-based methods can be used to reveal the 3D structure of the vessel anatomy. However, due to the constant improvement of MRA acquisition sequences, much of this work has become outdated. As shown, the use of contrast-enhanced MRA even allows immediate 3D surface-based visualization based on thresholding (Fig. 9.1).

9.3 Reformatted Techniques

Although 3D visualizations enhance the spatial perception of the vascular structure, none of the exoscopic views is free from artifacts. Therefore, reformatting the acquired image volume along a set of arbitrary planes will remain an important fallback option in MRA image display techniques. Actually, reformatting (or reslicing) consists of resampling the intensity values from the original measurement grid along a new grid. In this way, intensity values are assigned to the voxels of the new grid by interpolating the intensities of neighboring voxels of the original grid. A number of interpolation techniques exist. Reformatting is generally known as MPR (see Sect. 9.1). Although available for many years already, advances in computer hardware and image processing software have led to a number of different MPR appearances recently. Most of them are supported interactively in current image reading systems.

The best known occurrence of MPR involves reformatting a 3D volume data set along the three main orientations (transverse, sagittal, and coronal). This so-called orthoviewing is interactively manipulated by "cross-hair cursors" that allow two views to be updated by pointing out their intersection in a third. Figure 9.4, left, shows an example. This display method is most effective when processes with a limited spatial extent need to be assessed (e.g., a stenosis).

To cope with structures that require interpretation according to accumulating evidence over the entire acquisition volume (e.g., peripheral arteries, aortic dissection), so-called "3D reformatting" may be appropriate. In this case, the reader defines a bounding box, in 3D, enclosing the structure(s) of interest. The base plane of this box is most likely to be oblique with respect to the three main orientations. The location of the box is chosen to closely circumscribe the subvolume of interest. Then MPRs along planes parallel to the base plane are generated in order to scroll through the data set. Figure 9.4, right, shows an example.

We have already mentioned a final variation on the MPR theme, namely, C(urved)PR. Actually this is a generalization from 3D MPR, in which the "guiding line" perpendicular to the base plane of a bounding box is replaced by a true 3D curve. This curve is used as an access path into the 3D data set. While the reader "walks along" this path, reslices are generated, for example, perpendicular to the local tangent of the curve. 3D curves can be obtained most easily in the context of surface-based based descriptions of the vasculature (either manually or by medial axis transforms). Combining incomplete surface-based visualizations of the vasculature with CPR in this way might be a proper alternative to aiming for complete surface-based visualizations. Figure 9.5 illustrates this idea.

9.4 Virtual Endoscopy

The idea of using a 3D curve as an access path to image data is also prominent in a recent display technique termed "virtual endoscopy". Technically speaking, virtual endoscopy is only a specific application of surface or volume rendering. Indeed, instead of having the 3D scene virtual camera exoscopically, this camera is now submerged into the scene, hence generating endoscopic images. The 3D curve, for example, through a major artery, again needs to be delineated manually or by automated techniques. Although the virtual endoscopy techniques have been available since the late 1990s, more clinical studies are necessary to assess the value of this display technique for virtual angiography (e.g. Gobbetti et al. 1998). Figure 9.6 shows an example.

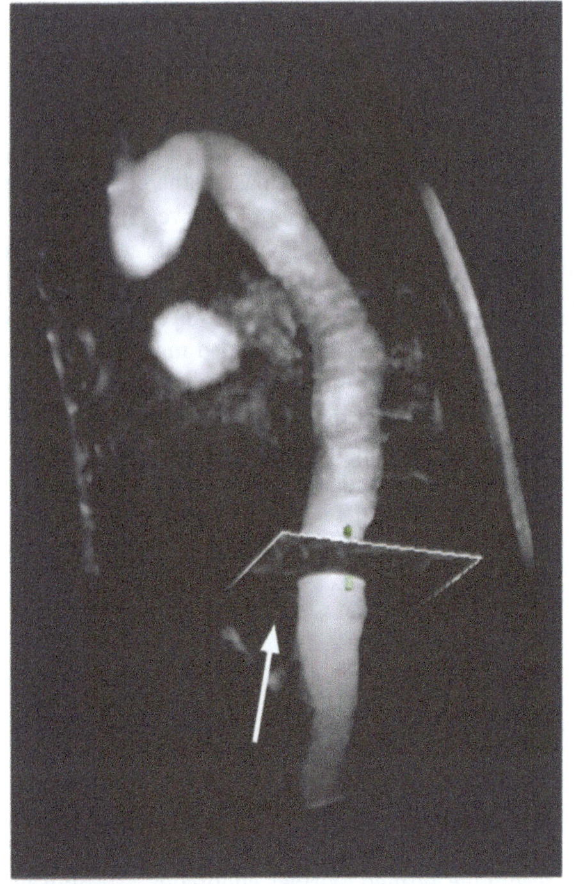
a

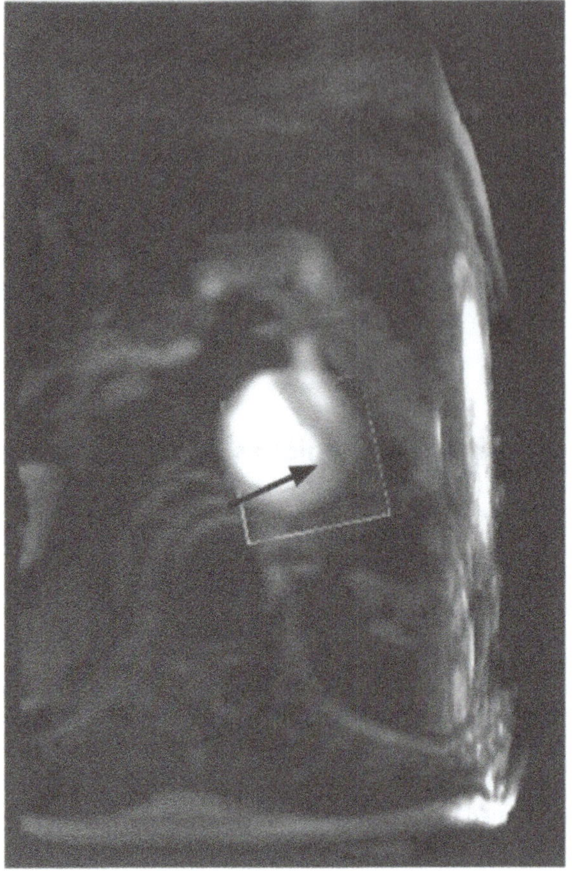
b

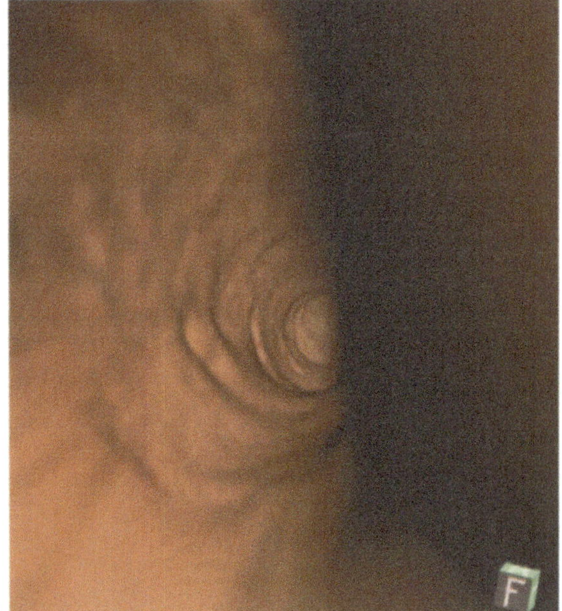
c

Fig. 9.6. Virtual endoscopy on the aortic dissection data set from Fig. 9.4. Similar to the approach in Fig. 9.5, a 3D curve is used to access the image data. However instead of using planar reslices, a virtual software camera is now flying through the aorta, in the direction pointed out on **a** (*arrow*). The descending dissection pointed out on **b**, is depicted as a huge wall on **c** (*arrow*; virtual endoscopic view courtesy of Dr. M. Thomeer, Leuven). Virtual endoscopic reading could be useful to assess the branching of thoracic and abdominal arteries with respect to the dissection

References

Anderson CM, Saloner D, Tsuruda JS, et al (1990) Artifacts in maximum-intensity-projection display of MR angiograms. AJR Am J Roentgenol 154:623–629

Cline HE, Dumoulin CL, Lorensen WE, et al (1991) Volume rendering and connectivity algorithms for MR angiography. Magn Reson Med 18:384–394

Gobbetti E, Pili P, Zorcolo A, Tuveri M (1998) Interactive virtual angioscopy. Proc IEEE Visualization, October 1998. IEEE Computer Society Press, Los Alamitos, CA, pp 435–438

Kalender WA, Prokop M (2000) 3D CT angiography. In: Udupa Jk, Herman GT (eds) 3D imaging in medicine, CRC Press, Boca Raton, 2nd edn. pp 265–283

Laub GA (1990) Display for MR angiography. Magn Reson Med 14:222–229

Li W, Haacke E, et al (1992) Automated local maximumintensity projection with three-dimensional vessel tracking. J Magn Reson Imaging 2:519–526

Lorensen WE, Cline HE (1987) Marching cubes: a high resolution 3D surface reconstruction algorithm. Computer Graphics 21:163–169

Pfister H, Hardenbergh J, Knittel J, Lauer H, Seiler L (1999) The VolumePro Real-Time Ray-Casting System Proceedings of Siggraph '99, August 1999. Addison Wesley, Los Angeles, pp 251–260

Saloner D, Hanson WA, Tsuruda JS, et al (1991) Application of a connected-voxel algorithm to MR angiographic data. J Magn Reson Imaging 1:423–430

Van Cleynenbreugel J, Verstreken K, Marchal G, Suetens P (1996) A flexible environment for image guided virtual surgery planning, VBC '96. Lecture notes in Computer Science 1131:501–510

Vandermeulen D, Delaere D, Suetens P, Bosmans H, Marchal G (1992) Local filtering and global optimisation methods for 3D magnetic resonance angiography (MRA) image enhancement. Proceedings Workshop on visualization in biomedical computing, October 13–16, 1992. Chapel Hill, North Carolina, pp 274–288

10 Quantification of Blood Flow

JÖRG F. DEBATIN

CONTENTS

10.1 Introduction

Magnetic resonance (MR) techniques can reach beyond the morphologic assessment of the cardiovascular system by allowing direct quantitative characterization of flow dynamics. Reflecting the inherent motion sensitivity of the MR imaging (MRI) experiment with regard to both amplitude and phase, two different MR techniques are available for flow measurements: one is based on the influence of motion on signal amplitude, the other on the influence of motion on signal phase. They can be combined with various gating schemes to achieve excellent temporal resolution throughout the cardiac cycle (PELC et al. 1991a). Compared to Doppler ultrasound, both techniques are less operator dependent and do not require the presence of an appropriate acoustic window.

J.F. DEBATIN, MD, MBA
Zentralinstitut für Röntgendiagnostik, Universitätsklinikum Essen, Hufelandstrasse 102, 45122 Essen, Germany

The amplitude technique exploits a time-of-flight effect. It is based on the application of a thin saturation band across the vessel of interest and tracks the flow-induced displacement of this band. This technique, referred to as bolus tracking, requires in-plane visualization of the vessel. While it has been shown to accurately measure flow velocities in the great thoracic vessels as well as the portal venous system (EDELMAN et al. 1989), the technique is handicapped by saturation phenomena, volume averaging, and insensitivity to slow flow, particularly in small vessels.

The phase technique provides velocity maps that directly determine the spatial mean velocity within each voxel across the lumen of a vessel. By analyzing the vessel of interest in cross section, it overcomes many of the limitations inherent to bolus tracking and Doppler ultrasound (PELC et al. 1991a). This is particularly true with regard to flow volume quantitation. Doppler ultrasound and MRI bolus tracking sample flow parameters only in a single plane of a vessel's cross-section. Quantitation of blood flow volume therefore requires the additional determination of the vessel's diameter as well as assumptions with regard to the actual flow pattern within the vessel being investigated. Although the characterization and classification of the frequently complex flow dynamics seen throughout the vascular system have been subject to some controversy, there is general agreement that physiologic velocity profiles usually constitute a mixture of different classic flow profiles (CARO et al. 1978). Modeling of in vivo flow is, hence, rather difficult and can potentially introduce considerable measurement error. Due to the voxel-based flow analysis inherent to MRI phase mapping, the phase contrast (PC) technique remains totally insulated from the ramifications of this discussion. Hence, accurate flow and velocity quantitation is possible throughout virtually all vascular structures with the phase-based flow mapping technique (PELC et al. 1991a).

Following technical refinements in gradient and sequence design, the phase technique has thus emerged as the method of choice for flow quantitation with MRI (HAACKE et al. 1991). This chapter will focus on the physical principles and clinical applications of this phase-based flow quantitation technique, referred to as PC flow mapping.

10.2 Technical Considerations

Despite the increasing availability of phase mapping techniques in virtually all newer MR systems, the clinical impact of MR-based flow quantitation has remained rather limited. This finding can at least partially be attributed to psychological aspects: radiologists are trained to evaluate morphology rather than function and are often fearful of numbers. A second factor has to with the technique's complexity, which provides ample possibility for operator errors to occur. Those can translate into considerable measurement errors, resulting in absurd and therefore discouraging results. Despite the investment of considerable effort to make the technique more user friendly, meaningful and accurate quantitative PC data are still predicated upon a thorough understanding of the physical principles underlying PC flow mapping and careful attention to detail in the performance of the technique.

10.2.1 Principle of Phase

Each MR image is based upon the transverse magnetization within each voxel, defined by both magnitude and direction (Fig. 10.1). The latter represents the phase of a particular spin. Phase contrast flow mapping exploits the fact that the precessing frequency of spins is dependent on the strength of the magnetic field. Spins moving through magnetic field gradients will therefore obtain a different processing frequency and thus a different phase. In fact, in the presence of a magnetic field gradient, constant velocity motion produces a change in phase (*f*) proportional to velocity (*v*):

$$f = v\,(g\,M_1) \qquad (1)$$

where M_1 is the first moment of the gradient wave form 'G(t)' evaluated at the time of the center of the echo and ' is the constant gyromagnetic ratio.

Phase information is not merely affected by velocity, but instead by many other factors such as magnetic field inhomogeneities, Eddy currents, and pulse sequence tuning. By obtaining two measurements with different velocity-induced phase shifts, an insensitivity to other sources of phase shift can be achieved, when they are subtracted from one another. This digital subtraction process is eminently important and is the reason for referring to this technique as "PC flow mapping." The two data sets with different first moments along one direction are acquired in an interleaved fashion. If two complete data sets are acquired, the difference in phase (Δf) in each voxel is:

$$\Delta f = v\,(g\,\Delta M_1) \qquad (2)$$

where ΔM_1 is the change in first moment and *v* is the velocity component traveling in the direction of ΔM_1. The moment change causes spins moving along the encoded direction to acquire a phase shift proportional to velocity (Pelc et al. 1991a). Since static structures exhibit no phase change, the subtraction eliminates undesired phase effects. Hence the resultant "PC" image merely reflects motion in the direction of ΔM_1. This concept can be generalized for the measurement of flow in any direction (Pelc et al. 1991b). For reasons of measurement accuracy it is crucial, however, that quantitative flow measurements are always performed in the slice select direction.

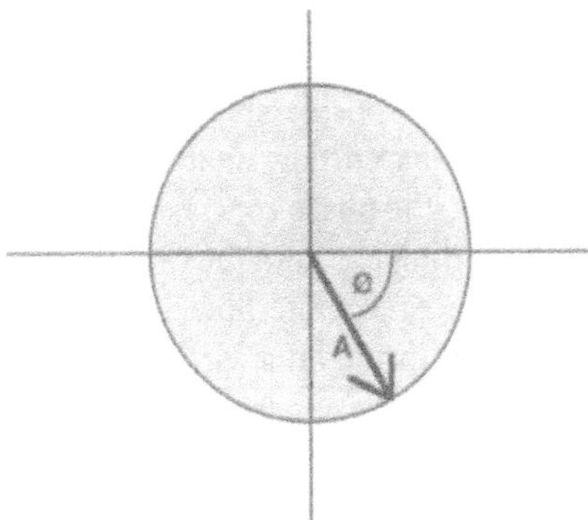

Fig. 10.1. Magnetization on the transverse plane – signal consists of an amplitude (*A*) and a direction (Ø=phase)

10.2.2 Flow Quantitation

Phase contrast images depict pixel values that are dependent only on motion in the slice select direction. By properly scaling the phase shift data, velocity images can be formed. Velocity data are expressed on a gray scale with negative values displayed dark, positive ones bright, and zero velocity as gray. By convention, flow from right to left, anterior to posterior, and superior to inferior is defined as "positive," whereas flow in the opposite direction is considered "negative." To suppress noise in regions of low signal, vascular images are frequently "magnitude masked" by multiplying the phase shift with the signal magnitude in each pixel (PELC et al. 1991a).

PC velocity measurements (cm/s) can be used directly, much like Doppler measurements. For flow that is oblique to the imaging plane, the velocity values must be corrected by cos(q), where q is the angle between the flow direction and the slice select direction. For through plane flow, the flow rate (ml/s) is defined by the product of measured flow velocity (cm/s) and pixel area (cm^2).

$$\text{velocity (cm/s)} \times \text{area (cm}^2\text{)} = \text{flow rate (ml/s)} \qquad (3)$$

The flow volume rate through any vessel can be obtained by adding up the flow rates in all pixels within the vessel lumen.

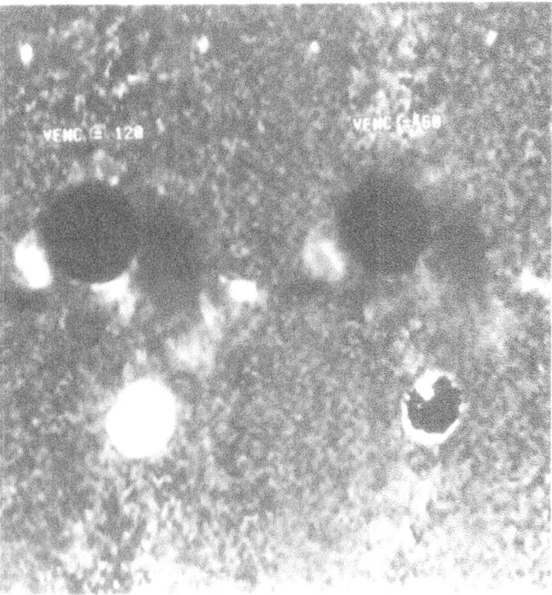

Fig. 10.2. The velocity encoding value (VENC) must be chosen appropriately to avoid aliasing. Defined as the velocity that produces a phase shift of p radians or 180°, VENC should always be chosen to exceed the expected maximal velocity within the vessel of interest

10.2.3 Flow Sensitivity Adjustment

The strength of the flow encoding gradient and hence the sensitivity of the PC technique to flow is controlled by DM_1. It can be characterized by the phase change per unit velocity and expressed as radians per centimeter per second. A more intuitive parameter is the velocity encoding value (VENC), defined as the velocity that produces a phase shift of p radians or 180°. Hence, VENC controls the dynamic range of velocities that can be measured.

Since phase is unique only over 360°, the phase shift computed from a different phase reconstruction is forced to lie in the ±180° range. Any actual phase shift outside this range is erroneously depicted by a multiple of 360°. A velocity of 1.1 VENC will hence be falsely depicted as -0.9 VENC. This phenomenon is referred to as velocity aliasing (Fig. 10.2) and must be considered analogous to spatial wrap-around artifacts in MRI. To avoid such aliasing, VENC should always be chosen to exceed the expected maximal velocity within the vessel of interest. The VENC chosen should, however, not be too high, since it is inversely proportional to the signal-to-noise ratio (SNR) in PC images (PELC et al. 1991b). Thus, EVANS et al. (1993a) suggest that VENC should be chosen to exceed the maximal expected velocity by not more than 25%.

10.2.4 Strategies for PC Synchronization

PC velocity data are temporal averages of instantaneous velocities. The degree of temporal averaging is determined by the length of the data acquisition window. For non-gated sequences, the latter is defined by the total imaging time. While this is sufficient for the quantitative characterization of constant flow found in much of the venous system, pulsatile arterial flow requires measurements at multiple points along the cardiac cycle. This can be achieved by combining the PC technique with various forms of cardiac gating.

Cine-PC imaging combines phase-modulation with gradient echo cine-imaging. Pulse repetition is independent of the ECG signal, which is monitored and used to increment the spatial phase encoding at the beginning of each cardiac cycle retrospectively. For a single section and a single flow encoding direction, two sequences with alternating first moments are interleaved during each cardiac cycle, yielding a two-dimensional velocity map in a vascular cross section. The temporal resolution is defined by twice the length of the repetition time (PELC et al. 1991b).

The number of cine-PC frames which can be obtained within a cardiac cycle is inversely proportional to the length of the repetition time and the subject's heart rate (PELC et al. 1991b). The data acquired in any one cardiac cycle can, however, be interpolated to the desired number of *n* frames (usually 16) regardless of the actual number of acquired phases. The total cine-PC scan time is determined by the product of desired phase encoding steps (128–256) and the length of the cardiac cycle.

To permit breath-held data acquisitions, the PC technique has been implemented in segmented k-space acquisitions (DEBATIN et al. 1994; FREDRICKSON and PELC 1994). These techniques use very short repetition times of around 8–10 ms. Several "bundled" phase encoding steps (views per segment) are acquired in rapid succession within each cardiac cycle. Since the bundled views in a single segment contribute to the reconstruction of the same phase image, the data acquisition time can be reduced by a factor corresponding to the number of views per segment (generally 4–8), without any sacrifice in spatial resolution. Compared to the retrospectively gated, slower cine-PC technique, segmented PC acquisitions have several disadvantages. Despite the use of very short TRs, the temporal resolution is sufficient only to collect between four and 12 quantitative data points throughout a cardiac cycle. The number of data points can be somewhat improved by employing "view-sharing," whereby new images are reconstructed based upon equal amounts of data from two neighboring images (FOO et al. 1993). The actual temporal resolution (i.e., data acquisition time for an individual image), however, remains unaffected. To improve temporal resolution and still permit data collection in apnea, ultrafast data acquisition strategies (DEBATIN et al. 1995a) can be employed. Using a multi-shot echo planar technique, flow could be accurately quantitated in vitro as well as in vivo (DEBATIN et al. 1995b, c). The technique provided as many as 20 phase images within a single cardiac cycle in a single breath-hold lasting merely 9 s. For quantitating flow in smaller vessels, the technique is still handicapped, however, by poor spatial resolution and pulsatility artifacts.

10.2.5 Flow Averaging Effects

Both temporal and spatial data averaging may adversely impact PC measurement accuracy. The number of data points necessary to properly characterize a flow profile is dependent on the degree of pulsatility. Flow volume measurements without sufficient temporal resolution may contain errors. These errors are unpredictable and may over- or underestimate true flow. Temporal resolution should therefore always be maximized, providing at least 16 to 20 phases for flow quantification in highly pulsatile vessels such as the aorta or superior mesenteric artery. To maximize temporal resolution, flow quantification should be limited to through-plane flow, encoded in a single direction in a single imaging location.

Spatial averaging effects are somewhat less intuitive. Intravoxel partial voluming occurs along the periphery of a vessel within voxels containing both static and flowing spins. Due to flow enhancement, the signal intensity of moving spins exceeds the signal intensity of static spins. For moving spins, the total signal intensity fraction is thus far greater than the pixel volume fraction. This results in an overestimation of true flow. The degree of error is directly proportional to the number of such peripherally located voxels relative to the total number of voxels containing flowing spins. Hence, the effect increases proportionally with increases of vessel angulation, slice thickness, or voxel size (PELC et al. 1991a).

Another form of spatial averaging occurs in vessels subject to motion perpendicular to their flow direction (DEBATIN et al. 1994). This applies particularly to the quantitative analysis of intraabdominal vessels such as the portal vein and renal arteries. Motion causes blurring of the target vessel, resulting in overestimation of the actual vessel size (Fig. 10.3). Around the vessel's periphery a number of voxels contain flowing and static spins for varying degrees of time. This, too, causes overestimation of the flow rate, the extent of which is dependent on the degree of motion relative to the vessel size (DEBATIN et al. 1994).

10.2.6 Optimal Quantitative Analysis

In order to maximize the accuracy of quantitative PC flow mapping analysis, a number of ground rules apply.

a. Repetition time (TR): the shortest possible repetition time should be chosen (20–40 ms) to assure maximal temporal resolution
b. Echo time (TE): the shortest possible echo time should be chosen to minimize dephasing artifacts (5–10 ms)
c. Flip angle: a flip angle of 30–45° renders a good intravascular signal, while preserving a sufficient signal in the stationary tissue does not exacerbate intravoxel partial volume effects. A smaller flip angle should be chosen for ultrafast turbo gradient PC sequences

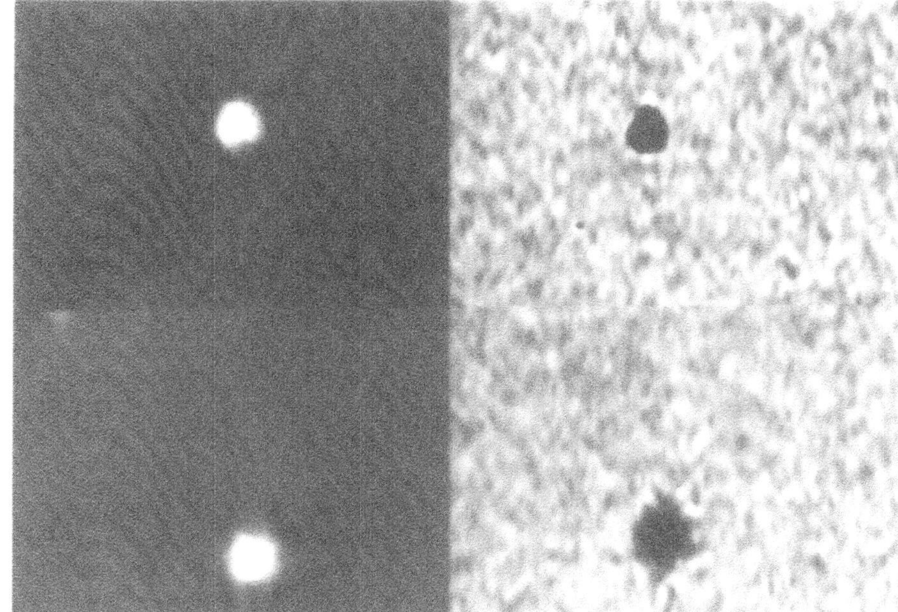

Fig. 10.3. Amplitude (*left*) and corresponding phase image (*right*) of a flow phantom acquired with (*top*) and without (*bottom*) simulated respiratory motion. Motion induces blurring of the vessel margin, which results in an artifactual increase of vessel size

d. Imaging plane: to maximize measurement accuracy and precision, vessels should be imaged perpendicular to their course. To assure an optimal PC imaging plane perpendicular to the vessel of interest, double oblique localizing strategies are imperative
e. Sectional thickness: to limit partial voluming, the sectional thickness chosen should be as thin as possible, while maintaining adequate SNR. A thickness of 3–6 mm is recommended
f. In-plane resolution: field of view and matrix should be chosen to assure a minimum of 12–16 pixels within the lumen of the vessel of interest
g. Temporal resolution: temporal resolution should be maximized by only mapping through-plane flow and encoding in a single direction
h. VENC: VENC should be chosen to exceed the maximum expected flow velocity by 25%. The values summarized below should be viewed as guidelines:
i. Frequency encoding direction: the frequency encoding direction should be chosen so as to avoid signal contamination in the vessel of interest of pulsatility artifacts
j. Saturation bands: phase artifacts from surrounding pulsatile structures may be reduced by the placement of spatial presaturation bands. These bands should be placed carefully to avoid inadvertent saturation of inflowing spins into the vessel of interest
k. Data acquisition strategy: fast data acquisition strategies, permitting data acquisition within a single breath-hold should be chosen to quantitate flow in vessels subject to respiratory motion. The associated reduction in temporal resolution is more than offset by the avoidance of respiration induced spatial partial voluming effects
l. Flow data analysis: flow data analysis needs to be performed carefully. To reduce noise, the measurement ROI should be defined carefully to only include the vessel volume. These definitions should be performed separately for each frame on the magnitude images, using a threshold approach based on the maximal intravascular signal intensity. While the correct threshold value depends on a variety of factors, including vessel size, velocity profile, and signal intensity of the surrounding tissues, it ranges between 30% and 50% of the maximal intraluminal signal intensity for most vascular structures

10.3 Clinical Applications

The number of clinical applications for quantitative PC imaging has been growing. The ensuing discussion will be limited to representative examples and must by no means be considered comprehensive.

10.3.1 Cerebrovascular System

In the nondiseased state, the majority of the clinically important arteries of the head and neck are characterized by a laminar flow profile and are only mildly pulsatile. These favorable conditions make them ideally suited for quantitative PC flow mapping (Fig. 10.4), complementing the already well established vascular MRI methods. In contrast to other quantitative techniques, such as stable xenon computed tomography, single photon emission tomography, and positron emission tomography, which yield total or regional cerebral blood flow (Fazekes et al. 1988), the PC technique allows for the assessment of individual vessels. Localized disease can thus be detected. Furthermore, it allows for the comprehensive evaluation of patients with subclavian steal syndrome. In addition to quantifying the degree of subclavian steal, PC flow mapping can assess the efficacy of vascular reconstructive surgery.

PC flow analysis has considerable potential in the evaluation of flow-restrictive extracranial lesions and also intracranial lesions. Beyond distinguishing the two, PC flow analysis may help determine the degree of flow compromise and might by used to evaluate the progression or stability of disease.

With regard to vascular malformations, potential goals of PC flow analysis include the identification of typical hemodynamics and the assessment of therapeutic interventions. Marks et al. (1992) noted carotid arterial flow to be increased bilaterally in 16 patients with large AVNs. Following embolization of the AVNs, repeat flow analyses revealed considerable reductions in total cerebral blood flow (Marks et al. 1992).

PC techniques have also been used to measure flow in the sagittal sinus (Jordan et al. 1992). By using a combination of MRA and PC flow analysis techniques, it may be possible to determine the degree of venous compromise and to evaluate the flow rate through the affected venous channel.

10.3.2 Cardiac Applications

10.3.2.1 Overall Cardiac Function

PC MRI provides an ideal means for the quantitative assessment of cardiac function through flow volume measurements of the ascending aorta (left ventricular function) or the main pulmonary artery (right ventricular function), corresponding to cardiac output (Fig. 10.5). The imaging plane (perpendicular to the vessel) and VENC (150 cm/s in the aorta; 60 cm/s in the pulmonary artery) must be chosen carefully. PC-based velocity and flow volume determinations have been found to be highly accurate (Evans et al. 1993b). To avoid dephasing artifacts, the measurement plane in the ascending aorta must be somewhat distal to the valve plane. Coronary flow is thus not accounted for, resulting in a slight underestimation of true aortic flow (Evans et al. 1993b).

10.3.2.2 Valvular Heart Disease

Valvular heart disease, including aortic regurgitation, has been studied extensively using the PC technique (Dulce et al. 1992; Honda et al. 1993). The amount of antegrade and retrograde flow in the ascending aorta can be quantified with PC flow analysis (Fig. 10.5). Retrograde diastolic flow in the aorta represents a combination of normal regurgitant coronary flow, estimated at between 2% and 6% of cardiac output (Dulce et al. 1992), and blood escaping retrograde into the left ventricle through the aortic valve (Honda et al. 1993). Patients with aortic insufficiency will have increased retrograde flow during diastole regardless of whether the aortic regurgitation is isolated or part of a complex multivalvular disease process.

In patients with severe mitral valve insufficiency (Mohiaddin et al. 1991) the PC flow profile across the mitral valve is altered. Instead of the normal biphasic antegrade flow, these patients have reverse flow in the pulmonary veins during systole (Mohiaddin et al. 1991).

Flow patterns in patients with valvular stenosis contain higher-order-motion terms causing complex flow in and distal to the area of stenosis (Sondergaard et al. 1992). Peak systolic jet velocities of up to 5.6 m/s and 2.4 m/s have been seen in patients with aortic and mitral stenosis, respectively (Eichenberger et al. 1993). By aligning a short-axis PC imaging plane perpendicular to the aortic jet within 1 cm of the aortic valve, one investigating group reports encouraging results with regard to quantification of aortic flow (Eichenberger et al. 1993). The initial VENC was set at 500 cm/s and adjusted upwards if aliasing occurred. Based on PC-measured maximum instantaneous aortic jet velocities, pressure gradients can be calculated by using the simplified Bernoulli equation. PC-based gradient determinations correlated closely with Doppler and cardiac catheterization measurements, both in normal subjects and patients with aortic stenosis (Eichenberger et al. 1993).

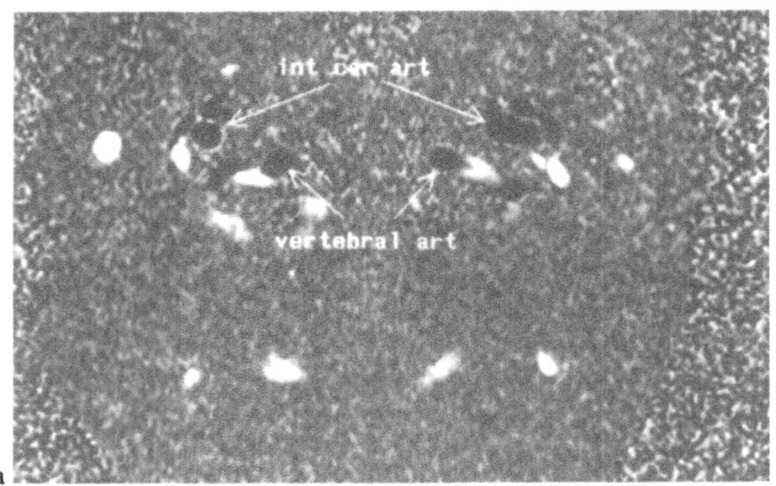

a

FLOW PLOT Legend: b F4 avg
a F3 avg

ml/min
Trigger Delay (msec)

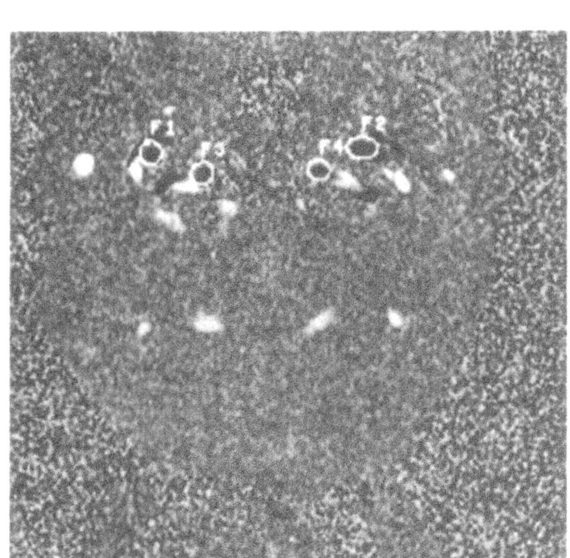

Flow Rate / Cycle (ml/min)

	F3	F4
b Avg:	−101.4	−122.3

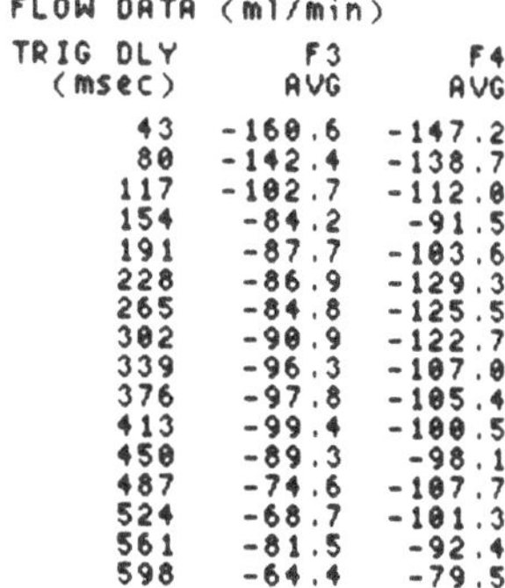

FLOW DATA (ml/min)

TRIG DLY (msec)	F3 AVG	F4 AVG
43	-160.6	-147.2
80	-142.4	-138.7
117	-102.7	-112.0
154	-84.2	-91.5
191	-87.7	-103.6
228	-86.9	-129.3
265	-84.8	-125.5
302	-90.9	-122.7
339	-96.3	-107.0
376	-97.8	-105.4
413	-99.4	-100.5
450	-89.3	-98.1
487	-74.6	-107.7
524	-68.7	-101.3
561	-81.5	-92.4
598	-64.4	-79.5

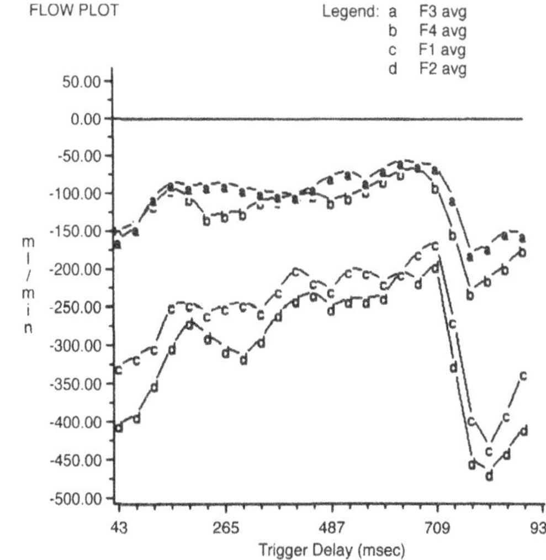

c

Fig. 10.4a–c. Internal carotid arteries (ICA) and vertebral arteries (VA) In a normal subject: SI encoded phase contrast images shortly above the carotid bifurcation (**a**) demonstrating the regions of interest for the ICA and VA flow measurement (**b**, *left*). Tables showing average flow rates (right VA 100 ml/min, left VA 122 ml/min) and flow data as well as volume flow rates plot (F1=right ICA, F2=left ICA, F3=right VA, F4=left VA) (**c**)

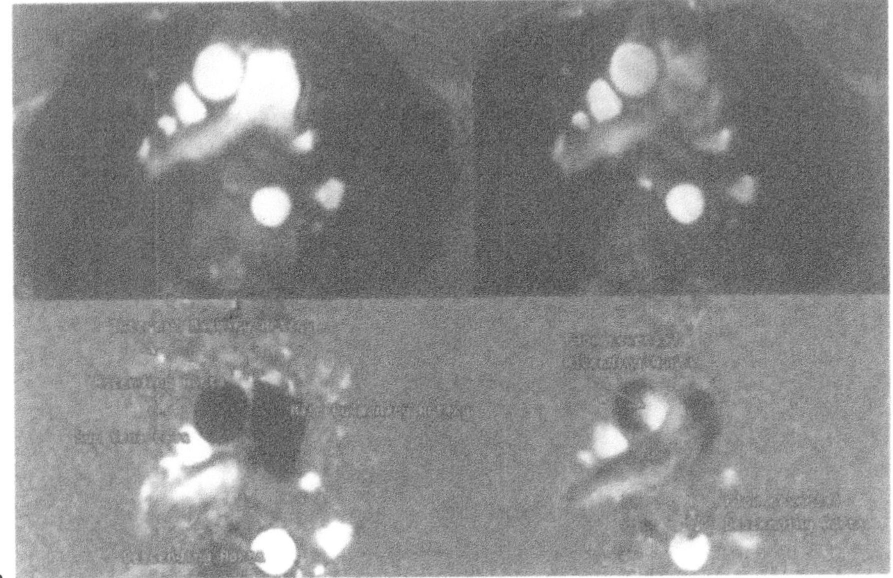

a

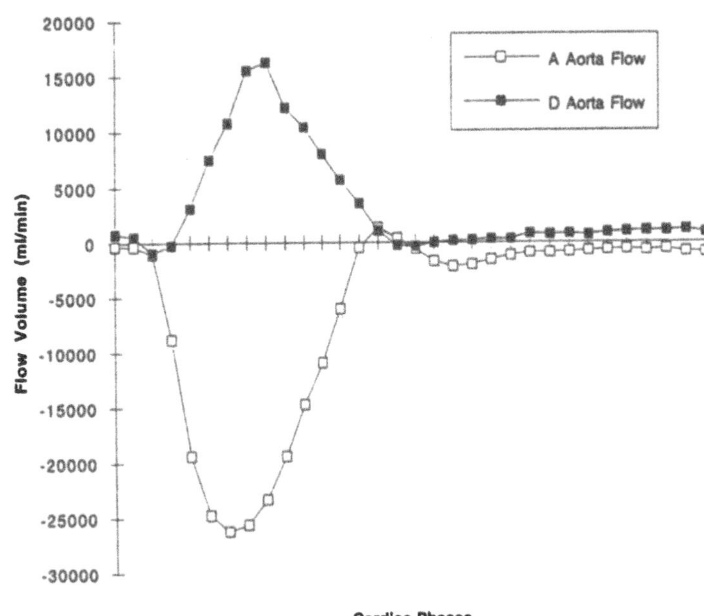

b

Fig. 10.5a, b. Ascending and descending aorta in a normal subject: axial cine-PC acquisition at the level of the pulmonary artery bifurcation, using ECG triggering and a velocity encoded value of 150 cm/s. Magnitude and SI encoded phase contrast images of two frames acquired in early systole (**a**, *left*) and mid-diastole (**a**, *right*) are displayed with the flow volume profiles (**b**). Maximal flow in the ascending aorta occurs during early systole at which time it is homogeneously antegrade. Toward the end of systole and during diastole, a channel of retrograde flow develops in the ascending aorta along the left posterior wall (**a**, *right*), while there is continued antegrade flow along the anterior wall

10.3.2.3
Congenital Heart Disease

The noninvasive evaluation of postsurgical patients with congenital heart disease is clearly desirable. Shunt volumes can be easily assessed by determining right and left ventricular outputs (Pelc et al. 1991a; Fig. 10.6).

Ideal evaluation of surgical shunts should go beyond the determination of patency. PC imaging provides an ideal means for the quantitative measurement of flow in surgical shunts. Shunt volume determinations over time as well as in differing physiologic conditions provides the most valuable clinical information (Kilner et al. 1991; Sieverding et al. 1992; Fig. 10.7). Surgical grafts must be sufficiently well localized to permit a PC imaging plane perpendicular to the conduit clear of any metallic clips, which may induce dephasing artifacts.

10.3.2.4
Coronary Arteries and Veins

Much emphasis has recently been placed on the noninvasive measurement of coronary flow. Using a segmented k-space technique, Sakuma et al. (1997)

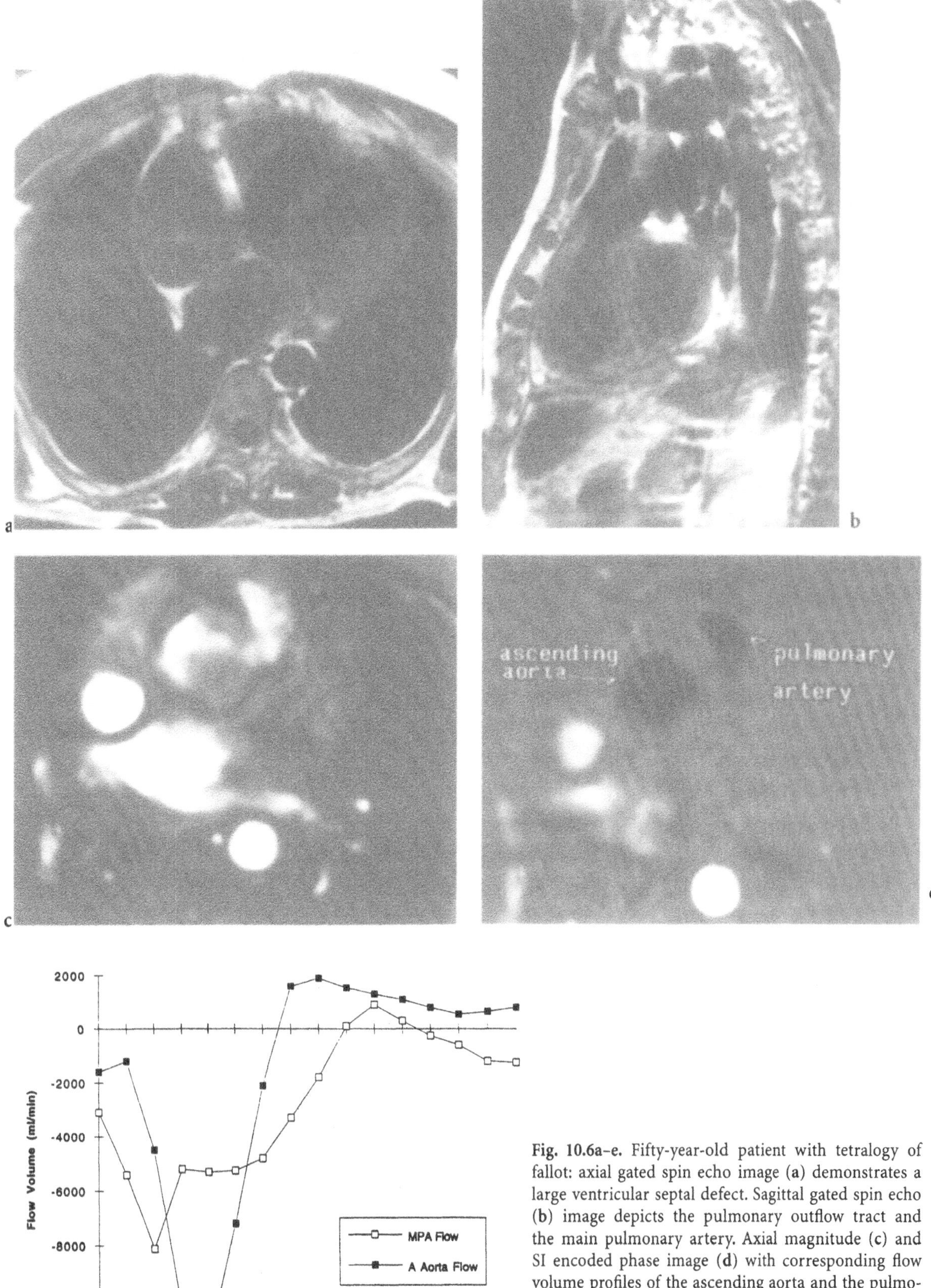

Fig. 10.6a–e. Fifty-year-old patient with tetralogy of fallot: axial gated spin echo image (**a**) demonstrates a large ventricular septal defect. Sagittal gated spin echo (**b**) image depicts the pulmonary outflow tract and the main pulmonary artery. Axial magnitude (**c**) and SI encoded phase image (**d**) with corresponding flow volume profiles of the ascending aorta and the pulmonary artery (**e**) show these to be dissimilar, favoring the aorta. This represents a shunt reversal (right to left shunt) due to pulmonary hypertension. Furthermore, flow in both the aorta and pulmonary artery is reversed during diastole indicating valvular insufficiency

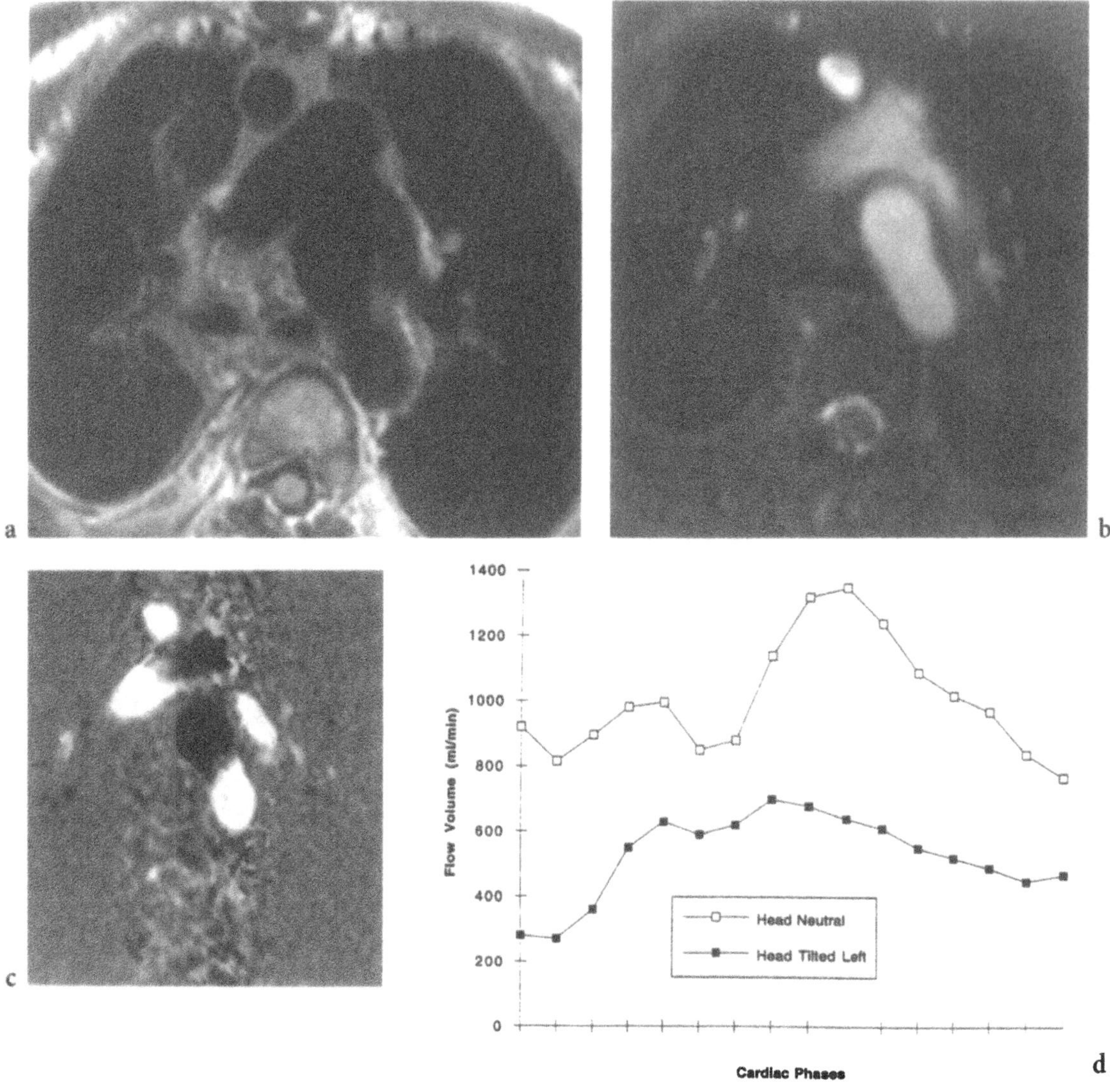

Fig. 10.7a–d. Fifteen-year-old patient with complex congenital heart disease, status post placement of a surgical jugulocaval shunt for obliteration of the superior vena cava. At the time of the examination, the patient presented with positional transient ischemic attacks. Axial spin echo image at the level of the pulmonary artery bifurcation (**a**) depicts the graft located posterior to the sternum. On the magnitude (**b**) and corresponding phase contrast image (**c**) of an axial SI flow encoded cine-PC acquisition, obtained at a comparable level, the conduit is shown to contain flow in the SI direction. At this level, cine-PC acquisitions were performed with the patient's head neutral and tilted to the left. Compared to graft flow with the patient's head in a neutral position, flow in the left-side down position (**d**) was markedly reduced. Positional kinking of the graft at the site of anastomosis was surgically confirmed

demonstrated PC flow quantitation of flow volume in the left anterior descending artery to be accurate when compared to sonographic flowmetry in a dog study, before and after stimulation with dipyridamole. The coronary flow profile differs considerably from the normal arterial flow pattern: flow is less pulsatile and maximal during diastole, when the intramyocardial pressures are lower. The authors emphasize the need to collect the data in a double oblique plane perpendicular to the course of the coronary artery (Sakuma et al. 1997). Clarke et al. (1996) showed in an experimental study that the temporal resolution needs to be sufficient to permit the acquisition of at least six frames spaced equally throughout the cardiac cycle for accurate coronary flow measurements.

In conjunction with pharmacological stress testing, PC flow measurements also permit determination of the coronary flow reserve (CFR; Davis et al. 1997). PC flow measurements of the left anterior descending coronary artery in ten healthy volunteers before and after administration of dipyridamole revealed a mean CFR of 5.0±2.6 (Fig. 10.8; DAVIS et al. 1997). Since flow limiting stenoses have already induced vasodilatation to maintain flow, the response to vasoactive stimulation in stenosed vessels can be expected to be dampened.

Small vessel size and cardiac as well as respiratory motion complicate PC analysis of coronary flow. It has, therefore, been proposed to measure flow in the coronary sinus (VAN ROSSUM et al. 1992). PC measurements of mean blood flow in normal subjects are reported at 144 ml/min with a mean velocity of 2.1 cm/s and a mean cross-sectional vessel area of 1.2 cm^2. The flow pattern in the coronary sinus is described as biphasic: the first peak occurs in systole and a second peak in early diastole (VAN ROSSUM et al. 1992). This approach potentially provides a global assessment of left ventricular perfusion and, thus, total coronary flow. If combined with pharmacologic stress testing, these data may in fact permit determination of total CFR. At this time, the clinical relevance of such measurements remains doubtful: in any case, the inability to attribute any CFR reduction to a particular coronary artery must be considered a significant limitation of this technique.

10.3.2.5
Coronary Artery Grafts

Both saphenous and internal mammary grafts can be assessed in a quantitative manner with PC techniques (DEBATIN et al. 1993; ZÜND et al. 1997). Flow wave forms in grafted internal mammary arteries (IMAs) are significantly different from those in native vessels (Fig. 10.9), as shown in a study evaluating IMA coronary bypass grafts in 15 patients. Flow is less

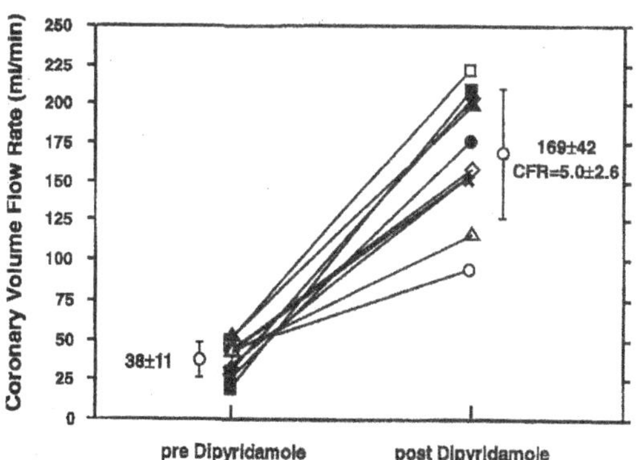

Fig. 10.8. The individual changes in volume flow rates of the left anterior descending (LAD) coronary artery coronary. Flow data were collected based on a breath-held segmented k-space acquisition. Dipyridamole increased coronary volume flow rates (*CFR*)at rest to at least 2.1 times in each volunteer

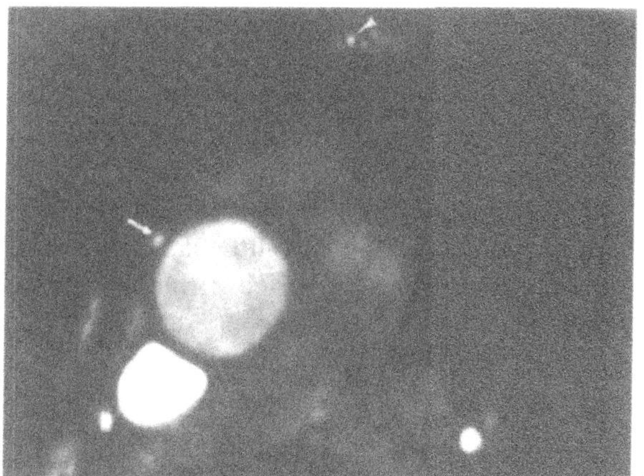
a

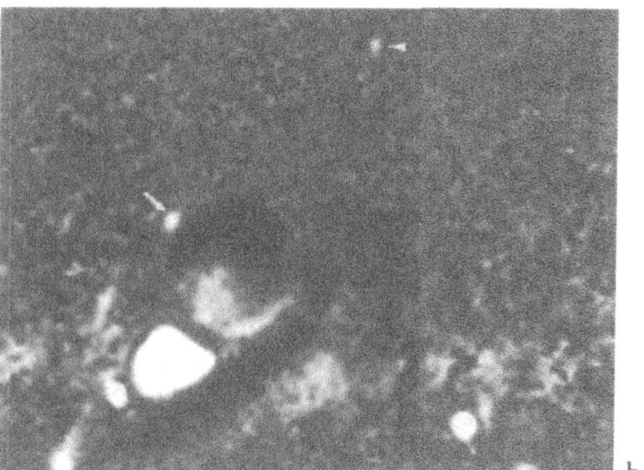
b

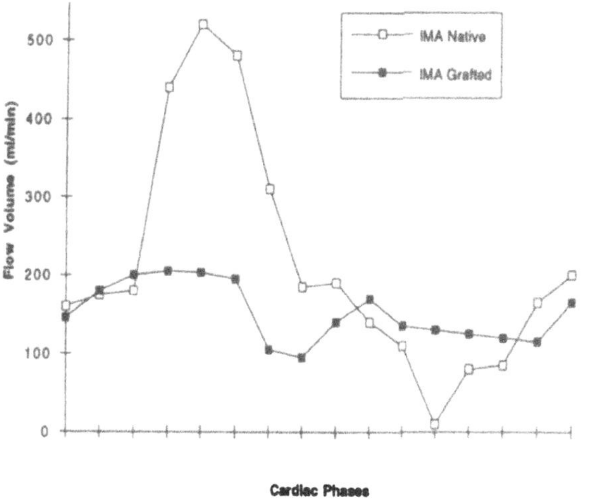

c

Fig. 10.9a–c. Internal mammary artery (IMA) bypass graft: axial cine-PC acquisition obtained at the level of the pulmonary artery bifurcation in a recently post-operative patient. Magnitude (**a**) and SI encoded phase contrast images (**b**) of a single systolic frame demonstrate a right-sided IMA bypass graft in cross section. Flow volume plots (**c**) compare the native right-sided IMA with the grafted vessel on the left. Peak systolic flow volume was lower in the graft than in the native vessel, reflecting assimilation of graft flow to coronary flow patterns. The patent IMA graft carried 110 ml/min to the left anterior descending coronary artery

pulsatile with lower peak systolic velocities (31 cm/s in grafted IMAs vs. 49 cm/s in native IMAs; DEBATIN et al. 1993). There is greater flow during diastole, which frequently exceeds systolic flow. This flow pattern reflects simulation by the IMA graft of coronary flow dynamics, which are characterized by maximal flow during diastole and only little flow during systole. Flow in the IMA grafts varied considerably, from 28 ml/min to 164 ml/min (mean=80.3 ml/min; DEBATIN et al. 1993). Through serial follow-up, PC flow mapping may aid in the early detection of graft disease, enhancing the ability to successfully intervene.

10.3.3 Pulmonary Arteries

PC flow mapping has been shown to provide accurate and reproducible pulmonary flow measurements (EVANS et al. 1993a; CAPUTO et al. 1991; KONDO et al. 1992). PC-based flow quantification of the right and left pulmonary arteries is employed in the assessment of patients with pulmonary branch stenosis as well as following the creation of surgical shunts (HATABU et al. 1991). Comparative analysis of differential pulmonary perfusion between PC MRI and radionuclide studies has revealed excellent correlation in a recent prospective study involving 40 preoperative lung transplant patients (SILVERMAN et al. 1993). While radionuclide lung scanning merely provides relative perfusion data, PC flow mapping is capable of calculating blood flow to each lung in addition to reliably determining the cross-sectional area of the central pulmonary vessels. In order to help determine which lung should be transplanted, the accurate measurement of flow to each lung is particularly useful in the planning stages of single lung transplantation (LEVINE et al. 1990). Such measurements may also be useful for postoperative follow-up as well as in the assessment of a wide variety of pulmonary disease states (CAPUTO et al. 1991).

Flow profiles in patients with pulmonary arterial hypertension differ from those in normal subjects (Fig. 10.10). Both pulmonary peak systolic velocities

a

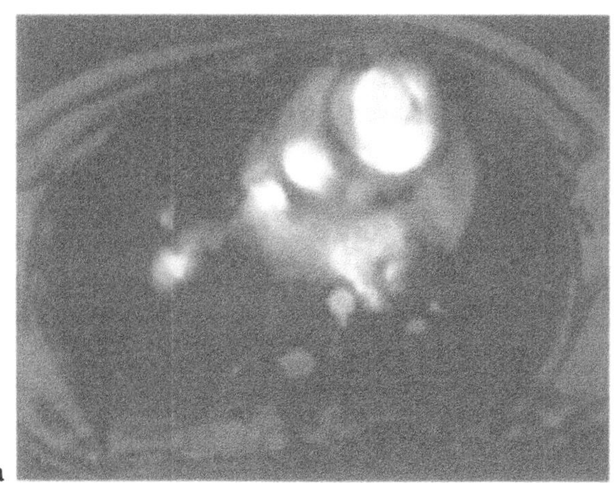

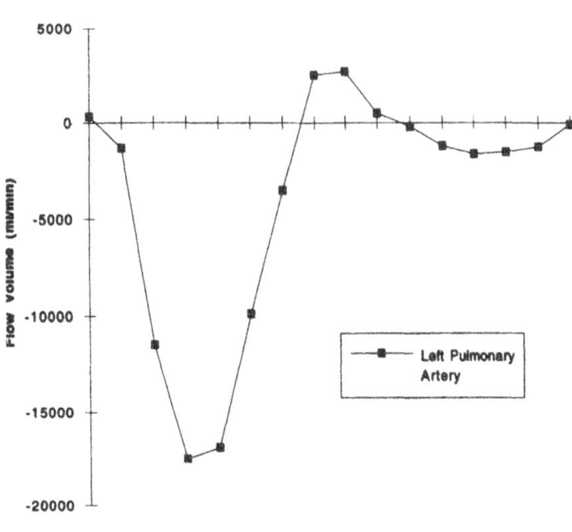

c

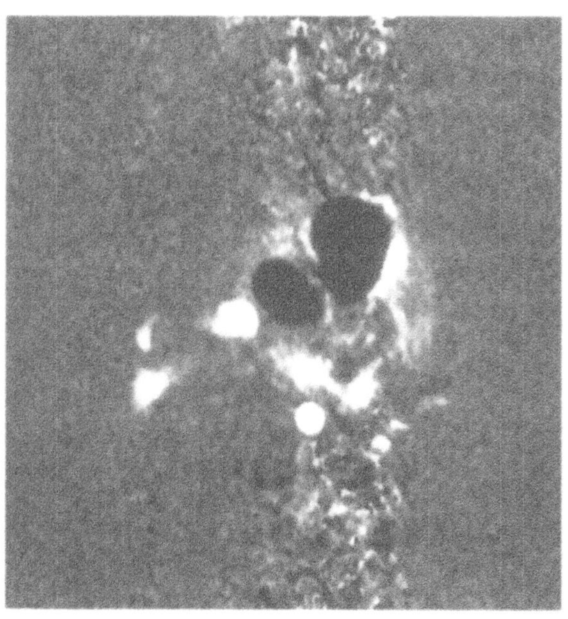

b

Fig. 10.10a–c. Forty-year-old woman with primary pulmonary arterial hypertension. Axial cine-PC acquisition obtained at the level of the pulmonary outflow tract. Magnitude (**a**) and SI encoded phase contrast images (**b**) of a single systolic frame demonstrate a significantly dilated pulmonary outflow tract (*arrow*). The flow pattern of the pulmonary outflow tract and the left pulmonary artery is abnormally pulsatile, reflecting the increased pulmonary pressures (**c**). There is merely minimal flow during diastole. Flow reversal during early diastole indicates a small component of pulmonary valvular insufficiency

and blood flow have been shown to be significantly lower in patients with pulmonary arterial hypertension (30 cm/s vs. 59 cm/s and 48 ml vs. 63 ml) despite similar cardiac outputs (KONDO et al. 1992). Furthermore, in patients with pulmonary hypertension, blood flow at peak systole was significantly more heterogeneous, with wide differences reported between maximum central and spatial mean velocities (KONDO et al. 1992). Finally, the percentage of retrograde flow in patients with pulmonary arterial hypertension is significantly greater than that of healthy subjects (17.3% vs. 3.3%). The retrograde channel occurs along the right posterior wall of the main pulmonary artery in mid-late systole or early diastole (KONDO et al. 1992). While these observations appear promising, the exact sensitivity and specificity of these abnormal flow characteristics with regard to the identification and classification of pulmonary arterial hypertension are still unclear.

10.3.4 Aorta

The velocity-dependent contrast inherent to PC imaging can differentiate between fast and slow flow as well as thrombus (PELC et al. 1991a). As a result, PC flow mapping offers enhanced characterization of aortic flow patterns in the chest and the abdomen. While flow in the suprarenal aorta is homogeneously antegrade, flow in the infrarenal aorta has a retrograde component, resulting in more pulsatility. The retrograde flow component in the infrarenal aorta is absorbed by the renal arteries, which are characterized by high diastolic flow volumes.

Some experience has been reported with cine-PC evaluation of patients with aortic coarctation (ENGVALL et al. 1995; JULSRUD et al. 1997). PC flow quantification can be used to determine the maximal flow velocity within the stenosis itself. High flow velocities within the stenosis mandate use of a maximal VENC. Such measurements have been shown to slightly underestimate flow velocity determinations with echocardiography (ENGVALL et al. 1995). If combined with flow velocity measurements just proximal to the coarctation, the simplified Bernoulli equation can be employed to determine the systolic, diastolic, and mean pressure gradient. Beyond providing rudimentary pressure gradient data, PC techniques permit indirect assessment of the hemodynamic significance of an aortic coarctation, by comparing flow volume measurements proximal and distal to the stenotic region (JULSRUD et al. 1997). Differences favoring flow volumes in the distal descending aorta reflect collateral flow predominantly via the intercostal arteries. Good correlation with surgical findings has been documented (JULSRUD et al. 1997).

PC techniques may also aid in the analysis of aortic dissections. Flow volumes can easily determined in the true and false channels of aortic dissections (CHANG et al. 1991; Fig. 10.11). In a study of six patients with type B dissections (CHANG et al. 1991), both peak and average velocities in the false lumen were noted to be significantly lower than those in the true lumen . In contrast, flow volume per cardiac cycle was not significantly different. The clinical significance of different flow profiles in false lumina of aortic dissections is yet to be determined. It is conceivable, however, that their hemodynamic characterization over time may emerge as a useful predictor of the likelihood of thrombosis.

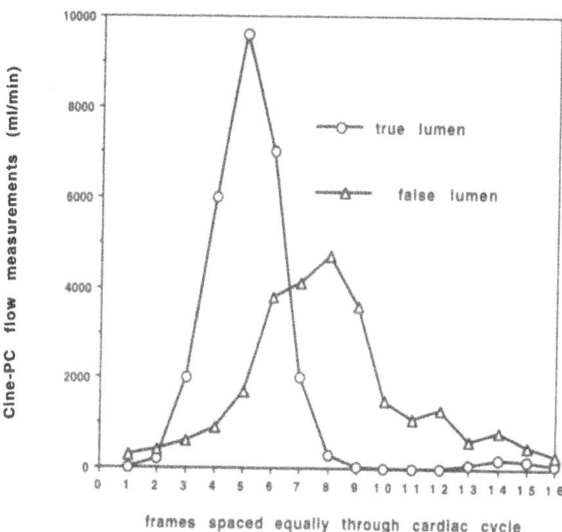

Fig. 10.11. A 41-year-old patient with an aortic dissection. The flow profiles of the two lumen are plotted for the 16 acquired frames. Overall the flow in the false lumen is lower than in the true lumen

10.3.5 Renovascular Disease

Compromise of renal arterial blood flow has long been recognized as a cause of hypertension (HILLMAN 1989) and end-stage renal disease (RIMMER and GENNARI 1993). Despite considerable efforts, reliable identification of these patient subgroups is still imperfect. Most imaging methods hitherto employed in the diagnosis of renovascular disease, including the accepted gold standard catheter angiography, rely on the morphologic assessment of renal arteries.

These techniques are limited by their inherent inability to predict the hemodynamic importance of a particular arterial lesion. PC flow mapping promises to overcome this deficit, by complementing morphologic renal arterial MR imaging strategies (Debatin et al. 1991).

Prerequisite to any PC-based diagnosis of renovascular disease, however, is the ability to accurately quantitate renal arterial flow. In vitro and in vivo analysis has shown that accurate renal flow measurements are only possible if based upon fast real time or breath-held data acquisitions (Debatin et al. 1994; Bock et al. 1998; Sommer et al. 1998). Relative to renal blood flow measurements obtained by means of para-aminohippurate (PAH) clearance, conventional non-breath-held cine-PC imaging unpredictably overestimated flow, reflecting artifactual enlargement of the actual vessel size (Fig. 10.12). Accurate flow measurements, on the other hand, could be obtained with TRIADS-PC (time-resolved imaging with automatic data segmentation; Fredrickson and Pelc 1994), a view-order selection technique permitting the acquisition of six equally spaced PC frames in 37 s (Fig. 10.12). With ultrashort TRs, segmented k-space techniques can provide a similar temporal resolution (Debatin et al. 1994). Even better temporal resolution can be achieved with a recently described interleaved gradient echoplanar imaging (IGEPI) sequence.

As pointed out in the technique section, it is important to acquire the PC data in a plane as perpendicular as possible to the vessel of interest. An accurate localizing sequence thus needs to be collected prior to PC imaging. The recent implementation of new ultrafast contrast-enhanced 3D MRA techniques (Leung et al. 1996) now permits a thorough assessment of the renal arterial morphology (Fig. 10.13). Breath-held contrast-enhanced 3D MRA allows for a thorough visualization of the renal arterial morphology and pathology (Prince et al. 1995). Due to the three-dimensional nature of the data, the correct scan plane, perpendicular to the renal artery and proximal to its first bifurcation, is easily identified. In addition, accessory renal arteries are readily seen. For accurate renal flow quantitation, it is important to measure flow in all vessels supplying a single kidney. Flow in supernumerary renal arteries must thus be measured as well.

Renal arteries are characterized by a fairly homogeneous flow profile. Systolic peaks are low and diastolic flow is high, reflecting the retrograde flow component in the infrarenal aorta during diastole. In analogy to Doppler sonography, increases in systolic flow velocities associated with decreased diastolic flow have been associated with the presence of renal artery disease (Bock et al. 1998). Preliminary results suggest that the presence of a renal artery stenosis can indeed be detected based on the velocity flow profile (Bock et al. 1998).

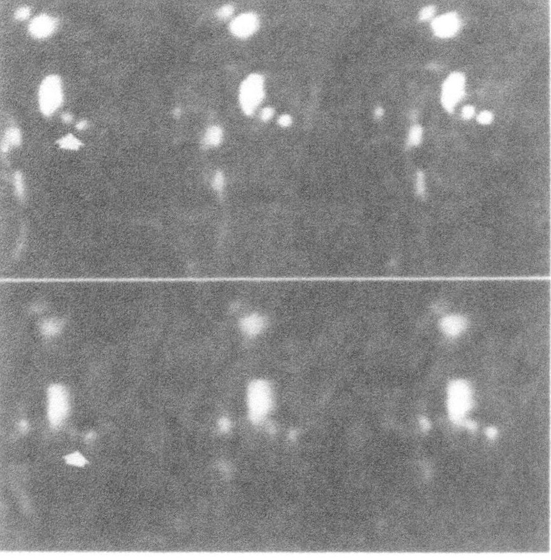

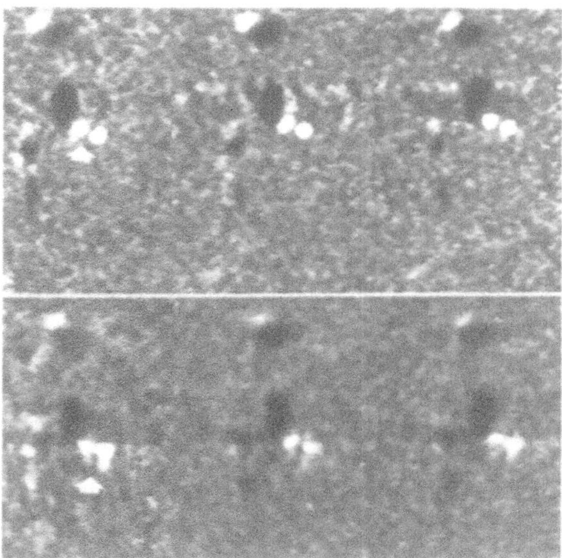

Fig. 10.12. Magnitude (**a**) and phase contrast (PC) (**b**) images of three frames equally spaced throughout the cardiac cycle of breath-held TRIADS-PC (*upper rows*) and non-breath-held cine-PC (*lower rows*). The subject is known to have two left renal arteries. Both vessels are clearly identified as such on both image sets. On the cine-PC images, the vessels are less well defined and characterized by blurred margins due to respiratory motion

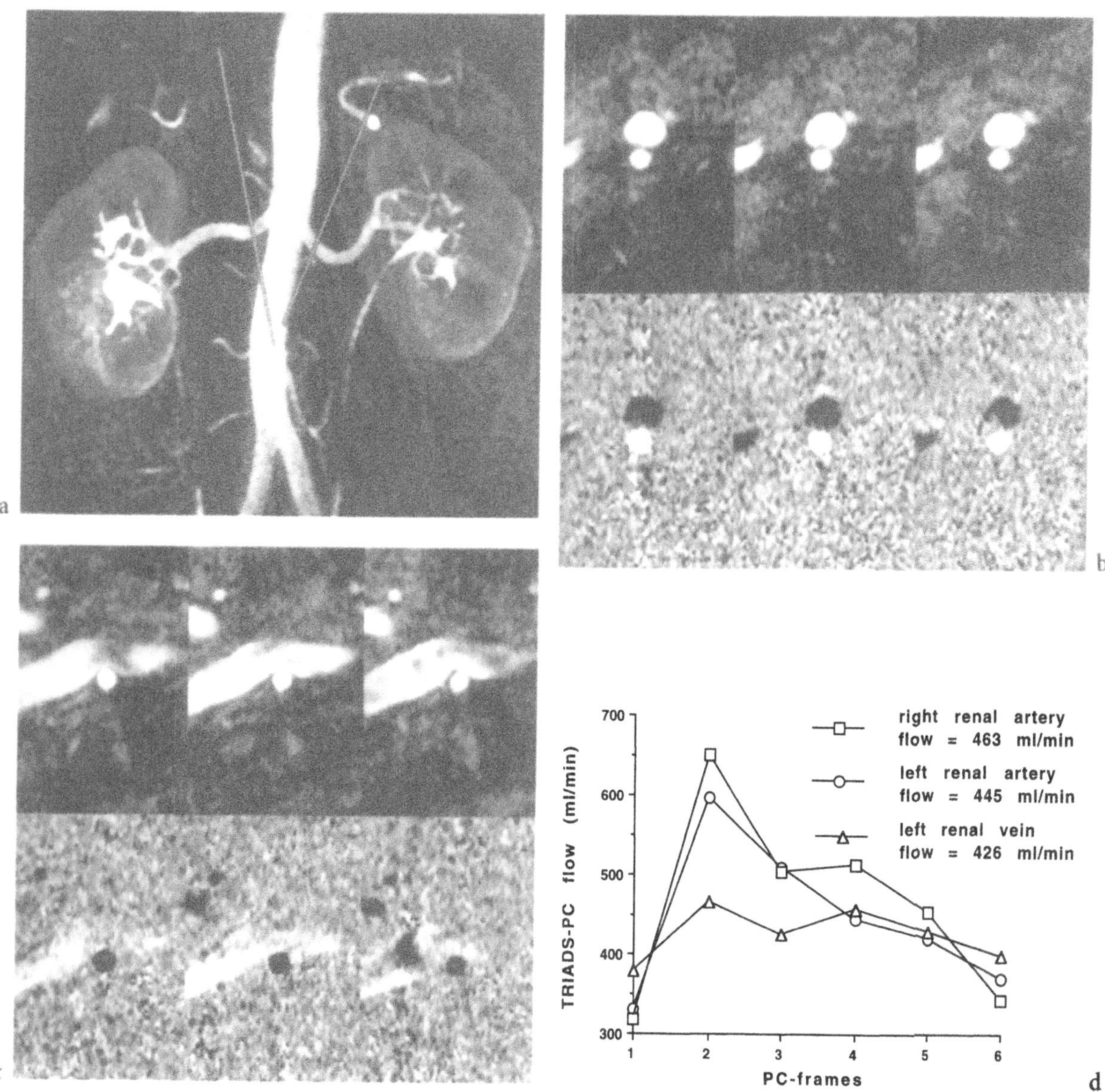

Fig. 10.13. Maximum intensity projection of a contrast-enhanced 3D MR angiogram displaying normal renal arteries (**a**). The 3D data set consists of 44 contiguous 2-mm sections, collected over a convenient breath-hold lasting 23 s. The 3D morphologic images are well suited as a basis for planning the PC acquisition transecting the renal artery in a plane perpendicular to its course and proximal to the take-off of the first branch vessel. Breath-held segmented k-space PC acquisitions acquired perpendicular to the left (**b**) and right renal artery (**c**) show the magnitude images on *top* and the corresponding phase contrast images on the *bottom*. Based on their respective flow directions, the left renal artery (*arrow*) is displayed bright, while the left renal vein and right renal artery are shown as black on the PC images. Renal flow volumes of this subject are plotted over a cardiac cycle (**d**). There is good correlation between left and right renal arterial flow as well as left arterial and left venous flow

Beyond the ability of any other noninvasive technique, including Doppler sonography, PC MRI can accurately quantitate renal arterial flow volume. Due to the inherent anatomic variance in renal position and size, the value of absolute flow volume numbers is limited. Two measurements over time, however, permit relative comparisons. Thus, the therapeutic effect of various interventions, for example, percutaneous transluminal angioplasty (PTA), can be quantitated (Fig. 10.14). Furthermore, the effect of various vasoactive agents on renal arterial flow volume can be measured with PC flow mapping.

Renal blood volume can also be related to renal tissue volume. In a recent study renal flow volumes were determined with PC MRI in 20 patients (40 kidneys). Arterial flow was normal to 28 kidneys and

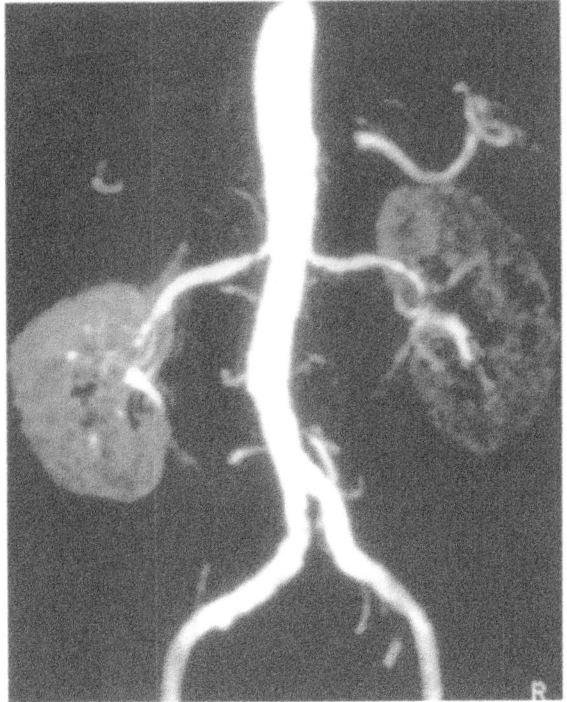

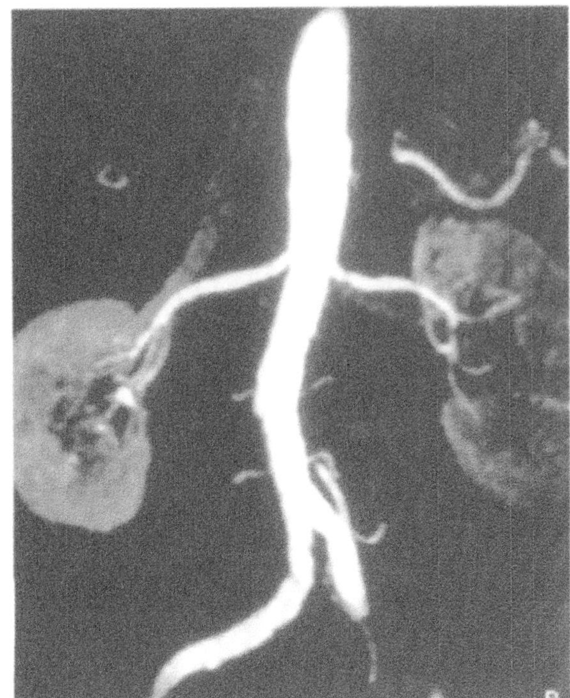

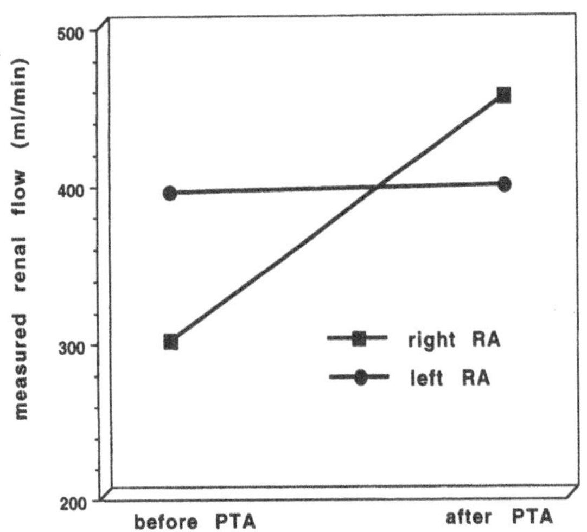

Fig. 10.14. Contrast-enhanced 3D MRA exams, performed in a patient with a right-sided renal artery stenosis before (**a**) and after percutaneous transluminal angioplasty (*PTA*; **b**) demonstrate near complete reduction of the stenosis. PC flow volume measurements acquired before and after PTA of a significant renal artery stenosis reveal a vast PTA-induced increase in renal flow volume (**c**)

impaired due to the presence of a stenosis in 12 kidneys (C. Binkert M.D., personal communication). Analysis of the flow volume data reveals a significant difference between kidneys with normal arterial flow and those with an impaired arterial supply. These data suggest the existence of a critical cut-off value beyond which renal ischemia will indeed be induced (Fig. 10.15). Such a value may be able to aid in the differentiation between significant and nonsignificant renal arterial disease. Clearly, further study is warranted to explore this exciting quantitative means for assessing the renal arterial vascularity.

10.3.6 Mesenteric Ischemia

Mesenteric ischemia remains a frequently perplexing diagnostic dilemma. Chronic mesenteric ischemia is caused by a deficiency of the blood supply to the intestine due to stenosis or occlusion of the splanchnic arteries. Despite the high incidence of celiac and mesenteric artery stenosis in patients with advanced atherosclerotic disease, the syndrome of mesenteric ischemia is rare. This observation reflects the presence of a rich collateral network in the form of vascu-

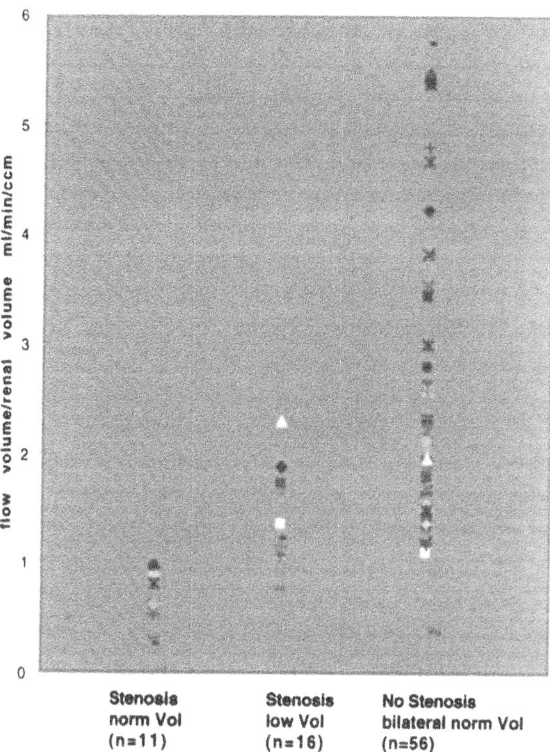

Fig. 10.15. Scatter diagram plotting renal flow volumes per renal mass (ml/cm³). A significant difference ($P<0.05$) is seen in renal flow between kidneys with impaired arterial flow and those with normal arterial supply. There remains, however, some overlap

(Prince et al. 1995). The high incidence of visceral artery stenosis in an asymptomatic population makes it difficult to determine the clinical significance of any morphologic finding. In this regard, PC MRI may complement morphologic imaging.

PC MRI has been employed to assess flow volumes in the SMA and superior mesenteric vein (SMV; Li et al. 1994). To avoid respiratory motion, flow measurements of the SMA should be performed close to the vessel's origin. For maximal diagnostic efficacy, measurements should be made in the fasting state as well as following caloric stimulation. Postprandial flow in the SMA has been shown to increase over 100% in normal volunteers (Fig. 10.16). This postprandial hyperemia was significantly reduced (51%) in patients with high-grade (>50%) stenosis (Li 1998; Dalman et al. 1996). The percentage change in SMA blood flow 30 min after food intake provided the best distinction between healthy subjects and asymptomatic and symptomatic patients. In a limited number of patients with hemodynamically less significant stenoses (>50%) the postprandial flow increase was indistinguishable from that seen in normal volunteers. The same investigators reported that increased postprandial blood flow within the SMV out of proportion to SMA blood flow is another marker for mesenteric ischemia. Discrepantly increased SMV flow reflects recruitment of collateral flow, induced by the presence of a significant SMA stenoses (Li et al. 1994).

lar arcades which readily compensate for stenosis or occlusion of a single splanchnic artery. Patients generally do not develop symptomatic mesenteric ischemia unless blood flow in at least two of the three visceral arteries is severely compromised.

Because of the risks associated with arterial catheterization, the clinical diagnosis of mesenteric ischemia is generally one of exclusion. Delays in diagnosis are compounded by the propensity for symptoms of mesenteric ischemia to overlap with and mimic those of more common intestinal disorders such as peptic ulcer disease, chronic cholecystitis, and pancreatic carcinoma. Establishing the diagnosis of mesenteric ischemia is highly desirable, however, as surgical endarterectomy, re-implantation, or transluminal angioplasty of the diseased vessels offer primary success rates varying between 80% and 100% and 50% and 75% for long-term clinical improvement.

Contrast-enhanced 3D MRA has been shown to provide comprehensive morphologic analysis of the superior mesenteric artery (SMA) and celiac trunk

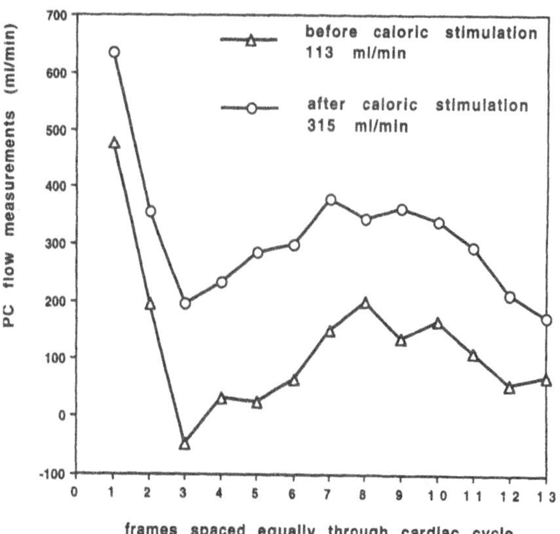

Fig. 10.16. Flow volumes of the superior mesenteric artery measured with PC-MRI over a cardiac cycle in a healthy volunteer before and after stimulation with a standard (475 kcal) calorie meal. Following caloric stimulation, flow increased 80% relative to the fasting baseline

10.3.7 Portal Hypertension

The measurement accuracy of PC flow mapping with regard to quantitation of portal venous flow is well documented (Burkart et al. 1993a, b; Thomsen et al. 1993). Reflecting the relatively homogeneous flow profile of the portal vein, ungated PC techniques can be employed. This reduces acquisition times considerably to about 15 s. Portal venous flow is markedly influenced by the state of respiration. Breath-holding influences intrathoracic and intraabdominal pressures, thereby significantly altering portal flow volumes. Portal venous PC data should thus be collected while the patient is breathing shallowly.

PC flow mapping permits the quantification of the postprandial increase in portal flow (Thomsen et al. 1993). Similarly, changes induced by therapeutic interventions can be quantified. Thus, the effect of TIPS placements on mean portal venous flow can be assessed with PC techniques. Following TIPS, portal flow volume increased by 96% to 1946±910 ml/min. Shunts that were found to be patent 7 days after TIPS placement revealed higher increases in portal flow (134±149%) than those which were found to be occluded within the first week (10.0 and 2.8%; Debatin et al. 1996; Fig. 10.17).

Hemorrhage from gastroesophageal varices is the main complication in patients with portal hypertension (Galambos 1979). Since gastroesophageal collaterals drain into the azygos system, measurement of blood flow therein reflects the magnitude of blood flow in the collateral circulation (Mahl and Groszmann 1990). Since the magnitude of collateral flow appears to influence the course of variceal bleeding, azygos flow may be a predictor of variceal hemorrhage. This was verified by Bosch et al. (1985), who demonstrated in a study encompassing 100 patients that azygos flow was markedly increased in patients with portal hypertension and revealed an association between the risk of variceal hemorrhage and highly elevated azygos flow.

Flow in the azygous venous system can be quantitated with PC MRI (Debatin et al. 1996; Wu et al. 1996). A conventional PC sequences can be used as respiratory motion does not affect these small paravertebral vessels. Cardiac triggering is useful, as flow in the azygos veins does reflect the varying right atrial pressures. Good results can be achieved with an axial cine-PC acquisition traversing the T6/7 intervertebral disc space. Since the vessels are rather small, thin sections (3–5 mm) should be combined with high in-plane resolution (0.5+0.5 mm). A superior spatial saturation band can be applied to eliminate signal contamination from pulsatility artifacts emanating from the aorta.

Mean azygos flow, measured in ten volunteers, amounted to 86±21 ml/min. Considerably higher

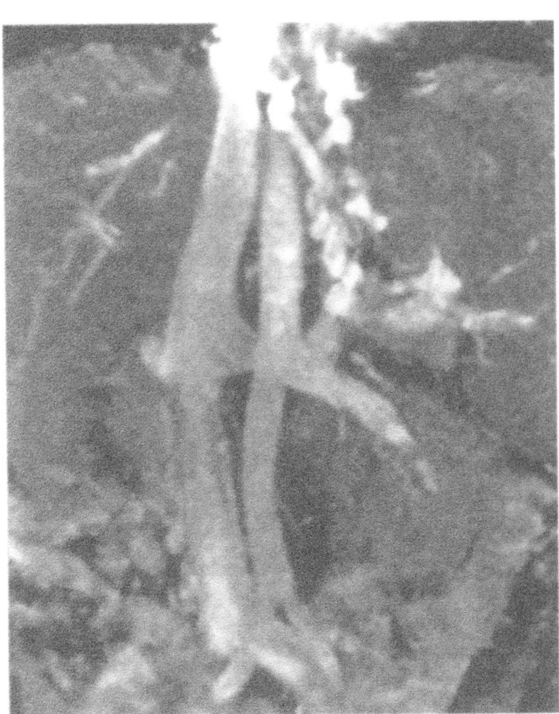

a

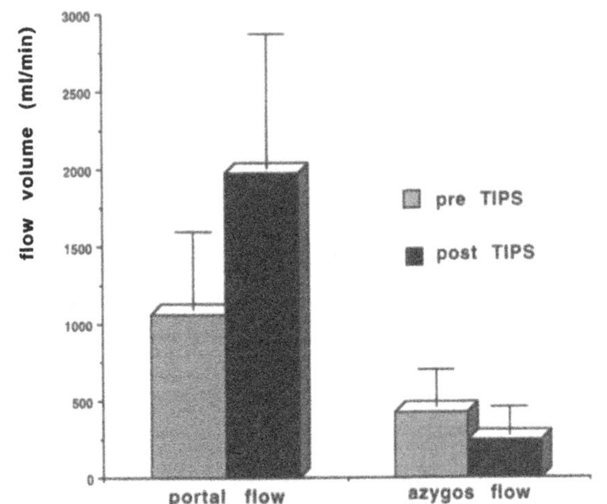

b

Fig. 10.17. Coronal GRE maximum intensity projection image (MIP) (**a**) in a patient with portal hypertension displaying extensive gastroesophageal varices before TIPS. Portal venous pressures were reduced from 32 mmHg to 12 mmHg following placement of TIPS. Graphic display of the TIPS-induced hemodynamic changes (**b**) reveals an increase in portal venous flow and a significant reduction in azygos flow

azygos flow volumes were found in patients with portal hypertension, where mean flow amounted to 424±238 ml/min (range 151–869 ml/min). The nonparametric Mann-Whitney U test showed azygos flow in patients with portal hypertension to be significantly higher than flow in normal volunteers ($P<0.001$).

The therapeutic effect of TIPS on azygos flow and thereby on the flow volume in gastroesophageal varices can also be quantitated with PC MRI. TIPS placement reduced azygos flow on average by 46±42.3% (range 14%–88%) in patients with patent shunts (Debatin et al. 1996). These data suggest that PC blood flow measurements of the azygos system might indeed reflect therapeutic effectiveness (Fig. 10.18).

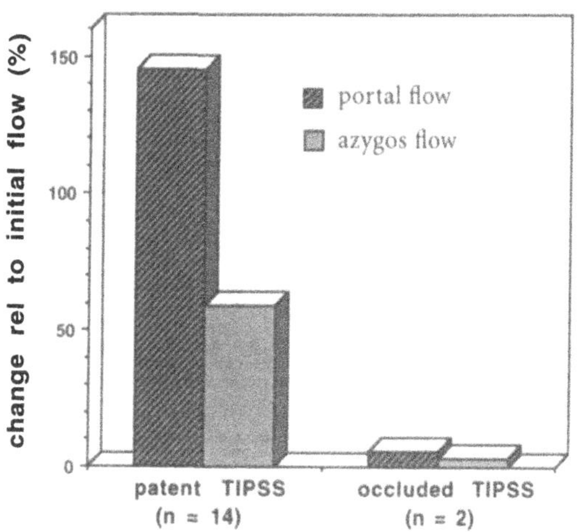

Fig. 10.18. Mean relative changes in flow volume quantitated with cine-PC. In patients with patent shunts (n=18) mean portal flow increased while azygos flow decreased. Only minimal changes in portal and azygos flow volumes were seen in two patients with invasively documented shunt occlusion. *TIPSS*, z

10.3.8 Arterial System in the Lower Extremities

The flow pattern throughput the arteries of the lower extremities is typically triphasic. It is characterized by one systolic and two diastolic components (AbuRahma and Diethrich 1988).

Normal flow volume in the lower extremities is highly variable. In a study of eight normal subjects cine-PC flow determinations of pedal flow, defined as the sum of flow in the trifurcation vessels measured at the level of the talotibial joint, ranged from 32 to 183 ml/min (mean 91 ml/min; Debatin et al., to be published). Flow measurements over time in the same normal subjects showed considerable intrasubject variability. It can be as high as 100% in individual vessels (Debatin et al., to be published). This predominantly reflects nonstandardized subject and environmental factors, such as limb temperature and recent exercise, affecting the degree of vasodilatation. Attempts should, therefore, be made to standardize patient and environmental conditions at the time of quantitation, particularly if measurements are performed to assess flow volume over time.

The response to ischemia is a progressive loss of the triphasic flow character and the development of a more monophasic pattern (Fig. 10.19). Arterial lesions of hemodynamic significance cause the period of early diastolic flow reversal to decrease and ultimately disappear as the lesion becomes more severe. This pattern is attributed to the progressive dilatation and recruitment of peripheral arterioles within the distal vascular bed paralleled by the development of collaterals.

Abnormal wave forms above and below hemodynamically significant popliteal artery stenosis have been demonstrated with PC flow mapping (Caputo et al. 1992). The return to a normal triphasic pattern following percutaneous angioplasty, although rare, due to the frequent presence of concomitant lesions, has also been shown (Caputo et al. 1992). At this time it is unclear how accurate analysis of PC flow profiles will be with regard to identification and classification of the severity of stenotic lesions. Combined contrast-enhanced 3D MRA (Ho et al. 1998) and cine-PC imaging above and below morphologically detected stenoses can provide both anatomic information and the physiologic flow data.

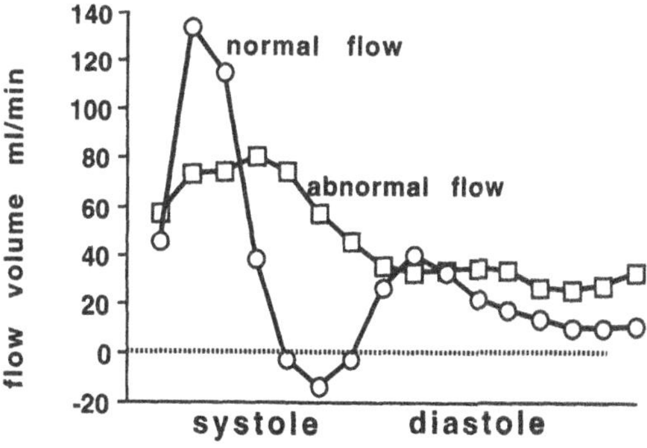

Fig. 10.19. Flow volume plot comparing normal triphasic with abnormal monophasic and biphasic flow profiles. The abnormal pattern is characterized by reduced peak systolic velocity diastole with diastolic flow velocities reaching 30%–50% of peak systolic values. This pattern is attributed to the progressive dilatation and recruitment of peripheral arterioles within the distal-vascular bed paralleled by the development of collaterals

References

AbuRahma AF, Diethrich EB (1988) Current noninvasive vascular diagnosis. PSG Publishing Company

Bock M, Schoenberg SO, Schad LR, Knopp MV, Essig M, van Kaick G (1998) Interleaved gradient echo planar (IGEPI) and phase contrast CINE-PC flow measurements in the renal artery. J Magn Reson Imaging 8:889–895

Bosch J, Mastai R, Kravetz D, Bruix J, Rigau J, Rodés J (1985) Measurement of azygos venous blood flow in the evaluation of portal hypertension in patients with cirrhosis. Clinical and haemodynamic correlations in 100 patients. J Hepatol 1:125–139

Bosch J, Mastai R, Kravetz D, Navasa M, Rodes J (1986) Hemodynamic evaluation of the patient with portal hypertension. Sem Liver Dis 6:309–317

Bosch J, Pizcueta P, Feu F, Fernández M, García-Pagán JC (1992) Pathophysiology of portal hypertension. Gastroenterol Clin North Am 21:1–14

Burkart DJ, Johnson CD, Ehman, RL, Weaver AL, Ilstrup DM (1993a) Evaluation of portal venous hypertension with cine phase-contrast MR flow measurements: high association of hyperdynamic portal flow with variceal hemorrhage. Radiology 188:643–648

Burkart DJ, Johnson CD, Morton MJ, Wolf RL, Ehman RL (1993b) Volumetric flow rates in the portal venous system: measurement with cine phase-contrast MR imaging. AJR Am J Roentgenol 160:1113–1118

Caputo GR, Kondo C, Takayuki M, et al (1991) Right and left lung perfusion: in vitro and in vivo validation with oblique-angle, velocity-encoded cine MR imaging. Radiology 180:693–698

Caputo GR, Masui T, Gooding GAW, Chang J-M, Higgins CB (1992) Popliteal and tibioperoneal arteries: feasibility of two-dimensional time-of-flight MR angiography and phase velocity mapping. Radiology 182:387–392

Caro CG, Pedley TJ, Schroter RC, Seed WA (1978) The mechanics of the circulation. Oxford University Press, New York

Chang J-M, Friese K, Caputo GR, Kondo C, Higgins CB (1991) MR measurement of blood flow in the true and false channel in chronic aortic dissection. JCAT 15:418–423

Clarke GD, Hundley WG, McColl RW, Eckels R, Smith D, Chaney C, Li HF, Peshock RM (1996) Velocity-encoded, phase-difference cine MRI measurements of coronary artery flow: dependence of flow accuracy on the number of cine frames. J Magn Reson Imaging 6:733–742

Dalman EL, Li KC, Moon WK, Chen I, Zarins CK (1996) Diminished postprandial hyperemia in patients with aortic and mesenteric arterial occlusive disease. Quantification by magnetic reonance flow imaging. Circulation 94 [Suppl 2]:206–210

Davis CP, Liu PF, Hauser M, Goehde SC, von Schulthess GK, Debatin JF (1997) Coronary flow and coronary flow reserve measurements in humans with breath-held magnetic resonance phase contrast velocity mapping. Magn Reson Med 37:537–544

Debatin JF, Spritzer CE, Grist TM, et al (1991) Imaging of the renal arteries: value of MR angiography. AJR Am J Roentgenol 157:981–990

Debatin JF, Strong JA, Sostman HD (1993) MR characterization of blood flow in native and grafted internal mammary arteries. J Magn Reson Imaging 3:443–450

Debatin JF, Ting RH, Wegmüller H, Sommer FG, Fredrickson JO, Brosnan TJ, Bowman BS, Myers BD, Herfkens RJ, Pelc NJ (1994) Renal artery blood flow: quantitation with phase-contrast MR imaging with and without breath holding. Radiology 190:371–378

Debatin JF, Leung DA, Wildermuth S, Holtz D, McKinnon GC (1995a) Advances in vascular echoplanar imaging. Cardiovasc Intervent Radiol 18:277–287

Debatin JF, Wildermuth S, Leung DA, Botnar R, Felblinger J, McKinnon GC (1995b) Flow quantitation with eco-planar phase-contrast velocity mapping: in vitro and in vivo evaluation. J Magn Reson Imaging 5:656–662

Debatin JF, Davis CP, Felblinger J, McKinnon GC (1995c) Evaluation of ultrafast phase contrast imaging in the thoracic aorta. MAGMA 3:59–66

Debatin JF, Zahner B, Meyenberger C, Romanowski B, Schöpke W, Marincek B, Fuchs WA (1996) cine-Pc MR quantitation of azygos blood flow in volunteers and patients with portal hypertension before and after tips. Hepatology 24:1109–1115

Debatin JF, Dalman R, Herfkens RJ, Harris EJ, Pelc NJ (to be published) Cine phase-contrast MRI assessment of pedal blood flow. Eur Radiol

Dulce M-C, Mostbeck GH, O'Sullivan M, et al (1992) Severity of aortic regurgitation: interstudy reproducibility of measurements with velocity-encoded Cine MR imaging. Radiology 185:235–240

Edelman RR, Mattle HP, Kleefield J, Silver MS (1989) Quantification of blood flow with dynamic MR imaging and presaturation bolus tracking. Radiology 171:551–556

Eichenberger AC, Jenni R, von Schulthess GK (1993) Aortic valve pressure gradients in patients with aortic valve stenosis: quantification with velocity-encoded Cine MR imaging. AJR Am J Roentgeol 160:971–977

Engvall J, Sjoqvist L, Nylander E, Thuomas KA, Wranne B (1995) Biplane transoesophageal echocardiography, transthoracic Doppler, and magnetic resonance imaging in the assessment of coarctation of the aorta. Eur Heart J 16:1399–1409

Evans AJ, Iwai F, Grist TA, et al (1993a) Magnetic resonance imaging of blood flow with a phase subtraction technique: 'in vitro' and 'in vivo' validation. Invest Radiol 28:109–115

Evans AJ, Fumiharu I, Grist TA, et al (1993b) Magnetic resonance imaging of blood flow with a phase subtraction technique. In vitro and in vivo validation. Invest Radiol 28:109–115

Fazekes F, Niederkom K, Schmidt R, et al (1988) White matter signal abnormalities in normal individuals: correlation with carotid ultrasonography, cerebral blood flow measurements, and cerebrovascular risk factors. Stroke 19:1285–1288

Foo TK, Bernstein T, Aisen A, Hernandez RJ, Collick BD, Pavlik G (1993) High temporal resolution breath-held Cine cardiac imaging using view sharing. In: Book of abstracts. Society of Magnetic Resonance in Medicine,p 1269

Fredrickson JO, Pelc NJ (1994) Time-resolved MR imaging by automatic data segmentation. J Magn Reson Imaging 4:189–196

Galambos JT (1979) Evaluation and therapy of portal hypertension. In: Galambos JT (ed) Cirrhosis. Saunders, Philadelphia, pp 253–287

Haacke EM, Smith AS, Lin W, Lewin JS, Finelli DA, Duerk JL (1991) Velocity quantification in magnetic resonance imaging. Top Magnetic Reson Imaging 3:34–49

Hatabu H, Gefter WB, Konishi J, Kressel HY (1991) Magnetic resonance approaches to the evaluation of pulmonary vascular anatomy and physiology. Magn Reson Q 7:208–225

Hillman BJ (1989) Imaging advances in the diagnosis of renovascular hypertension. AJR Am J Roentgenol 153:5–14

Ho KY, Leiner T, de Haan MW, Kessels AG, Kitslaar PJ, Engelshoven JM (1998) Peripheral vascular tree stenoses: evaluation with moving bed infusion-tracking MR angiography. Radiology 206:683–692

Honda N, Machida K, Hashimoto M (1993) Aortic regurgitation: quantitation with MR imaging velocity mapping. Radiology 186:189–194

Jordan J, Pelc NJ, Enzmann D (1992) Velocity imaging and flow quantitation in the superior sagittal sinus and dural venous sinuses with ungated and Cine gated 2D phase contrast MR. Presented at the 30th ASNR Meeting, St. Louis Mo. Book of Abstracts, ASNR Meeting: 58

Julsrud PR, Breen JF, Felmlee JP, Warnes CA, Connolly HM, Schaff HV (1997) Coarctation of the aorta: collateral flow assessment with phase-contrast MR angiography. AJR Am J Roentgenol 169:1735–1742

Kilner P, Firmin D, Simon R, et al (1991) Valve and great vessel stenosis: assessment with MR jet velocity mapping. Radiology 178:229–235

Kondo C, Caputo GR, Masui T, et al (1992) Pulmonary hypertension: pulmonary flow quantification and flow profile analysis with velocity-encoded Cine MR imaging. Radiology 183:751–758

Leung DA, McKinnon GC, Davis CP, Pfammatter T, Krestin GP, Debatin JF (1996) Breathheld contrast-enhanced 3D MR angiography. Radiology 201:569–571

Levine SM, Gibbons WJ, Bryan CL, et al (1990) Single lung transplantation for primary pulmonary hypertension. Chest 98:1107–1115

Li KC (1998) Mesenteric occlusive disease Magn Reson Imaging Clin North Am 6:33–50

Li KCP, Whitney WS, McDonnell CH, Fredrickson JO, Pelc NJ, Dalman RL, Jeffrey RB Jr (1994) Chronic mesenteric ischemia: evaluation with phase-contrast Cine MR imaging. Radiology 190:175–179

Mahl TC, Groszmann RJ (1990) Pathophysiology of portal hypertension and variceal bleeding. Surg Clin North Am 70:251–266

Marks M, Pelc NJ, Ross M, Enzmann D (1992) Determination of cerebral blood flow with a phase contrast Cine MR imaging technique: evaluation of normal subjects and patients with arteriovenous malformations. Radiology 182:467–476

Mohiaddin RH, Amanuma M, Kilner PJ, et al (1991) MR phase-shift velocity mapping of mitral and pulmonary venous flow. JCAT 15:237–243

Pelc NJ, Herfkens RJ, Shimakawa A, Enzmann DR (1991a) Phase contrast cine magnetic resonance imaging. Magn Reson Q 7:229–254

Pelc NJ, Bernstein M, Shimakawa A, Glover G (1991b) Encoding strategies for three-direction phase contrast MR imaging of flow. J Magn Reson Imaging 1:405–413

Prince MR, Narasimhan DL, Stanley JC, et al (1995) Breath-hold gadolinium-enhanced MR angiography of the abdominal aorta and its major branches. Radiology 197:785–792

Rigau J, Bosch J, Bordas JM, Navasa M, Mastai R, Kravetz D, Bruix J, Feu F, Rodés J (1989) Endoscopic measurement of variceal pressure in cirrhosis: correlation with portal pressure and variceal hemorrhage. Gastroenterology 96:873–880

Rimmer JM, Gennari FJ (1993) Atherosclerotic renovascular disease and progressive renal failure. Ann Intern Med 118:712–719

Sakuma H, Saeed M, Takeda K, Wendland MF, Schwitter J, Szolar DH, Derugin N, Shimakawa A, Foo TK, Higgins CB (1997) Quantification of coronary artery volume flow rate using fast velocity-encoded cine MR imaging. AJR Am J Roentgenol 168:1363–1367

Sieverding L, Jung W, Kiose U, Apitz J (1992) Noninvasive blood flow measurement in quantification of shunt volume by cine magnetic resonance in congenital heart disease. Pediatr Radiol 22:48–54

Silverman JM, Julien PJ, Herfkens RJ, Pelc NJ (1993) Quantitative differential pulmonary perfusion: magnetic resonance imaging vs. radionuclide lung scanning. Radiology 189:699–701

Sondergaard L, Thomsen C, Stahlberg F, et al (1992) Mitral and aortic valvular flow: quantification with MR phase mapping. J Magn Reson Imaging 2:295–302

Thomsen C, Ståhlberg F, Henriksen O (1993) Quantification of portal venous blood flow during fasting and after a standardized meal – a MRI phase-mapping study. Eur Radiol 3:242–247

Van Rossum AC, Visser FC, Hofman MBM, et al (1992) Global left ventricular perfusion: noninvasive measurement with cine MR imaging and phase velocity mapping of coronary venous outflow. Radiology 182:685–691

Wu MT, Pan HB, Chen C, Chang JM, Lo GH, Wu SS, Yeung HN, Yang CF (1996) Azygos blood flow in cirrhosis: measurement with MRI and correlation with variceal hemorrhage. Radiology 198:457–462

Zünd G, Hauser M, Vogt P, Davis CP, Lachat M, Künzli A, Genoni M, Turina M (1997) New approach to patency and flow assessment after left internal thoracic artery hypoperfusion syndrome with additional saphenous vein graft to the left anterior descending artery with phase-contrast magnetic resonance angiography. J Thorac Cardiovasc Surg 114:428–33

11 Hardware Configurations

Klaus Scheffler

CONTENTS

11.1 Introduction

As with all other magnetic resonance (MR) imaging modalities, magnetic resonance angiography (MRA) techniques benefit from rapid gradient systems, low-noise coil and receiver components, and from a clever implementation of imaging sequences and postprocessing software. This chapter gives a brief overview on several hardware components that may influence the quality of MRA images. The most important technical improvement within recent years was the development of high-power gradient systems. A three-dimensional (3D) data set can now be acquired within a few seconds and the contrast-enhanced MRA technique has thus become routinely available on conventional MR scanners. In addition, local receiver coils such as multi-array coils have significantly improved the signal-to-noise ratio (SNR), and an increased image resolution is now possible even for a large field-of-view.

K. Scheffler, PhD
Radiologische Universitätsklinik Freiburg,
Sektion Bildgebende und Funktionelle Medizinische Physik,
Hugstetterstrasse 55, 79106 Freiburg, Germany

11.2 Magnetic Field Strength

11.2.1 Signal-to-Noise Ratio

The field strength of the main magnetic field B_0 has several impacts on basic MR imaging parameters. Most importantly, the available MR signal increases with increasing magnetic field strength. Depending on the particular hardware configuration, the MR signal and thus the SNR increase linearly with the main field, but can increase even quadratically with an optimized coil-receiver chain. This is true for all MR imaging and spectroscopy techniques. In particular, MRA techniques greatly benefit from high magnetic field strength, since for several applications, such as contrast-enhanced MRA (CE-MRA), the intrinsic SNR is reduced due to saturation effects and due to a limited time for data acquisition. In principle, the reduced SNR for low- to mid-field systems, i.e., 0.2–0.5 T, can be compensated with an increased scan time. However, the compensation for a reduction of SNR by a factor of 2 requires a fourfold increase in scan time. This may not be possible in terms of involuntary patient motion or for breath-hold techniques.

11.2.2 T1 Effects

The longitudinal relaxation time T1 also increases with higher magnetic field strength (Abragam 1961). For time-of-flight (TOF) and CE-MRA techniques, which are based on saturation of the background signal of stationary tissue, this will result in a high background signal for low-field applications. A particular problem is the saturation of fat signals which have relatively short T1 times in the order of 200–300 ms at 1.5 T and about 100 ms at 0.5 T. At low fields, fat saturation pulses are necessary for TOF and CE-MRA sequences.

11.2.3 Susceptibility Effects

Changes in the local field are induced at boundaries between different types of tissue, most importantly between air and tissue. The change in susceptibility does not depend on the magnetic field strength. However, the resulting discontinuity of the local field grows linearly with the applied main magnetic field. Most MRA sequences are basically T1-weighted gradient echo sequences and are thus more or less sensitive to field inhomogeneities, depending on the echo time. For low-field systems up to 0.3 T, signal losses at boundary regions between different tissues are greatly reduced compared with high-field systems. This effect can be compensated by using shorter echo times; however, the corresponding gradient system is in most cases not available on low-field systems.

11.2.4 Radiofrequency Power Absorption

Besides several disadvantages, the reduced radiofrequency (RF) power for spin excitation is one of the most important advantages of low-field systems. The required RF power increases quadratically with the main magnetic field. For example, if we assume that a 90° pulse requires 100 W at 0.2 T, the same pulse at 1.5 T would require 5.6 kW. As a consequence, for rapid 3D sequences as used with 3D CE-MRA, one may easily run into RF safety problems due to a very high specific absorption rate (SAR). The SAR can be reduced by increasing the duration of the excitation pulse, which, however, will increase the echo time (TE) and repetition time (TR).

11.3 Gradient Performance

Since the commercial introduction of magnetic resonance imaging in 1984, gradient amplifiers and gradient coil performance have improved in the order of one magnitude. The main driving force for the design of high-power gradient systems was initiated by the demands of echo planar imaging (EPI) technology. Nowadays, state-of-the-art gradient technology allows gradient pulses of 20–30 mT/m within a rise time of 100 μs.

Time-of-flight (TOF), phase-contrast (PC), and contrast-enhanced (CE) MRA techniques are based on gradient echo sequences. The amplitude of the refocused echo depends on the TE and on the T2* relaxation time. For CE-MRA, the T2* relaxation time becomes very short due to the infused contrast agent (CA). Assuming a 50-fold dilution of the CA, T2* will be reduced to about 8 ms for a 0.5-molar gadolinium-based CA and to about 6 ms for superparamagnetic ferumoxide particles (SPIO or USPIO agents). A very short TE, and therefore a high-gradient performance, is mandatory for CE-MRA techniques.

In addition, for first-pass CE-MRA the total scan time is limited to a short window between the arterial inflow and the venous return of the CA. Scan time is typically 10–15 s for the cerebral vasculature and about 20–40 s for peripheral vessels. Fast acquisition of high-resolution 3D data sets thus requires very short TRs, and therefore a very rapid gradient system.

11.3.1 Gradient Strength and Slew Rate

The performance of a gradient system is defined by its maximum gradient strength, G_{max}, maximum slew rate, *SR*, and gradient duty cycle, η.

The gradient amplitude is proportional to the current flowing through the gradient coil. Typically, a gradient strength of 1 mT/m requires a current of about 10 A. For any type of Fourier imaging, the required gradient strength during the readout period is inversely proportional to the product of the readout time, T_a, and the image resolution, Δx.

$$G_{\max} \propto \frac{1}{2\gamma \Delta x T_{\mathrm{a}}} \tag{1}$$

γ is the gyromagnetic ratio, which for protons is 42.577 MHz/T. In principle, high image resolution does not require high gradient amplitudes. However, for fast 3D sequences, the combination of a short TR and thus a short readout time, T_a, and high image resolution, Δx, results in gradient amplitudes of about 20–30 mT/m.

The slew rate (*SR*) of a gradient system is defined as the change in gradient strength per second, and is given in Tesla per meter per second (T/m/s). It depends on the gradient coil inductivity, *L*, and on the maximum available voltage of the gradient power supply. For example, to reach a gradient strength of 20 mT/m within 500 μs, the required loading voltage will be 500 V for a coil inductivity of L=1 mH. For rise times of 200 μs or below, conventional gradient amplifiers can no longer supply the required voltage of more than 1,000 V. So-called gradient or EPI boosters are used which provide a fixed voltage pattern and are switched on during the gradient ramps (Schmitt et al. 1998).

The capability of a gradient system to withstand the power applied to it is defined by its duty cycle, η. It is given by the ratio of the switched gradient time course divided by the maximum possible gradient area:

$$\eta = \frac{\int_0^T |G(t)|\,dt}{G_{\max}T} \tag{2}$$

Depending on the particular sequence design, ultrafast 3D sequences exhibit a gradient duty cycle of 60%–85%, which is considerably more than for conventional spin echo sequences.

11.3.2 Dependence of TE and TR on Gradient Strength and Slew Rate

Short echo times reduce intravoxel dephasing, flow-related dephasing, and signal loss due to CA-induced T2* shortening. The minimum TE which can be achieved for a conventional gradient echo sequence depends on the readout time, T_a (or bandwidth $bw = 1/T_a$), the image resolution, and finally on the maximum gradient strength and slew rate. As shown in Eq. 1, for a given image resolution, Δx, the minimal readout time is given by the maximum gradient strength. However, a short acquisition time or high bandwidth generally does not guarantee the shortest possible TE. Figure 11.1 illustrates the dependence of TE on the bandwidth for three different gradient systems.

Assuming an image resolution of 1 mm in readout direction, the shortest possible TE is 1.14 ms for a G_{max}=30 mT/m and SR=100 T/m/s gradient system, and 3.3 ms for a G_{max}=10 mT/m and SR=10 T/m/s gradient system.

The dependence of TE on the maximal gradient amplitude G_{max} and slew rate SR is shown in Fig. 11.2. It demonstrates that the minimum possible TE is mainly controlled by the gradient slew rate. For an image resolution of 1 mm, no significant reduction of TE can be achieved with gradient amplitudes beyond 25–30 mT/m.

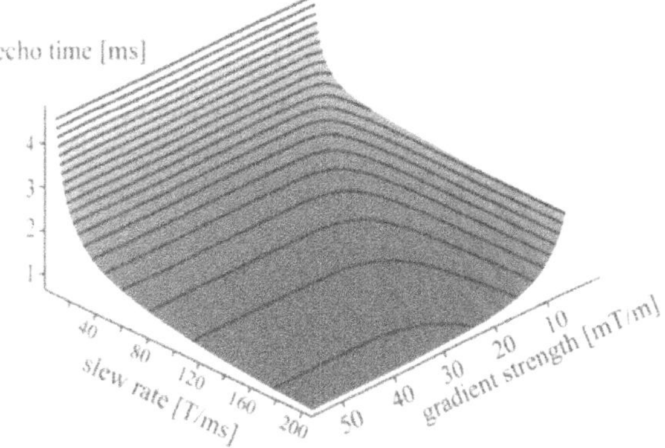

Fig. 11.2. Minimal possible TE as a function of the maximum gradient amplitude and slew rate. Calculations are based on fractional echo readout and readout resolution of 1 mm. For G_{max}=25 mT, the minimum TE is mainly influenced by the available slew rate

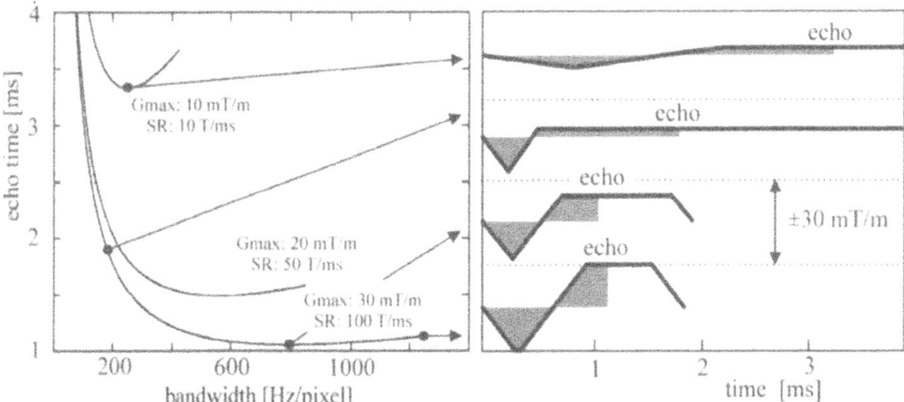

Fig. 11.1. *Left*: Echo time (TE) as a function of the readout bandwidth for three different gradient systems (G_{max}=10 mT/m, SR=10 T/m/s; G_{max}=20 mT/m, SR=50 T/m/s; G_{max}=30 mT/m, SR=100 T/m/s). The calculations are based on an asymmetric echo readout and a readout resolution of 1 mm. In general, the minimally possible TE corresponds to a bandwidth which is below the maximum possible bandwidth. The minimal TE gradient waveform for the G_{max}=30 mT/m SR=100 T/m/s system is shown in the *third row of the right panel*. Both higher and lower bandwidths will result in an increased TE (*second and fourth row*)

11.3.3 Limiting Side Effects of High-Power Gradient Systems

11.3.3.1 *Peripheral Nerve Stimulation*

According to Faraday's law, a change of the magnetic field flux creates an electric field E directly proportional to the rate of change of the B-field dB/dt. In a conductive surrounding, the change of B gives rise to electric currents. The fast switching pattern of gradients needed for MRA sequences can induce rapidly changing currents in the body that are potentially hazardous and can cause neuromuscular stimulation (Budinger et al. 1991). Experimental and theoretical evaluations have shown a linear relation between the applied magnetic flux B and the duration of the gradient stimuli. Safety considerations therefore limit the speed of the gradient system. Because of the different geometries of the three gradient coils, the stimulation hazard is worst for the z direction (i.e., the readout gradient for sagittal or coronal slice direction).

11.3.3.2 *Acoustic Noise*

With the introduction of ultrafast gradient systems, the acoustic noise produced by the imaging sequence can cause harm to patients and operators. The acoustic noise is generated by Lorentz forces which act perpendicular to the gradient current and main magnetic field. The Lorentz forces cause a deformation of the coil structure and generate vibrations similar to a loud speaker. The highest noise level will be generated when all three gradient axes are switched at the same time. The noise level of an ultrafast 3D sequence may reach sound pressure levels of about 90–120 dB SPL, and patients need to be protected by headphones (Hedeen and Edelstein 1997).

11.3.3.3 *ECG Gating*

A further problem of rapidly switched gradients is their disturbance of ECG signals. The ECG must be detected in violent electromagnetic surroundings, due to the gradient switching, which induce large peaks in the ECG, and due to the induced RF power during the excitation pulse. Dedicated fiber optics and pre-amplifiers may be useful in making the unwanted signals at least significantly smaller than the QRS peak to avoid false triggering. Therefore, the ECG triggering needs to be done very carefully and the ECG signal cannot be used as a monitoring signal.

11.4 Radiofrequency Coils

The signal-to-noise ratio (SNR) in MR imaging is given by:

$$\mathrm{SNR} \propto V_{voxel}\sqrt{NT_a} \tag{3}$$

where V_{voxel} is the volume of one image voxel, T_a is the readout time within each TR, and N is the total number of phase-encoding steps (Macovski 1996). For clinical applications, NT_a is always limited, either to minimize the risk of involuntary patient movement or due to the short time of the arterial phase of CA in first-pass CE-MRA techniques. CE-MRA, in particular, is hampered by a low SNR since the entire 3D k-space has to be collected within 10–30 s. The resulting decrease in SNR may be compensated by using CA with a high relaxivity, R_1 (the SNR is proportional to the square root of R_1). However, the most effective way to increase SNR is the use of local receive coils such as the head coil or phased array coils.

The dependence of SNR on the coil performance is given by:

$$\mathrm{SNR} \propto \sqrt{\frac{Q}{V_{eff}}} \tag{4}$$

where Q is the quality of a series resonant circuit and V_{eff} the effective volume received by the RF coil (Vlaardingerbroek and den Boer 1996). Multichannel coils are designed to study a large field-of-view (FOV) without needing to acquire the whole FOV with a single coil, which lowers the SNR. Each coil of an array coil receives another part of the FOV, and thus each coil gives a signal from a different region. Since signals come from coils with a small effective volume, V_{eff}, SNR will be increased. Figure 11.3 (left panel) compares the SNR of different types of coils, measured on a phantom at 1.5 T. The SNR of the body coil was set to an arbitrary value of 1.0. MRA of the abdominal region is a typical application of multichannel coils. The large region of interest of about 40×50 cm can be covered with a four-array coil. Figure 11.3 (right panel) shows two

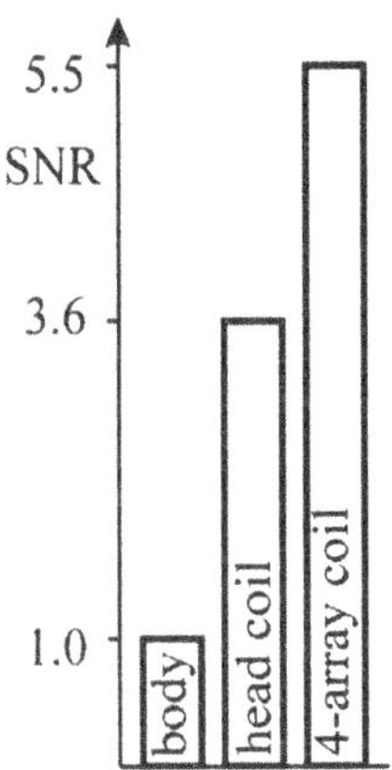

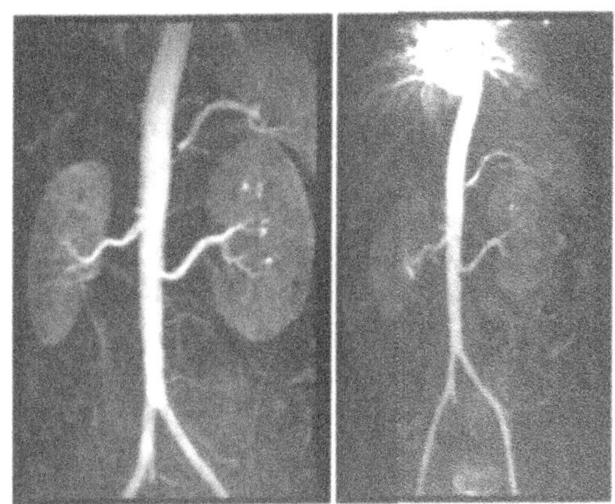

Fig. 11.3. *Left*: SNR measured for the body, head, and four-channel phased array coil (water phantom, 1.5 T Siemens Symphony). The multi-array coil shows a fivefold increase in SNR compared to the body coil. *Right*: Abdominal CE-MR angiogram measured with the multi-array coil (*left*, resolution 1+1+1 mm^3) and body coil (*right*, resolution 1+2+2 mm^3) (Courtesy of Dr. Matthias Boos, University Hospital, Basel, Switzerland). Although the image resolution differs by a factor of four, both images show a similar SNR

images of the same patient measured with the phased array coil and the body coil. Both images show a comparable SNR but the multichannel image (left) has a twofold higher image resolution than the body coil image (right).

The use of local array coils is mandatory for CE-MRA, and several approaches including the multichannel SMASH technique demonstrate an excellent SNR compared to the single coil technique.

11.5 Sequence Control

Most 3D imaging techniques acquire k-space in a row-by-row sampling pattern. The readout of one row of the 3D k-space is typically placed between two nested loops, the line loop and the partition loop. For stationary objects, the resulting image quality does not depend on the particular 3D acquisition scheme. For example, imaging of a water phantom using centric phase encoding versus linear phase encoding would give exactly the same result. Completely different results must be expected for non-stationary objects, as discussed in detail in Chap. 8. Variation of CA concentration and thus signal intensity during k-space acquisition will produce image artifacts which are directly related to the k-space acquisition scheme.

A very promising k-space acquisition strategy is spiral or elliptic sampling of the second (lines) and third (partitions) k-space coordinate, which ideally results in an isotropic blurring effect (see also Chap. 8).

Such "unconventional" k-space trajectories require high flexibility in the sequence control unit of the MR scanner. An example of a spiral-like acquisition scheme is shown in Fig. 11.4. The sequence was designed for CE-MRA of the carotid arteries and

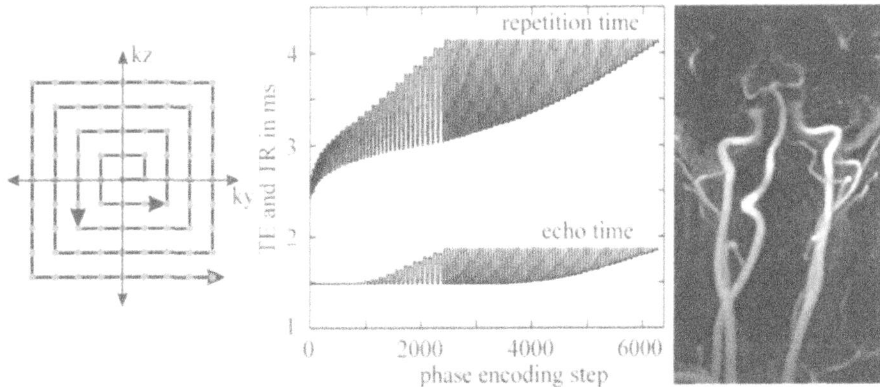

Fig. 11.4. Example of an elliptic reordered CE-MRA sequence with optimized TE and TR. The *left panel* shows the elliptic or spiral-like sampling of the in-plane (k_y) and through-plane (k_z) phase-encoding steps. The *middle panel* plots the resulting TE and TR for each phase-encoding step during image acquisition (128×50=6400 encoding steps). The total image time was 21.3 s (on a 1.5-T Siemens Symphony) compared to 28.2 s for a fixed TE and TR acquisition scheme. The *right panel* shows a CE-MR angiogram of the carotid arteries acquired with elliptic k-space sampling

consists of 128 in-plane phase-encoding steps (k_y) and 50 through-plane phase-encoding steps (k_z). In addition, the 3D sequence incorporates flexible TE and TR times which are automatically adjusted during run time to the particular phase-encoding position. Since encoding of the outerpart of k-space requires longer phase-encoding gradients, TE and TR slightly increase during image acquisition (as shown in the middle panel of Fig. 11.4). The right panel of Fig. 11.4 shows a CE-MRA of the carotid arteries based on the described 3D sequence.

This example demonstrates the need for a very flexible sequence control unit in order to cope with the requirements of time-critical CE-MRA sequences. A further example is the automatic or user-controlled change between 2D and 3D sequences as used, for example, in the fluoroscopic triggering technique (Wilman et al. 1998).

11.6 Data Storage and Image Calculation

Acquisition and calculation of 3D images require very large raw data storage and fast processors for reconstruction. For example, an imaging volume of 400+400+200 mm3 with a resolution of 1 mm in each dimension needs about 120 megabytes of free RAM memory. The use of multi-array coils, data oversampling and interpolation may easily result in RAM storage in the order of several gigabytes. The post-processing (i.e., fast Fourier transform, MPR, MIP) of such a huge amount of data within a short time definitely requires dedicated hardware, state-of-the-art workstations, and image display stations.

References

Abragam A (1961) The principles of nuclear magnetism. Oxford University Press, Oxford

Budinger TF, Fischer H, Hentschel D, Reinfelder HE, Schmitt F (1991) Physiological effects of fast oscillating magnetic flux gradients. J Comput Assist Tomogr 15:909–914

Hedeen RA, Edelstein WA (1997) Characterization and prediction of gradient acoustic noise in MR imagers. Magn Reson Med 37:7–10

Macovski A (1996) Noise in MRI. Mag Reson Med 36:494–497

Schmitt F, Stehling MK, Turner R (1998) Echo-planar imaging. Springer, Berlin Heidelberg New York

Vlaardingerbroek MT, den Boer JA (1996) Magnetic resonance imaging. Springer, Berlin Heidelberg New York

Wilman AH, Riederer SJ, Huston J III, Wald JT, Debbins JP (1998) Arterial phase carotid and vertebral artery imaging in 3D contrast-enhanced MR angiography by combining fluoroscopic triggering with an elliptic centric acquisition order. Magn Reson Med 40:24–35

12 Artifacts and Limitations

Rolf Vosshenrich and Peter Reimer

CONTENTS

12.1 Introduction

Magnetic resonance angiography (MRA) has emerged as a noninvasive technique for evaluating patients with different vascular diseases. However, with the standard two-dimensional (2D) time-of-flight (TOF) technique there are many difficulties in detecting stenoses and occlusions in diseased arteries because of a variety of flow-related artifacts (Brunereau et al. 1998). Therefore, alternative strategies have been studied to improve MRA (Atkinson et al. 1997), including cardiac gating, segmented fast gradient-echo MRA, and the phase-contrast (PC) technique with variable velocity encoding. A few years ago, three-dimensional (3D) contrast-enhanced (CE) MRA was introduced as a method for vascular imaging with short acquisition times. A thorough understanding of the underlying mechanisms, proper techniques, and artifacts is essential to fully exploit the diagnostics potentials of these methods and to avoid misinterpretations (Stringer 1997; Tsuruda et al. 1992). This chapter presents some of the artifacts, limitations, and pitfalls that may be encountered with MRA.

Rolf Vosshenrich, MD
Zentrum Radiologie der Universität, Röntgendiagnostik I, Robert-Koch-Strasse 40, 37083 Göttingen, Germany
Peter Reimer, MD
Professor, Zentrale Röntgendiagnostik, Städtisches Klinikum, Moltkestrasse 14, 76133 Karlsruhe, Germany

12.2 General Artifacts

12.2.1 Motion, Breathing, Peristalsis, and Pulsation

A variety of artifacts are relatively independent of the chosen technique, always to a variable degree, depending on the imaged region present. Motion and breathing artifacts are predominantly encountered in MRA of the chest and abdomen (Figs. 12.1, 12.2). A short acquisition time, such as that used in CE-MRA, is an easy way of circumventing these artifacts. Alternatively, advanced gating techniques such as navigator techniques may solve these problems as well. Pulsation artifacts (Fig. 12.3) are visible throughout the body; however, they are most severe in the chest with highest flow velocities in normal arteries. Although ECG gating is helpful in minimizing pulsation artifacts, it extends acquisition times. Peristalsis in the abdomen is best minimized by short acquisition times, as with CE-MRA. Gross motion by uncooperative patients (Fig. 12.4) or patients unable to sustain a breath-held acquisition (Fig. 12.2) may be circumvented by keeping the acquisition time as short as possible.

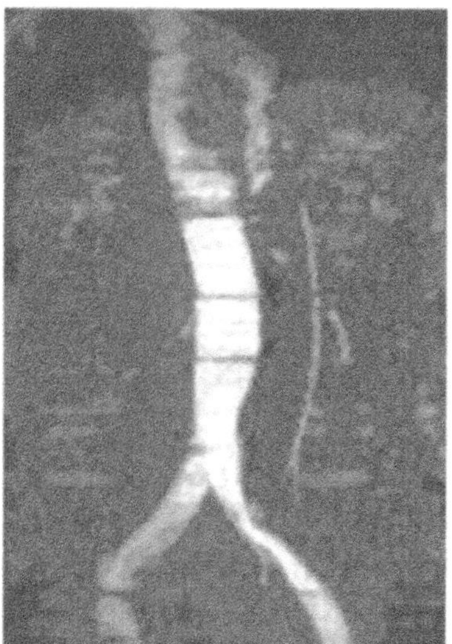

Fig. 12.1. Follow-up of an AV fistula by TOF MRA of the lower abdomen. Each slice was imaged during a separate breath-hold. The MIP shows multiple stepping artifacts due to motion and different breath-hold positions for the different positions

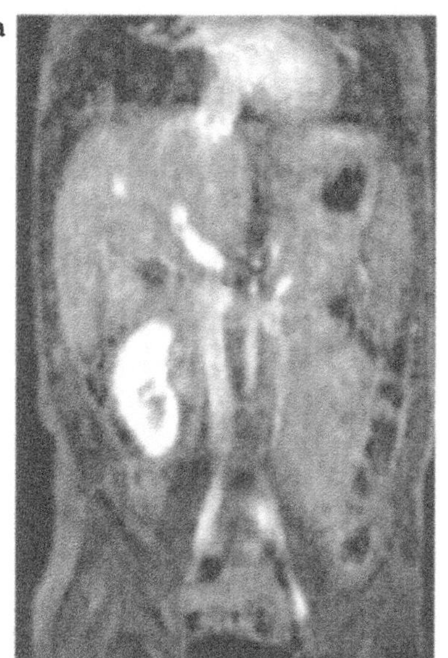

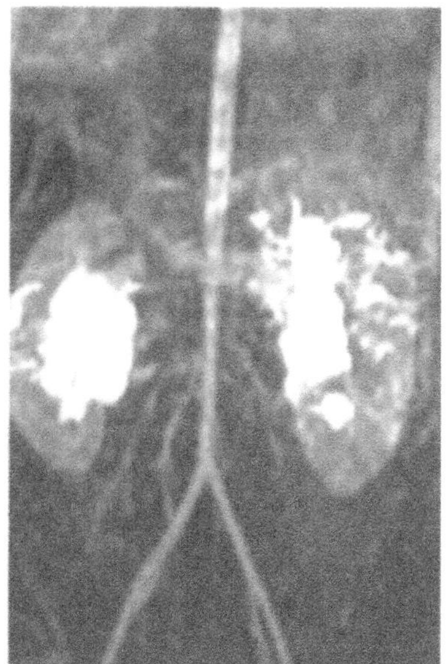

Fig. 12.2a, b. CE-MRA of the abdomen in a 9-year-old child with breathing during the acquisition and motion artifacts. The young patient was not able to sustain a breath-held acquisition. (**a**) coronal raw data image, (**b**) MIP

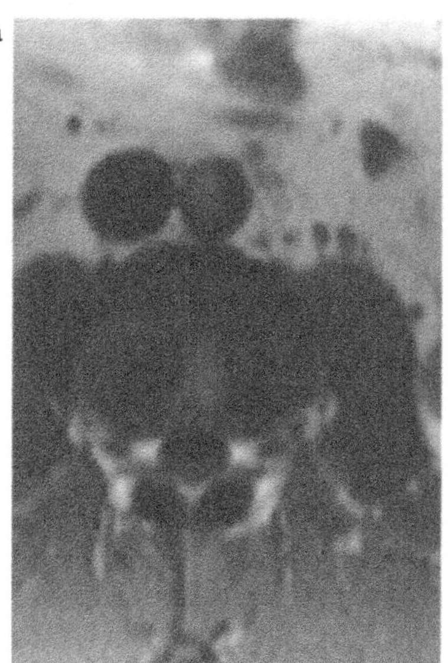

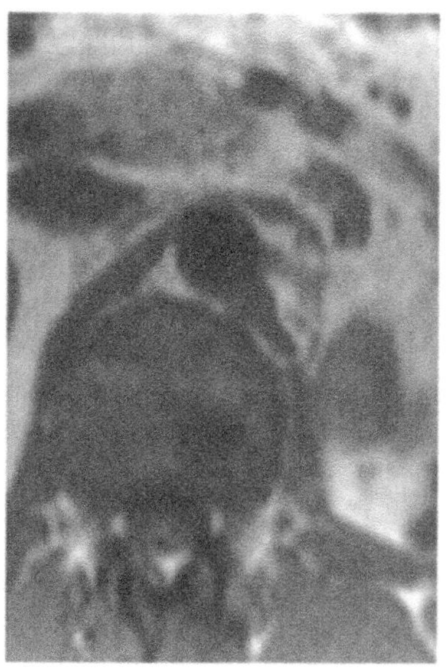

Fig. 12.3a, b. Two axial T1-weighted SE images (**a, b**) of the abdominal aorta demonstrate different signal within the aorta going along with round-shaped signal changes within the vertebral body. Pulsation artifacts cause the pseudolesions with ghosting along the phase-encoding direction

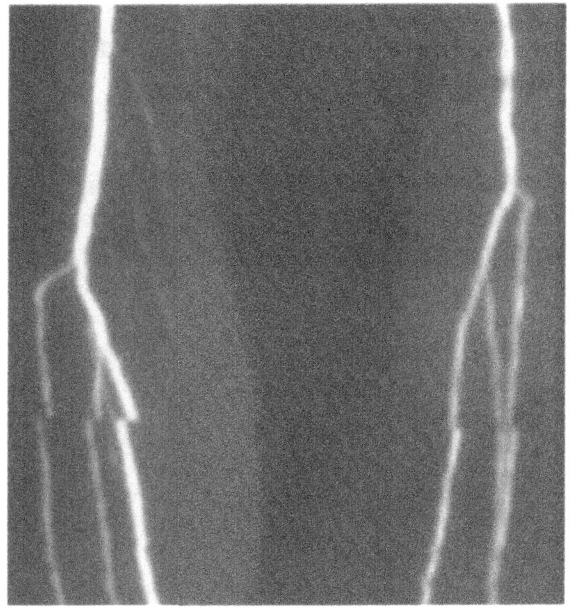

Fig. 12.4. The 2D TOF MRA of the right popliteal artery shows motion artifacts. The movements of the patient during the acquisition caused gross spatial misregistrations of the vessel

12.2.2 Hematoma

A short T1 relaxation time of tissue may mimic blood flow especially on TOF-MRA images. Signal from fat or bone marrow generates a background signal, which is typically visible on maximum intensity projection (MIP) images because of the incomplete suppression of signal. Signal from subacute to early chronic hematoma containing intracellular or extracellular methemoglobin may present a more difficult problem to solve. The signal intensity may be as high as from flowing blood and unless source data are carefully observed it may be overseen. A typical pitfall is a subacute thrombus within an aneurysm (Schmieder et al. 1999; Tsuruda et al. 1992). PC-MRA or CE-MRA can be applied in uncertain cases.

12.2.3 Slab Placement

Vessels excluded from the image slab can appear falsely occluded (Fig. 12.5). Typical regions are the brachiocephalic trunk or left subclavian artery when the supra-aortal region is imaged, or the femoral arteries or popliteal arteries during peripheral run-off studies. An image showing slab placement should always be demonstrated or printed to avoid this false positive diagnosis (Anderson et al. 1990).

12.2.4 Postprocessing

Similar problems may occur due to postprocessing of source data (Anderson et al. 1990; Schreiner et al. 1996). Typically, the data set is loaded and subsequently the displayed region centered onto the vessels of interest. Vessels may be cut off accidentally simulating false positive occlusions (Fig. 12.6). We recommend that an overview MIP be displayed to start with. Targeted MIPs are then created going along with the clinical referrals.

The MIP itself has substantial drawbacks (Stringer 1997). Areas with poor flow contrast, including the edges of blood vessels and small vessels with slow flow, may be obscured by an overlap with brighter stationary tissue. As a result, the apparent vessel lumen may be falsely narrowed and stenoses exaggerated. It is helpful to view the individual sections to determine the true diameter of the lumen or restrict the volume of interest for processing (targeted MIP).

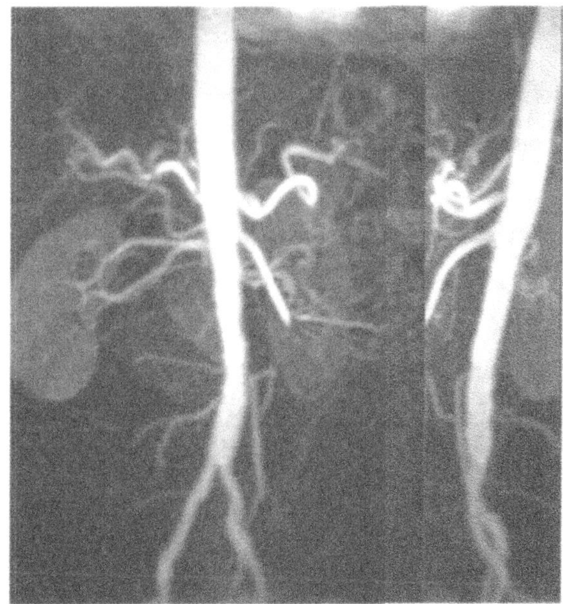

Fig. 12.5. CE-MRA [anteroposterior MIP (*left*) and lateral MIP (*right*)] of the upper abdomen shows a pseudo-occlusion of the SMA on the anteroposterior view (*left*). The image slab was placed below the entire course of the SMA just covering the proximal portion thus artificially cutting off the distal SMA. The lateral MIP (*right*) demonstrates the slab placement

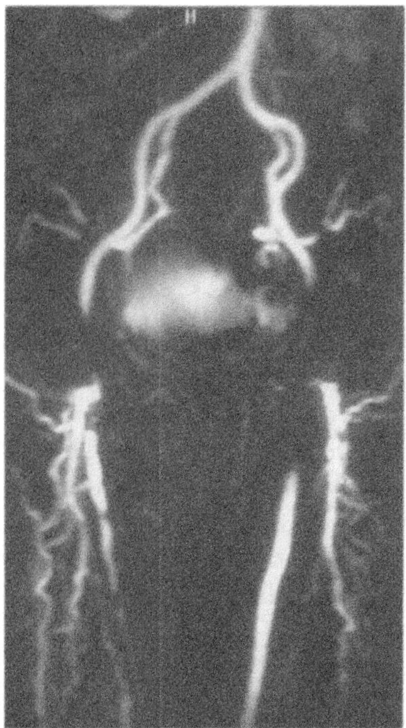

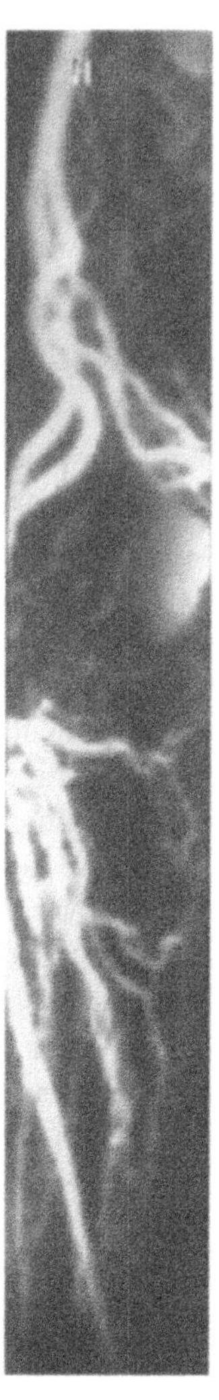

a,b

Fig. 12.6. The anteroposterior MIP (**a**) of a CE 3D MRA of the iliaco-femoral arteries demonstrates a signal loss within both proximal femoral arteries. The signal proximal and distal to the "occluded segments" appears completely normal. The sagittal MIP reconstruction (**b**) solves the problems by visualizing the proximal femoral vessels that were artificially excluded from the image slab during image processing and thus appeared occluded

12.3 Artifacts of Non-Contrast-Enhanced MR Angiography

When the course of a vessel causes blood to remain in the imaging slice for a sufficient time, progressive signal loss results because of saturation of the vascular spins by the same pulses that saturate signal from the stationary background tissue (WILCOCK et al. 1995). Signal loss in patent vessels from in-plane flow saturation is one of the most common pitfalls in 2D TOF MRA (FÜRST et al. 1995). This loss of signal may simulate an occlusion or higher grade of stenosis than present. Saturation of in-plane flow occurs typically in two anatomic areas: tortuous iliac arteries and the proximal anterior tibial artery (Figs. 12.7, 12.8). Signal loss is accentuated on MIPs, which do not distinguish between faint vascular signal and background signal. Strategies to overcome these problems include examination of the source images, cardiac gating, segmented acquisitions, and contrast enhancement (MIROWITZ 1993).

Signal loss also occurs when flow is turbulent, e.g., when distal to stenoses and bifurcations, or within aneurysms (Fig. 12.9). Because of complex flow in these areas, the velocities of blood vary extremely from voxel to voxel, which results in loss of vascular signal. These alterations of signal intensities are caused by intravoxel phase dispersion. This phenomenon contributes to the overestimation of the sever-

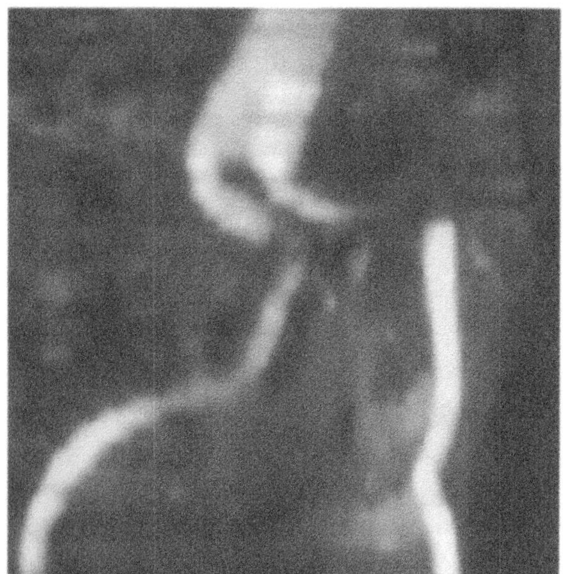

a

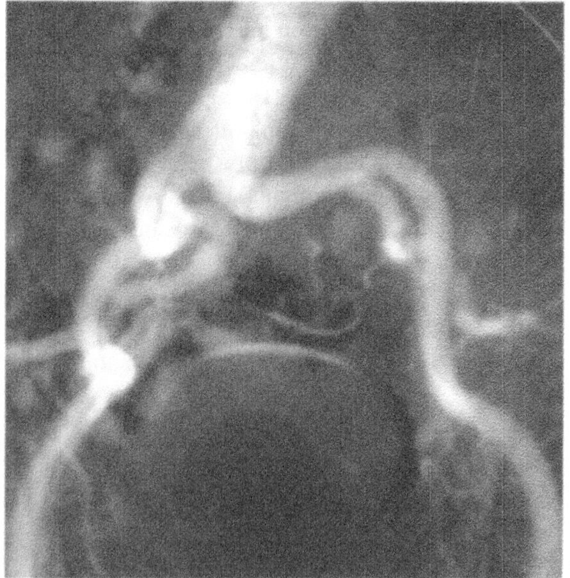

b

Fig. 12.7a, b. 2D TOF MRA (**a**) and DSA (**b**) of the aortoiliac arteries demonstrate tortuous iliac vessels. The TOF (**a**) image shows a short signal loss in both iliac arteries where the vessels take an almost horizontal turn. The corresponding DSA (**b**) shows no pathologies in both vessels segments indicating signal loss due to tortuous vessels, flow turbulence, and in-plane flow saturation

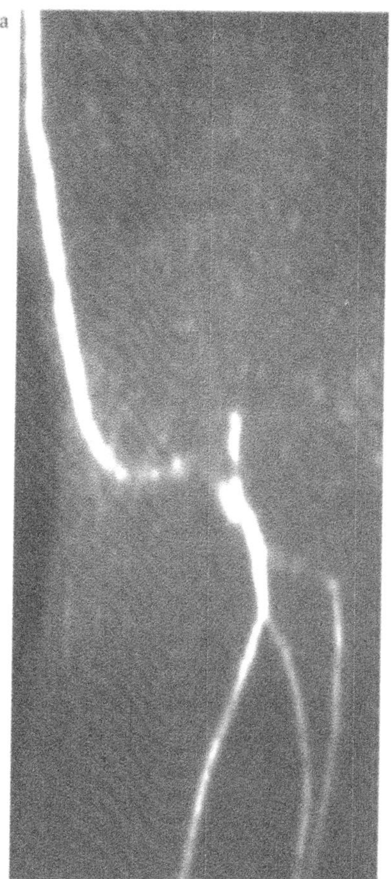

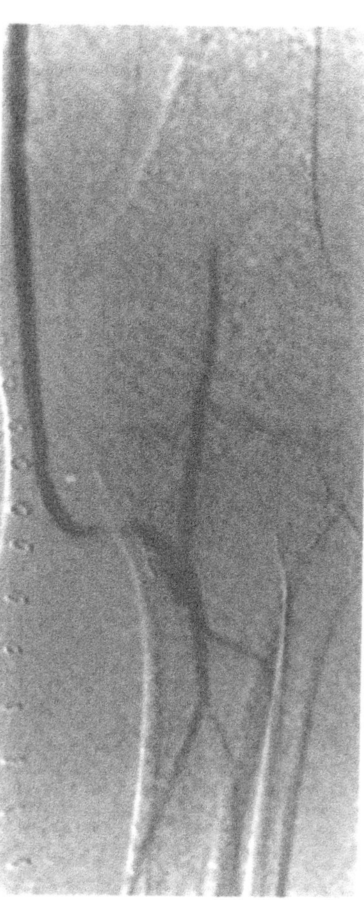

Fig. 12.8a,b. 2D TOF MRA (**a**) and DSA (**b**) demonstrate the popliteal artery with a femoropopliteal bypass. TOF-MRA shows in-plane flow in the distal anastomosis causing partial saturation of the flowing spins, resulting in diminished flow-related enhancement. The comparative DSA confirms this finding

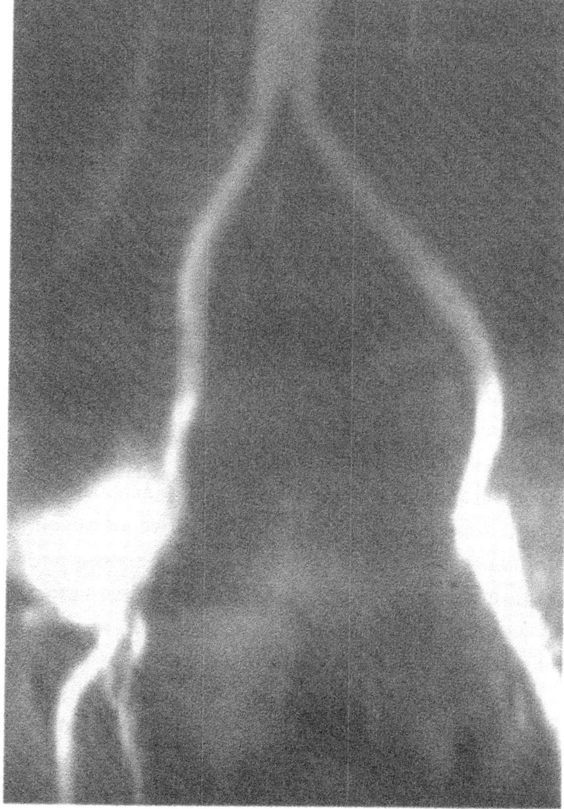

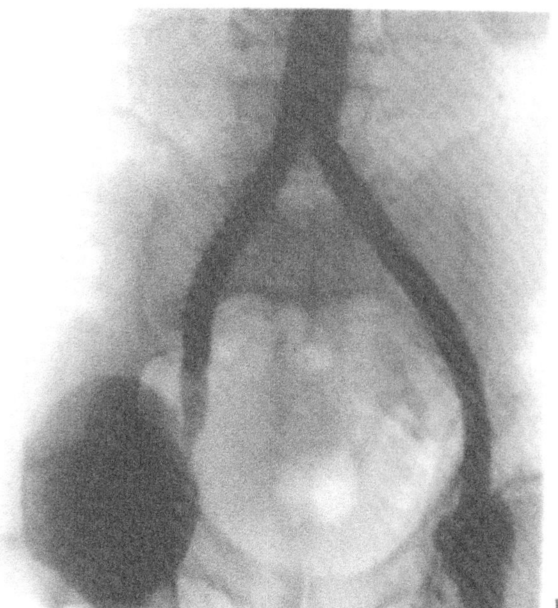

Fig. 12.9a, b. 2D TOF MRA (**a**) and DSA (**b**) of the iliac arteries demonstrate an aortobifemoral graft with large bilateral graft aneurysms. The aneurysms appear smaller with the TOF images because of slow turbulent flow resulting in spin saturation and an underestimation of the cavity. The corresponding DSA confirms this artifact

ity of stenoses (Fig. 12.10; Table 12.1). MIP algorithms intensify the apparent signal loss by ignoring the faint signal in these vessel segments (STRINGER 1997).

A tracking saturation band in the flow direction of the vein towards the artery is necessary in 2D TOF MRA to eliminate signal from veins. However, if the arterial flow passes through the saturation band before entering the imaging slice, it will also be come saturated. This problem is commonly observed in the pelvis, where the iliac arteries can be quite tortuous (Fig. 12.8). The coverage of peripheral artery occlusions may appear longer on 2D TOF MRA than in conventional angiography because retrograde flow in collateral vessels itself may be saturated by the inferior saturation band since this imitates the flow direction of the veins.

Table 12.1. Overestimation of stenoses by non-contrast-enhanced MRA

Stenosis overestimation by:	Effects	Reduce the caused effects by:
Flow acceleration	Dephasing during TE	Reduce TE (TOF)
Turbulent flow Vortex flow Stream separation distal to stenosis		Increase VENC(PC) Increase resolution, increase dose (CE-MRA)
Vessel turns	Flow void	CE-MRA
Overlay of vessels within one voxel (PC MRA)	Dephasing → signal loss	Small volume TOF or CE-MRA

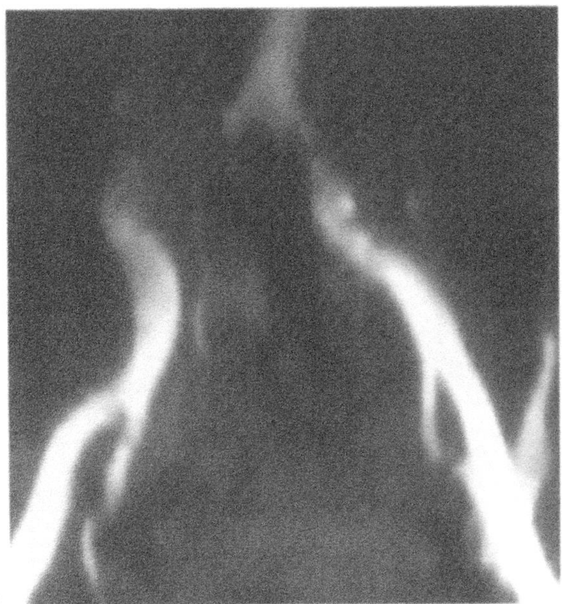
a

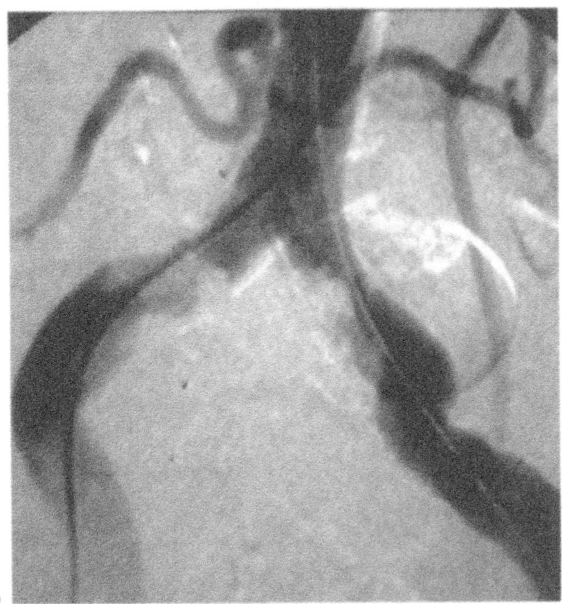
b

Fig. 12.10a, b. 2D TOF MRA (**a**) and DSA (**b**) of the iliac arteries demonstrate high-grade bilateral common iliac artery stenoses. The TOF image shows a short but complete signal loss within the stenoses mimicking occlusions. The DSA (**b**) explains the overestimation by the severity of stenoses in both vessels segments

Arterial flow in normal peripheral vessels is characteristically triphasic. The arterial blood flows antegrade through the imaging section during systole and continues into the saturation band. Later in the cardiac cycle, there is a brief period of retrograde flow that carries saturated blood into the imaging plane. This saturated blood has low signal intensity, and a dark stripe is seen on the corresponding MR angiogram. Increasing the separation between the saturation band and the imaging section eliminates this artifact (OWEN et al. 1993).

Flow distal to stenoses is frequently brighter and the vessels appear larger than in the corresponding normal vessels. First-order flow compensation is optimal for flow at a constant velocity, as seen distal to occlusive disease. Normal pulsatile flow is subject to signal loss because of the variability in the velocity and acceleration of blood during the cardiac cycle. As a result, vessels with poor signal intensity may be normal. Correlation with physical examinations and noninvasive studies is essential. Cardiac gating with imaging during diastole will minimize this artifact, but will increase the acquisition time (FRANK et al. 1995).

Pulsatile flow can cause ghosting artifacts in the phase-encoding direction. The wide range of pulsatile flow velocities induce phase variations in addition to phase encoding that results in multiple images of the same vessels. An important technical point in 2D TOF MRA of the lower extremity is to localize the phase encoding in the anterior-posterior direction. If severe ghosting artifacts occur, the best MIP reconstruction will be the direct coronal view because the artifact will not be visible from this perspective. Cardiac gating, smaller flip angles, or careful image post-processing can reduce these artifacts.

Motion artifacts can also simulate abnormalities in the vasculature. A patient's motion from section to section during the acquisition of 2D TOF angiogram results in the apparent offset of the vessel that can simulate a vascular lesion. The presence of motion can be verified by evaluation of the outer contour of the skin and each of the individual sections (Fig. 12.1).

Knowledge of prior vascular surgery is essential for the correct performance and interpretation of MRA in postoperative patients. Grafts may be located in places that normally do not contain major run-off arteries, such as cross-femoral or axillo-femoral grafts. These extra-anatomic grafts may require careful application of additional sequences to be imaged completely. Similarly, flow may be reversed in certain vessels as a consequence of bypass surgery.

It is also possible to use MRA to image the vasculature after percutaneous interventional treatments such as angioplasty or stenting. To document the technical result after angioplasty, 2D TOF MRA can be used. However, for the imaging of intravascular stents, the use of TOF MRA is limited.

Ferromagnetic vascular clips, joint prostheses, and foreign bodies (Fig. 12.11) can cause variable degrees of signal loss (Grieve et al. 1999; Schurmann et al. 1999; Shellock and Kanal 1998; Shellock 2000). Signal loss due to metal artifacts cannot be reliably detected on MIP images. The patient's history and reading of the source images and radiographs are necessary (Okamoto et al. 1997). Signal loss can also occur at tissue-air interfaces such as bowel loops overlying an iliac artery. A review of the axial slices and the localizer images may identify this artifact as the cause of unexpected signal loss (Kaufman et al. 1998).

PC-MRA is widely available with sequences allowing the visualization of a particular range of flow velocities, both with 2D and 3D techniques (Dumoulin et al. 1993). Basically, the amplitude and duration of the flow velocity-encoding gradient determine the sensitivity to flow velocity. Stronger gradients induce larger phase shifts for velocities and weaker gradients induce smaller phase shifts for velocities. The technique is also sensitive to slow flow showing venous overlay (Fig. 12.12), but there is a risk of aliasing as known from color duplex ultrasound. Other sources of artifacts are peristaltic motion and breathing motion close to vessels which may be minimized by the administration of scopolamine to suppress bowel motion (Dumoulin et al. 1993). Using a velocity-

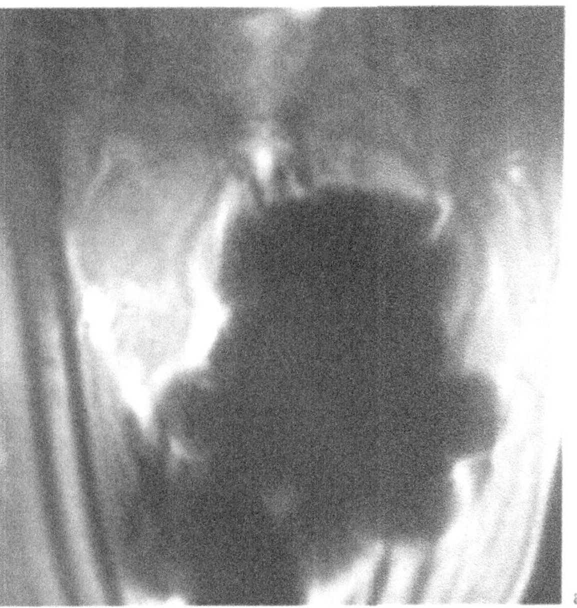
a

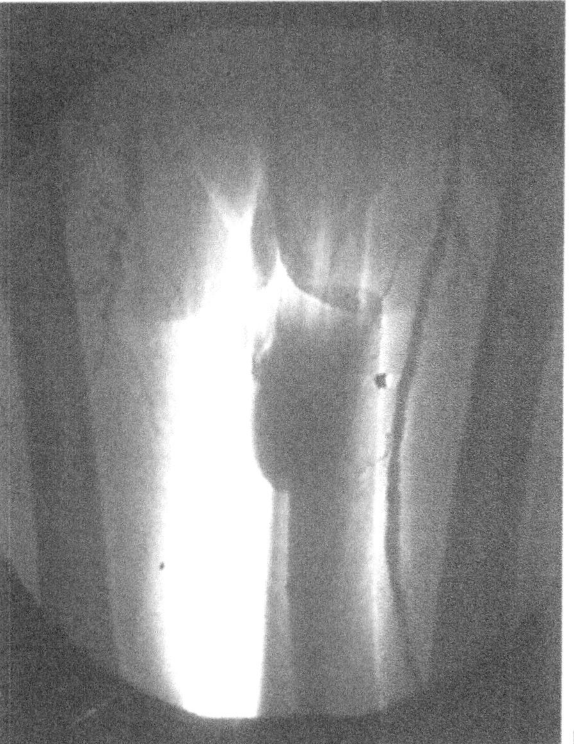
b

Fig. 12.11. A 2D FLASH localizer (**a**) of the lower limbs demonstrates a nearly complete signal loss within the left thigh. The corresponding DSA (**b**) shows small shrapnel causing the large susceptibility artifact

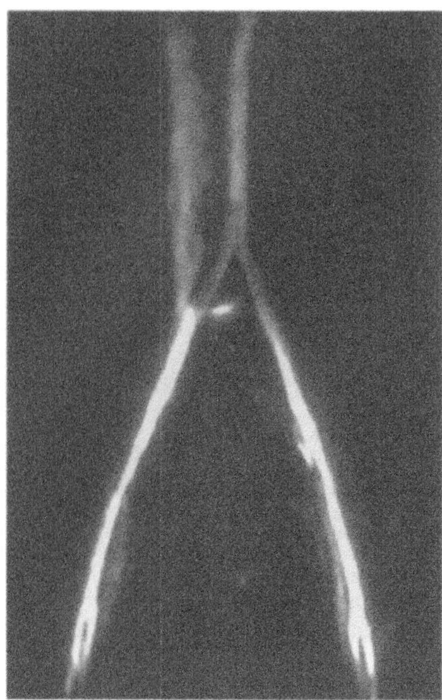

Fig. 12.12. The 2D PC MRA of the aortoiliac vessels shows the arteries with venous overlay by the iliac veins and inferior vena cava

encoding gradient sensitive for slow flow to image tibial vessels may result in the visualization of overlapping venous vessels. Both 2D PCA and 3D PCA combine certain advantages and disadvantages. 2D PCA has a shorter scan time, fewer saturation effects, improved background suppression, sensitivity to slow flow, and robustness against short T1. It is a projection technique with dephasing artifacts due to vessel overlap and is prone to aliasing. 3D PCA has fewer dephasing artifacts, and improved signal-to-noise ratio and resolution. Measurement is significantly longer and aliasing at low VENCs produces artifacts.

12.4 Artifacts of Contrast-Enhanced MR Angiography

12.4.1 Timing

The combination of short acquisition times of about 15–30 s for high-resolution CE-MRA and short contrast infusion times of about 2–15 s (10–30 ml of contrast material infused at 2–5 ml/s) requires precise bolus timing to achieve angiograms without venous enhancement (Boos et al. 1998). Several methods of ensuring accurate bolus timing have been developed. The easiest is the bolus timing method with a test bolus, typically 1 or 2 ml of contrast medium, to calculate for the bolus arrival time (BAT). The 3D scan is subsequently timed according to the BAT. This method does not require special hardware or software. Deviations in BAT among test scans and 3D scans may be due to inconsistent flow, volumes, or breathing. It is of utmost importance to keep all parameters (saline flush, contrast injection, breathing) constant. Alternative methods are semiautomatic techniques such as smart-scan (scan starts when a certain predefined level of signal increase is reached) or fluoroscopic triggering (real-time MR fluoroscopy to monitor contrast arrival) to initiate scanning during bolus arrival or rapid temporally resolved acquisitions (Schoenberg et al. 1999). Mistiming of the contrast bolus leads to a variety of artifacts (Maki et al. 1998).

12.4.2 Dose and Flow

The degree of T1 shortening depends on the intravascular concentration of contrast material. A low intravascular signal within major arteries may be caused by a slow flow rate. The bolus geometry depends on the parameters of the i.v. bolus injection (flow rate, dose and saline flush). An increased flow rate in the order of 2–4 ml/s, an increased saline volume (20–40 ml), and an increased saline flow (2–4 ml/s) can increase vessel contrast. Faster injections will mainly shorten the bolus without a significant effect on the resulting contrast. One potential pitfall is to acquire a high-resolution MRA scan with a bolus too short to cover the high-frequency k-lines at the outer k-space which defines image resolution. Therefore, the bolus geometry has to be consistent with all parameters to optimize for vessel contrast (Earls et al. 1996; Maki et al. 1998).

12.4.3 Venous Enhancement

When the data acquisition is initiated too late, depending on the scanned region, relevant venous enhancement may occur (Fig. 12.13). The carotid arteries and renal arteries with short arteriovenous circulation times often show venous enhancement in adjacent veins (internal jugular veins or renal veins).

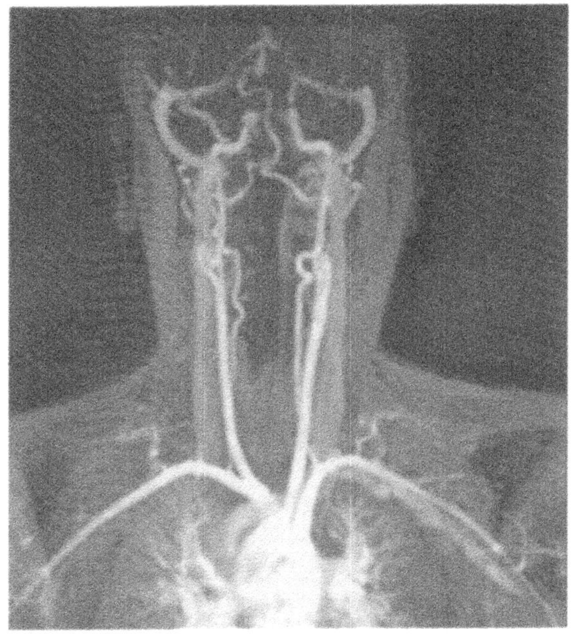

Fig. 12.13. CE-MRA of the supra-aortal arteries with the body phased array coil (flow rate 2 ml/s, 0.1 mmol Gd-DTPA/kg) and a high-resolution sequence (matrix 512+200, acquisition time 24 s) demonstrates complete venous enhancement due to the rapid venous return and long acquisition time

Venous enhancement may cause an overlay with the arteries hampering image interpretation. Although venous enhancement does not affect visualization of arteries on source data, it often degrades postprocessed images such as MIPs. This pitfall can be useful if information about venous vessels is also desired (Lebowitz et al. 1997). Data sets obtained during the venous phase subtracted from data sets obtained during the arterial phase may show a better venous contrast than postprocessed venous phase data sets alone. Another cause of peripheral venous enhancement is abnormal arteriovenous shunting, which may occur in up to 15% of patients at run-off studies (Fig. 12.14).

12.4.4 Maki Artifact

When the data acquisition is initiated too early, the central k-space lines are not "covered" by the maximum of contrast enhancement. Coronal source and MIP images show dark central vessels with bright edges or a stripe-like appearance near the vessel border (Fig. 12.15). The bolus arrives in the vessel after central contrast-determining low-frequency k-space lines have been collected while peripheral high spatial frequency lines that determine edge contrast are collected after contrast enhancement. This artifact is also called "Maki" artifact by some authors (Maki et al. 1996).

12.4.4.1 Mural or Extraluminal Pathology

Gadolinium-enhanced MRA displayed as postprocessed MIP images represents a visualization restricted to the vessel lumen (Lee et al. 2000). As on DSA, the caliber of aneurysms can be substantially underestimated if mural thrombosis results in a normal lumen diameter. Similarly, vasculitis and dissections or intramural hematomas can be missed. Imaging protocols of the major vessels or in case of referrals with suspected extraluminal pathology, therefore, must include unenhanced T1/T2-weighted sequences and possibly enhanced T1-

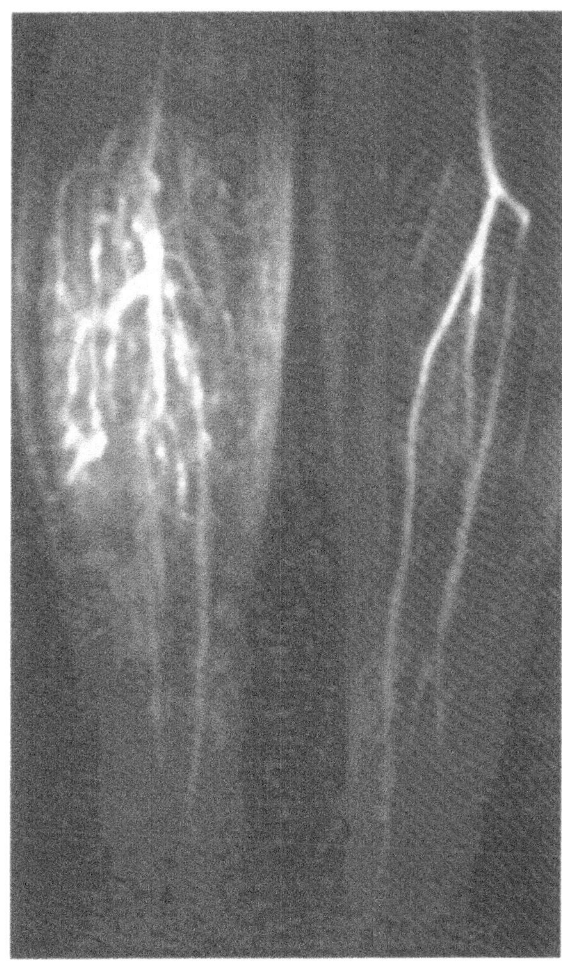

Fig. 12.14. CE-MRA run-off study of the pedal vessels demonstrates significant venous overlay most likely at least partially due to multiple AV fistulas

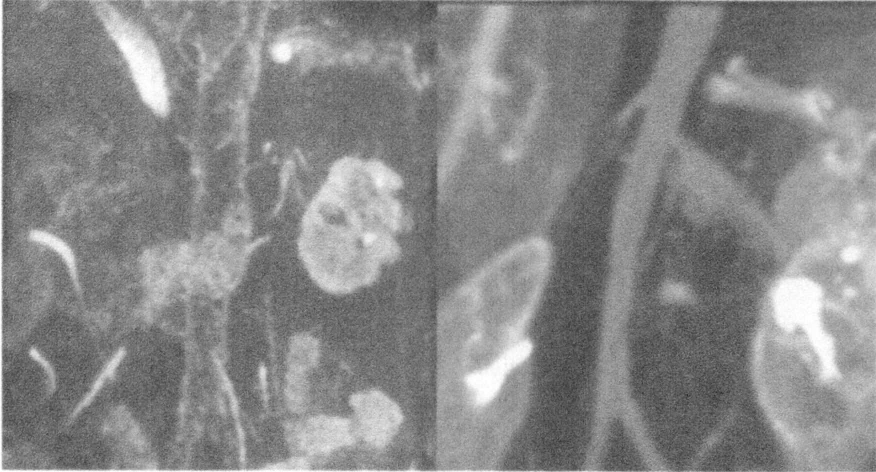

Fig. 12.15. Two CE-MRA studies of the abdomen with data acquisition of the middle of k-space before the contrast peak. The first example (*left*) shows almost complete dark bands within the aorta with little contrast and also significant shine-through artifacts of bright bowel content. The second example (*right*) demonstrates a thin dark band within the central lumen of the abdominal aorta

weighted sequences. Calcified atheromatous disease may be invisible on CE-MRA (Fig. 12.16).

12.4.4.2 Overestimation

Although to a lesser degree than with non-contrast-enhanced MRA techniques, CE-MRA also overestimates vascular stenoses because of spin dephasing by turbulent flow and partial volume effects. Standard voxel dimensions range in the order of =1 mm x≤2 mm x≤2 mm based upon a 128–512 matrix at a FOV of 300–500 mm. However, the remaining lumen within a stenotic segment may be smaller than 1 mm. The problem is aggravated on MIP images in which subtle vascular signal at a stenosis cannot be distinguished from background signal (Fig. 12.16). Therefore, grading of hemodynamic relevant stenoses should rely on assessment of source data (Hoogreveen et al. 1998; Lee et al. 2000).

12.4.4.3 Underestimation

Although to a lesser degree than overestimation, underestimation of stenoses may also occur due to partial volume effects, spatial resolution, and contrast resolution of 3D acquisitions (Lee et al. 2000). Again, the problem is aggravated on MIP images and grading is improved by the assessment of source data.

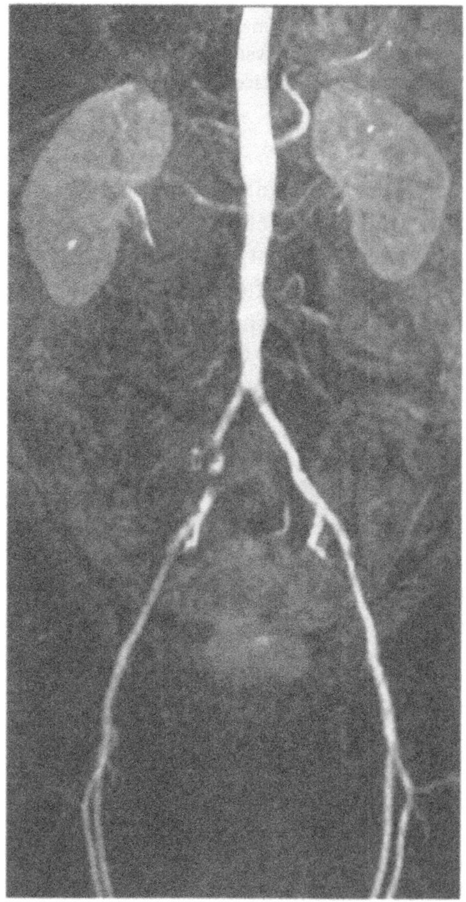

Fig. 12.16. CE-MRA of the aortoiliac region demonstrates small vessel segments with absent signal. These high-grade calcified stenoses are also overestimated by CE-MRA. Also relevant for CE-MRA, image interpretation requires the assessment of original data sets

12.4.5 Pseudodisease

Low image resolution [lower with large voxel dimensions (2 mm) relative to vessel size (renal arteries or small pedal arteries)] may result in an inaccurate display of vessels and assessment of vessel caliber. A stairstep or beaded vessel contour may result mimicking pathology such as fibromuscular dysplasia or vasculitis. Therefore, a higher resolution should be used for small vessels (LEE et al. 2000).

12.4.6 Image Filtering

Some vendors offer dedicated filter software for additional postprocessing of MRA data sets. With this software, data sets or already postprocessed data sets may be either smoothed or edge enhanced. This feature is primarily used to artificially enhance vessel background contrast and make signal within vessels more homogeneous. However, the physician using this particular postprocessing tool may also smooth vascular pathology and thus underestimate disease (Fig. 12.17). Therefore, these postprocessing steps should only be performed when the diagnosis has been made based on the original data set, the overview MIP, and targeted MIPs to highlight imaging results and impress our medical colleagues.

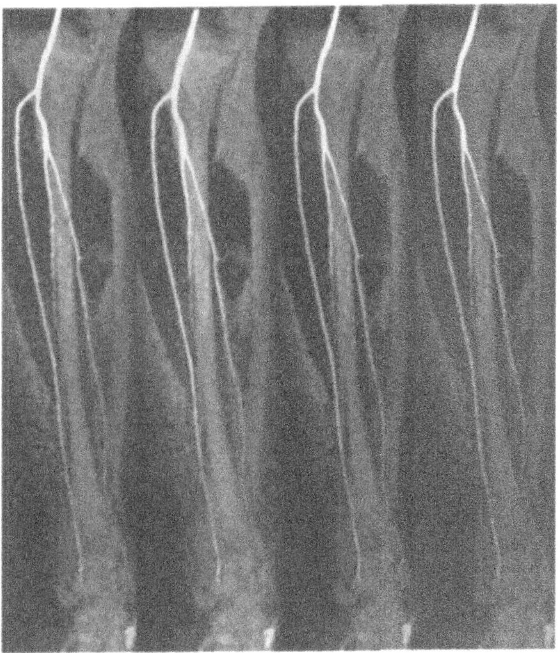

Fig. 12.17. Different filter algorithms [*from left to right*: raw data, smooth, intermediate (smooth/sharp), and sharp] are applied to the same CE-MRA data set. The images of the pedal vessels demonstrate that filtering modifies the visibility, appearance, and conspicuity of vessels. Signal within vessels and the entire images become more homogeneous while small irregularities of the vessel wall are less conspicuous. Image interpretation requires the assessment of original data sets prior to filtering. Filtered images are nevertheless preferred by clinicians. The images also demonstrate shine through artifacts from bone marrow and fat

12.4.7 Metallic Artifacts

Susceptibility artifacts from metallic stents, joint prostheses, surgical clips, and shrapnel may cause signal loss within a vessel mimicking stenoses or occlusions (Figs. 12.18, 12.19). Careful reviewing of source data and clinical history are essential. Newer stent design, such as with some stents with thin nitinol structures, allows for an assessment of the stent lumen (BAUM et al. 2000; HILFIKER et al. 1999).

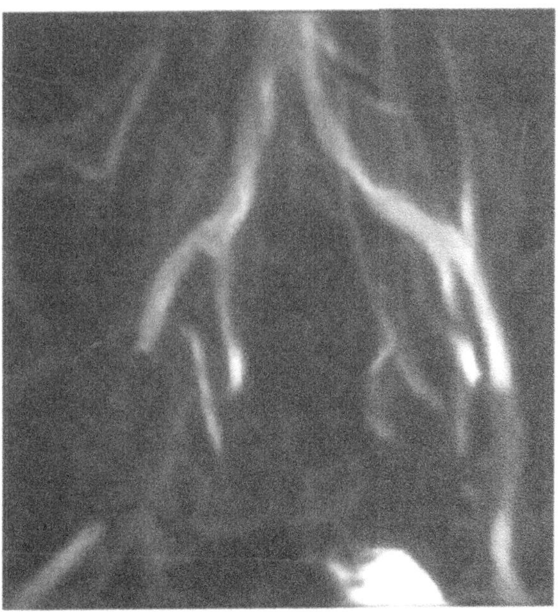

Fig. 12.18. CE 3D MRA of the pelvic arteries after stent implantation. Complete signal loss in the right external iliac artery is caused by a stainless steal stent (Palmaz-Stent). Partial signal loss in the left external iliac artery is caused by a nitinol stent (Memotherm-Stent)

12.4.8 Inflow Artifacts

Gadolinium is typically injected into one cubital vein. Residual concentrated gadolinium contrast material may remain in central veins causing susceptibility artifacts in ipsilateral veins (LEE et al. 1999). The T2* artifact may cause adjacent signal loss and create a

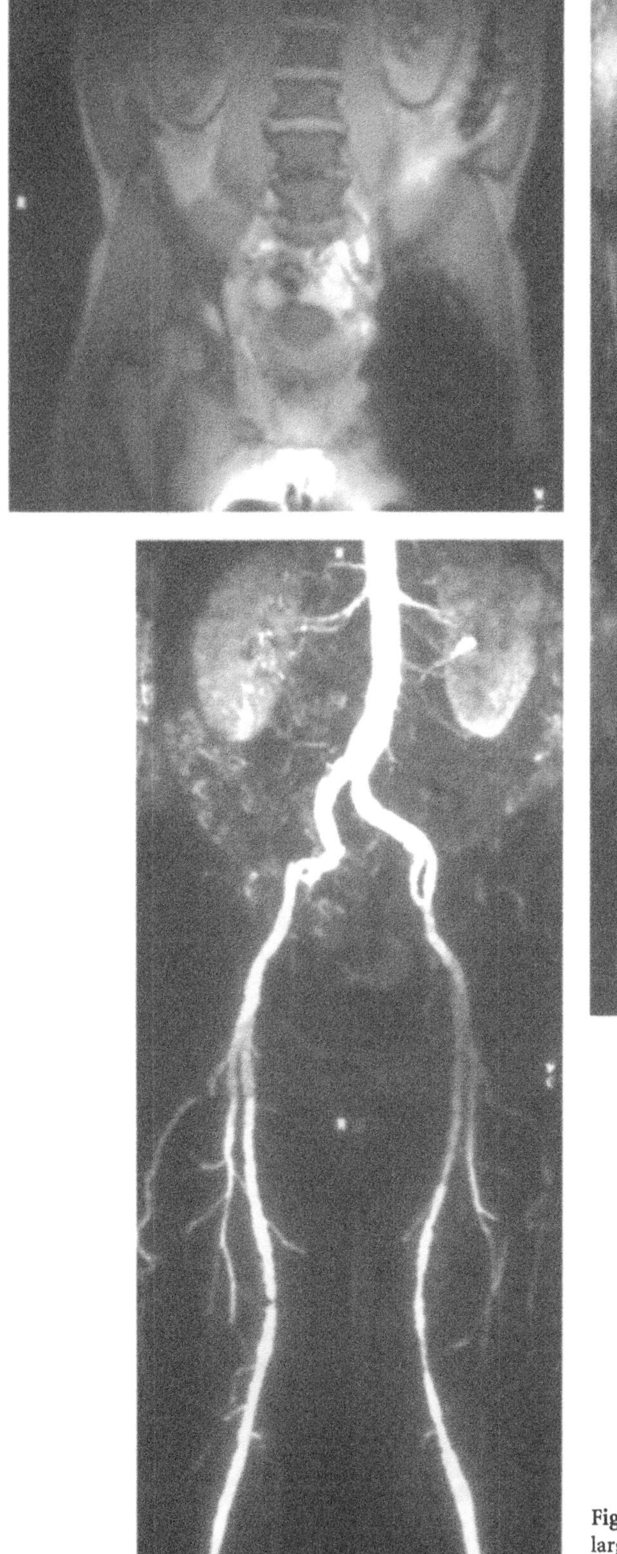

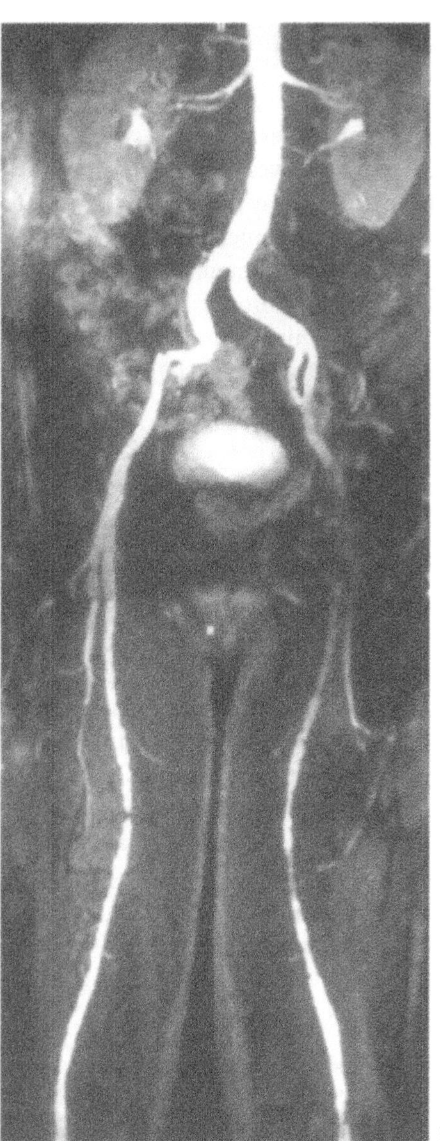

a b c

Fig. 12.19. A 2D FLASH localizer (**a**) of the pelvis shows a large susceptibility artifact caused by a left-sided hip prosthesis. Unsubtracted CE 3D MRA (**b**) demonstrates a markedly reduced signal intensity of left external iliac artery and proximal femoral artery. The use of a subtraction technique (**c**) leads to better diagnostic image quality

false positive stenosis or occlusion when veins and arteries are in close proximity. Since the left brachiocephalic vein crosses not only the left-sided arterial vessels but also the central arterial vessels, a right-sided injection is recommended when the supra-aortal vasculature is imaged. Delayed imaging may resolve uncertain cases (KRINSKY et al. 1998).

12.4.9 Subtraction

Subtraction of data sets is a tool to increase vessel contrast (LEBOWITZ et al. 1997). Typically, a plain data set and a contrast-enhanced data set are obtained and subtracted from each other (Fig. 12.19). The subtracted data set is then postprocessed. This also applies to arterial and venous phase data sets. Inconsistent filling of all vessels with contrast medium may result in an incomplete signal within vessels mimicking pathology.

12.4.10 Fat Suppression

Tissues with short T1 relaxation times (fat, bone marrow, hemorrhage, and bowel content) will also have high signal intensity on MRA images and may interfere with image interpretation. Again, the problem is aggravated on MIP images, and image interpretation is improved by the assessment of source data (Figs 12.15, 12.17). Fat-suppression techniques or image subtraction techniques, or both, can be used to improve vessel visualization (LEE et al. 2000).

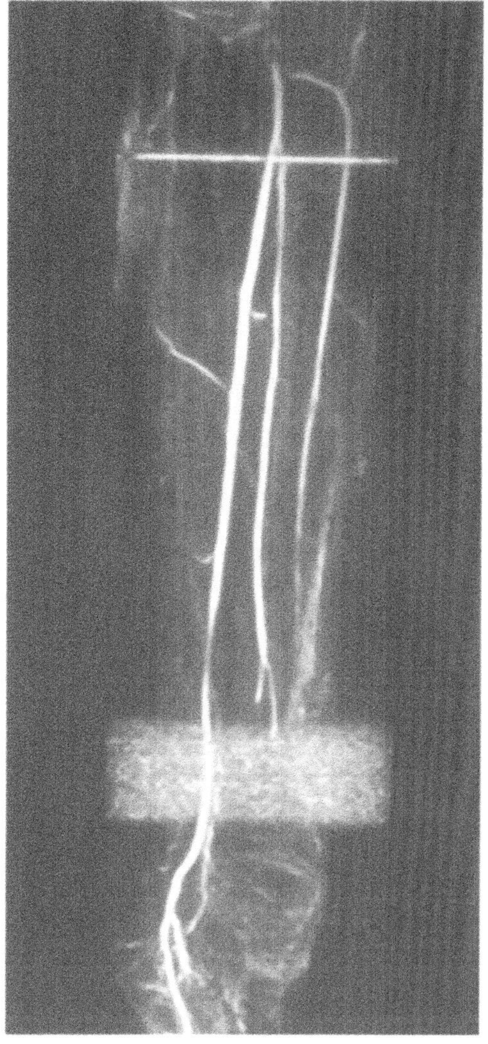

Fig. 12.20. CE 3D MRA of the lower limb showing banding artifacts. A defect in the cabin door isolation caused the artifacts

12.5 Tips – Source Data, Overview MIP, and Targeted MIP

Many misinterpretations can be avoided my evaluating the MRA data sets with a vigorous routine (Fig. 12.20). We recommend that the interpreting physician analyze the quality of source data sets before an overview MIP is generated by the technician. A careful analysis of the source data set detects most of the general and specific artifacts encountered in the particular technique used. The responsible physician should then process targeted MIP images going along with the clinical question and the specific findings of the particular study. For the final diagnosis, all available imaging data consisting of the source data set, the overview MIP, and the targeted MIPs should be utilized.

References

Anderson CM, Saloner D, Tsuruda J, Shapeero L, Lee R (1990) Artifacts in maximum-intensity projection display of MR angiograms. AJR Am J Roentgenol 154: 623–629

Atkinson DJ, Vu B, Chen DY, Duerinckx A, Bradley WG (1997) First pass MRA of the abdomen: ultrafast, non-breath-hold time-of- flight imaging using Gd-DTPA bolus. J Magn Reson Imaging 7:1159–1162

Baum F, Vosshenrich R, Fischer U, Castillo E, Grabbe E (2000)

Stent artifacts in 3D MR angiography: experimental studies. Rofo Fortschr Geb Rontgenstr Neuen Bildgeb Verfahr 172:278–281

Boos M, Lentschig M, Scheffler K, Bongartz GM, Steinbrich W (1998) Contrast-enhanced magnetic resonance angiography of peripheral vessels. Different contrast agent applications and sequence strategies: a review. Invest Radiol 33:538–546

Brunereau L, Bousson V, Arrive L, Levy C, Marsot-Dupuch K, Tubiana JM (1998) Artifacts in magnetic resonance angiography. J Radiol 79:849–859

Dumoulin CL, Steinberg FL, Yucel EK, Darrow RD (1993) Reduction of artifacts from breathing and peristalsis in phase-contrast MRA of the chest and abdomen. J Comput Assist Tomogr 17:328–332

Earls J, Rofsky N, DeCorato D, Krinsky G, Weinreb J (1996) Breath-hold single-dose gadolinium-enhanced three-dimensional MR angiography. Usefulness of a timing examination and MR power injector. Radiology 201:705–710

Frank A, Selby K, van Tyen R, Nordell B, Saloner D (1995) Cardiac-gated MR angiograms of pulsatile flow. K-space strategies. J Magn Reson Imaging 5:297–307

Fürst G, Hofer M, Sitzer M, Kahn T, Muller E, Modder U (1995) Factors influencing flow-induced signal loss in MR angiography: an in vitro study. J Comput Assist Tomogr 19:692–699

Grieve JP, Stacey R, Moore E, Kitchen ND, Jager HR (1999) Artefact on MRA following aneurysm clipping: an in vitro study and prospective comparison with conventional angiography. Neuroradiology 41:680–686

Hilfiker PR, Quick HH, Schmidt M, Debatin JF (1999) In vitro image characteristics of an abdominal aortic stent graft: CTA versus 3D MRA. Magma 8:27–32

Hoogreveen R, Bakker C, Viergever M (1998) Limits of accuracy of vessel diameter measurement in MR angiography. J Magn Reson Imaging 8:1228–1235

Kaufman J, Mc Carter D, Geller S, Waltman A (1998) Two-dimensional time-of-flight MR angiography of the lower extremities: artifacts and pitfalls. AJR Am J Roentgenol 171:129–135

Krinsky G, Maya M, Rofsky N, Lebowitz J, Nelson PK, Ambrosino M, Kaminer E, Earls J, Masters L, Giangola G, Litt A, Weinreb J (1998) Gadolinium-enhanced 3D MRA of the aortic arch vessels in the detection of atherosclerotic cerebrovascular occlusive disease. J Comput Assist Tomogr 22:167–178

Lebowitz J, Rofsky N, Krinsky G, Weinreb J (1997) Gadolinium-enhanced body MR venography with subtraction technique. AJR Am J Roentgenol 169:755–758

Lee V, Martin D, Krinsky G, Rofsky N (2000) Gadolinium-enhanced MR angiography: artifacts and pitfalls. AJR Am J Roentgenol 175:197–205

Lee Y, Chung T, Joo J, Chien D, Laub G (1999) Suboptimal contrast-enhanced carotid MR angiography from the left brachiocephalic venous stasis. J Magn Reson Imaging 10:503–509

Maki J, Pronce M, Londy F, Chenevert T (1996) The effects of time varying intravascular signal intensity and K-space acquisition order on three-dimensional MR angiography image quality. J Magn Reson Imaging 6:642–651

Maki JH, Prince MR, Chenevert TC (1998) Optimizing three-dimensional gadolinium-enhanced magnetic resonance angiography. Invest Radiol 33:528–537

Mirowitz SA (1993) Apparent vascular occlusion on cranial TOF MRA with peripheral presaturation technique. J Comput Assist Tomogr 17:927–931

Okamoto K, Ito J, Furusawa T, Sakai K, Tokiguchi S (1997) "Pseudoocclusion" of the internal carotid artery: a pitfall on intracranial MRA. J Comput Assist Tomogr 21:831–833

Owen R, Baum R, Carpenter J, Holland G, Cope GA (1993) Symptomatic peripheral vascular disease: selection of imaging parameters and clinical evaluation with MR angiography. Radiology 187:627–635

Schmieder K, Falk A, Hardenack M, Heuser L, Harders A (1999) Clinical utility of magnetic resonance angiography in the evaluation of aneurysms from a neurosurgical point of view. Zentralbl Neurochir 60:61–67

Schoenberg SO, Wunsch C, Knopp MV, Essig M, Hawighorst H, Laub G, Prince MR, Allenberg JR, Van Kaick G (1999) Abdominal aortic aneurysm. Detection of multilevel vascular pathology by time-resolved multiphase 3D gadolinium MR angiography: initial report. Invest Radiol 34:648–659

Schreiner S, Paschal CB, Galloway RL (1996) Comparison of projection algorithms used for the construction of maximum intensity projection images. J Comput Assist Tomogr 20:56–67

Schurmann K, Vorwerk D, Bucker A, Neuerburg J, Grosskortenhaus S, Haage P, Piroth W, Hunter DW, Gunther RW (1999) Magnetic resonance angiography of nonferromagnetic iliac artery stents and stent-grafts: a comparative study in sheep. Cardiovasc Intervent Radiol 22:394–402

Shellock F (2000) Pocket guide to MR procedures and metallic objects:update 2000. Raven Press, New York

Shellock F, Kanal E (1998) Aneurysm clips: evaluation of MR imaging artifacts at 1.5 T. Radiology 209:563–566

Stringer WA (1997) MRA image production and display. Clin Neurosci 4:110–116

Tsuruda J, Saloner D, Norman D (1992) Artifacts associated with MR neuroangiography. AJNR Am J Neuroradiol 13:1411–1422

Wilcock DJ, Jaspan T, Worthington BS (1995) Problems and pitfalls of 3-D TOF magnetic resonance angiography of the intracranial circulation. Clin Radiol 50:526–532

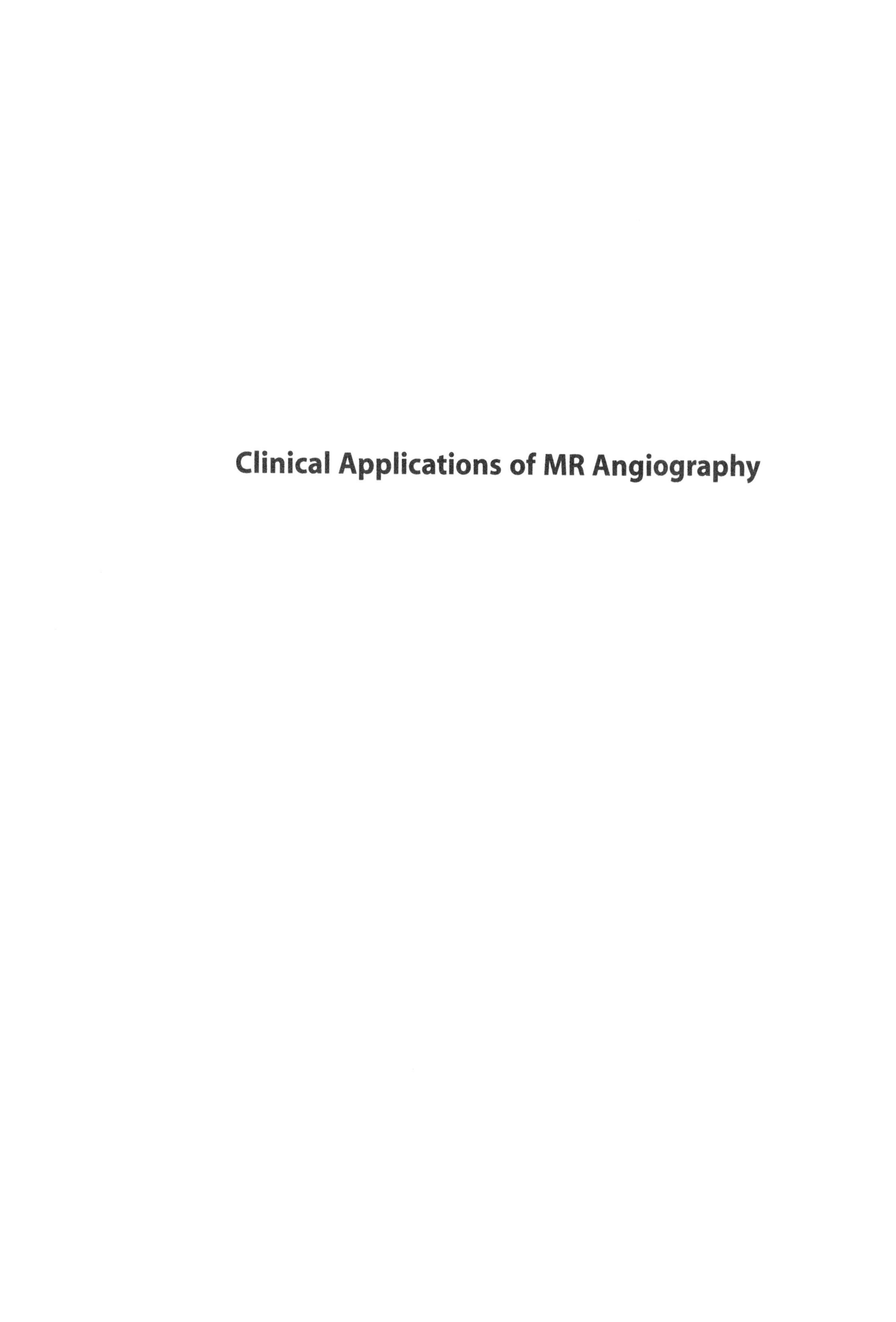

Clinical Applications of MR Angiography

13 Intracranial Vessels

GUIDO WILMS, GUY MARCHAL, HILDE BOSMANS

CONTENTS

13.1 Introduction

X-ray angiography remains the gold standard for the study of the intracranial vessels, (BRANT-ZAWADZKI et al. 1983). For some time now, conventional cut film angiography has been replaced by digital subtraction techniques. After the initial over-enthusiasm for the intravenous application of digital subtraction angiography, the method was rapidly abandoned due to insufficient vessel contrast, superimposition of vascular territories and the requirement of good patient co-operation (WILMS et al. 1983). Nowadays the intra-arterial selective and superselective study of the intracranial vessels with digital subtraction is routinely used for the visualisation of the intracranial vessels (BRANT-ZAWADZKI et al. 1983).

The morphological information obtained from these studies offers exquisite anatomical detail with visualisation of very small distal cortical or deep branches, especially if a matrix of 1024×1024 is used. The venous anatomy and drainage both of normal brain and of pathological conditions is very well demonstrated. Besides the morphological information, some flow information is obtained due to the temporal character of the technique, with sequential image acquisition during the arterial, capillary and venous phase. This allows visualisation of local or generalised flow changes, such as an increase or decrease, asymmetry between the hemispheres, and steal phenomena or venous shunting (BRANT-ZAWADZKI et al. 1983). In addition, the development of very small and flexible microcatheters now allows superselective catheterization of distal cerebral arteries, permitting detailed study of the contributing arteries to arteriovenous malformations or tumours (VINUELA et al. 1989).

Similarly, the treatment during interventional angiography of cerebral aneurysms, arteriovenous malformations, arteriovenous fistulas, and even stenotic disease based on vasospasm or atherosclerosis is part of the routine practice of many centres (VINUELA et al. 1989). Unfortunately, even in experienced hands, angiography remains an invasive method, with the possibility of severe neurological and even life-threatening complications (WAUGH and SACHARIAS 1992). The risk of a neurological event is estimated at 4%, with permanent deficit in 1% (HANKEY et al. 1990). Furthermore, the information obtained by angiography is mostly indirect, both for vascular and non-vascular diseases. The exact size of an aneurysm can be underestimated, haemorrhage in an arteriovenous malformation is not detected, etc. The absence of soft tissue information in angiography is a

G. WILMS, MD
Professor, Department of Radiology, University Hospitals K.U. Leuven, Herestraat 49, 3000 Leuven, Belgium
G. MARCHAL, MD, PhD
Professor, Department of Radiology, University Hospitals K.U. Leuven, Herestraat 49, 3000 Leuven, Belgium
H. BOSMANS, PhD
Professor, MR Physicist, Department of Radiology, University Hospitals K.U. Leuven, Herestraat 49, 3000 Leuven, Belgium

major drawback, which necessitates additional cross-sectional techniques, such as computed tomography (CT), or magnetic resonance imaging (MRI).

Transcranial Doppler, particularly in combination with colour Doppler, is a valuable non-invasive alternative for the functional study of the cerebral vessels, but unfortunately with poor morphological performance (De Bray et al. 1988; Mursch et al. 2000; Schminke et al. 2000). It allows the detection and follow-up of flow alterations in the major cranial vessels and the evaluation of the intracranial vascular reserve during carotid compression, and can even be performed as a bed-side examination. In comparison with angiography and ultrasonography (US), the most important advantage of newer techniques such as MRA (Blatter et al. 1992; Huston and Ehman 1993; Marchal et al. 1990, 1992; Pernicone et al. 1990, 1992; Ruggieri et al. 1992), and recently CTA (Schwartz et al. 1994), is the integrated display of both vessels and soft tissues. In addition, magnetic resonance angiography (MRA) allows the quantification of intracranial flow

13.2 Technical Considerations

Both flow-dependent and flow-independent MRA techniques can be used for the visualisation of the intracranial vessels. The use of flow-dependent techniques is possible, as throughout the cardiac cycle there is a substantial inflow effect. In addition, the intracranial vessels are confined to a small volume of interest, which can be studied with high-performance coils. Furthermore, the effects of the most common causes of MR artefacts, such as respiration, cardiac motion, and susceptibility changes are minimal. Moreover, the clinical experience with MRA of the intracranial vessels is rapidly increasing.

There is still no single robust time-of-flight sequence that can be used for all intracranial MRA applications. It is clear that the techniques will differ for the study of arterial or venous disease. The quality of venous MR angiograms is strongly determined by the saturation phenomenon. Arterial MR angiograms are less degraded by saturation, but flow-induced dephasing may be highly undesirable.

In the following sections we shall discuss the different techniques being explored today that can be used for visualisation of intracranial vessels. A sequence protocol will be provided, and the advantage of using multiple acquisitions to clarify unexpected signal behaviour will be stressed. We will then focus on ultrafast contrast-enhanced MRA of intracranial vessels, proposing possible parameter settings.

13.2.1 Cerebral Arteriography

13.2.1.1 Time-of-Flight Acquisitions

Although successful two-dimensional (2D) MRA examinations of intracranial arterial diseases have been reported, the acquisition of true 3D data is preferred since they provide more detailed angiograms that can be viewed from any projection direction. Three-dimensional (3D) time-of-flight (TOF) techniques are often used to study intracranial arteries. An example of a 3D TOF acquisition of a normal young volunteer is shown in Fig. 13.1a. In clinical practice, the vessel detail is often inferior to this example due to saturation. This effect commonly arises in patients with a reduced cardiac output or lesions with impaired arterial flow. Therefore, the MR parameters should always be carefully adjusted (Ruggieri et al. 1989; Haacke et al. 1990). In addition, many of the techniques developed to reduce saturation and to increase the signal-to-noise ratio between the blood vessels and the stationary tissues have to be applied whenever possible. This is especially true if high-resolution acquisitions are performed.

13.2.1.1.1 TONE

To overcome saturation in transverse MRA acquisitions of the brain, a first technique is the use of "tilted optimised non-saturating excitation" (TONE) radiofrequency (RF) pulses. These pulses provide flip angles that are variable along the slice selection direction. Typically, low flip angles are applied at the entrance side of the arteries in the volume of interest to delay the saturation phenomenon. The flip angle is then steadily increased along the cranial direction. Using increasing flip angles maximally recovers the remaining signal of the flowing blood (Tkach et al. 1992; Atkinson 1994). In Fig. 13.1a and b, we compare the MR angiograms obtained with a regular RF pulse and a TONE RF excitation pulse (10° at the entrance side of the intracranial arteries and 30° near the top of the 3D volume). The peripheral branches are better visualised by using TONE excitation pulses.

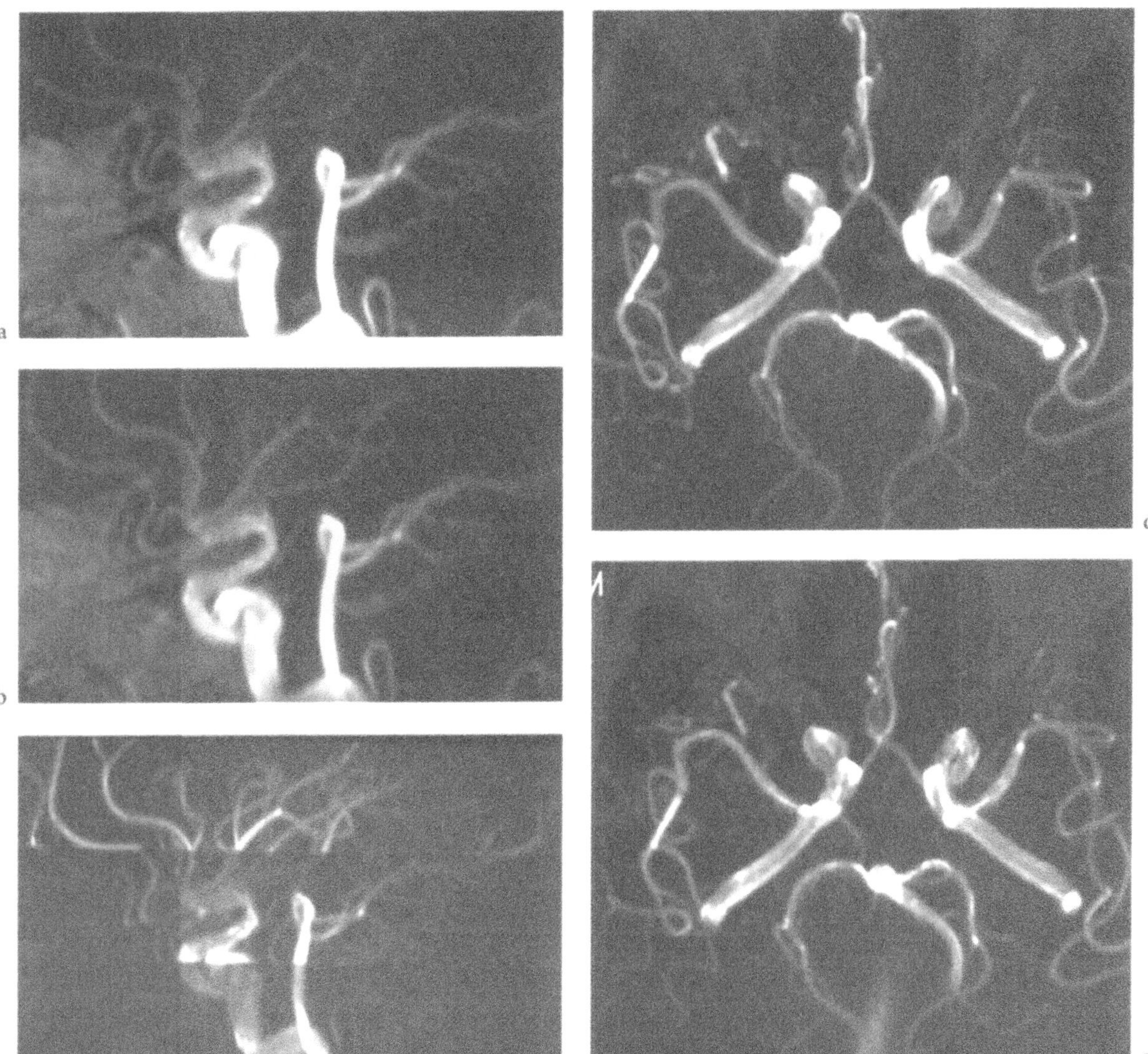

Fig. 13.1a–e. High-resolution TOF MRA of a normal young volunteer, TR/TE/Fl 24 ms/7 ms/20°, rectangular FOV 158×250 mm. **a** Sagittal projection, single volume. **b** Identical acquisition, TONE RF excitation pulse. **c** Acquisition using multiple thin slabs. **d** Transverse projection, multiple thin slab acquisition (MOTSA), TONE RF excitation pulse. **e** Identical acquisition as in **d**, but with magnetisation transfer preparation pulse (TR 40 ms). As the different techniques are added, the quality of the MR angiograms steadily increases

13.2.1.1.2
Multiple Overlapping Thin Slab Acquisition (MOTSA)

Theoretically, all the intracranial vessels can be examined with a single transverse, sagittal or coronal 3D TOF acquisition using a slab thickness of 128 mm/128 partitions. With this technique, however, there is obvious signal decrease in the blood vessels that are distal in the volume. In order to reduce the saturation, the number of excitations for the spins in the vessels has to be reduced. This can be done by acquiring multiple consecutive 3D TOF acquisitions restricted to a smaller part of the brain, using for example a slab thickness of 32 mm/32 partitions. If the acquisition volume is oriented transversally, the saturation of the blood is minimised. Because the slab excitation profiles in the slice selection direction are never ideal, these multiple 3D acquisitions have to be mutually overlapping. MR angiograms are calculated from a single data set that is composed of images obtained during the different consecutive acquisitions (Marchal et al. 1990; Blatter et al. 1991; Lewin et al. 1991). If the MRA data are projected along an axis different from the slice selection direction, the transitions between the different slabs remain visible in the angiograms (Fig. 13.1c). Increasing the slab overlap and reducing the number of partitions can reduce this "Venetian blind artefact". Blatter et al. (1993) propose MRA acquisitions using 16 partitions, 50% slab overlap and a post-processing algorithm that combines the overlapping slabs from each adjacent slab by selecting on a pixel-by-pixel basis the brightest of the spatially coincident pixels.

13.2.1.1.3
Prepulses

Another way to cope with saturation in the intracranial arteries with 3D TOF acquisitions is the suppression of the signal of the stationary tissues (Edelman et al. 1992; Lin et al. 1993; Atkinson 1994). Fat suppression prepulses can be applied. However, this requires a well-shimmed system that is free of eddy currents. If spins of the blood have a precessional frequency matching the resonance frequency of the fatty tissue before entering the volume of interest, they are saturated by the fat suppression prepulse. In addition, in the brain, the contribution of fatty signal is small. Superposition of fatty tissue in the maximum-intensity-projections (MIPs) can largely be avoided by means of a targeted MIP, which is available on routine scanners. Therefore, this prepulse is not often used in routine MRA protocols for intracranial vessels.

The use of magnetisation transfer (MT) prepulses is more widespread (Mathews et al. 1999). In brain MRA, this technique mainly suppresses the signal of the brain tissue. The benefits of MT prepulses are more obvious than those of fat saturation pulses. Besides, this application does not put extreme requirements on the system hardware. The minimal repetition time (TR) is, however, shorter. A comparison of a 3D TOF with TONE RF excitation and with and without MT prepulse is shown in Fig. 13.1d and e. The contrast-to-noise ratio between vessel and brain tissue is significantly improved and therefore small vessels are better visualised.

13.2.1.1.4
Contrast Enhancement

Another method to reduce saturation in a 3D TOF MRA image is the intravenous injection of a contrast agent that shortens the T1 of the blood (Yano et al. 1997; Mathews et al. 1999). The veins and small arterial branches are better visualised on a CE TOF study than in a plain MRA study. The disadvantages of the use of contrast agents with TOF techniques are the more invasive character of the technique and an increased cost. It is impossible to separate arteries from veins by means of saturation pulses. Finally, soft tissues may enhance and superimpose on the angiogram.

13.2.1.1.5
Targeted MIP

In the MIP, the contrast-to-noise ratio of the vessels may be poor. This is due to superposition of high signal intensities of subcutaneous tissues. A postprocessing procedure that nulls the signal of the subcutaneous tissues before projection provides angiograms with better contrast-to-noise ratio. Theoretically, with targeted MIP (Fig. 13.2) the same result could

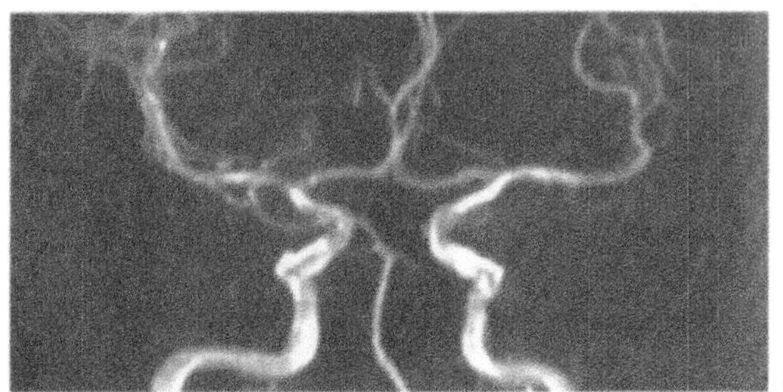

a

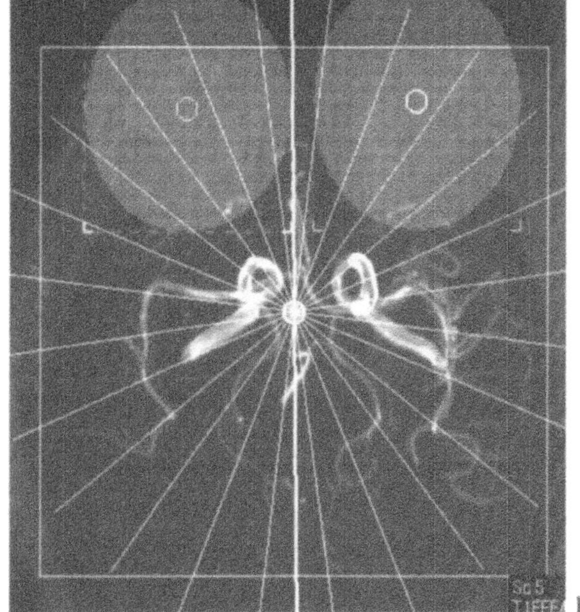

b

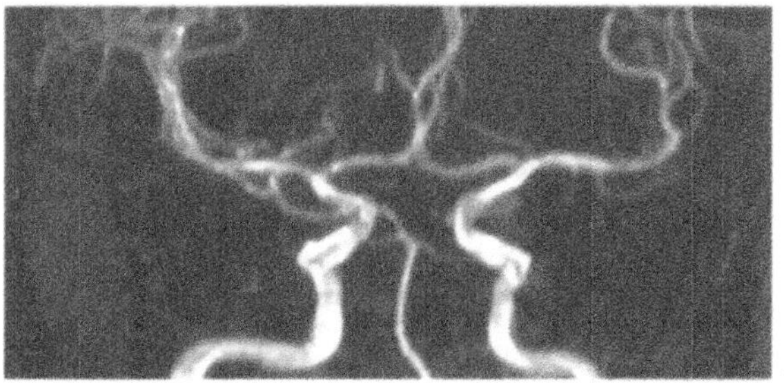

c

Fig. 13.2a–c. TOF acquisition in a normal young volunteer (TR/TE/Fl 40 ms/7 ms/20°, FOV 250 mm, slab thickness 32 mm/32partitions, matrix 192×512). **a** Coronal projection. **b** Transverse overview showing the subvolume that was projected and the two volumes of which the signal intensities were excluded from the MIP. **c** Targeted MIP shows improved vessel detail

be obtained. However, contouring the tissues may be time-consuming. Automation of this procedure may be helpful.

13.2.1.1.6
Gadolinium-Enhanced Dynamic 3D MRA

Dynamic 3D MRA after bolus injection of gadolinium uses ultrashort TR (±6 ms) and TE (±2 ms) without flow compensation to obtain ultrafast MRA of the intracranial vessels (Lang et al. 1998; Parker et al. 1998; Isoda et al. 2000; Metens et al. 2000) (Fig. 13.3). Typically, three consecutive acquisitions of 18 s are obtained. This allows a very accurate study of the intracranial vasculature without signal-intensity losses due to turbulence or flow-saturation effects. The very short acquisition time of the sequence makes it more suitable for use with uncooperative patients (Metens et al. 2000). In the MRA study of arteriovenous malformations, it allows dynamic information to be obtained by the consecutive acquisition of images in the arterial and venous phase.

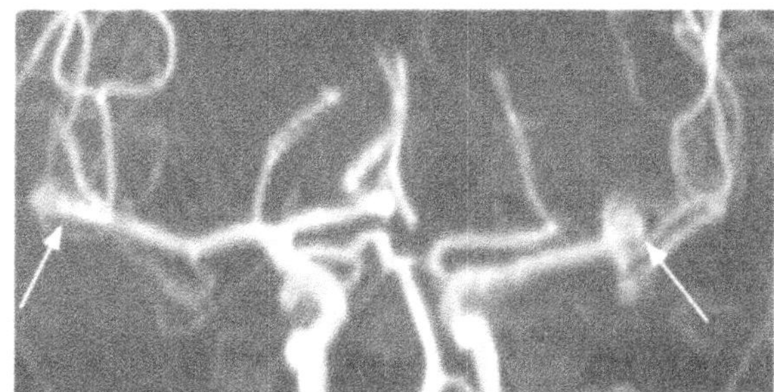

a

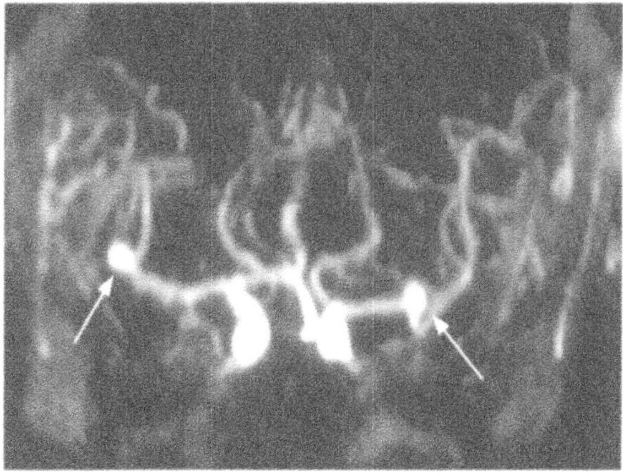

b

Fig. 13.3a, b. Dynamic contrast-enhanced MRA in a patient with bilateral aneurysms of the middle cerebral artery. **a** 3D TOF MRA (TR/TE/Fl 39 ms/7 ms/20°, FOV 150+200, matrix 192+256, acquisition time of 12 min). Bilateral ("mirror") aneurysms of the middle cerebral artery (*arrows*). **b** Dynamic contrast-enhanced MRA after bolus injection of 15 ml of gadolinium-DTPA (TR/TE/Fl 3.2 ms/1.1 ms/25°, matrix 96×120, interpolation along k_z, acquisition time of 17 s). Confirmation of the bilateral middle cerebral artery aneurysms (*arrows*). Note lower resolution

13.2.1.2
Phase-Contrast Acquisitions

Three-dimensional phase-contrast (PC) acquisitions are another means of overcoming the saturation (Pernicorne et al. 1990). The choice of an appropriate velocity-encoding gradient (VENC) can be difficult in arterial disease, as both extremely low and very rapid flow can be present, e.g., in arteriovenous malformations. A major advantage of the PC technique is that the quality of the angiograms is largely independent of the orientation of the acquisition volume. In the sagittal 3D PC acquisition (Fig. 13.4), saturation is still present but the blood vessel signal remains significantly higher than the background signal. Using the PC acquisition, arteries and veins can be studied by the same procedure. The image detail is lower than that achieved with a CE (high-resolution) TOF acquisition, but the latter suffers from superimposition of enhancing soft tissues. The use of PC acquisitions is also indicated in patients with acute thrombosis and bleeding associated with vascular malformations. In contrast to

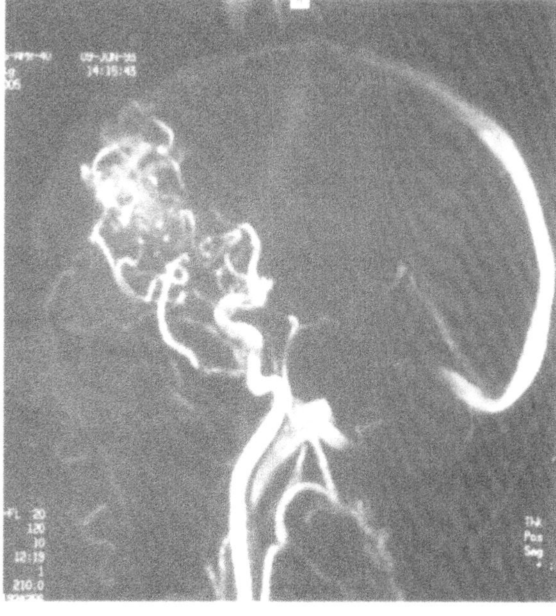

Fig. 13.4. PC acquisition in a patient with an AVM in the frontal lobe (TR/TE/Fl 30 ms/10 ms/20°, VENC 35 cm/s, FOV 210 mm, matrix 192×256, slab thickness 64 mm/32 partitions, sagittal acquisition volume, acquisition time of 12 min). This PC acquisition shows the feeder arteries coming from both the internal and external carotid artery, the nidus, and some draining veins

TOF acquisitions, all stationary tissue signals, including those from high signal intensity blood, are suppressed.

13.2.1.3
Flow-Induced Turbulence

Flow-induced dephasing is a very fundamental problem in both TOF and PC MRA. It consists of a signal dropout frequently seen in the knee of the middle cerebral arteries, in the carotid siphon, in hyperdynamic flow situations, and in aneurysms. It occurs with any bright-blood acquisition technique that fails to refocus the flowing spins at the echo time. For the reduction of flow-induced dephasing, a first approach is to use sequences in which the amplitude and the duration of the applied gradients are minimised (Schmalbrock et al. 1990; Evans et al. 1993). MR imagers with more powerful gradient systems perform better in this regard. A second approach is to increase the image resolution. Theoretically, smaller voxels contain a smaller range of flow velocities. Hence, the intravoxel dispersion is reduced. This effect is well known from comparative studies of 2D and 3D acquisitions: 2D acquisitions that use thicker slices to improve the signal-to-noise ratio frequently enhance flow-induced dephasing. This phenomenon is illustrated in Fig. 13.5. A patient with a stenosis in

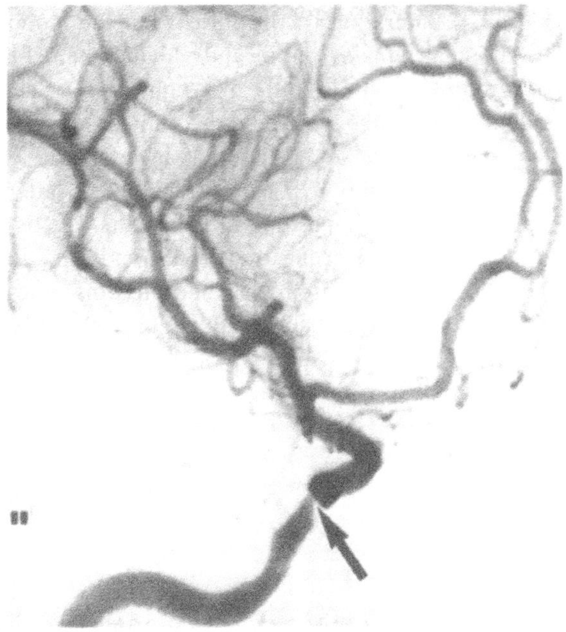

a

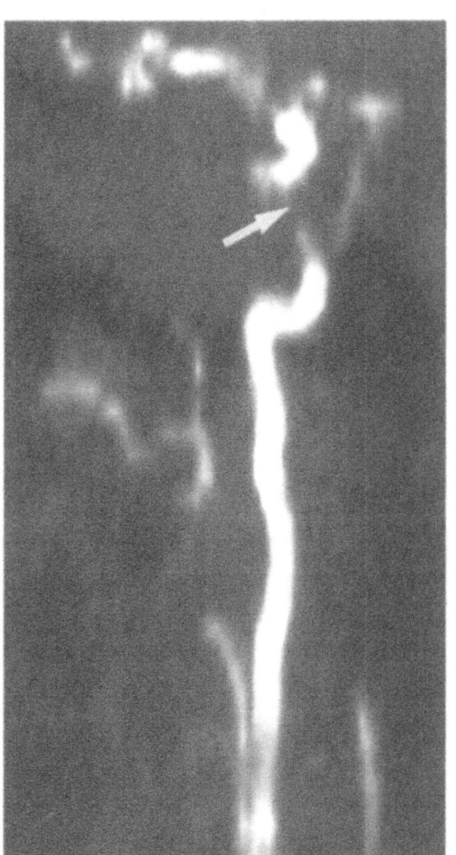

b

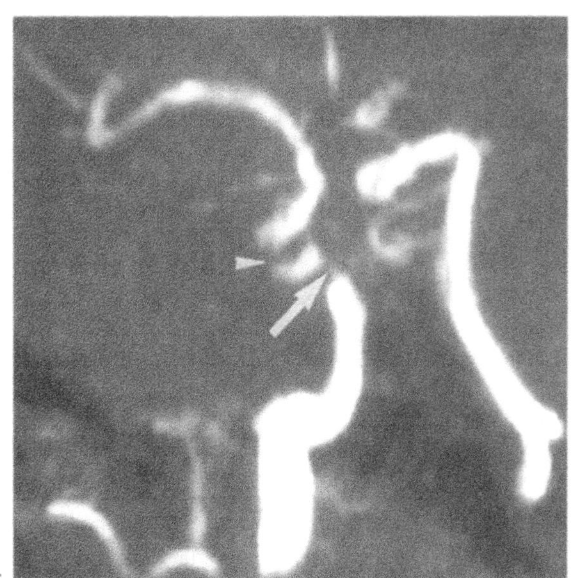

c

Fig. 13.5a–c. Comparative digital subtraction angiography (DSA) and TOF study in a patient with a stenosis in the petrosal portion of the carotid artery. **a** DSA examination shows stenosis of proximal carotid siphon (*arrow*). **b** 2D TOF acquisition, TR/TE/Fl 40 ms/10 ms/35°, FOV 200 mm, slice thickness 3 mm, venous presaturation, transverse slices. **c** 3D high-resolution TOF study, TR/TE/Fl 42 ms/11 ms/25°, FOV 200 mm, slab thickness 52 mm/64 partitions, matrix 192×512, transverse acquisition volume. The stenosis (*arrow*) is detected in both the 2D and the 3D TOF acquisition. The stenosis is overgraded in the 2D TOF study and accurately visualised in the 3D TOF study. Flow-induced signal voids in the carotid siphon are seen in the 3D study (*arrowhead*)

the cranial portion of the carotid siphon was examined with a 2D TOF and a 3D high-resolution TOF acquisition. The lesion was seen in both acquisitions but the degree of stenosis was overestimated in the 2D TOF acquisition whereas it was correctly visualised in the 3D TOF study.

A comparison between a lower resolution acquisition with field of view (FOV) 210 mm, matrix 192×256, slab thickness 52 mm/64 partitions and a higher resolution acquisition with matrix 192×512 is shown in Fig. 13.6. The flow-induced dephasing in the carotid siphon is more obvious in the high-resolution study than in the lower resolution acquisition.

Another way to cope with the spin dephasing is to perform non-refocused black-blood acquisitions. In these sequences, all flowing spins cause signal voids, particularly in vessels with turbulent flow. The simplest black-blood sequence is a regular spin-echo acquisition with thin slices and parallel saturation volumes to null the signal of inflowing spins (Edelman et al. 1990a; Bosmans et al. 1990).

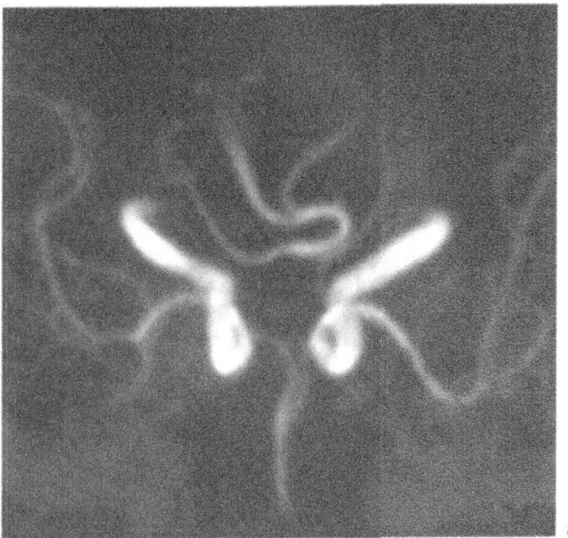

a

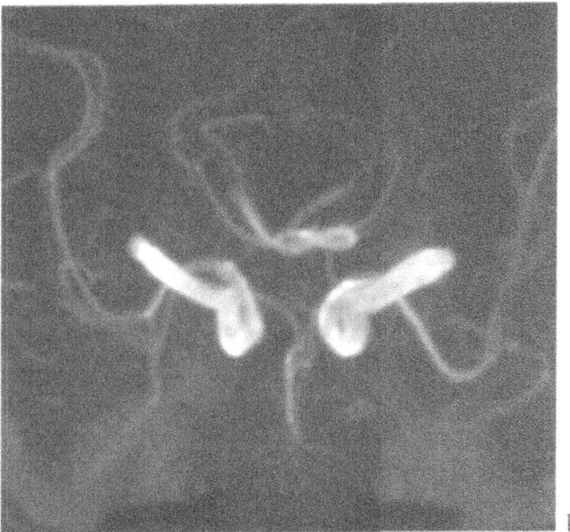

b

Fig. 13.6a, b. Comparative study of a low- and high-resolution TOF acquisition in a normal volunteer (TR/TE/Fl 42 ms/7 ms/20°, FOV 210 mm, slab thickness 52 mm/64 partitions, acquisition time of 8 min). **a** Matrix 192×256; **b** matrix 192×512. The vessel delineation is sharper in the high-resolution acquisition. However, flow-induced dephasing due to higher order flow in, for example, the carotid siphon causes increased signal voids

13.2.2 Cerebral Venography

The MRA protocol for the study of the cerebral veins is heavily determined by the slow flow in these vessels. Whereas 3D TOF techniques are considered a standard sequence for MRA acquisitions of intracranial arteries, they are not optimal for the visualisation of the venous structures. As an example, the signal intensity in the sagittal sinus is maximal where it enters the imaged slab. This signal gradually decreases lower down in the slab. The signal disappears first near the sinus wall, where the velocities are the slowest, and later in the middle of the sinus. The transverse sinus is not interpretable with this technique and smaller veins are not visualised.

In the following sections, the specific techniques that can be used to cope with the saturation effects in cerebral MRA venography are discussed.

13.2.2.1 Time-of-Flight Acquisitions

The first way to reduce the number of excitations that the flowing spins are subjected to is to reduce the thickness of the imaged volume or slice. In plain MRA, 2D TOF rather than 3D TOF acquisitions should be performed to visualise the veins (Mattle et al. 1991). Furthermore, to be optimal, a 2D slice has to be oriented as perpendicular as possible to the veins.

Saturation of venous signal can suggest venous thrombus. A disadvantage of the plain 2D TOF acquisition mode is the limited resolution in the MIP projections for projection directions that significantly differ from the slice selection direction. Even with slightly overlapping slices, the staircase aspect of the vessels in the MR angiograms is present. Better venous detail can be obtained with CE TOF acquisitions.

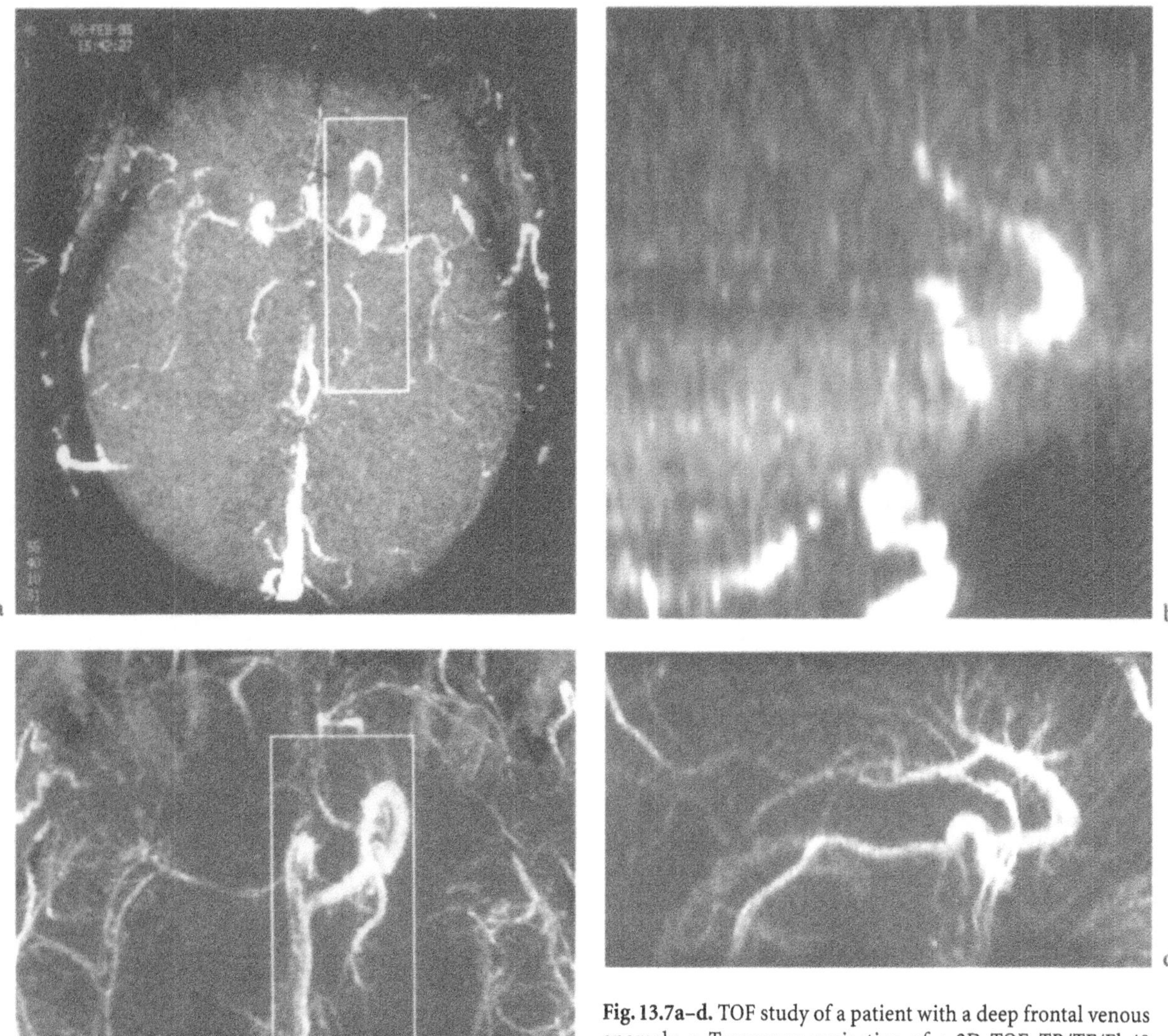

Fig. 13.7a–d. TOF study of a patient with a deep frontal venous anomaly. **a** Transverse projection of a 2D TOF, TR/TE/Fl 40 ms/10 ms/35, slice thickness 3 mm, FOV 220 mm, matrix 256×256, transverse slices. **b** Sagittal projection of a small region of interest. **c** Transverse projection of a 3D TOF study after the injection of 0.1 mmol/kg Gd-DTPA. TR/TE/Fl 43 ms/10 ms/20°, slab thickness 60 mm/64 partitions, FOV 220 mm, matrix 256×5 12, transverse acquisition. **d.** Sagittal projection of a small region of interest. The lesion was detected with the 2D TOF acquisition but the quality of the MR angiogram is poor. The MR angiogram of the CE 3D TOF study nicely shows the collector vein and the smaller medullary veins of the lesion

In Fig. 13.7 we compare a 2D TOF acquisition, (slice thickness 3 mm, matrix 256×256) and a CE 3D TOF acquisition (slab thickness 60 mm/64 partitions, matrix 256×5 12) in a patient with a venous anomaly. Whereas no small veins are visualised with the 2D TOF acquisition, the 3D CE TOF acquisition provides a detailed picture of the venous anomaly. The benefits of the injection of contrast agents for this kind of pathology are obvious. Besides a reduction of the saturation effects, the improved signal-to-noise ratio allows the use of 3D sequences for a more detailed venous anatomy to be obtained.

13.2.2.2 Phase-Contrast Acquisitions

Phase-contrast acquisitions, in which the signal of the stationary tissues is subtracted, provide generally good venous detail. Although the venous signal also decreases due to saturation after a series of excitation pulses, it remains significantly higher than the background signal and therefore the veins remain well visible in the images. The VENCs have to be adapted to the averaged velocities of the veins. In practice, a VENC of 5–30 cm/s can be used to study the sagittal sinus. The long acquisition time is an important drawback of PC techniques. This is particularly true for high-resolution acquisitions or when acquisitions with different VENCs have to be performed. It should be stressed, however, that slice or slab orientations can be chosen more freely than in 2D TOF. PC acquisitions can be applied along the axis of the vessel. A single sagittal acquisition volume with a total acquisition time of 12 min can be applied to visualise the sagittal sinus.

13.3 Normal Intracranial Vascular Anatomy

13.3.1 General Anatomy

13.3.1.1 The Internal Carotid Artery

The cervical internal carotid artery (ICA) enters the skull through the carotid canal in the petrous bone. After a short vertical course, the artery courses medioventrally towards the cavernous sinus. Here the course is vertical up to the sellar floor (presellar segment) where the artery shows an S-shaped configuration. Therefore this juxtasellar segment is called the "carotid siphon".

Small branches arising from the intracavernous portion of the ICA are never seen in normal patients. At the level of the anterior clinoid process, the artery traverses the dura of the cavernous sinus and becomes the supraclinoid segment. Ventrally, the ophthalmic artery arises. More cranially, the posterior communicating artery originates and runs posteriorly to join the posterior cerebral artery. A few millimetres more distally, the anterior choroidal artery arises, courses around the brain stem, and enters the choroid plexus. This artery supplies important portions of the internal capsula. At the top of the supraclinoid segment the ICA bifurcates in the middle and anterior cerebral arteries.

13.3.1.2 Circle of Willis

The circle of Willis is a vascular ring connecting the internal carotid and vertebral arteries with each other. The anterior portion is formed by the horizontal segments of both anterior cerebral arteries, connected by the anterior communicating artery. This portion is connected with the posterior cerebral arteries by the posterior communicating arteries.

13.3.1.3 The Anterior Cerebral Artery

The anterior cerebral artery (ACA) first shows a horizontal segment called the CA1 segment. At this point medial lenticulostriate arteries arise, the largest of which is called the recurrent artery of Heubner. These small arteries supply parts of the internal capsula and of the basal ganglia. The anterior communicating artery joins the two anterior cerebral arteries.

The anterior cerebral artery first gives off two branches (the orbitofrontal and frontopolar arteries). Just at the level of the corpus callosum, the artery divides into the pericallosal artery, running around the corpus callosum and the callosomarginal artery, running within the cingulate gyrus. Both arteries supply the medial aspect of the brain: the callosomarginal artery the frontal region and the pericallosal artery the parietal region. Cortical branches run over the cerebral hemisphere and anastomose with the middle cerebral artery (MCA) and posterior cerebral artery (PCA).

13.3.1.4 The Middle Cerebral Artery

The MCA takes a horizontal course under the frontal lobe. Here the lateral lenticulostriate arteries arise, supplying parts of the internal capsula and of the basal ganglia. Then the MCA courses around the island of Reil and extends into the fissure of Sylvius. The end arteries show an inward bend reaching the top of the sylvian fissure. All these arteries are aligned along the sylvian line. Since the sylvian fissure runs posterosuperiorly, a triangle is described in the lateral view, called the sylvian triangle.

After giving rise to a small branch, the anterior temporal artery, the MCA mostly bifurcates into an anterior and a posterior trunk. The arteries arising from the anterior trunk supply the rolandic sensorimotor region and Broca's area. The posterior trunk supplies the postrolandic parietal region and a large portion of the temporal lobe.

13.3.1.5 The Posterior Cerebral Artery

The PCA originates from the distal basilar artery and runs laterally around the brain stem. In the proximal part perforating arteries arise, supplying the thalamus. The most important branches of the ambient segment are the medial and lateral posterior choroidal arteries. The former supplies the thalamus and the choroid plexus, while the latter supplies parts of the cerebral peduncle and the basal ganglia.

The terminal branches of the posterior cerebral artery supply the visual cortex (calcarine artery) and the surrounding parieto-occipital cortex.

13.3.1.6 The Vertebrobasilar System

The intracranial vertebral arteries enter the foramen magnum ventrally and converge in front of the medulla to form the basilar artery. Before the junction they give off the anterior spinal artery, which descends in front of the medulla oblongata, the posterior inferior cerebellar artery (PICA), which courses around the medulla and supplies the inferior vermis and parts of the cerebellum, and a posterior meningeal artery for the tentorium.

The basilar artery runs ventrally of the brain stem and bifurcates in the interpeduncular cistern. Smaller pontine branches are usually invisible even with angiography. The inferior cerebellar artery (AICA) originates proximally and runs laterally over the pons to the cerebellopontine angle.

The superior cerebellar arteries run in the perimesencephalic cistern to supply the cerebellar hemisphere and the middle and superior cerebellar peduncle.

13.3.1.7 Normal Variants of the Arterial Anatomy

The internal carotid artery can be hypoplastic or absent. In these cases, the petrous and sellar segment are frequently absent. In other cases, the ascending pharyngeal artery takes over the cervical portion and joins the petrous portions of the carotid canal by means of intratympanic anastomoses. This is incorrectly called an aberrant intratympanic course of the ICA.

The most frequent variations of the circle of Willis are a "foetal" origin of the posterior cerebral artery, where the posterior cerebral artery arises directly from the carotid artery and the proximal PCA is hypoplastic (15% of cases); hypoplasia of one CA1 segment, with a hypoplastic anterior communicating artery, joining the two cerebral arteries arising from the other side (25%); and hypoplasia of the posterior communicating artery (20%). Duplication of these arteries is described in about 5% of the cases.

Foetal remnants of anastomoses between the carotid arteries and the vertebral system can persist. The most frequent is the persistent trigeminal artery, originating from the junction of the presellar and juxtasellar ICA and joining the basilar artery through the cavernous sinus. The terminal branches of the ACA, PCA and MCA are extremely variable.

13.3.1.8 Venous Anatomy

The most important veins of the brain are the dural venous sinuses, the superficial veins, and the deep cerebral veins. Bone and meninges are drained by diploic and meningeal veins. The most important dural sinuses are: the superior sagittal sinus, the inferior sagittal sinus, the straight sinus, the transverse and sigmoid sinuses, and the cavernous and the petrosal sinuses.

The superior sagittal sinus runs in the midline in a duplication of the falx. At the junction of the superior sagittal, straight, and transverse sinuses, a slight dilatation, the torcular Herophili, is found.

The inferior sagittal sinus runs in the inferior free edge of the falx. At the junction of the vein of Galen and the inferior sagittal sinus, the straight sinus is formed and runs between the leaves of the joining falx and tentorium. The transverse sinus runs laterally over the tentorium. The sigmoid sinus then courses inferolaterally towards the internal jugular vein.

The inferior and superior petrosal sinuses extend from the cavernous sinus to the jugular bulb and the sigmoid sinus, respectively. The sphenoparietal sinus is formed by meningeal and superficial middle cerebral veins and drains into the cavernous sinus. Both cavernous sinuses, lying next to the sphenoid bone and containing the ICA and cranial veins III, IV, V1, V2 and VI, are connected via intercavernous sinuses.

The superficial or cortical veins drain the cortex. Two constant veins are seen. The vein of Labbé, draining posteriorly into the transverse sinus, and the vein of Trolard, draining into the superior sagittal sinus in the parietal region.

Medial and lateral subependymal veins, the largest of which (the thalamostriate and septal veins) join to form the internal cerebral vein, form the deep venous system. The basal vein of Rosenthal, running along the brain stem, joins the internal cerebral vein behind the brain stem to form the vein of Galen. This vein courses around the splenium of the corpus callosum, where it joins the straight sinus in the incisura tentorii.

13.3.1.9
Normal Variants of the Venous Anatomy

Variants of the venous anatomy are very frequent. The most frequent anomaly is a hypoplasia of one of the transverse sinuses. The torcular can be connected to the jugular bulb by a midline occipital sinus. The superficial veins considerably differ in calibre. Sometimes the vein of Trolard is very large with a small vein of Labbé, in other patients the opposite is true. The anatomy of the small subependymal vein is very variable.

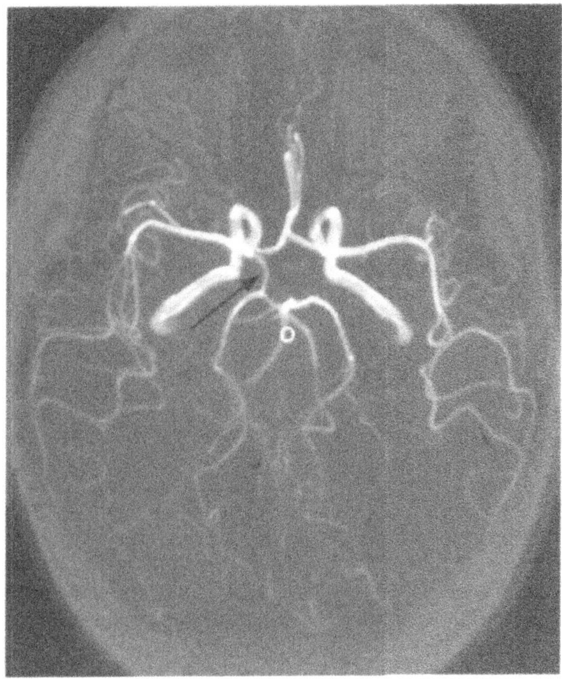

Fig. 13.8. Normal anatomy of circle of Willis. Transverse MIP of 3D TOF MRA sequence. TR/TE/Fl 35 ms/7.2 ms/20°, magnetisation transfer preparation pulse and TONE RF excitation, rectangular FOV 150×200 mm, slab thickness 82 mm, matrix 200×512, acquisition time 6.44 min, number of excitations (Nex) = 1. Anterior part of circle of Willis is formed by the horizontal segments of the anterior cerebral arteries. The right posterior communicating artery (*arrow*) is hypertrophic. The left posterior communicating artery is not visualised. Note that branches of the middle and posterior cerebral arteries are well visualised

13.3.2
MRA Display of the Anatomy and MRA Limitations

The major intracranial arterial branches are well visualised on MRA images. Routinely, the transverse projection is used for the display of arteries (Fig. 13.7, 13.8). Though this is quite an unusual projection in comparison to conventional angiography, it allows one to study the vessels of both hemispheres and/or of distal branches separately without superposition. Selective information for one hemisphere in the lateral projection can be obtained either by selective acquisition of one hemisphere or by projecting a single hemisphere out of the global angiogram by targeted MIP (Fig. 13.9a) (Mattle and Wentz 1992).

Routinely, the major intracranial arteries are easily displayed: in their proximal course this includes the carotid siphon, the anterior and middle cerebral artery and their branches. The degree of visualisation of the distal branches not only depends on the imaging parameters used but also widely varies among patients, depending on their cardiovascular status. Since the flow in the vascular system is dependent on cardiac output, it is not surprising that the visibility of the distal intracranial arteries decreases with age (Kusinoki et al. 1999). Therefore MR angiograms are generally better in children than in adults. Very small arteries, such as the lenticulostriate arteries and the anterior choroidal arteries, are routinely visualised in children but rarely visible even in young adults.

The application of the maximum intensity algorithm to extract an angiogram out of a 3D data set further reduces the conspicuousness of small vessels (Anderson et al. 1990). This is particularly true for the study of the circle of Willis, where the intensity of the small posterior communicating artery is further reduced by volume averaging effects with the low-intensity CSF. Therefore if these arteries are the focus of the study, a careful review of the native images is mandatory.

The anterior communicating artery is best visible on coronal projections (Fig. 13.10). Persistent foetal branching of the posterior communicating artery from the supraclinoid portion of the carotid artery is a frequent finding and is always obvious on axial projections (Fig. 13.11). The respective contributions of the different vessels to the cerebral territories can be deduced from selective MR angiograms with placement of spatial saturation volumes (Mattle and Wentz 1992).

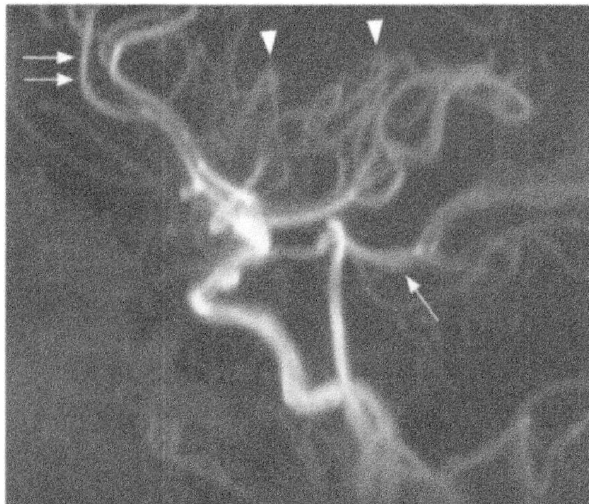

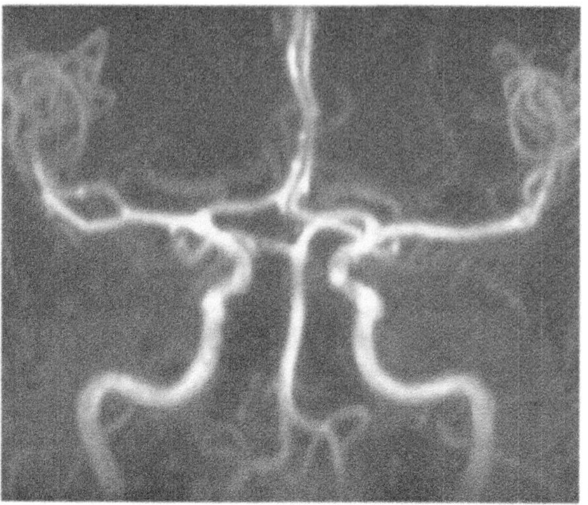

a b

Fig. 13.9. a Normal anatomy of the brain vessels. Same patient as in Fig. 13.8a. Sagittal MIP of the same sequence. The anterior cerebral artery (*double arrow*) with the pericallosal and callosomarginal artery is well seen. The insular branches of the middle cerebral artery (*arrowhead*) are well visualised. Visualisation of the posterior cerebral artery (*arrow*), and its terminal cortical branches. **b** Frontal MIP of same sequence. Excellent visualisation of the normal anatomy

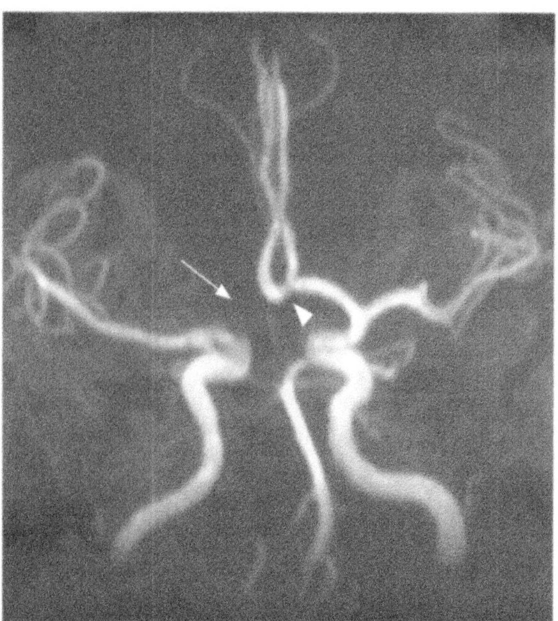

Fig. 13.10. Normal variant of circle of Willis. Coronal MIP of 3D TOF MRA sequence. TR/TE/Fl 35 ms/7.2 ms/20°, magnetisation transfer preparation pulse and TONE RF excitation, rectangular FOV 150×200 mm, slab thickness 82 mm, matrix 200×512, acquisition time 6.44 min, Nex=1. Note aplasia of the right CA1 segment of the anterior cerebral artery (*arrow*). Both CA2 segments fill via the left internal carotid artery, over the anterior communicating artery (*arrowhead*)

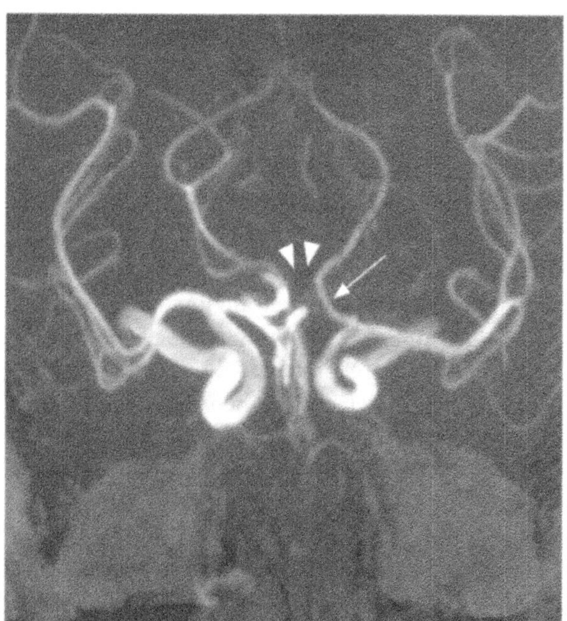

Fig. 13.11. Persistent foetal branching of posterior communicating artery. Note the large posterior communicating artery (*arrow*) originating immediately from the supraclinoid portion of the internal carotid artery and giving rise directly to the posterior cerebral artery. There is aplasia (*arrowheads*) of proximal posterior cerebral artery (P1 segment). Semicoronal MIP of 3D TOF MRA sequence. TR/TE/Fl 35 ms/7.2 ms/20°, magnetisation transfer preparation pulse and TONE RF excitation, rectangular FOV 150×200 mm, slab thickness 82 mm, matrix 200×512, acquisition time 6.44 min, Nex=1

Coronal projection offers the best view of the anterior cerebral arteries, the anterior communicating artery and the horizontal segment of the middle cerebral artery as well as the confluence of the vertebral arteries and the basilar artery (Fig. 13.9b). The carotid siphons are best seen on the sagittal projections.

Stereoscopic viewing, closed vessel projection and surface shaded rendering (Anderson et al. 1990) eliminate spatial ambiguity.

The main dural venous sinuses are well visualised. Due to the different anatomical orientation, the projection will have to differ according to the sinus being studied. The superior sagittal and straight sinuses are best evaluated in the sagittal projection (Fig. 13.12), and the transverse and sigmoid sinuses in the transverse, frontal, or oblique projection. The smaller deep venous circulation is best visualised on gadolinium-enhanced venograms, in the sagittal and axial plane (Fig. 13.12) (Marchal et al. 1992). The cavernous sinus can be studied in the transverse and the frontal projection.

Outpouching arachnoid granulations (Fig. 13.13) can cause pseudoimages of thrombus in the dural sinuses.

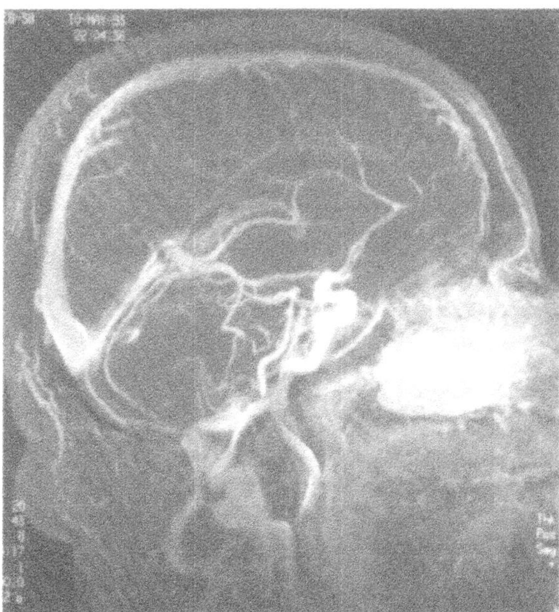

Fig. 13.12. Normal venous anatomy. Sagittal MIP of 3D TOF acquisition TR/TE/Fl 42 ms/8 ms/20°, FOV 250 mm, matrix 384×512, slab thickness 64 mm/64 partitions, acquisition time 16 min. Gd-DTPA-enhanced study. Excellent demonstration of deep and superficial cerebral veins

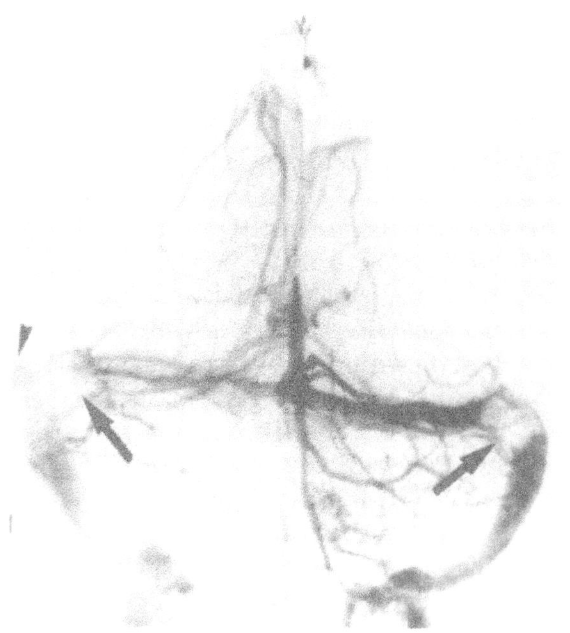

a

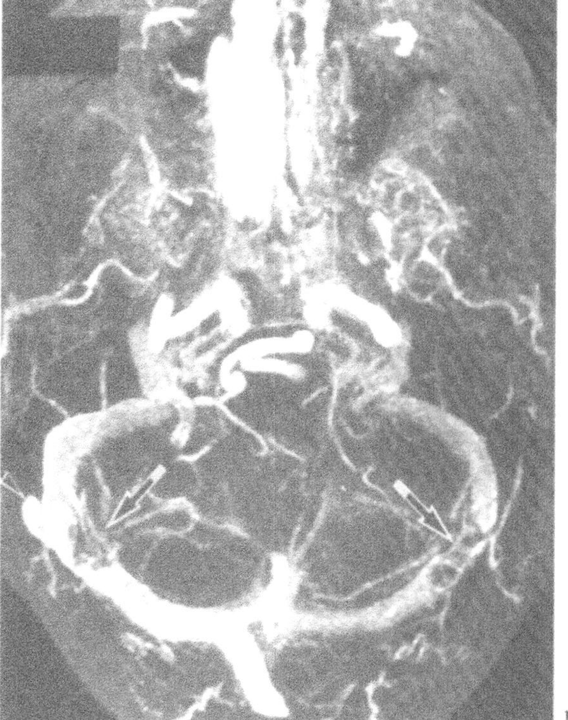

b

Fig. 13.13a, b. Venous aneurysm and venous filling defects caused by arachnoid (Paccioni's) granulation. **a** Selective intra-arterial DSA of the left vertebral artery. Anteroposterior projection. A lateral venous aneurysm is seen on the *right* (*arrowhead*). Bilateral intraluminal filling defects (*arrows*) are present at the transition of the transverse and sigmoid sinus, caused by arachnoid granulations. **b** Transverse MIP of 3D contrast-enhanced TOF MRA sequence. The venous aneurysm is well visualised (*arrowhead*). Filling defects (*arrows*) in the transverse sinus are well depicted on both sides. TR/TE/Fl 42 ms/10 ms/20°, magnetisation transfer preparation pulse, rectangular FOV 152×210 mm, slab thickness 52 mm/64 partitions, matrix 192×512, acquisition time 8 min, Nex=1

13.4 Pathology

13.4.1 Arterial Stenosis and Occlusion

The most common manifestation of acute intracranial vascular obstruction is stroke, a sudden neurological deficit, most commonly occurring in the sensorimotor or visual cortex. The symptoms can be limited or transient (transient ischaemic attacks or reversible ischaemic neurological deficits). However, very frequently cerebral infarction is massive and is the immediate cause of death. In case of survival severe neurological disability is common.

The most frequent cause of stroke is embolism originating in the extracranial neck vessels, with obstruction of distal branches or the main stem of the middle cerebral artery. The prognosis largely depends on the availability of the intracranial collaterals.

Besides stenosis or obstruction of cerebral vessels, stroke can be due to other causes, such as intraparenchymal haemorrhage and subarachnoid haemorrhage.

The detection of haemorrhage is important with respect to patient's management and therapy.

Intracranial atheromatous stenoses mostly occur at the level of the carotid siphon, the basilar artery (Fig. 13.14) or the main stem of the middle cerebral artery. Peripheral stenoses are far less common. The importance of their detection increases if the extracranial vessels are normal. Failure of surgery of the neck vessels is commonly due to associated distal lesions.

In young patients the main causes of intracranial stenoses are infections or auto-immune based arteritis (Fig. 13.15) (Heiserman et al. 1992), sickle cell anaemia, dissection or vasospasm either traumatic or caused by aneurysm rupture (Goldberg 1992; Vogl et al. 1992; Zimmerman et al. 1992; Wiznitzer et al. 1990; Gillams et al. 1998). In children, moyamoya disease and basal occlusion by osteopetrosis or achondroplasia have to be considered (Vogl et al. 1992; Lisovoski and Rosseaux 1993).

Total vascular obstruction is readily demonstrated by MRA. The impact of the demonstration of a vascular occlusion by MRA is increasing since effective thrombolytic treatment is now available for these patients (Ohue et al. 1998).

Low to moderate stenoses without major effect on the local flow pattern are also usually well demonstrated by MRA techniques (Pernicone et al. 1990,

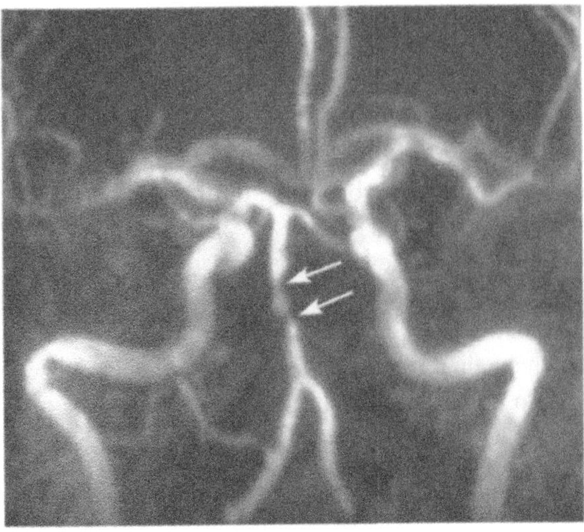

Fig. 13.14. Stenosis of the basilar artery. Coronal MIP of 3D TOF MRA sequence. TR/TE/Fl 35 ms/7.2 ms/20°, magnetisation transfer preparation pulse and TONE RF excitation, rectangular FOV 150×200 mm, slab thickness 82 mm, matrix 200×512, acquisition time 6.44 min, Nex=1. Note double stenosis of the basilar artery (*arrows*)

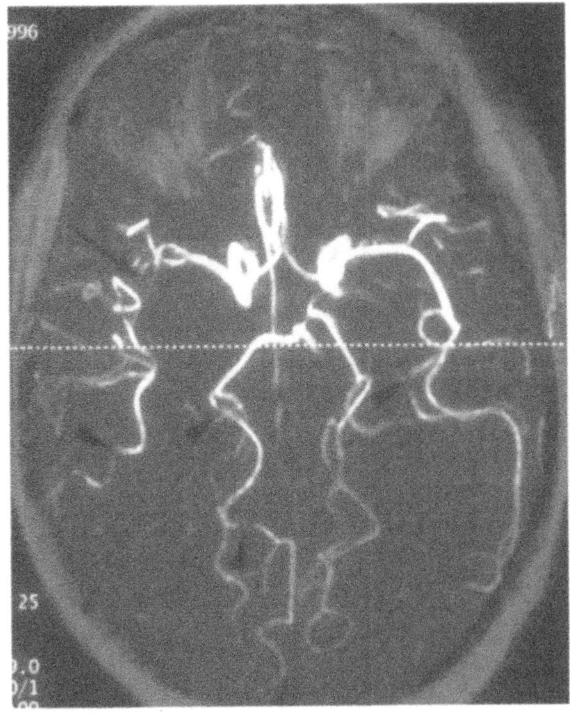

Fig. 13.15. Vasculitis of the intracranial arteries. Transverse MIP of 3D TOF MRA sequence. TR/TE/Fl 35 ms/7.2 ms/20°, magnetisation transfer preparation pulse and TONE RF excitation, rectangular FOV 150×200 mm, slab thickness 82 mm, matrix 200×512, acquisition time 6.44 min, Nex=1. Note multiple stenotic lesions of the middle and posterior cerebral arteries (*arrows*)

1992; OELERICH et al. 1998). On the other hand, stenoses which induce important local flow disturbances are generally overestimated both in diameter and in length because of incomplete flow rephasing in these areas (Fig. 13.16). Tight stenoses can simulate total obstruction, particularly on 3D TOF MRAs, because of saturation of the slow-flowing blood distal to the stenosis (Fig. 13.16) (MASARYK et al. 1991; KATZ et al. 1989).

In general, saturation can be overcome by the injection of gadolinium since it makes the vascular signal less flow dependent (RUNGE et al. 1993; CREASY et al. 1990; MARCHAL et al. 1992; METENS et al. 2000). Another approach consists of the application of consecutive 2D acquisitions perpendicular to the post-stenotic vessel (BOSMANS et al. 1992). One can only conclude that total obstruction is present if the previously mentioned methods fail to demonstrate any distal vessels (Fig. 13.16).

Besides the basal occlusions, the hypertrophic collaterals in the basal ganglia are the most striking feature of moya-moya disease (Fig. 13.17) (YAMADA et al. 1992). However, these collaterals together with associated infarcts in the cerebral parenchyma are often already visible on plain spin-echo images.

Intracranial dissection is usually an extension of an extracranial carotid dissection (GELBERT et al. 1991). The spontaneous hyperintense aspect of the thrombus can mimic flowing blood on the MIP. Therefore correlation with the spin-echo images or the applications of PC sequences is frequently needed (GELBERT et al. 1991).

Although vasospasm can be detected by transcranial Doppler (MURSCH et al. 2000), morphological information can help in the selection of patients who could benefit from interventional neuroradiological procedures, such as angioplasty, papaverine infusion or selective underlying aneurysm embolisation, and

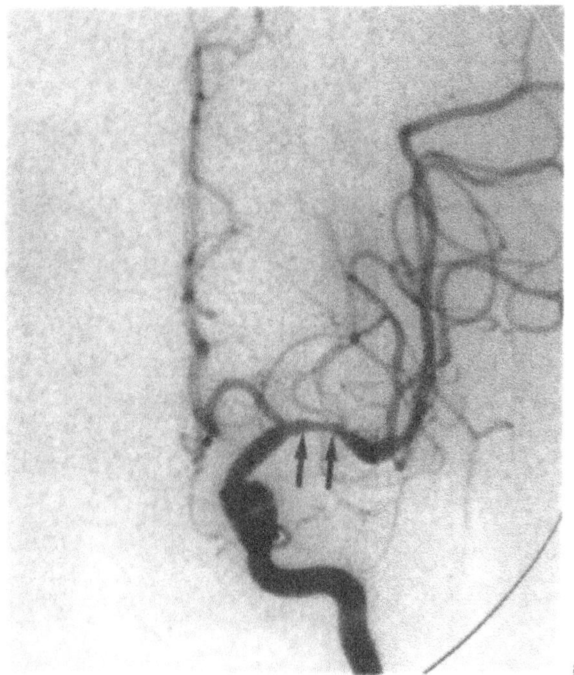

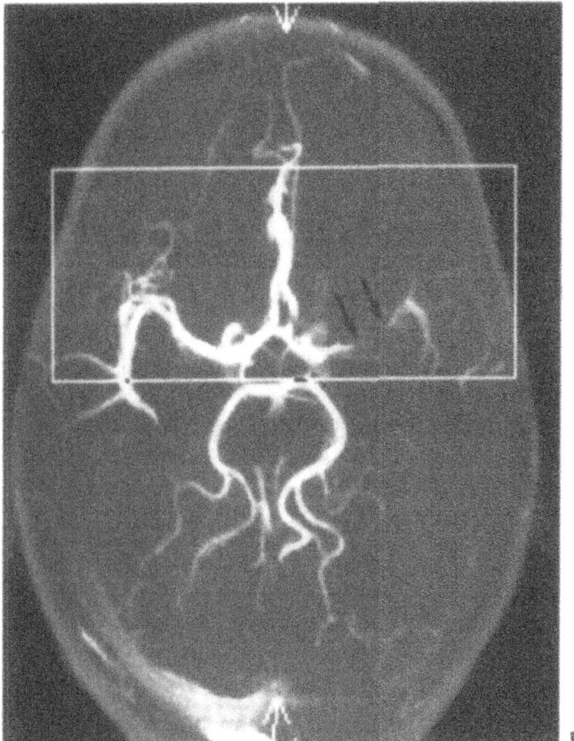

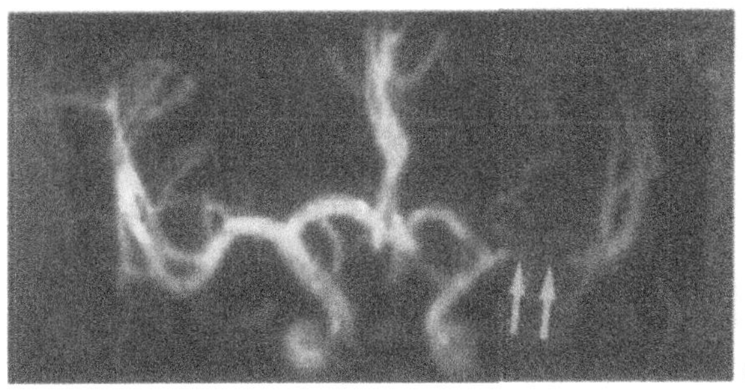

Fig. 13.16a–c. Middle cerebral artery stenosis. Presumed arteritis in a 3-year-old child. **a** Selective intra-arterial DSA of the left internal carotid artery. Anteroposterior projection. Moderate (50%–60%) stenosis (*arrows*) of the horizontal middle cerebral artery main stem. Note the involvement of proximal 0.5 cm of a lateral lenticulostriate artery, originating at the site of maximal stenosis. **b** Transverse and **c** Coronal MIP of 3D TOF MRA sequence. TR/TE/Fl 40 ms/10 ms/20°, magnetisation transfer preparation pulse and TONE RF excitation, rectangular FOV 150×200 mm, slab thickness 52 mm/64 partitions, matrix 192×256, acquisition time 8 min, Nex=1. There is severe overestimation of the degree of stenosis (*arrows*), with total disappearance of the signal at the level of the lesion due to turbulence. The presence of signal in the distal part of the middle cerebral artery indicates that the artery is not occluded. Stenosis of the lenticulostriate artery is not seen

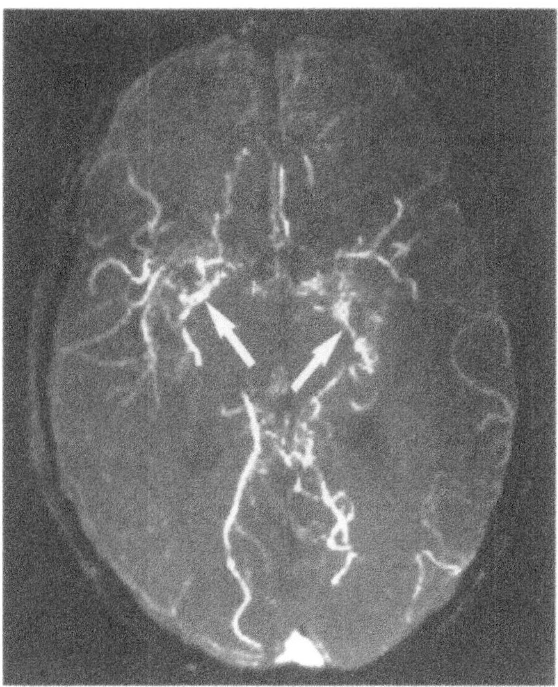

Fig. 13.17. Moya-moya disease in a 5-year-old child. Transverse MIP of 3D TOF MRA sequence (1.5-T MR system). TR/TE/Fl 40 ms/7 ms/20°, FOV 230 mm, MOTSA, slab thickness 32 mm/32 partitions, mutual overlap of 6 mm, total of 5 slabs; matrix 256×256, acquisition time 5×5 min, Nex=1. The carotid siphon and the main stem of middle cerebral, anterior, and posterior cerebral arteries are not visualised, pointing to basal occlusion. There is visualisation of extensive collateral circulation (*arrows*) in the basal ganglia

in defining the optimal time for intervention (Mathurin et al. 1993).

In patients with eclampsia, reversible signal changes of the brain parenchyma as well as reversible stenoses are seen (Koyama 1997).

As already mentioned, the prognosis of vascular occlusive disease both of the intra- and extracranial vessels largely depends on the available collateral circulation. Of the various possible collateral pathways, only the circle of Willis, which is close to the major vessels, can be adequately studied by MRA (Masaryk et al. 1989). Leptomeningeal collaterals can be only indirectly seen by virtue of asymmetry of the distal circulation.

13.4.2 Aneurysms

Most cerebral aneurysms are congenital and originate around the circle of Willis. They occur in 1%–14% of the population (Osborn 1994). More distal localisations are far less common and can be of septic origin. Populations at risk are patients with a strong family history of aneurysm, Marfan's disease, renal polycystic disease, aortic coarctation, fibromuscular disease, collagen vascular disease, or multiple meningiomas (Osborn 1994).

Most intradural aneurysms manifest themselves by rupture with subarachnoid haemorrhage. Extradural lesions, such as carotid-ophthalmic or cavernous sinus aneurysms, are often large and give rise to compressive phenomena with cranial nerve palsy or visual disturbances.

The risk of aneurysm rupture is estimated at 2% a year so that more than 50% of the lesions will ultimately rupture. When rupture occurs, 75% of the patients die within 3 days. Therefore, an undetected aneurysm poses a life-threatening risk. Hence an accurate, non-invasive screening technique is essential (Osborn 1994), especially since operation of an unruptured aneurysm causes low morbidity (4%) and mortality (Weir 1990). Furthermore, endovascular treatment with detachable coils is now widely used as a less invasive alternative for surgery (Vinuela et al. 1997; Cognard et al. 1998).

In the diagnostic work-up of a patient with a suspected intracranial aneurysm, several questions have to be answered using catheter angiography, spiral CT, or MRA (Keogh and Vhora 1998). The aneurysm has to be detected or the absence of an aneurysm has to be confirmed with certainty. It has to be kept in mind that aneurysms can be multiple (Fig. 13.17). The exact topographic location has to be determined, including the vessel of origin, demonstration of the aneurysm neck, and clarification of the relationship to neighbouring vessels. The morphology and size of the aneurysm must be demonstrated. In the case of multiple aneurysms, it may be necessary to demonstrate which lesion has bled. Finally, vasospasm has to be ruled out.

Neurosurgical therapy for intracranial aneurysm involves clipping the aneurysmal neck or in the case of absence of a surgical neck "wrapping" of the aneurysmal dome. Endovascular techniques were formerly only used for certain locations, less accessible with neurosurgery, such as the basilar tip or the cavernous sinus. Nowadays, endovascular treatment of cerebral aneurysms with detachable coils (GDC: Guglielmi detachable coils) has become the method of first choice in most centres (Vinuela et al. 1997; Cognard et al. 1998). For giant aneurysms with a broad neck, parent vessel occlusion with detachable balloons or coils can be performed.

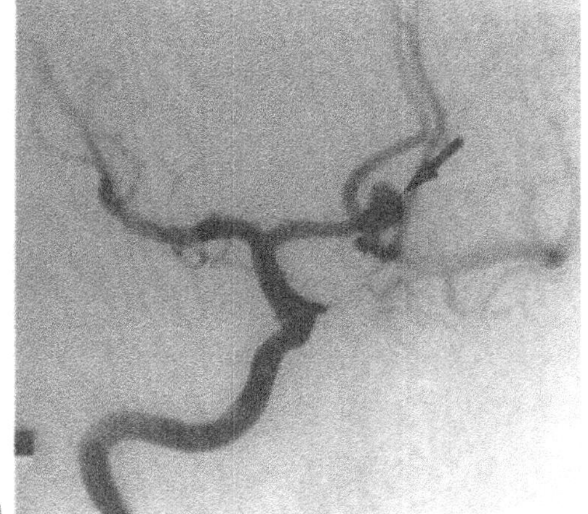

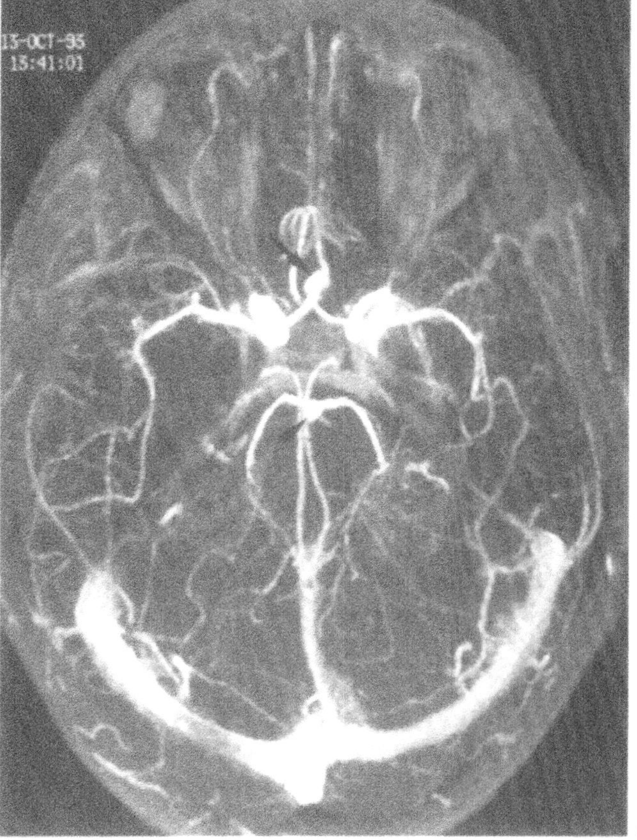

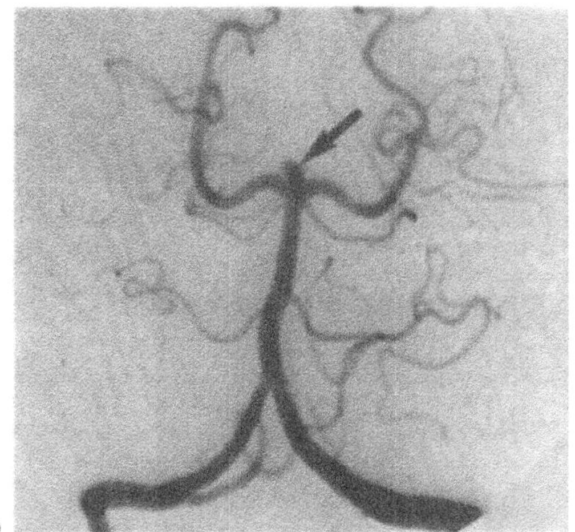

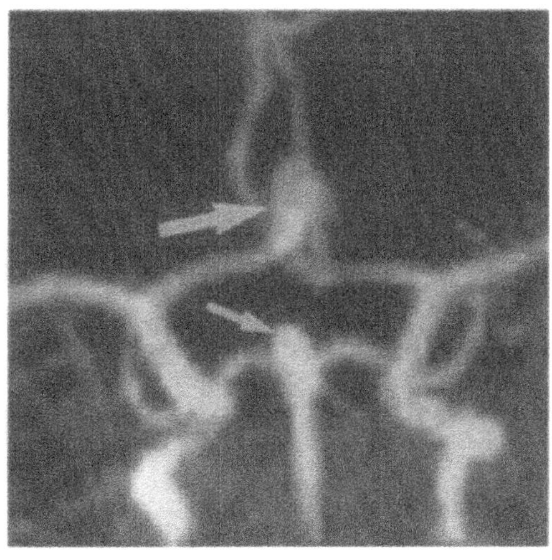

Fig. 13.18a–d. Aneurysm of the anterior cerebral artery and of the basilar tip, in the same patient. **a** Selective intra-arterial DSA of the right internal carotid artery. Right anterior oblique projection. An aneurysm (*arrow*) of the anterior communicating artery is seen, with a diameter of 6 mm. **b** Selective intra-arterial DSA of the left vertebral artery in the anteroposterior projection, showing a 3-mm aneurysm (*arrow*) of basilar tip. **c** Transverse MIP of 3D TOF MRA sequence, immediately after the injection of 0.2 mmol/kg Gd-DTPA. TR/TE/Fl 42 ms/10 ms/38°, magnetisation transfer preparation pulse, FOV 153×210 mm, slab thickness 52 mm/64 partitions, matrix 192×512, acquisition time 8 min, Nex=1. A lesion of anterior communicating artery is easily recognised (*arrow*). The aneurysm of basilar tip (*arrowhead*) cannot be differentiated from vascular loop of the basilar artery. **d** Frontal MIP of 3D TOF MRA sequence, second acquisition after contrast enhancement. TR/TE/Fl 42 ms/10 ms/30°, magnetisation transfer preparation pulse, FOV 156×210 mm, slab thickness 52 mm/64 partitions, matrix 192×256, acquisition time 8 min, Nex=1. There is excellent visualisation of both lesions (*arrows*)

Larger aneurysms can be easily detected with conventional spin-echo MRI. However, differentiation of small aneurysms from vascular loops and of signal void from dense bone from the anterior clinoid process can be difficult (Fig. 13.18).

Depending on the techniques used, MRA in combination with MRI has a detection rate of approximately 90%–95% for aneurysms as small as 3–4 mm (Fig. 13.18) (Curnes et al. 1993; Sevick et al. 1990; Schuierer et al. 1992; Ross et al. 1990; Zamani 1997; Keogh and Vhora 1998; Wardlaw and White 2000). The high diagnostic accuracy of MRA makes it an ideal method for screening of cerebral aneurysms in patients with polycystic kidneys and in patients with a positive familial history (Geevarghese et al. 1999; Roberts et al. 1999).

Since small aneurysms are easily missed because of superimposition of the carrier vessels, a careful analysis of the MRA in multiple projections and of the native images is mandatory (Fig. 13.18).

Local turbulence often occurs in larger aneurysms and can simulate intraluminal thrombus or lead to an underestimation of the volume of the lesion (Figs. 13.19–13.21).

Saturation due to slow flow in larger aneurysms will reduce the signal in the lesion and the distal vessels (Fig. 13.20). Here, too, injection of gadolinium allows recovery of the vascular signal (Marchal et al. 1992). However, after gadolinium injection, the

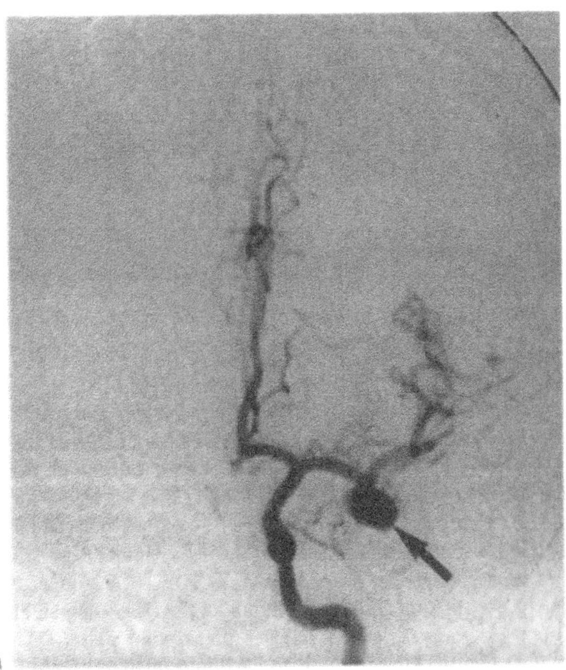

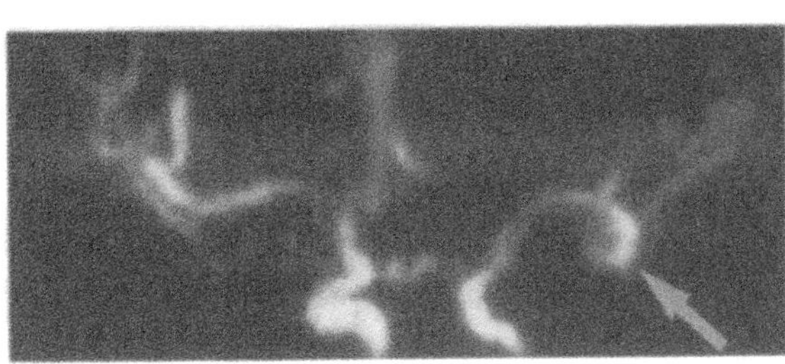

Fig. 13.19a, b. Middle cerebral artery aneurysm: signal loss due to turbulence. **a** Selective intra-arterial DSA of left internal carotid artery. Anteroposterior projection. A large aneurysm (diameter 1 cm) (*arrow*) of the left middle cerebral artery is seen. **b** Coronal MIP of 3D PC MRA sequence, performed 1 week later. TR/TE/Fl 30 ms/10 ms/20°, FOV 210 mm, VENC 30 cm/s, slab thickness 40 mm/32 partitions, matrix 192×256, acquisition time 12 min, Nex=1. There is central signal drop out in the aneurysmal sac (*arrow*) due to turbulence

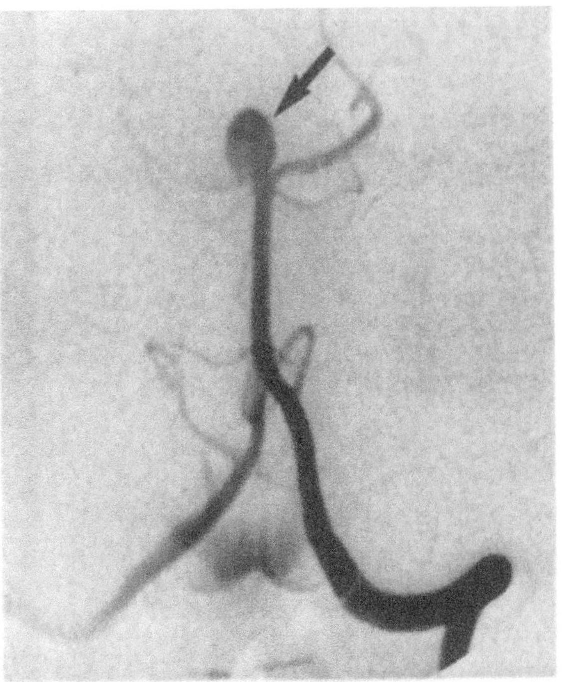

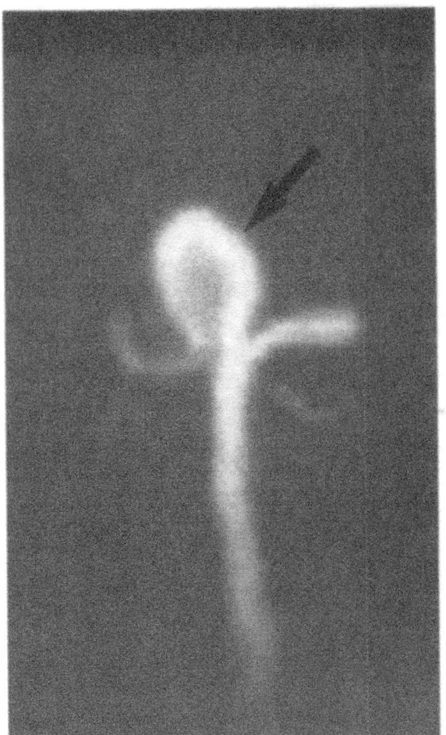

Fig. 13.20a, b. Basilar tip aneurysm: signal loss due to turbulence. **a** Selective intra-arterial DSA of the left vertebral artery. Anteroposterior projection, early arterial phase: a basilar tip aneurysm (*arrow*) is shown. Turbulence within the aneurysmal sac is well depicted. **b** Coronal MIP of 3D TOF MRA sequence. TR/TE/Fl 40 ms/7 ms/20°, magnetisation transfer preparation pulse and TONE RF excitation, rectangular FOV 165×220 mm, slab thickness 52 mm/64 partitions, matrix 192×256, acquisition time 8 min, Nex=1. The aneurysm (*arrow*) of the basilar tip is very well visualised. Intra-aneurysmal turbulence causes signal loss

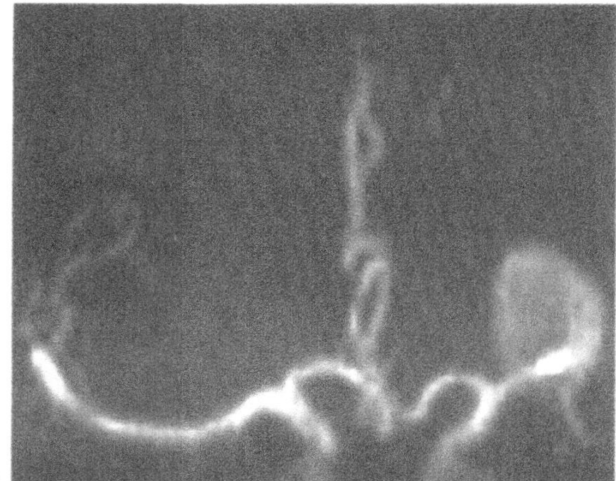

a

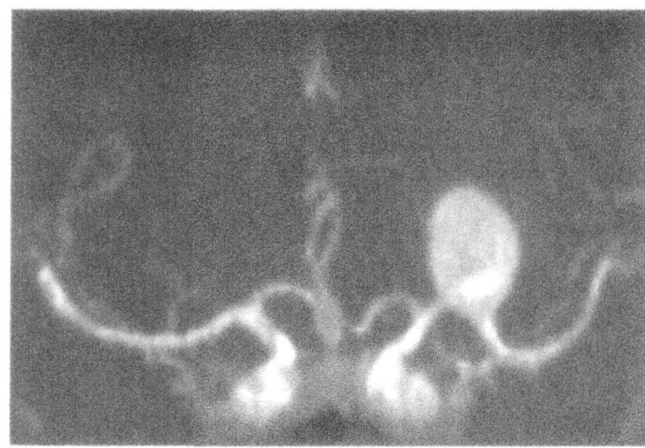

b

Fig. 13.21a, b. Middle cerebral artery aneurysm. Transverse MIP of 3D TOF acquisition, TR/TE/Fl 40 ms/10 ms/20°, FOV 220 mm, matrix 256×256, slab thickness 64 mm/64 partitions, acquisition time 10 min. **a** MIP of pre-Gd-DTPA study shows flow-induced turbulence and saturation in the middle cerebral artery. **b** MIP of contrast-enhanced TOF study shows filling of the aneurysm and good filling of the middle cerebral artery

enhancement of the venous plexus in the region of the cavernous sinus can obscure intracavernous lesions. High signal from partial thrombosis or haemorrhage interferes with TOF angiograms, causing blurring of the aneurysm outline or overestimation of the patent lumen (Fig. 13.22) (Gouliamos et al. 1992). In these cases correlation with the spin-echo images and/or PC acquisitions will accurately demonstrate the exact size of the aneurysm (Pernicone et al. 1990; Huston and Ehman 1993). In the same way, in giant unruptured aneurysms, 3D TOF gives optimal images. For haemorrhagic, thrombosed or distal aneurysms and for the study of the different components of the aneurysms, as for instance thrombus, haemorrhage or patent residual lumen, 2D MRA with presaturation is more informative (Brugières et al. 1998). Besides the diagnosis of aneurysms, MRA, by virtue of its ability to yield multiple projections, allows very accurate evaluation of the anatomical implantation, the origin of the lesion, and the neck of the aneurysm. The transverse projections are of particular value in many cases of eccentrically developed aneurysms. As mentioned above, accompanying vasospasm is readily diagnosed and can easily be followed up by sequential MRA studies.

In dissecting aneurysms of the intracranial arteries, MRA will not demonstrate an aneurysmal sac but evolving irregularities of the arterial wall on serial examinations (Lamino et al. 1997).

Given the high sensitivity of MRA in the detection of intracerebral aneurysms, one might propose that patients be screened with this technique to select those who require further angiographic set-up. After therapy, with surgical clipping, it is impossible to follow up the lesion due to susceptibility artefacts from the implanted material (Fig. 13.23). After endovascular therapy with detachable coils, patients can adequately be followed up with 3D TOF MRA, since the platinum coils are not ferromagnetic (Brunereau et al. 1999). After parent vessel occlusion, spin-echo MRI and MRA will confirm the occlusion of the parent vessel and confirm the progressive disappearance of the lesion (Tsuruda et al. 1992). MRA is very well suited to the follow-up of patients with untreated aneurysms or after failure of endovascular therapy to assess whether morphological changes in the aneurysmal configuration indicate new therapeutic approaches to be appropriate.

With dynamic gadolinium-enhanced 3D MRA, the detection of cerebral aneurysms is even better than with 3D TOF or PC MRA (Fig. 13.24). In a series of 23 aneurysms, Metens et al. (2000) reported a 100% detection rate of the lesions with a mean size of 6 mm, the smallest measuring 2 mm in diameter, whereas 3D TOF missed one and 3D PC seven of the 23 aneurysms. Using consecutive acquisitions of two perpendicular volumes, with a coronal arterial phase followed by a transverse venous phase acquisition, the authors were able to cover a large region where the overwhelming majority of saccular aneurysms present.

The relationship between the aneurysm and the parent vessel and the size of the aneurysmal neck are adequately depicted. In this way, one can decide to treat the patient with detachable coils or with surgery.

The very short acquisition time allows satisfactory images, even in restless patients after subarachnoid haemorrhage. Metens et al. (2000) stress the fact that in giant aneurysms, differentiation between mural trombus and slow flow is easy with dynamic gado-

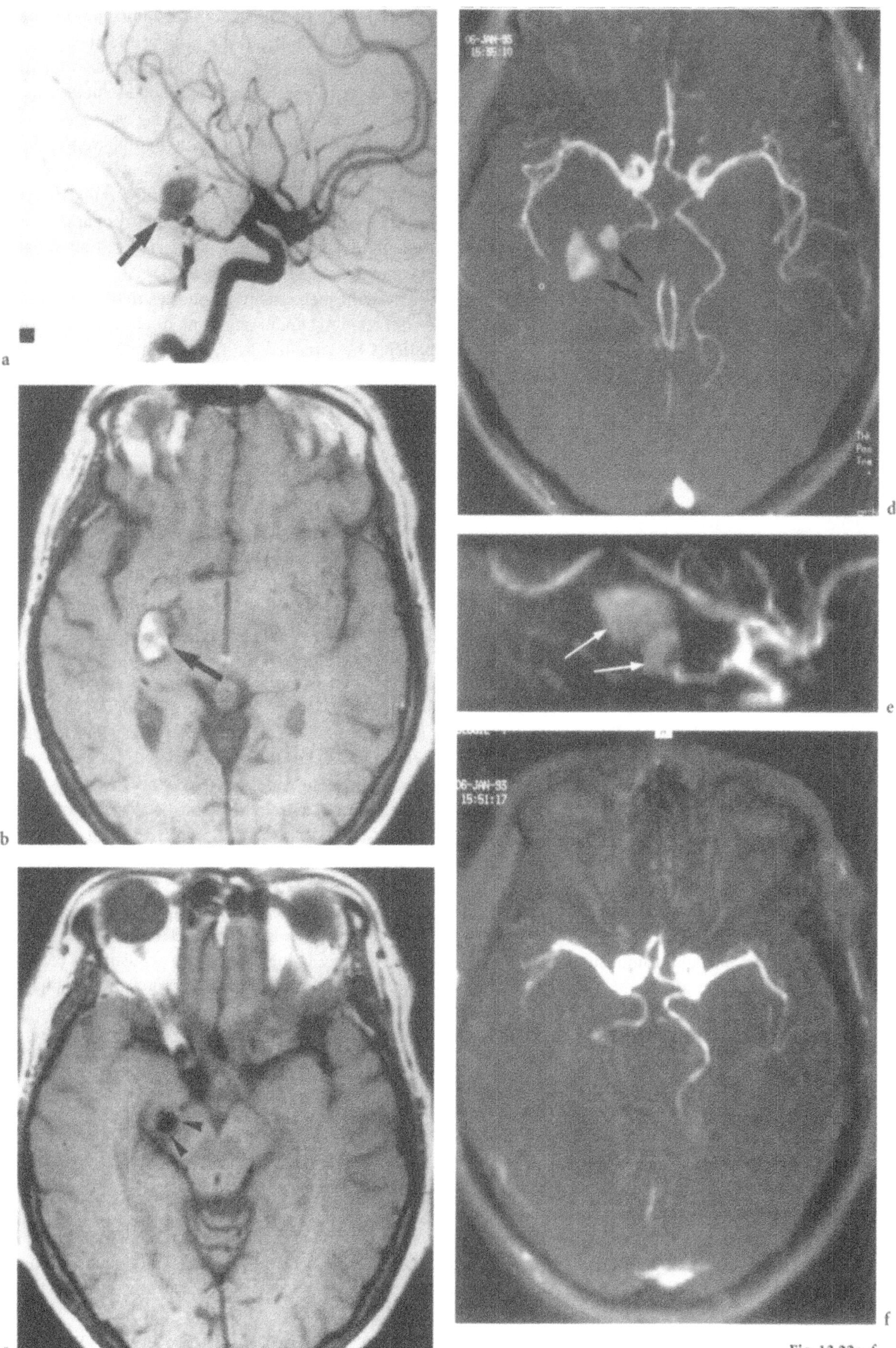

Fig. 13.22a–f

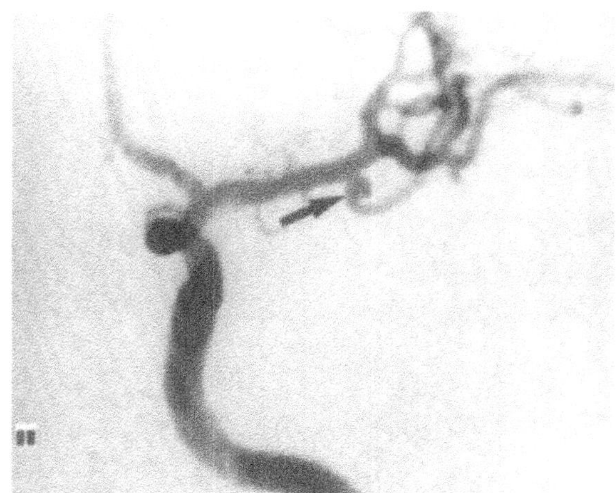

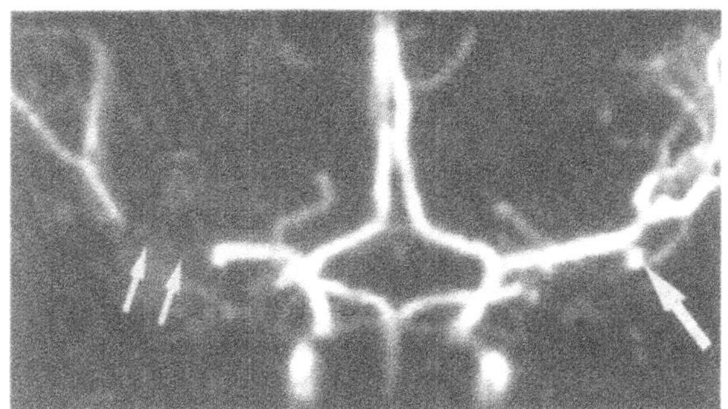

Fig. 13.23a, b. Small middle cerebral artery aneurysm. **a** Selective intra-arterial DSA of the left internal carotid artery. Anteroposterior submental projection. There is a small (diameter 3 mm) aneurysm (*arrow*) of temporal branch of left middle cerebral artery. **b** Coronal MIP of 3D TOF MRA sequence. TR/TE/Fl 40 ms/ 10 ms/20°, magnetisation transfer preparation pulse and TONE RF excitation, FOV 153×210 mm, slab thickness 52 mm/64 partitions, matrix 192×256, acquisition time 8 min, Nex=1. The small aneurysm (*arrow*) is well visualised. Note the signal drop out in right middle cerebral artery due to a metallic clip (*double arrow*)

Fig. 13.22a–f. Posterior cerebral artery aneurysm, probably mycotic: superposition of recent haemorrhage. **a** Selective intra-arterial DSA of the right internal carotid artery. A large (diameter 8 mm) aneurysm (*arrow*) of the perimesencephalic portion of the right posterior cerebral artery is visualised. **b, c** Transverse T1 weighted (TR=456 ms; TE=40 ms, 1 acq.) spin-echo MR sequence. Hyperintense haemorrhage (*arrow*) is located posteriorly to aneurysm (*arrowheads*) presenting signal void. **d** Sagittal and **e** transverse MIP of 3D TOF MRA sequence. TR/TE/Fl 43 ms/8 ms/20°, magnetisation transfer preparation pulse and TONE RF excitation, FOV 165×220 mm, slab thickness 32 mm/32 partitions, matrix 256×256, acquisition time 6 min, Nex=1. Both the aneurysm and the haemorrhage (*arrows*) are depicted as hyperintense. **f** Posterior cerebral artery aneurysm, probably mycotic: supTransverse MIP of 3D PC MRA sequence. TR/TE/Fl 45 ms/ 8 ms/20°, FOV 260 mm, VENC 30 cm/s, slab thickness 32 mm/32 partitions, matrix 192×256, acquisition time 9 min, Nex=1. Stationary tissue of haemorrhage is subtracted. The size of the aneurysm is underestimated due to increased dephasing effects of flow turbulence in the PC MRA sequence

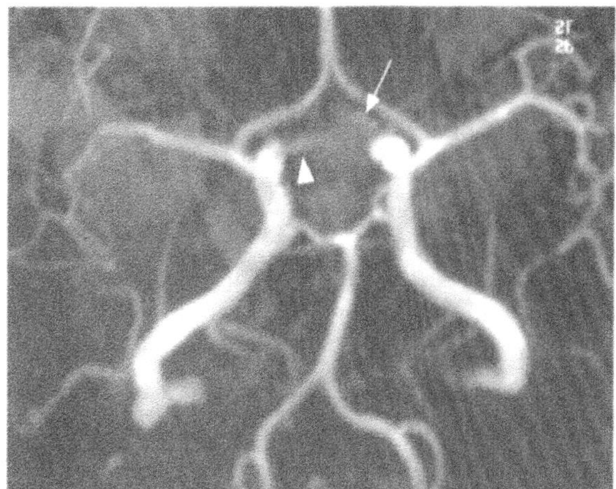

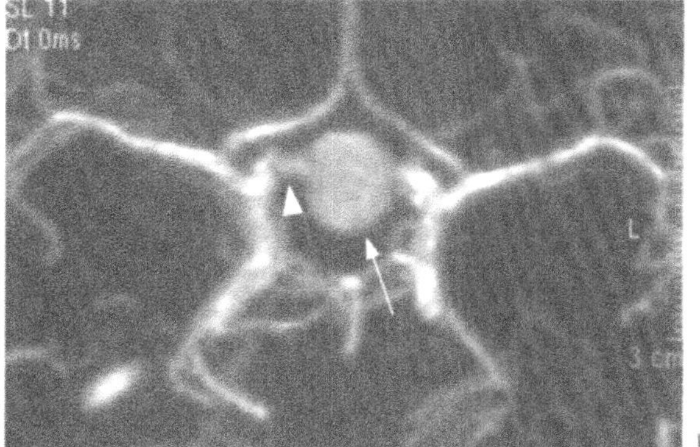

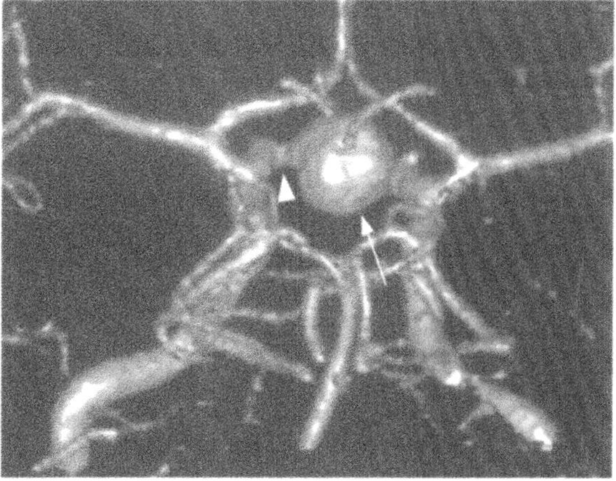

Fig. 13.24a–c. Value of dynamic contrast-enhanced MRA on slow-flow aneurysms. **a** Semicoronal MIP of a 3D TOF MRA sequence. TR/TE/Fl 35 ms/7,2 ms/20°, magnetisation transfer preparation pulse and TONE RF excitation, rectangular FOV 150×200 mm, slab thickness 82 mm, matrix 200×512, acquisition time 6,44 min, Nex=1. The aneurysm (*arrow*) is poorly visualised due to extremely slow flow within the aneurysmal sac. Note the small neck of the aneurysm (*arrowhead*). **b** Dynamic contrast-enhanced MRA sequence in the same patient. MIP in an identical projection. 3D FFE, TR/TE/Fl 4.3 ms/1.5 ms/45°, FOV 250 mm, matrix, 256×256, acquisition time 14 s, slice thickness 1,2 mm. The sac of the aneurysm (*arrow*) and the aneurysmal neck (*arrowhead*) are nicely demonstrated. **c** 3D surface rendered image of the dynamic contrast-enhanced MRA sequence in the same projection. Excellent visualisation of the aneurysm (*arrow*) and the aneurysm neck (*arrowhead*)

linium-enhanced 3D MRA, since a trombus is never hyperintense on the arterial images.

13.4.3 Arteriovenous Malformations

Intracranial arteriovenous malformations (AVMs) represent the most common type of cerebral vascular malformation. AVMs consist of a cluster or nidus of multiple arteriovenous shunts, fed by one or more hypertrophic arteries and drained by tortuous hypertrophic veins. Aneurysms, which occur on the feeding arteries and draining veins as well as in the nidus, are the source of frequently fatal haemorrhagic complications (TURJMAN et al. 1994). AVMs are usually large and visible on plain spin-echo MRI (GRAVES and DUFF 1990).

The most severe clinical manifestation is haemorrhage, which has a high morbidity and mortality rate. However, many patients will develop substantial morbidity due to the lesion, even in the absence of haemorrhage. Most frequent manifestations are epilepsy or cranial nerve deficits. Considering the potential risk of bleeding even asymptomatic lesions are more aggressively treated nowadays.

Therapeutic possibilities include surgery, endovascular embolisation and radiotherapy. Combination of therapies is not uncommon. Angiography is not necessary for the diagnosis of cerebral AVMs since they are already well depicted on contrast-enhanced CT or spin-echo MR images. The choice of therapy can be made solely on the basis of topography and size. Angiography has to demonstrate the number, size and location of the feeding arteries, the size of the nidus, the presence of intranidal arteriovenous shunts and the size and course of the draining veins. Aneurysms on the feeding arteries, in the nidus or on the draining veins also have to be visualised considering the important prognostic implications.

Because of the high flow in the feeding arteries, they are generally well visualised on 3D TOF MRA or PC MRA (Fig. 13.25, Fig. 13.27) (NÜSSEL et al. 1991; EDELMAN et al. 1989; KESAVA and TURSKI 1998). However, in some larger lesions, the hyperdynamic character of the flow in these feeding vessels can lead to severe local turbulences leading to signal loss (Fig. 13.26). Therefore small aneurysms on the feeding arteries are frequently missed. On the other hand, in many cases both the nidus and the draining veins will be only partially visualised due to saturation. Here again, the injection of gadolinium or the application of less saturating sequences (2D/3D MOTSA)

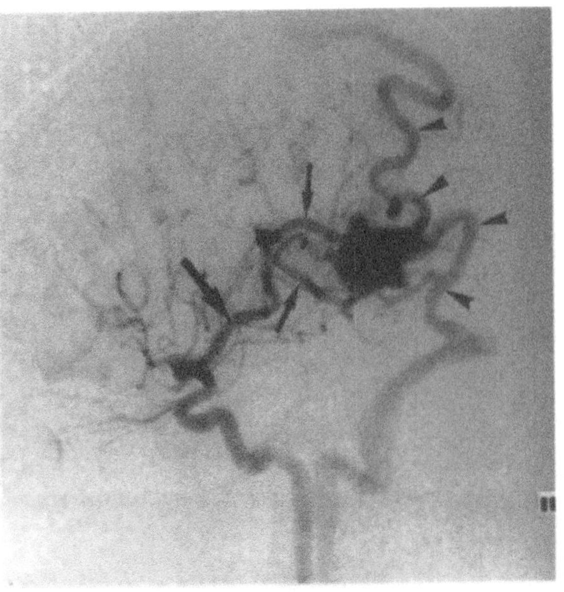

a

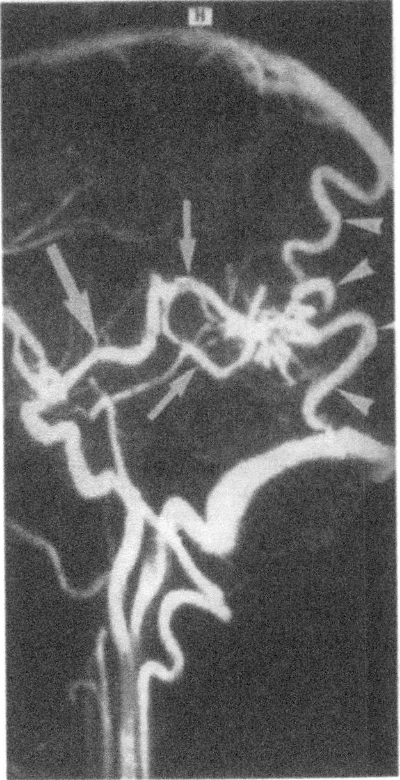

b

Fig. 13.25a, b. Left temporo-occipital AVM. **a** Selective intra-arterial DSA of the left internal carotid artery. Lateral projection. The nidus is located in the temporo-occipital region. The posterior branch of the middle cerebral artery is hypertrophic (*arrow*). The hypertrophic angular and posterior temporal branches (*thin arrows*) feed the AVM. The lesion is drained by cortical veins (*arrowheads*) draining to the superior sagittal sinus and to the transverse sinus. **b** Sagittal MIP of 3D PC MRA sequence. TR/TE/Fl 30 ms/10 ms/20°, FOV 210 mm, VENC 30 cm/s, 2 sagittal overlapping thin 3D acquisitions, slab thickness 42 mm/32 partitions, matrix 192×256, acquisition time 2×12 min. Hypertrophic feeding arteries, nidus and draining veins are well visualised. *Arrows* correspond to *arrows* in **a**

can be very helpful (Blatter et al. 1991, 1992). With high-resolution 3D gradient-echo sequences with a long echo time, exquisite venous anatomy can be visualised. This allows better detection of small AVMs (Essig et al. 1999). Due to susceptibility artefacts, this method is less suited for the study of AVMs close to the skull base or having suffered from previous bleeding.

A main disadvantage of MRA is the lack of temporal selectivity. This might be overcome by time-resolved projection MRA, using a slice-selective snapshot FLASH sequence with a time resolution of two images per second after bolus injection of gadolinium-DTPA. This gives information on the haemodynamics of vascular malformations (Klish et al. 2000). The same temporal information might be obtained with dynamic gadolinium-enhanced 3D MRA (Parker et al. 1998).

Despite the spectacular images produced by MRA, in most patients selective and superselective angiography remains necessary when deciding which therapy is best for the patient. For the planning of radiosurgery, MRA seems to provide information on irregular AVM shape and is superior to MRI for defining the AVM nidus (Bednarz et al. 2000). MRA can be used to follow up cerebral arteriovenous malformations after radiosurgery or embolisation (Kauczor et al. 1993; Quisling et al. 1991).

Developmental venous anomalies (DVAs) or the so-called venous angiomas are considered to be congenital variants of the venous drainage of the brain and are mostly asymptomatic. In rare cases they are seen in patients with intracerebral haemorrhage. The lesions are easily seen on gadolinium-enhanced MRI (Marchal et al. 1992; Wilms et al. 1991). MRA can be useful to study the confluence of the draining vein of the lesion in the dural venous sinuses (Fig. 13.7). Stenoses at the confluence seem to be frequent and are believed to be at the origin of bleeding in these venous angiomas.

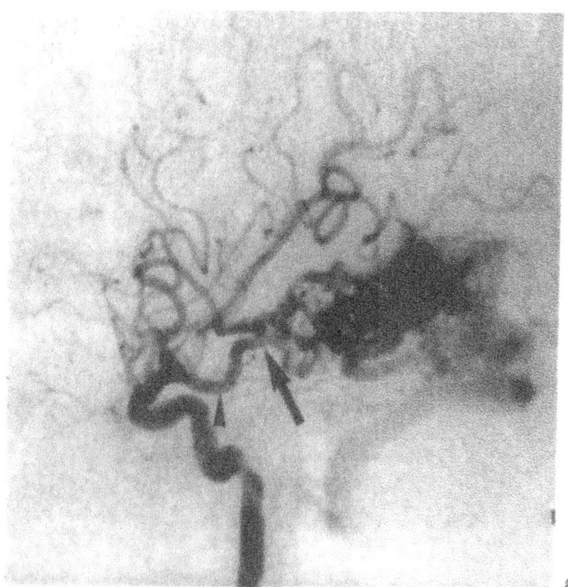

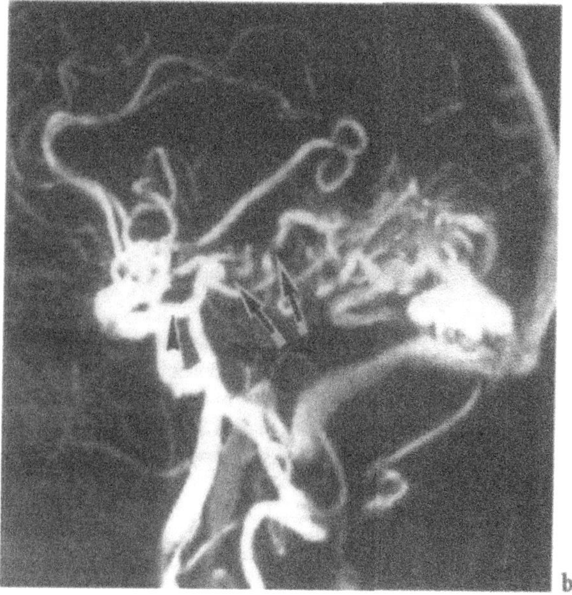

Fig. 13.26a, b. Left occipital arteriovenous malformation. **a** Selective intra-arterial DSA of the left internal carotid artery. Lateral projection. A huge nidus is present in the left occipital lobe. The lesion is fed by hypertrophic feeding arteries (*arrows*) arising from the posterior cerebral artery. There is embryonal branching of the left posterior cerebral artery of the left internal carotid artery via a hypertrophic "embryonal" posterior communicating artery (*arrowhead*). Venous drainage via hypertrophic cortical veins towards the transverse sinus. **b** Sagittal MIP of 3D PC MRA sequence. TR/TE/Fl 30 ms/10 ms/20°, FOV 210 mm, VENC 30 cm/s, two sagittal overlapping thin 3D acquisitions, slab thickness 48 mm/32 partitions, matrix 192×256, acquisition time 2×12 min, 1 Nex. There is excellent visualisation of the nidus. The posterior communicating artery is also well visualised (*arrowhead*). The perimesencephalic portion of the posterior cerebral artery and the proximal parieto-occipital artery show some interruption (*arrows*) due to turbulent flow. Venous drainage is well visualised

13.4.4 Tumours

The symptomatology of brain tumours is extremely variable and will largely depend on the location of the tumour.

The role of angiography in the study of cerebral tumours has dramatically changed since the advent of CT and, in particular, MRI. Since then, angiography has ceased to be used for the detection of a brain tumour or for the specification of its nature. Angiography is used to supply preoperative information on the vascular anatomy of the brain, the vascularity of the tumour, and the course of the cerebral veins in order to allow a decision on the surgical approach. In patients with extra-axial tumours, the external carotid artery supply needs to be visualised. Just as conventional angiography (Fig. 13.28a, b), MRA offers mostly indirect information by the visualisation of vessel displacement (Fig. 13.28c–e) (Wilms et al. 1995; Van Hemert 1997). The evaluation of the tumoral vascularity is beyond the scope of MRA. If the tumour enhances after injection of gadolinium, the relationship of the tumour with the vessels can be determined more exactly (Fig. 13.28f–h). In most patients, however, assessment of tumour size, location and vascularity is equally well diagnosed by CE spin-echo MRI. On the other hand, the venous anatomy is more effectively studied by MRA, especially after injection of gadolinium. The visualisation of the superficial cortical veins together with the cortical

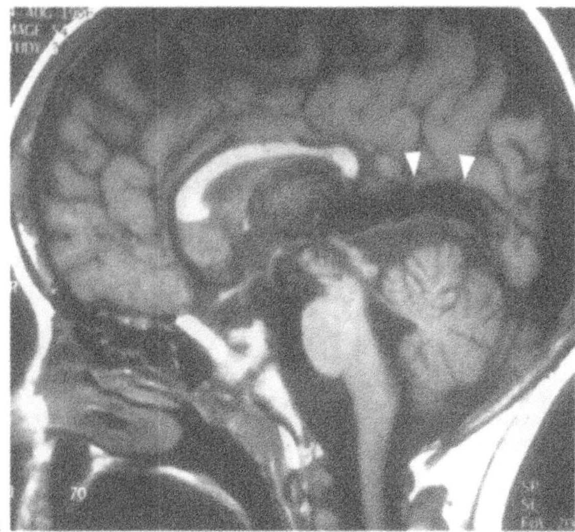

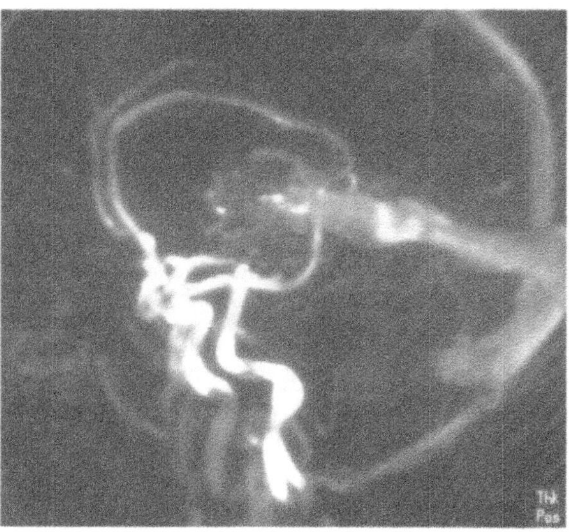

Fig. 13.27a, b. Aneurysmal malformation of the vein of Galen. **a** Sagittal T1-weigthed spin-echo sequence (TR=600 ms, TE=14 ms, 1 acq). Flow voids are seen in the thalamus. Note the enlarged falcine sinus (*arrowheads*). **b** Sagittal MIP of a 3D TOF MRA sequence. TR/TE/Fl 43 ms/8 ms/20°, magnetisation transfer preparation pulse and TONE RF excitation, FOV 165×220 mm, slab thickness 32 mm/32 partitions, matrix 256×256, acquisition time 6 min, Nex=1. Nice demonstration of the hypertrophic feeding choroidal vessels. The enlarged and abnormally coursing falcine sinus is well seen

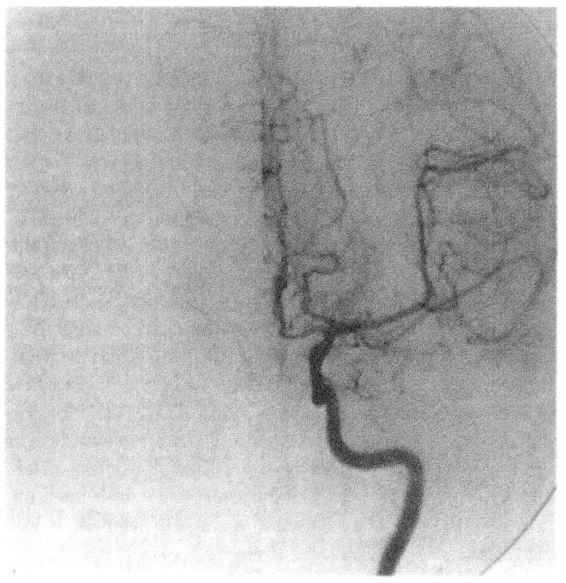

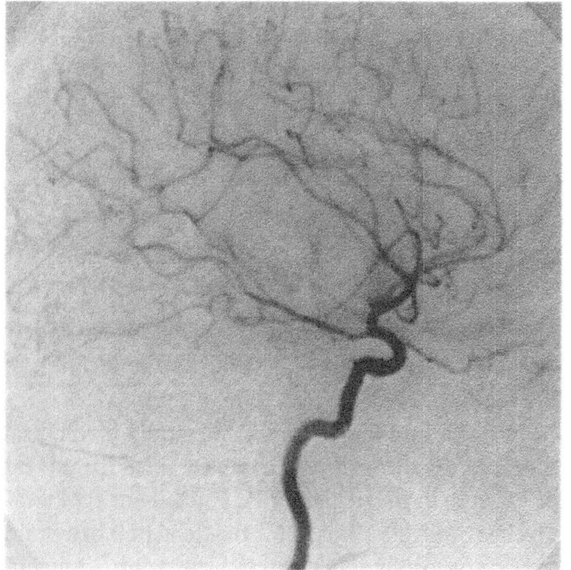

Fig. 13.28a,b →

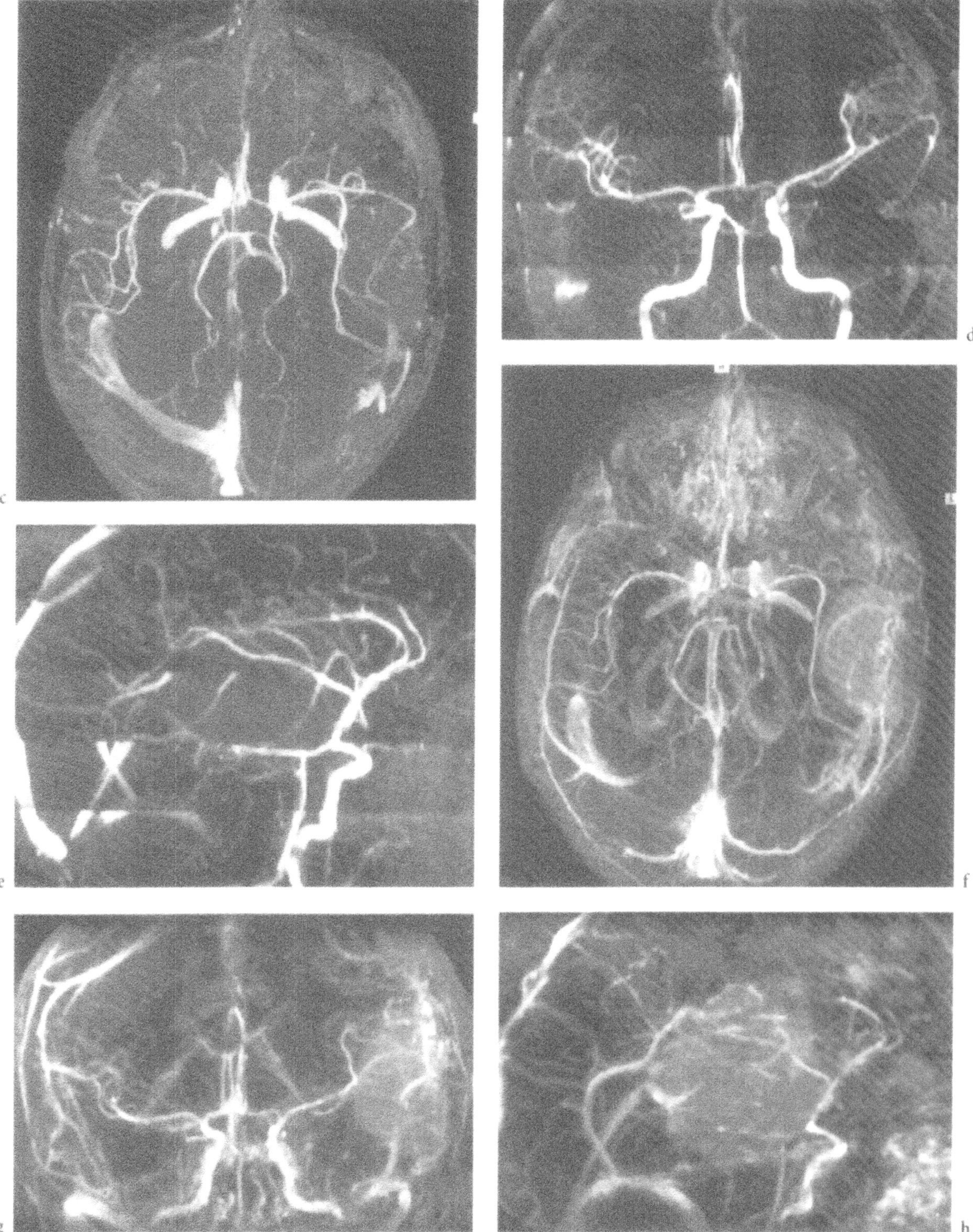

Fig. 13.28a–h. Left temporal glioblastoma. **a** Anter oposterior and **b** lateral projection of selective intra-arterial DSA of the left internal carotid artery. Elevation of the vascular branches of the middle cerebral artery is evident. Tumoral vessels with hypervascularisation and tumoral blush are present in the temporal region. **c** Transverse, **d** coronal and **e** sagittal MIP of unenhanced 3D TOF MRA sequence. TR/TE/Fl 43 ms/10 ms/20°, magnetisation transfer preparation pulse and TONE RF excitation, FOV 200 mm, MOTSA, slab thickness 32 mm/32 partitions, mutual overlap of 6 mm at each side, matrix 256×256, acquisition time 5×6 min, Nex=1. There is good visualisation of vascular displacement of the left middle cerebral artery branches. Tumoral vessels are not visualised. **f** Transverse, **g** coronal and **h** sagittal MIP of 3D TOF MRA sequence after gadolinium enhancement. TR/TE/Fl 43 ms/10 ms/20°, magnetisation transfer preparation pulse and TONE RF excitation, single thick slab acquisition 120 mm/128 partitions, matrix 192×256, acquisition time 18 min, Nex=1. The tumoral mass enhances and can be perfectly be located. Enhancing tumour somewhat obscures vessels of the middle cerebral artery. Visualisation of tumoral vessels is questionable

anatomy can be sufficient for the decision on the surgical approach.

Finally, the combination of MRI and MRA is used to increase the safety of stereotactic procedures by selecting the target point and defining the safest needle trajectory and approach (Michiels et al. 1995).

13.4.5 Venous Pathology

The clinical signs and symptoms of cerebral venous occlusive disease are often non-specific, with acute neurologic deterioration, due to cortical venous infarction and petechial perivascular haemorrhages. It is most commonly due to spread of infection, dehydration, haematological disorders, coagulopathies, trauma or tumours. The most frequently involved sinus is the superior sagittal sinus, followed by the transverse, sigmoid and cavernous sinuses. The superficial cortical veins that drain into the superior sagittal sinus are the most commonly occluded veins.

Many acute to subacute thromboses are already diagnosed on unenhanced T1 SE images by virtue of the hyperintense character of the fresh thrombus (Fig. 13.29c). The purpose of angiography is to confirm the CT or spin-echo MR diagnosis of cerebral venous occlusion and the evaluation of the extent of the venous occlusion (Flotho et al. 1999).

In MRA the presence of a thrombus is seen as a filling defect within the lumen (Nadel et al. 1990; Padayachee et al. 1991; Finn et al. 1993). High-intensity fresh thrombi can also cause false-negative images on TOF sequences (Fig. 13.29a). In these cases, PC methods and the application of saturation pulses can be necessary (Fig. 13.29b,d). One has to be aware of possible false-positive results related to saturation in 2D TOF MRA sequences (Fig. 13.30). An appropriate choice of scan planes is therefore mandatory. In thrombosis of the deep cerebral veins, the deep veins can be hyperintense on T1-weigthed spin-echo images. On T2-weigthed spin-echo images, both thalami will show hyperintensity. MRA demonstrates absence of filling of the deep venous system (Lafitte et al. 1999) (Fig. 13.31). In Fig. 13.32 the compression of the sagittal sinus by a small meningioma is illustrated.

As mentioned above, giant arachnoid granulations can cause filling defects mimicking intraluminal thrombus in the dural venous sinuses (Fig. 13.13).

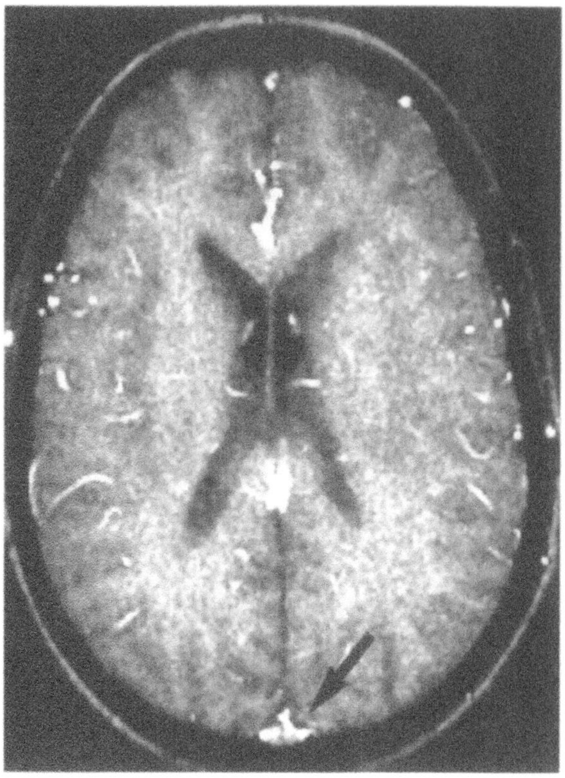

a

Fig. 13.29a–e. Superior sagittal sinus thrombosis. **a** Transverse single slice 2D TOF MRA acquisition. TR/TE/Fl 40 ms/10 ms/90°, FOV 230 mm, slice thickness 4 mm, matrix 256×256, acquisition time 10 s, Nex=1. Hyperintense signal (*arrow*) is present in arteries and in the superior sagittal sinus.

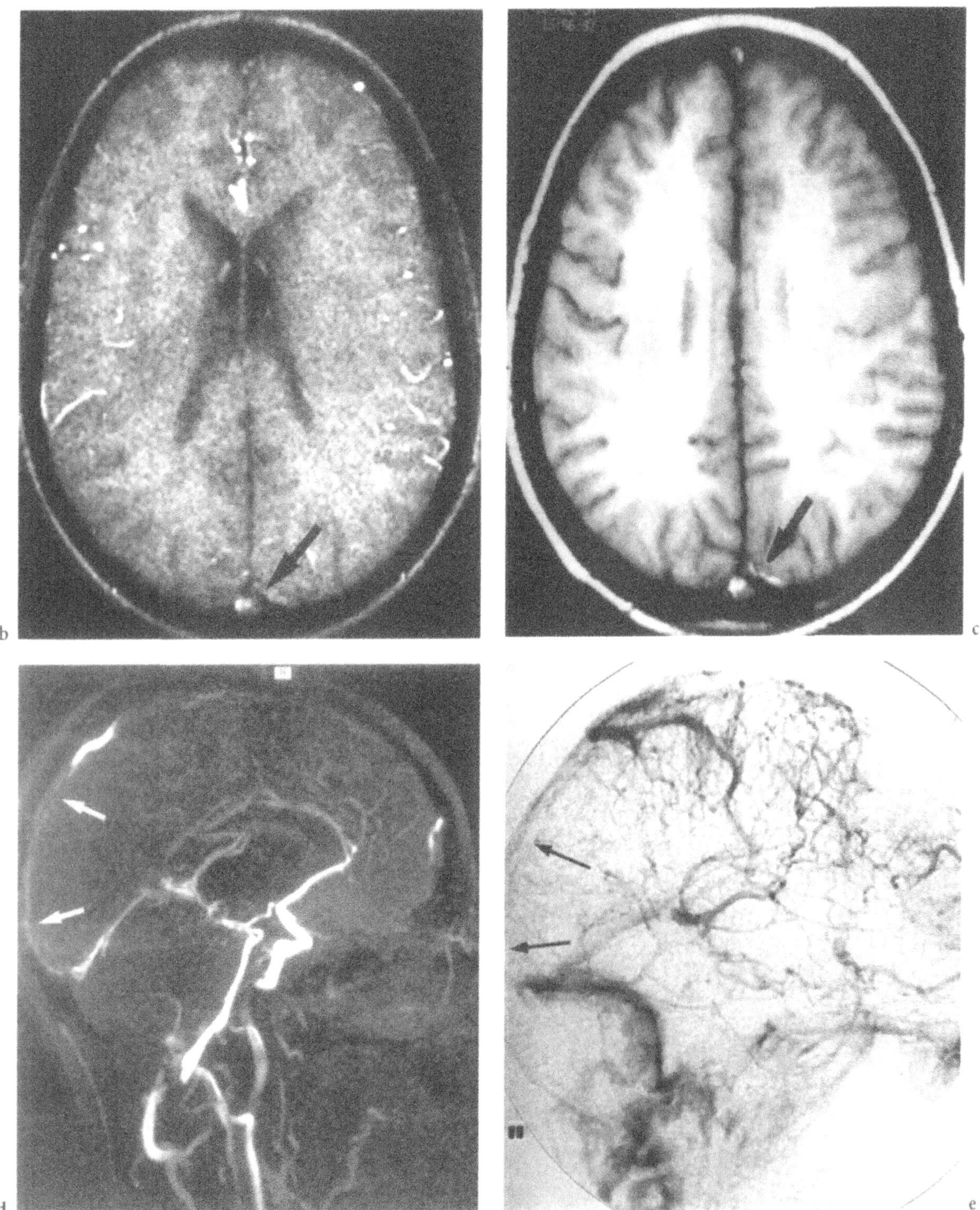

Fig. 13.29a–e. (Continued) Superior sagittal sinus thrombosis. **b** Identical acquisition with venous presaturation. Most of the hyperintense signal (*arrow*) in the superior sagittal sinus persists, pointing to venous thrombus. **c** Transverse T1-weighted spin-echo sequence at the same level. Thrombus is hyperintense (*arrow*). **d** Sagittal MIP of 3D PC MRA sequence. TR/TE/Fl 30 ms/10 ms/20°, FOV 210 mm, VENC 30 cm, slab thickness 45 mm/32 partitions, matrix 192×256, acquisition time 12 min, Nex=1. The superior sagittal sinus (*arrows*) is only partially patent in the most distal third. **e** Selective intra-arterial DSA of the left internal carotid artery. Lateral projection; venous phase. The superior sagittal sinus is occluded. Some patency (*arrows*) of the distal one third, above the torcular Herophili

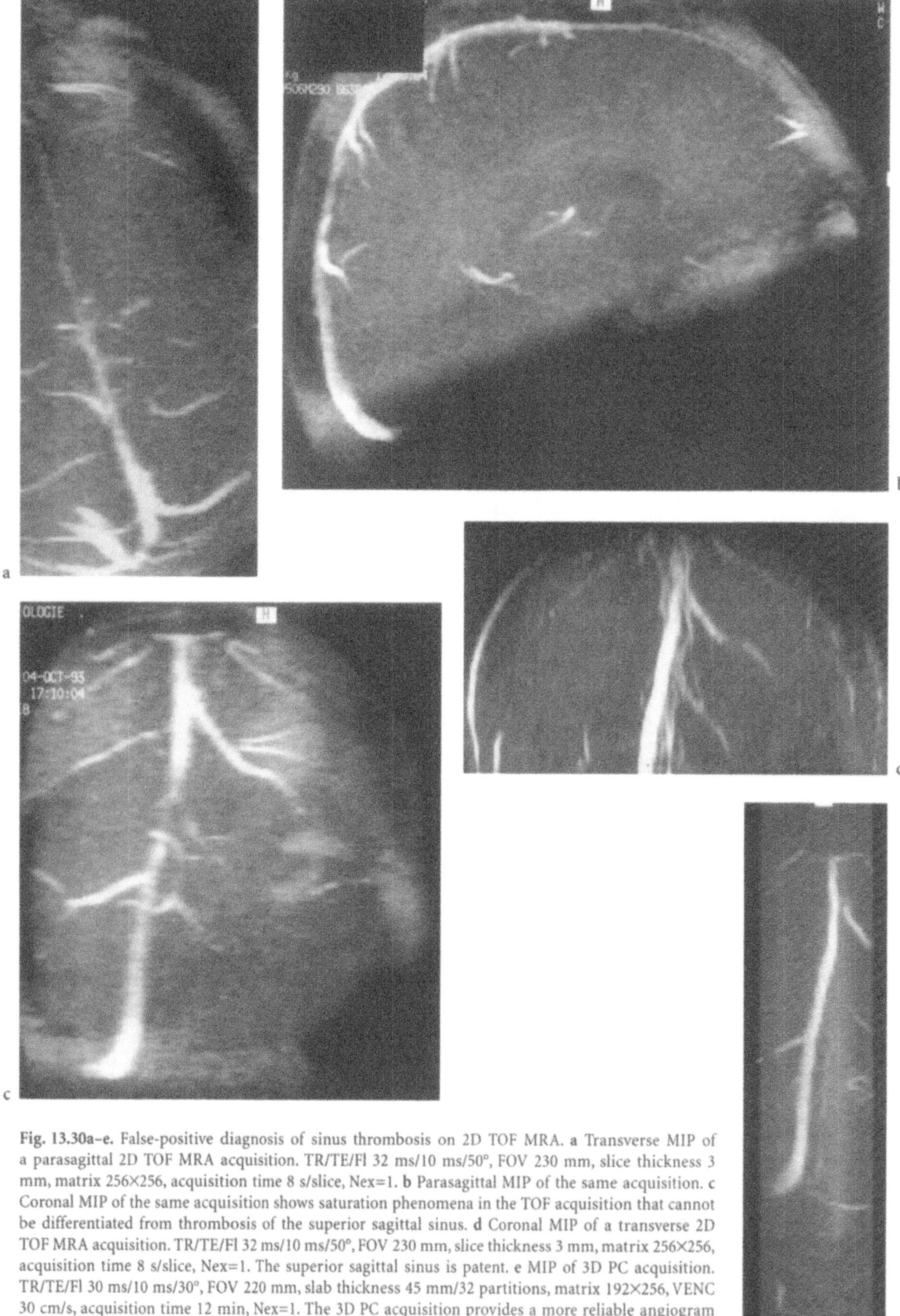

Fig. 13.30a–e. False-positive diagnosis of sinus thrombosis on 2D TOF MRA. **a** Transverse MIP of a parasagittal 2D TOF MRA acquisition. TR/TE/Fl 32 ms/10 ms/50°, FOV 230 mm, slice thickness 3 mm, matrix 256×256, acquisition time 8 s/slice, Nex=1. **b** Parasagittal MIP of the same acquisition. **c** Coronal MIP of the same acquisition shows saturation phenomena in the TOF acquisition that cannot be differentiated from thrombosis of the superior sagittal sinus. **d** Coronal MIP of a transverse 2D TOF MRA acquisition. TR/TE/Fl 32 ms/10 ms/50°, FOV 230 mm, slice thickness 3 mm, matrix 256×256, acquisition time 8 s/slice, Nex=1. The superior sagittal sinus is patent. **e** MIP of 3D PC acquisition. TR/TE/Fl 30 ms/10 ms/30°, FOV 220 mm, slab thickness 45 mm/32 partitions, matrix 192×256, VENC 30 cm/s, acquisition time 12 min, Nex=1. The 3D PC acquisition provides a more reliable angiogram and does so independently of the projection direction

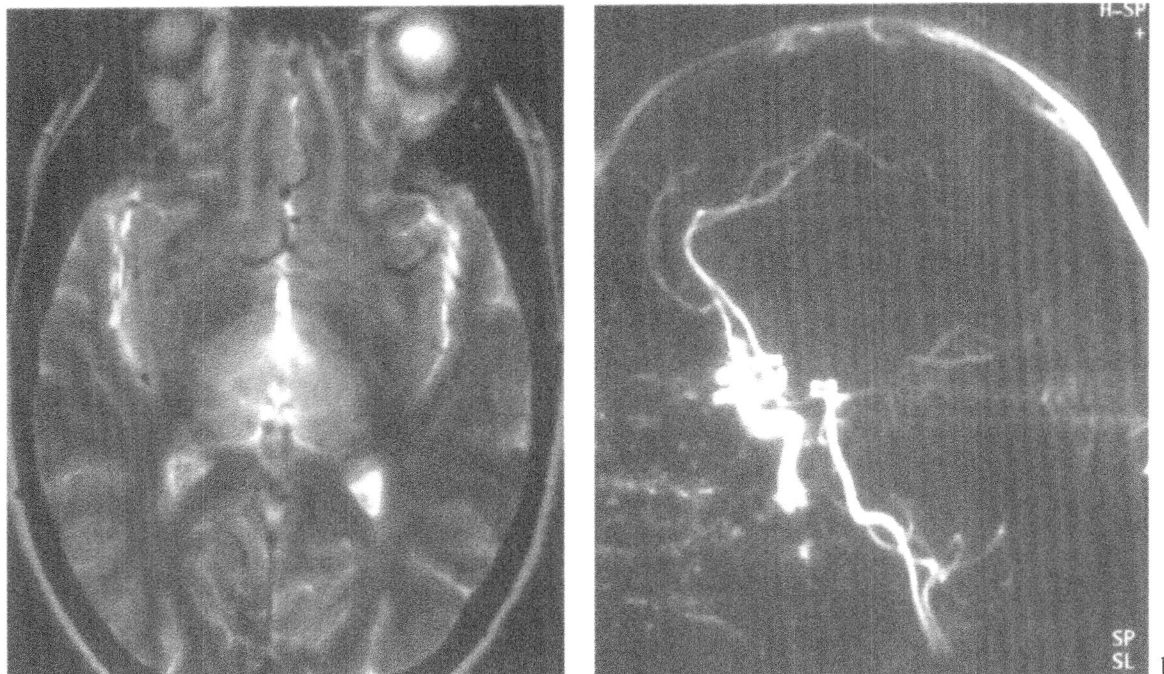

Fig. 13.31a, b. Thrombosis of the deep cerebral veins. **a** Transverse T2-weighted spin-echo image (TR=2500 ms, TE=90 ms, 1 acq.). Bilateral swelling and hyperintensity of the thalami, pointing to venous infarction. **b** Sagittal MIP of 3D PC MRA sequence (TR/TE/Fl 30 ms/10 ms/30°, FOV 220 mm, slab thickness 45 mm/32 partitions, matrix 192×256, VENC 30 cm/s, acquisition time 12 min, Nex=1). Note absence of visualisation of the deep cerebral veins and of the straight sinus

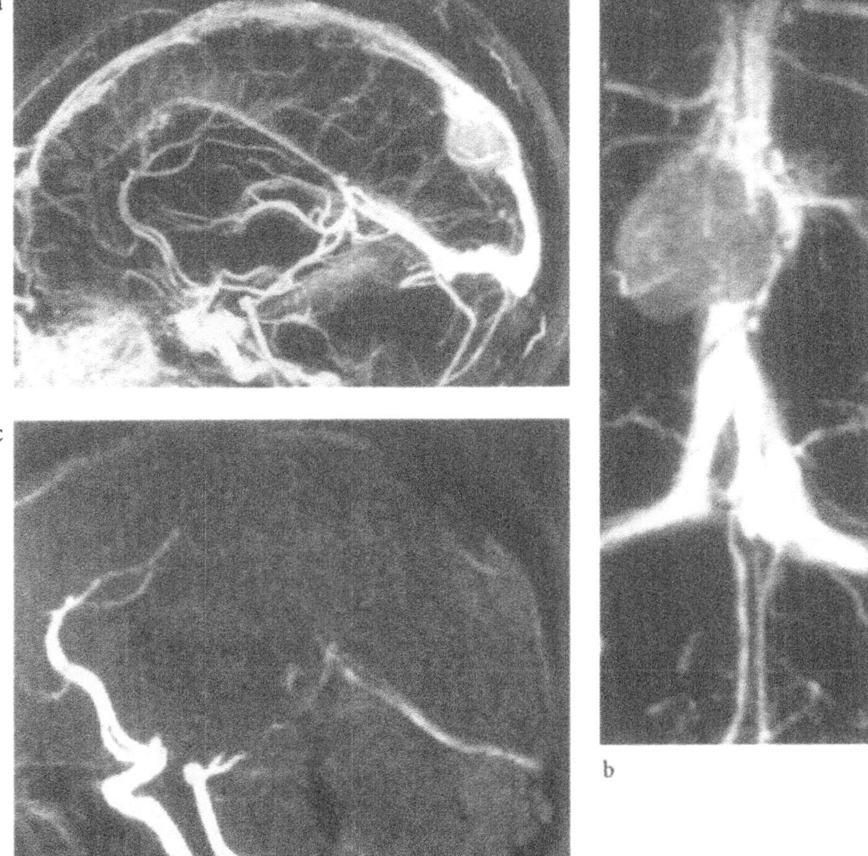

Fig. 13.32a–c. Meningioma with compression of the superior sagittal sinus. **a** Sagittal and **b** coronal MIP of 3D contrast-enhanced sagittal TOF MRA sequence. TR/TE/Fl 42 ms/11 ms/38°, magnetisation transfer preparation pulse, FOV 230 mm, slab thickness 52 mm/64 partitions, matrix 192×512, acquisition time 8 min, Nex=1. There is considerable narrowing of the superior sagittal sinus by the tumour. Collateral veins are visualised. **c** Sagittal MIP of 3D PC MRA sequence. Absence of signal in the superior sagittal sinus indicates reduced flow. TR/TE/Fl 30 ms/10 ms/20°, FOV 230 mm, VENC 30 cm/s, slab thickness 40 mm/32 partitions, matrix 192×256, acquisition time 12 min, Nex=1

13.4.6
Vascular Compression

Vascular loops can cause compression of cranial nerves. The classical example is the compression of the facial nerve in the cerebellopontine angle by loops of the anterior inferior cerebellar artery (AICA), causing facial nerve palsy or neuralgia (Felber et al. 1992). An elongated basilar artery can cause trigeminal neuralgia. The role of angiography consists of the visualisation of the compressing vascular loops. The tortuosity of the basilar artery and the AICA can be visualised with MRA and appropriate techniques. By correlation with the spin-echo sequences the diagnosis of vascular compression can be made.

13.5
Imaging Protocols

13.5.1
Imaging Protocols for Intracranial MRA of the Arteries

A 3D TOF acquisition through the suspected region is a quick and reliable first technique in many indications for intracranial MRA. However, frequently, unresolved questions remain that require additional approaches. A typical example is recent thrombus causing spontaneously hyperintense signal that interferes with the TOF angiogram. A T1-weighted (spin-echo) acquisition can be added to prove the presence of a tissue with short T1. Another approach is the use of a PC acquisition that subtracts the signal of the stationary tissues, including the blood clot, and therefore provides a more correct angiogram. In case of suspected aneurysms with bleeding, it is even suitable to start the study with a PC acquisition.

A second common problem is the signal loss in blood vessels. An additional contrast-enhanced TOF or a 2D TOF study can then be performed to differentiate between saturation-induced signal loss (in which case the signal loss disappears) and flow-induced phase effects (in which signal loss is not overcome).

In the preoperative study of patients with brain tumours or in the work up of patients with AVMs it might be necessary to visualise all the vessels of the brain. The whole brain can be imaged by means of multiple overlapping small 3D TOF acquisitions. A second contrast-enhanced acquisition can be added to improve the visualisation of the veins. PC acquisitions may be performed instead of TOF acquisitions. Though high-resolution PC angiography is time consuming, it can be advantageously used if the volumes of interest are limited. Occasionally, a PC study has to be repeated with different VENCs.

13.5.2
Imaging Protocols for Intracranial MRA of the Veins

In case of suspected sagittal sinus thrombosis, a 2D TOF or a PC acquisition is an appropriate first MRA sequence. With 2D TOF, one must realise that both inflowing blood and tissues with short T1 produce hyperintense signals. Furthermore, slices have to be oriented as perpendicular as possible to the veins. A T1-weighted spin-echo acquisition is necessary to rule out thrombus with short T1 if the 2D TOF examination is negative. 3D PC acquisitions can be performed to visualise the suspected regions with better resolution. This acquisition offers the additional advantage that the signal of thrombi is suppressed. In a contrast-enhanced TOF acquisition, saturation is also overcome and improved blood vessel detail can be obtained. It must be remembered that extracranial tissues and lesions with an abnormal blood–brain barrier will also be enhanced.

Venous anomalies can also be demonstrated with MRA. 2D TOF or 2D PC acquisitions can be used as localizers. 3D PC with low VENC or contrast-enhanced 3D TOF acquisitions provide the most detailed angiograms.

Similarly, the best visualisation of the venous drainage in larger intracranial lesions, including AVMs and tumours, is obtained with 3D PC imaging or 3D contrast-enhanced TOF acquisitions.

References

Anderson CM, Saloner D, Tsuruda JS, Shapeero LG, Lee R (1990) Artefacts in maximum-intensity-projection display of MR angiograms. AJR Am J Roentgenol 154:623–629

Atkinson D, Brant-Zawadzki M, Gillan G, Purdy D, Laub G (1994) Improved MR angiography: magnetisation transfer suppression with variable flip angle excitation and increased resolution. Radiology 190:890–894

Bednarz G, Downes B, Werner-Wasik M, Rosenwasser RH (2000) Combining stereotactic angiography and 3D time-of-flight magnetic resonance angiography in treatment planning for arteriovenous malformation radiosurgery. Int J Radat Oncol Biol Phys 46:1149–1154

Blatter DD, Parker DI, Robinson RO (1991) Cerebral MR

Angiography with multiple overlapping thin slab acquisition. I. Quantitative analysis of vessel visibility. Radiology 179:805–811
Blatter DD, Parker DL, Ahn SS, Bahr AL, Robinson RO, Schwartz RB, Jolesz FA, Boyer RS (1992) Cerebral MR Angiography with multiple overlapping thin slab acquisition. II. Early clinical experience. Radiology 183:379–389
Blatter DD, Bahr AL, Parker DL, Robison RO, Kimball JA, Perry DM, Horn S (1993) Cervical carotid MR angiography with multiple overlapping thin-slab acquisitions: comparison with conventional angiography. AJR Am J Roentgenol 161:1269–1277
Bosmans H (1992) Optimization procedures for magnetic resonance angiography acquisitions. PhD Thesis, KU Leuven, Belgium
Bosmans H, Marchal G, Van Hecke P, Vandermeulen D, Suetens P (1990) Magnetic resonance angiography: techniques, prospects and limitations. Frontiers in European Radiology 7:69–86
Bosmans H, Marchal G, Van Hecke P, Vanhoenacker P (1992) MRA review. Clin Imag 16:152–167
Bosmans H, Marchal G, Lukito G, Yicheng N, Wilms G, Laub G, Baert AL (1995) Contrast enhanced time-of-flight MR angiography of the brain: comparison of acquisition techniques in healthy volunteers. AJR Am J Roentgenol 164:161–167
Brant-Zawadzki M, Gould R, Norman D, Newton TH, Lane B (1983) Digital subtraction cerebral angiography by intraarterial injection: comparison with conventional angiography. AJR Am J Roentgenol 140:347–353
Brugières P, Blustajn J, Le Guerinel C, Meder JF, Thomas P, Gaston A (1998) Magnetic resonance angiography of giant intracranial aneurysms. Neuroradiology 40:96–102
Brunereau L, Cottier JP, Sonier CB, Medioni B, Bertrand P, Rouleau P, Sirinelli D, Herbreteau D (1999) Prospective evaluation of time-of-flight MR angiography in the follow-up of intracranial saccular aneurysms treated with Guglielmi detachable coils. J Compt Assist Tomogr 23:216–223
Campi A, Rodesch G, Scotti G, Lasjaunias P (1998) Aneurysmal malformation of the vein of Galen in three patients: clinical and radiological follow-up. Neuroradiology 40:816–821
Chakeres DW, Schmalbrock P, Brogan M, Yuan C, Cohen L (1991) Normal venous anatomy of the brain: demonstration with gadopentetate dimeglumine in enhanced 3-D MR angiography. AJR Am J Roentgenol 156:161–172
Cognard C, Weill A, Castaings L, Rey A, Moret J (1998) Intracranial berry anuerysms: angiographic and clinical results after endovascular treatment. Radiology 206:499–510
Creasy JL, Price RR, Presbrey T, Goins D, Partain CL, Kessler RM (1990) Gadolinium-enhanced MR-angiography. Radiology 175:280–283
Curnes JT, Shogry MEC, Clark DC, Elsner H (1993) MR angiographic demonstration of an intracranial aneurysm not seen on conventional angiography. AJNR Am J Neuroradiol 14:971–977
De Bray JM, Joseph PA, Jeanvoine H, Maugin D, Dauzat M, Plassard F (1988) Transcranial Doppler evaluation of middle cerebral artery stenosis. J Ultrasound Med 7:611–616
Dumoulin CL, Souza SP, Walker MF (1989) Three-dimensional phase-contrast angiography. Magn Reson Med 9:139–149
Edelman RR, Wentz KU, Mattle HP, O'Reilly GV, Candia G, Liu C, Zhao B, Kjellberg RN, Davis KR (1989) Intracerebral arteriovenous malformations: evaluation with selective MR angiography and venography. Radiology 173:831–837
Edelman RR, Mattle HP, O'Reilly GV, Wentz KU, Liu C, Zhao B (1990a) Magnetic resonance imaging of the flow dynamics in the circle of Willis. Stroke 21:56–66
Edelman RR, Mattle HP, Wallner B, Bajakian R, Kleefield J, Kent C, Skillman JJ, Mendel JB, Atkinson DJ (1990b) Extracranial carotid arteries: evaluation with 'BlackBlood' MR angiography. Radiology 177:45–50
Edelman RR, Ahn SS, Chien D, Li W, Goldmann A, Mantello M, Kramer J, Kleefield J (1992) Improved time-of-flight MR angiography of the brain with magnetization contrast. Radiology 184:395–403
Essig M, Reichenbach JR, Schad LR, Schoenberg SO, Debus SO, Kaiser WA (1999) High-resolution MR venography of cerebral arteriovenous malformations. Magn Reson Imaging 17:1417–1425
Evans AJ, Richardson DB, Tien R, MacFall JR, Hedlund LW, Heinz ER, Boyko C, Sostman HD (1993) Poststenotic signal loss in MR angiography: effects of echo time, flow compensation and fractional echo. AJNR Am J Neuroradiol 14:721–729
Felber S, Birbamer G, Aichner F, Poewe W, Kampfl A (1992) Magnetic resonance imaging and angiography in hemifacial spasm. Neuroradiology 34:413–416
Finn JP, Zisk JHS, Edelman RR, Wallner BK, Hartnell GG, Stokes KR, Longmaid HE (1993) Central venous occlusion: MR angiography. Radiology 187:245–251
Flotho E, Druschky KF, Niederstadt T (1999) Diagnostic value of combined magnetic resonance imaging and magnetic resonance angiography in sinus thrombosis. Fortschr Neurol Psychiatr 67:95–103
Gao J-H, Holland SK, Gore JC (1988) Nuclear magnetic resonance signal from flowing nuclei in rapid imaging using gradient echoes. Med Phys 15:809–814
Geevarghese SK, Powers T, Marsh JW, Pinson CW (1999) Screening for cerebral aneurysms in patients with polycystic liver disease. South Med J 92:1167–1170
Gelbert F, Assouline E, Hodes JE, Reizine D, Woimant F, George B, Hagueneau M, Merland JJ (1991) MRI in spontaneous dissection of vertebral and carotid arteries: 15 cases studied at 0.5 Tesla. Neuroradiology 33:111–113
Gillams AR, McMahon L, Weinberg G, Carter AP (1998) MRA of the intracranial circulation in asymptomatic patients with sickle cell disease. Pediatr Radiol 28:283–287
Goldberg HT (1992) Angiography of extra- and intracranial occlusive cerebrovascular disease. Neuroimaging Clin N Am 2:487–507
Gouliamos A, Gotsis E, Vlahos L, Samara C, Kapsalaki E, Rologis D, Kapsalakis Z, Papavasiliou C (1992) Magnetic resonance angiography compared to intra-arterial digital subtraction angiography in patients with subarachnoid haemorrhage. Neuroradioogy 35:46–49
Graves VB, Duff TA (1990) Intracranial arteriovenous malformations: current imaging and treatment. Invest Radiol 25:952–960
Grieve JP, Stacey R, Moore E, Kitchen ND, Jager HR (1999) Artefact on MRA following aneurysm clipping: an in vitro study and prospective comparison with conventional angiography. Neuroradiology 41:680–686
Guglielmi G, Vinuela F, Duckwiler G, Dion J, Lylyk P, Berenstein A, Strother C, Graves V, Halbach V, Nichols D (1992) Endovascular treatment of posterior circulation aneurysms by electrothrombosis using electrically detachable coils. J Neurosurg 77:515–524
Haacke EM, Masaryk TJ, Wielopolski PA, Zypman FR, Tkach

JA, Amartur S, Mitchell J, Clampitt M, Paschal C (1990) Optimizing blood vessel contrast in fast three-dimensional MRI. Magn Reson Imaging 14:202–221

Hankey GJ, Warlow CP, Sellar RJ (1990) Cerebral angiographic risk in mild cerebrovascular disease. Stroke 21:209–222

Hausmann R, Lewin JS, Laub G (1991) Phase-contrast MR angiography with reduced acquisition time: new concepts in sequence design. J Magn Reson Imaging 11:415–422

Heiserman JE, Drayer BP, Keller PJ, Fram EK (1992) Intracranial vascular stenosis and occlusion: evaluation with three-dimensional time-of-flight MR angiography. Radiology 185:667–673

Huston J III, Ehman RL (1993) Comparison of time-of-flight and phase-contrast MR neuroangiographic techniques. Radiographics 13:5–19

Isoda H, Takehara Y, Isogai S, Masunaga H, Takede H, Nozaki A, Sakahara H (2000) MRA of intracranial aneurysm models: a comparison of contrast-enhanced three-dimensional MRA with time-of-flight MRA. 24:308–315

Katz BH, Quencer RM, Kaplan JO, Hinks RS, Post JD (1989) MR imaging of intracranial carotid occlusion. AJNR Am J Neuroradiol 10:345–350

Kauczor HU, Engenhart R, Layer G, Gamroth AH, Wowra B, Schad LR, Semmler W, van Kaick G (1993) 3D TOF MR angiography of cerebral arteriovenous malformations after Radiosurgery. J Comput Assist Tomogr 17:184–190

Keogh AJ, Vhora S (1998) The usefulness of magnetic resonance angiography in surgery for intracranial aneurysms that heve beld. Surg Neurol 50:122–129

Kesava PP, Turski PA (1998) MR angiography of vascular malformations. Neuroimaging Clin N Am 8:349–370

Klish J, Strecker R, Hennig J, Schumacher M (2000) Time-resolved MRA: clinical apllication in intracranial vascular malformations. Neuroradiology 42:104–107

Koyama M, Tsuchiya K, Hanaoka H, Hachiya J, Karube M, Koyama N, Nakamura Y (1997) Reversible intracranial changes in eclampsia demonstrated by MRI and MRA. Eur J Radiol 25:44–46

Kusinoki K, Oka Y, Saito M, Sadamoto K, Sasaki S, Miki H, Nagasawa K (1999) Changes in visibility of intracranial arteries on MRA with normal ageing. Neuroradiology 41:813–819

Lafitte F, Boukobza M, Guichard JP, Reizine D, Woimant F, Merland JJ (1999) Deep cerebral venous thrombosis: imaging in eight cases. Neuroradiology 41:410–418

Lang EW, Steffens JC, Link J, Mehdorn HM (1998) The utility of contrast-enhanced MR angiography for posterior fossa giant cerebral aneurysm management. Neurol Res 20:705–708

Lanzino G, Kaptain G, Kallmes DF, Dix JE, Kassell NF (1997) Intracranial dissecting aneurysm causing subarachnoid hemorrhage: the role of computerized tomographic angiography and magnetic resonance angiography. Surg Neurol 48:477–481

Laub GA, Kaiser WA (1988) MR angiography with gradient motion refocusing. J Comput Assist Tomogr 12:377–382

Lewin JS, Laub G, Hausmann R (1991) A direct comparison of three time-of-flight techniques. AJR Am J Neuroradiol 12:1133–1139

Lin W, Tkach JA, Haacke EM, Masaryk TJ (1993) Intracranial MR angiography: application of magnetization transfer contrast and fat saturation to short gradient-echo, velocity-compensated sequences. Radiology 186:753–761

Lisovoski F, Rosseaux P (1993) Cerebral infarction in young people, a study of 148 patients with early cerebral angiography. J Neurol Neurosurg Psychiatry 50:609–614

Marchal G, Bosmans H, Van fraeyenhoven L, Wilms G, Van Hecke P, Plets C, Baert AL (1990) Intracranial vascular lesions: optimization and clinical evaluation of three-dimensional time-of-flight MR angiography. Radiology 175:443–448

Marchal G, Michiels J, Bosmans H, Van Hecke P (1992) Contrast-enhanced MRA of the brain. J Comput Assist Tomogr 16:25–29

Masaryk TJ, Modic MT, Ross JS,. Masaryk TJ, Modic MT, Ross JS, Ruggieri PM, Laub GA, Lenz GW, Haacke EM, Selman WR, Wiznitzer M, Harik SI (1989) Intracranial circulation: preliminary clinical results with three-dimensional (volume) MR angiography. Radiology 171:801–806

Masaryk AM, Ross JS, DiCello M, Modic MT, Paranandi L, Masarynk TJ (1991) 3DFT magnetic resonance angiography of the carotid bifurcation: potential and limitations as a screening examination. Radiology 179:797–804

Mathews VP, Ulmer JL, White ML, Hamilton CA, Reboussen DM, Elster AD (1999) Depiction of intracranial vessels with MRA: utility of magnetization transfer saturation and gadolinium. J Comput Assist Tomogr 23:597–602

Mathurin P, Hammer F, Duprez T, Goffette P, Grandin C (1993) Survey of intracerebral vasospasm after subarachnoid hemorrhage with 3D MR angiography. Presented at the XIXth Congress of the ESNR, September 8–11, 1993

Mattle HP, Wentz KU (1992) Selective magnetic resonance angiography of the Head. Cardiovasc Intervent Radiol 15:65–70

Mattle HP, Wentz KU, Edelman RR, Wallner B, Finn JP, Barnes P, Atkinson DJ, Kleefield J, Hoogewoud HM (1991) Cerebral venography with MR. Radiology 178:453–458

Metens TH, Fatima R, Balériaux D, Roger TH, David PH, Rodesch G (2000) Intracranial aneurysms: detection with gadolinium-enhanced dynamic three-dimensional MR angiography. Initial results. Radiology 216:39–46

Michiels J, Bosmans H, Nuttin B, Knauth M, Verbeeck R, Vandermeulen D, Wilms G, Marchal G, Suetens P, Gybels J (1995) The use of magnetic resonance angiography in stereotactic neurosurgery. J Neurosurg 82:982–987

Mursch K, Bransi A, Vatter H, Herrendorf G, Behnke-Mursch J, Kolenda (2000) Blood flow velocities in middle cerebral artery branches after subarachnoid hemorrhage. J Neuroimaging. 10:157–61

Nadel L, Braun IF, Kraft KA, Jensen ME, Laine FJ (1990) MRI of intracranial sinovenous thrombosis: the role of phase imaging. Magn Reson Imaging 8:315–320

Nadel L, Braun IF, Kraft KA, Fatouros PP, Laine FJ (1991) Intracranial vascular abnormalities: value of MR phase imaging to distinguish thrombus from flowing blood. AJR Am J Roentgenol 156:373–380

Nüssel F, Wegmüller H, Huber P (1991) Comparison of magnetic resonance angiography, magnetic resonance imaging and conventional angiography in cerebral arteriovenous malformation. Neuroradiol 33:56–61

Oelerich M, Lentschig MG, Zunker P, Reimer P, Rummeny EJ, Schuierer G (1998) Intracranial vascular stenosis and occlusion: comparison of 3D time-of-flight and 3D phase-contrast MR angiography. Neuroradiology 40:567–573

Ohue S, Kohno K, Kusunoki K, Sadamoto K, Ohta S, Ueda T, Sakaki (1998) Magnetic resonance angiography in patients with acute stroke treated by local thrombolysis. Neuroradiology 40:536–540

Osborn A (1994) Intracranial aneurysm in diagnostic neuroradiology. Mosby, St Louis, Baltimore, pp 248–283

Padayachee TS, Bingham JB, Graves MJ, Colchester AC, Cox TC (1991) Dural sinus thrombosis: follow-up by magnetic resonance angiography and imaging. Neuroradiology 33:165–167

Parker DL, Tsuruda JS, Goodrich KC, Alexander AL, Buswell HR (1998) Contrast-enhanced magnetic resonance angiography of cerebral arteries. Invest Radiol 33:560–572

Pernicone JR, Siebert JE, Potchen EJ, Pera A, Dumoulin CL, Souza SP (1990) Three-dimensional phase-contrast MR angiography in the head and neck: preliminary report. AJNR Am J Neuroradiol 11:457–466

Pernicone JR, Thorp KE, Ouimette MV, Siebert JE, Potchen EJ (1992) Magnetic resonance angiography in intracranial vascular disease. Semin Ultrasound CT MR 13:256–273

Quisling RG, Peters KR, Friedman WA, Tart RP (1991) Persistent nidus blood flow in cerebral arteriovenous malformation after stereotactic radiosurgery: MR imaging assessment. Radiology 180:785–791

Roberts G, Nanra J, Phillips J (1999) Screening for familial intracranial aneurysm: resource implications. Br J Neurosurg 13:395–398

Ross JS, Masaryk TJ, Modic MT, Ruggieri PM, Haacke EM, Selman WR (1990) Intracranial aneurysms: evaluation by MR angiography. AJNR Am J Neuroradiol 11:449–456

Ruggieri PM, Laub GA, Masaryk TJ, Modic MT (1989) Intracranial circulation: pulse sequence considerations in three-dimensional (volume) MR angiography. Radiology 171:785–791

Ruggieri PM, Masaryk TJ, Ross JS, Modic MT (1992) Intracranial magnetic resonance angiography. Cardiovasc Intervent Radiol 15:71–81

Runge VM, Krisch JE, Lee C (1993) Contrast-enhanced MR angiography. J Magn Reson Imaging 3:233–239

Schmalbrock P, Yuan C, Chakeres DW, Kohli J, Pelc NJ (1990) Volume MR angiography: methods to achieve very short echo times. Radiology 175:861–865

Schminke U, Motsch L, von Smekal U, Griewing B, Kessler C (2000) Three-dimensional transcranial color-coded sonography for the examination of the arteries of the circle of Willis. J Neuroimaging 10:173–176

Schuierer G, Huk WJ, Laub G (1992) Magnetic resonance angiography of intracranial aneurysms: comparison with intra-arterial digital subtraction angiography. Neuroradiol 35:50–54

Schwartz RB, Tice HM, Hooten SM, Hsu L, Stieg Ph (1994) Evaluation of cerebral aneurysms with helical CT: correlation with conventional angiography and MR angiography. Radiology 192:717–722

Sevick RJ, Tsuruda JS, Schmalbrock P (1990) Three-dimensional time-of-flight MR angiography in the evaluation of cerebral aneurysms. J Comput Assist Tomogr 14:874–881

Tkach JA, Masaryk TJ, Ruggieri PM, Ross JS, et al (1992) The use of tilted optimized nonsaturating excitation (TONE) RF pulses and MTC to improve the quality of MR angiograms of the carotid bifurcation. 11th Annual scientific meeting of the SMRM. Aug 8–14, 1992, Berlin, 3905

Tsuruda JS, Shimakawa A, Pelc NJ, Saloner DL (1991) Dural sinus occlusion: evaluation with phase sensitive gradient-echo MR imaging. AJNR Am J Neuroradiol 12:481–488

Tsuruda JS, Sevick RJ, Halbach VV (1992) Three-dimensional time-of-flight MR angiography in the evaluation of intracranial aneurysms treated by endovascular balloon occlusion. AJNR Am J Neuroradiol 13:1129–1136

Turjman F, Massoud TF, Vinuela F, Sayre JW, Guglielmi G, Duckwiler G (1994) Aneurysms related to cerebral arteriovenous malformations: Superselective angiographic assessement in 58 patients. AJNR Am J Neuroradiol 15:1601–1605

Van Hemert RL (1997) MRA of cranial tumors and vascular compressive lesions. Clin Neurosci 4:146–152

Vinuela F, Dion J, Lylyk P, Duckwiler G (1989) Update on interventional neuroradiology. AJR Am J Roentgenol 153:23–33

Vinuela F, Duckweiler G, Mawad M (1997) Guglielmi detachable coilembolisation of acute intracranial aneurysms: perioperative anatomical and clinical outcome in 403 patients. J Neurosurg 86:475–482

Vogl TJ, Balzer JO, Stemmler J, Bergman C, Egger E, Lissner J (1992) MR angiography in children with cerebral neurovascular diseases: findings in 31 cases. AJR Am J Roentgenol 159:817–823

Wallner B, Weidenmaier W, Vogel J, Bargon G (1991) Darstellung zerebraler Flussdynamik mit MR Angiographie und selektiver Vorsättigung: erste Erfahrungen. Fortschr Röntgenstr 155:460–464

Wardlaw JM, White PM (2000) The detection and management of unruptured intracranial aneurysms. Brain 123:205–221

Waugh JR, Sacharias N (1992) Arteriographic complications in the DSA era. Radiology 182:243–246

Wilms G, Baert AL, Smits J, De Somer F (1983) Digital intravenous and intraarterial subtraction angiography. Fortschr Röntgenstr 138:140–147

Wilms G, Demaerel P, Marchal G, Baert AL, Plets C (1991) Gadolinium-enhanced MR imaging of cerebral venous angiomas with emphasis on their drainage. J Comput Assist Tomogr 15:199–206

Wilms G, Bosmans H, Marchal G, Demaerel Ph, Goffin J, Plets C, Baert AL (1995) Magnetic resonance angiography of supratentorial brain tumors: comparison with selective digital subtraction angiography. Neuroradiology 37:42–47

Wiznitzer M, Ruggieri PM, Masaryk TJ, et al (1990) Diagnosis of cerebrovascular disease in sickle cell anemia by magnetic resonance angiography. J Pediatr 117:551–555

Wolpert JM, Caplan LR (1992) Current rate of cerebral angiography in the diagnosis of cerebrovascular disease. AJR Am J Roentgenol 159:191–197

Yamada I, Matsushima Y, Suzuki S (1992) Moyamoya Disease: diagnosis with Three-dimensional time-of-flight MR angiography. Radiology 184:773–778

Yano T, Kodama T, Suzuki Y, Watanabe K (1997) Gadolinium-enhanced 3D time-of-flight MR angiography. Experimental and clinical evaluation. Acta Radiol 38:47–54

Zamani A (1997) MRA of intracranial aneurysms. Clin Neurosci 4:123–129

Zimmerman RA, Bogdan AR, Gusnard DA (1992) Pediatric magnetic resonance angiography: assessment of stroke. Cardiovasc Intervent Radiol 15:60–64

14 Carotid and Vertebral Arteries

STEPHAN WETZEL and GEORG M. BONGARTZ

CONTENTS

14.1 Introduction

14.1.1 Clinical Aspects

After cancer, cardiovascular disease represents the most important cost factor in health care in the Western world, with the number of cerebrovascular disorders growing steadily (KIDO and MORAN 1994; MASARYK and OBUCHOWSKI 1993). The main indication for examination of the supra-aortic vessels by magnetic resonance angiography (MRA) is the evaluation of carotid artery steno-occlusive disease caused by an atherothrombotic process. Atherothrombotic disease is a common cause of transient ischemic attacks and ischemic stroke. Compared with distal cerebral arteries, the carotids are much more commonly affected by atherosclerosis – and their impact on health care is far more important due to their surgical approachability. A number of controlled randomized studies with a large number of patients were performed to evaluate the benefit of surgical endarterectomy versus medical therapy such as anticoagulation or inhibition of thrombocytic aggregation (antiplatelet drugs) for treatment of carotid atherothrombotic disease. The effectiveness of carotid endarterectomy for patients with severe symptomatic stenosis of the internal carotid artery (70%–99 %) was proved in the NASCET study (Collaborators North American Symptomatic Carotid Endarterectomy Trial 1991; BARNETT et al. 1998) and in the ECST study (European Carotid Surgery Trialists' Collaborative Group 1998), and for patients with asymptomatic carotid stenosis of over 60% in the ACAS study (Executive Committee for the Asymptomatic Carotid Atherosclerosis Study 1995). For the correct treatment of patients, the aim of imaging the supra-aortic vessels is not only to prove the presence of a carotid artery stenosis, but moreover to provide a reliable grading of the steno-occlusive process. Furthermore, single or tandem lesions must be recognized and documented, contralateral vessels must be evaluated, and other reasons for flow reduction have to be demonstrated if present.

The correct recognition of dissections of the cervical vessels can be considered the second important task of MRA, as it is assumed that this disease accounts for up to 20% of ischemic strokes in younger patients (CRONQVIST et al. 1986; BOGOUSSLAVSKY and REGLI 1987). In such cases, MRA has not only the potential of depicting signs of vessel narrowing, but also of demonstrating the vessel wall hematoma, thus enabling the precise determination of the extent of the dissection.

S. WETZEL, MD
Department of Radiology, University Hospital, Kantonsspital, Petersgraben 4, 4031 Basel, Switzerland
G.M. BONGARTZ, MD
Professor, Department of Radiology, University Hospital, Kantonsspital, Petersgraben 4, 4031 Basel, Switzerland

14.1.2 Clinical Imaging of the Carotid and Vertebral Arteries

A variety of imaging techniques can be applied for investigation of the cervical vessels to recognize vessel stenosis, occlusion, dissection, or other reasons for flow reduction. These techniques provide either morphological or functional information about the vessels, and delineate either the vessel lumen or the vascular wall itself. From a technical viewpoint, the modalities for imaging of the cervical vessels can be divided into the invasive intra-arterial digital subtraction angiography (DSA) technique, and the noninvasive or minimally invasive studies of ultrasonography, CT angiography (CTA), and MRA.

Among the imaging techniques for the carotid arteries, DSA is still the most generally accepted method and is considered to be the standard of reference. The technique offers an excellent spatial resolution with matrix sizes of 1024×1024 available on most modern DSA units, which is not only advantageous for display of the cervical vessels but also for the delineation of the simultaneously investigated small-sized intracranial vessels. Furthermore, the high temporal resolution provides an assessment of the hemodynamic information. DSA strictly relates to the intraluminal part of the vessel due to partial replacement of the blood by contrast media. Estimation of the lumen is achieved by means of at least two projections of the injected vessel. Of course, this is not the same as an exact demonstration of the real lumen. Wall irregularities can be missed or overestimated as a result of limited projections (Schild 1994). The information on the vessel is acquired on the basis of the contrast media density in a specific vascular region. In addition, an estimation of the projective depth is obtained, this being the third dimension in the angiogram. Typically, DSA is performed by intra-arterial contrast media injection via a transfemoral catheter approach. Nonselective (aortic arch) and selective injection into each common carotid and/or vertebral artery must be differentiated since the reliability of the results and the possible side effects differ. Nonselective injection into the aortic arch allows an assessment of the proximal cervical vessels; however, selective injections into the supra-aortic vessels enable a more accurate diagnosis of each investigated vessel (Fig. 14.1a). The need for noninvasive imaging of the cervical arteries is based on the known side effects in angiography. The overall risk that transient neurological complications occur with selective catheter angiography is approximately 1%, the risk for permanent neurological deficit 0.3%. However, the subgroup of patients with transient ischemic attacks or stroke, in particular, were shown to be at a higher risk, with transit deficits occurring in 3% and permanent deficits in 0.7% with this purely diagnostic tool (Cloft et al. 1998). Besides the risk, the method is time-consuming, expensive, and patients and investigators are exposed to X-rays.

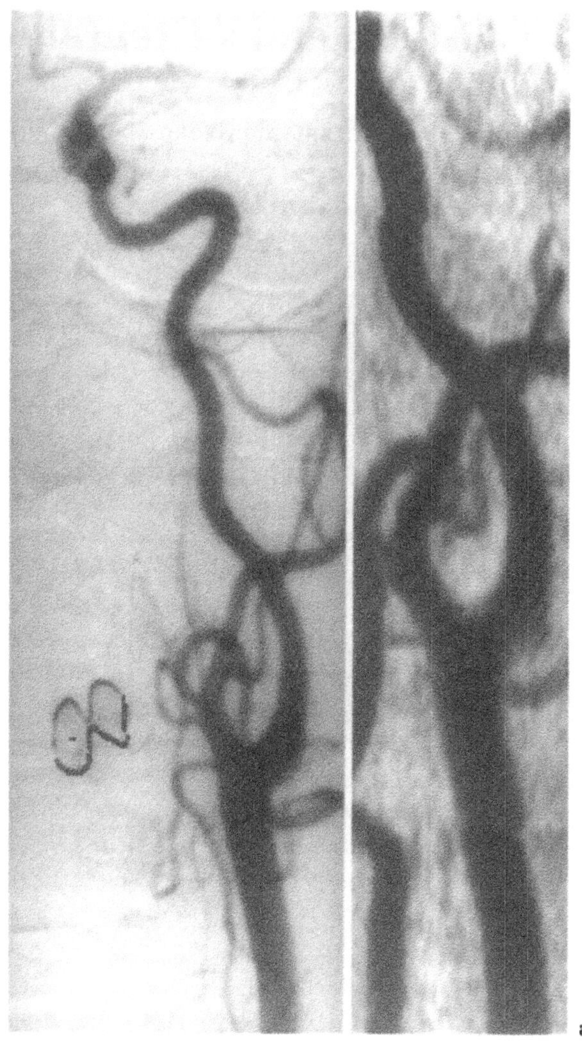

Fig. 14.1. a Intra-arterial selective DSA of the left common carotid artery in a patient with sonographic suspicion of a moderate to severe stenosis of the internal carotid artery. A minimally dilated carotid bulb is found in an otherwise normal vessel. **b** Correlative MRA of the same patient using the MOTSA technique displays a minor signal decay at the carotid bulb due to flow dephasing in the bifurcation. No pathological alteration was detected. The projection of the MRA is displayed black on white to make it similar to the correlative DSA investigation

Ultrasonography represents a challenging alternative to DSA in the work-up of carotid artery disease.

The method provides information on the structural changes of the cervical vessels and the hemodynamic aspect. Ultrasound images are constructed from echo-amplitude analysis of the tissue components. The brightness-modulated image (B-mode scan) is thereby displayed on a two-dimensional (2D) gray-scale display. Hemodynamic information is obtained by measuring the difference in frequency between two successive echos – the Doppler shift – indicating the velocity and direction of the moving blood cells. By use of a continuous wave Doppler with a two-part (emitting, receiving) transducer, a broad range of flow velocities can be detected. The pulse wave Doppler allows the determination of the depth of the insonated vessels and then their identification. With the introduction of color-coded duplex sonography it became possible to obtain simultaneously a B-mode scan in real time and to visualize the blood flow within the vessel. The direction of blood is thereby coded in a color, depending on the direction towards or away from the transducer, and the flow velocity correlates with the saturation. This technique improves the identification of the vascular structures and allows an assessment of the vessel wall. Ulcerations and intramural hemorrhage can be recognized as well as thrombotic material attached to the vessel wall. Color Doppler energy (CDE)-coded duplex-sonography allows a visualization of the ultrasound energy of moving components and thus an area measurement of carotid stenosis (Lyrer et al. 1999), while contrast-enhanced ultrasound, based on the application of galactose-based microbubble suspensions, is helpful in distinguishing occluded or sub-occluded arteries (Calliada et al. 1999). Ultrasound methods can be considered as an ideal tool for the noninvasive evaluation of the cervical vessels. However, the method is operator-dependent and allows only an incomplete delineation of the carotid arteries (especially of the intracranial part), with problems arising in the presence of calcified plaques. In numerous studies, color duplex ultrasound was found to have a peak accuracy of 90% or greater in the diagnosis of carotid arterial disease, despite the fact that a wide range of Doppler ultrasound thresholds were applied in these studies. Grant et al. (2000) reported that Doppler ultrasound was correct in classifying stenoses as above or below 70% in about 90% of cases. However a stenosis subclassification was not found to be reliable due to the wide range of Doppler ultrasound values for a given degree of arteriographically determined stenosis.

CTA has been introduced with the growing availability of spiral CT scanners. After intravenous injection, a bolus of contrast agent is tracked through the cervical arteries by using continuous table motion through the CT gantry as the X-ray tube spins continuously. The acquired data set can be displayed as 2D images in the form of axial source images or as multiplanar reconstructions in various planes. Three-dimensional (3D) reconstructions include maximum intensity projection (MIP) reconstructions and the shaded surface display. As the axial images provide a cross-sectional view, the percentage of area reduction can be precisely measured, and eccentricities of the vascular lumen can be identified. Furthermore, by use of pixel density determination, fat, fibrosis, and calcium of a carotid plaque can be differentiated. The current limitations are the relatively complicated postprocessing procedures for 3D data sets, because bones and calcified structures must be segmented prior to angiographic reconstruction. The second drawback is the limitation of scan volume due to tube heating in single-slice technology. A depiction of the entire course of the supra-aortic vessels with a single contrast agent bolus at a sufficiently high resolution is only possible with modern multi-array CT scanners.

In a recent study by Sameshima et al. (1999) investigating 128 carotid bifurcations, a high correlation was found between the degree of carotid stenosis estimated by conventional angiography and by 3D CTA MIP images: only five mild or moderate stenoses were overestimated by one category with CTA according to the NASCET classification. To date, CTA offers a superior spatial resolution compared with MRA.

MRA techniques based on natural flow effects require no radiation or contrast agent and therefore may be easily repeated several times to cover larger areas of the carotid system (Fig. 14.1b). If contrast-enhanced methods are applied, the coverage of the entire carotid system can be accomplished by use of a single contrast agent bolus. Like CTA, it is a cross-sectional approach, with the advantage over DSA of not having to rely on projection images. Unlike with CTA, 3D reconstruction methods are fairly easy to perform because of invisible bony structures of the neck and skull base, and especially with dynamic contrast-enhanced techniques, information on flow dynamics is readily available. MRA of the carotid arteries is gaining widespread acceptance, as this technique proved to provide a high accuracy for the detection as well as for the grading of carotid stenosis (see Sect. 14.4.2).

14.2 Technical Considerations

14.2.1 Flow Pattern in the Carotid System

The proximity to the heart, the elastic arterial wall, and the straight course of the vessel are the reasons for the strong forward flow in the carotid arteries. The constant positive pressure throughout the carotid cycle is guaranteed by the Windkessel function of the aorta, but may be altered in pathological states such as severe aortic regurgitation.

The easiest unidirectional flow pattern in a straight vessel is the so-called laminar flow. Laminar conditions describe the concentric composition of multiple layers of a flow profile, each with a specific velocity. The most central layer is the fastest, while the one neighboring the vascular wall is the slowest. The adhesive interactions of the different layers result in a velocity increase from the outer to the inner tube while the gradient between adjacent layers decreases.

The flow pattern in every vessel is strongly affected by the inner surface of the vessel wall, the velocity, the pulsatile character, and the direction. If any of these factors is changed under strongly laminar conditions, the flow pattern can alter to turbulent flow.

Upon the onset of turbulent conditions, the laminar character is suspended by the destruction of the adhesive interactions between the separate layers. In straight vessels a uniform flow pattern results, with all layers having more or less identical velocities (plug flow). With respect to MRA, the inflow effect is maximized in plug flow conditions.

A further increase in velocity destroys the unidirectional flow. The vectors representing the microscopic flow point in various directions. Nevertheless, the macroscopic flow direction remains unchanged. With the next step in turbulence, the macroscopic coherence of the flow direction is also altered, and within certain parts of the vessel, different flow directions exist simultaneously. This condition is called eddy flow or vortex flow. In the carotid artery, vortex flow exists at the bifurcation, behind prominent plaques, or distal to stenoses. In the carotid bifurcation, reversed flow or stagnant flow can be found which physiologically forms the carotid bulb (Bongartz et al. 1991).

MRA techniques based on natural flow effects are strongly affected by different flow conditions. Fast but laminar flow is the optimal condition for inflow MRA (time-of-flight technique). Plug flow enables even stronger inflow of "fresh" magnetization and results in further signal increase; however, plug flow is an unstable condition and is only demonstrable over a small range of velocities.

Microscopic turbulence causes considerable dephasing within the voxel. The effect is related to voxel size and gradient strength and can be partially compensated by flow rephasing gradients additionally implemented into the sequence. The worst conditions for MRA in general are found in the case of flow eddies or macroscopic turbulence. These conditions affect not only dephasing of the magnetization but also saturation of the spins (time-of-flight technique). This stage of turbulence cannot be completely compensated by means of gradient rephasing and always results in signal voids (Urchuk and Plewes 1992). The effects are minimized by shortening TE.

Contrast-enhanced techniques are not as sensitive to turbulent flow conditions as they rely mainly on the T1 shortening effect of a intravenously administered contrast agent. Because sequences with an ultrashort TE (1.5–2 ms) are applied with these methods, intravoxel dephasing is markedly decreased for a given voxel size. However, turbulence dephasing also exists, and must be considered a source of artifacts, especially if the voxel size is reduced (high-resolution MRA).

14.2.2 Time-of-Flight MRA

Inflow MRA is based on the differences in saturation between the extravascular signal and intravascular signal (moving blood). While signal intensities of static tissue (extravascular) are progressively suppressed by repetitive RF pulses, inflow enhancement in the investigated vessel produces the angiographic effect. The area or volume which is covered by the time-of-flight (TOF) sequence is of major importance for the MRA result, because flow saturation directly correlates with the visible length of the vessel within that volume. The longer the blood remains within the investigated volume, the more RF pulses are experienced, inducing a stronger saturation effect. In slow flow conditions, the volume covered must therefore be kept very small.

Optimized inflow conditions in TOF MRA are achieved by orientating the imaging plane perpendicular to the vascular flow direction (Fig. 14.2). This orientation, however, has the disadvantage that only a shorter part of the vessel can be covered. In several studies (as in most early investigations), a sagittal

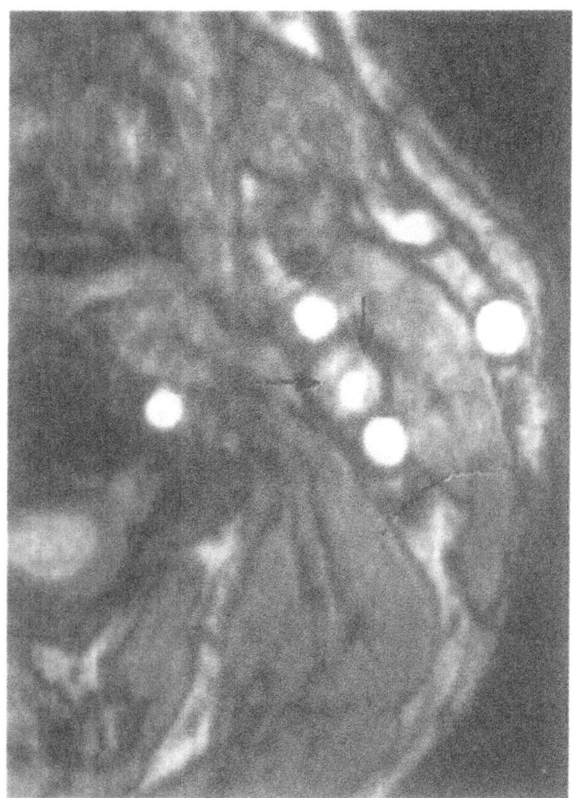

Fig. 14.2. Display of the original slice of a 3D data set through the neck, acquired in axial plane. The left internal carotid artery shows a moderate stenosis with a cicular but asymmetric thickening of the vascular wall. The atheroma shows inhomogeneous signals with bright foci at the anterior aspect, suspicious for lipoid infiltration or fresh thombotic material *(arrows)*

or a coronal approach has been chosen. Theoretically, this enables the delineation of the entire carotid system from its aortic origin up to the carotid siphon, even including the circle of Willis. The most important drawback is the saturation effect, which not only usually destroys the vascular signal far below the skull base, but also exaggerates poststenotic flow voids (Masaryk et al. 1991). From a technical point of view, the limitation of the RF pulses to the investigated volume must be considered. In transaxial volume imaging, the RF power is restricted to the investigational volume. In coronal or sagittal imaging, RF is also supplied to all tissues above and below the imaging field - including the thorax and the heart. Presaturation of the blood in the thorax will negatively affect the signal in the carotid arteries. Therefore, RF supply must be limited to the volume of interest by applying axial volumes or by using dedicated neck coils with transmit and receive capacities. This will prevent the RF pulses from reaching the areas downstream of the carotid arteries, thereby preserving the entire longitudinal magnetization for the inflow MRA.

The fast carotid flow encourages the application of volume inflow MRA because of the extremely high flow rates, with peak systolic values of about 100 cm/s. In 3D TOF, one single volume (slab) is excited and segmented into small slices by a second-phase encoding gradient, while in 2D TOF multiple single slices are acquired sequentially. Based on this different technical approach, both methods have specific advantages and disadvantages (Fig. 14.3):

1. Resolution: a major benefit of 3D TOF acquisition is the optimized resolution in all directions. With 3D techniques, slice thickness can be reduced to below 1 mm, while in 2D techniques slice thickness usually varies between 2 and 3 mm.
2. Saturation effects: the 2D method, compared with the 3D technique, shows an improved sensitivity

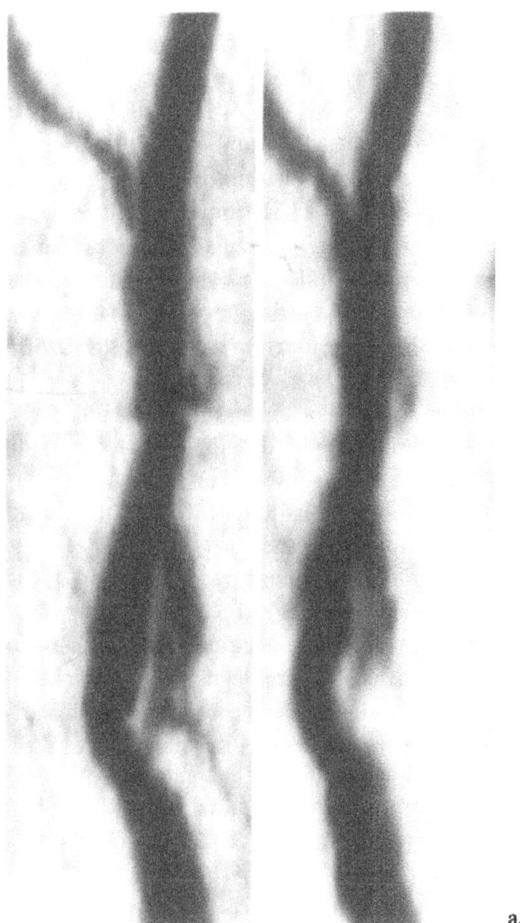

a,b

Fig. 14.3. Direct comparison of a small-voxel 3D acquisition (**a**) and a larger voxel 2D acquisition (**b**) in a patient with a severe stenosis at the origin of the external carotid artery. In the 2D technique, the turbulence in the stenosis causes more severe signal voids than the 3D technique

for inflowing magnetization based on minimized flow saturation effects: in sequential acquisitions each slice of the data set represents an "entry" slice with the strongest possible intravascular signal. This enables a slightly higher flip angle and as a consequence an overall improvement in SNR. Therefore, this technique is well suited for the detection of slow laminar flow conditions. However, depending on the larger voxel size and the higher flip angle applied in 2D techniques, saturation effects are enhanced for flowing spins that run within an imaging plane instead of crossing it perpendicularly. In the case of the carotid and vertebral arteries, in-plane saturation is rarely expected with transaxial MRA applications. Only in cases of vascular kinking or coiling does a notable problem occur (HUSTON et al. 1993). In cases of severe coiling with reversed flow direction, the problem is even pronounced.

3. Dephasing effects: pulsatile flow causes turbulences already under physiological conditions and marked turbulences causing spin dephasing are encountered poststenotically. Under these conditions, the larger voxel size of 2D TOF methods is disadvantageous: as the number of different possible phases increases within the voxel, the signal voids increase (Fig. 14.3). Conversely, the smaller voxel size with 3D TOF enhances the signal in areas of minor turbulences, owing to the reduced phase dispersions per single voxel, making the technique favorable for clinical MRA of the carotid arteries.

To reduce saturation effects in 3D acquisitions, different techniques were developed. PARKER et al. (1991) introduced the combination of multiple overlapping thin-slice acquisitions (MOTSA) to carotid imaging. Multiple, separately acquired 3D data sets are combined to yield a single reconstruction of the entire vessel. The volumes are acquired sequentially in order to prevent any saturation effect. Due to impairment of the slice profile at the boundaries of the volumes, the signal varies throughout each individual volume from the outer to the central slices. Therefore, a considerable overlap of one-third to one-quarter at each side of the volume is recommended. MOTSA techniques enable the investigation of the entire carotid artery without suffering from saturation effects. The disadvantages are the problem of incorrect matching of the separate volumes due to gross patient motion and signal variation at the volume boundaries because of residual saturation effects, leading to a slab boundary or "venetian blind" called artifact on the MRA MIP image.

A new and interesting alternative to the MOTSA technique has recently been introduced, whereby the slab "walks" continuously along the Z-direction, while acquiring data in an interleaved fashion in the k_y direction. This technique, termed SLINKY (sliding interleaved k_y) acquisition, showed a reliable mapping of vascular anatomy without the "venetian blind" artifact in a preliminary report (LIU et al. 1998).

Another technique to minimize saturation effects in transaxial volume TOF MRA is the adjustment of the RF profile (and thus the flip angle) along the carotid flow direction. The strong signal at the entry side of the volume requires a smaller flip angle as compared to the very distal part of the carotid artery, where saturation already strongly affects the signal. The presaturated arterial magnetization can still deliver signal when the flip angle is sufficiently large. Thus, the RF profile for 3D acquisitions can be altered such that a small flip angle is used at the proximal carotid artery while a much larger flip angle recalls the weaker signal distally. This technique is referred to as TONE (titled optimized non-saturating excitation) and was introduced by PURDY et al. (1992). The gradient of the TONE pulse (or ramped flip angle) directly depends on the velocity. In normal carotid flow, the gradient applied is 1:2 for a slab thickness of 8 cm up to 12 cm. As a side effect, S/N significantly decreases with larger slab thickness.

With recent hardware and software, in-plane matrices of 512 are most commonly used. The smaller voxel size shows benefits in areas of turbulence due to reduced intravoxel dephasing. Moreover, recognition of details like plaque morphology is improved.

In standard TOF sequences, a presaturation pulse is implemented into the sequence. This saturation pulse is placed parallel and directly superior to the imaging plane, nulling the cephalocaudad (venous) flow. If reversed flow occurs, the opposed arterial flow direction is affected simultaneously.

Typical parameter settings for axial 3D TOF carotid artery MRA are shown in Table 14.1.

Table 14.1. Typical parameter settings for axial 3D time-of-flight MRA of the carotid arteries

Parameter	multivolume (MOTSA)	single volume (TONE)
TR	30 ms	28 ms
TE	7 ms	6 ms
Flip angle	30°	20°
Slab thickness	1 mm	1.25 mm
Number of partitions	4×32	64 (128)
Time	4×1.30 min	5 min (10 min)

14.2.3 Phase-Contrast MRA

Phase-contrast MRA is based on the application of a bipolar gradient pulse pair producing a phase shift depending on the velocity component along the gradient. The technique is very flow sensitive and provides a full background suppression but requires a relatively long acquisition time if flow is encoded in all three spatial directions (3D phase-contrast MRA). Moreover, a variety of velocities occur in the carotid artery, complicating the correct selection of the velocity-encoding gradient (VENC). Thus, the method is not as widely used for depiction of carotid artery stenosis as the TOF technique.

Projective 2D PC, on the other hand, can be acquired quickly (<1 min) and easily. This technique is therefore often used to determine the topographic location of the cervical arteries in a coronal direction, enabling a correct placement of the volume to be investigated by contrast-enhanced MRA methods.

The possibility to measure flow velocity and volumetric flow rates by phase-contrast techniques allows information on the hemodynamical impact of a carotid stenosis to be obtained (Vanninen et al. 1995). However, these measurements are not commonly used in clinical practice.

14.2.4 Contrast-Enhanced MRA

The TOF MRA technique with its easy and robust set-up and high resolution can still be considered as the most frequently applied technique for evaluation of the cervical vessels by MRA at present. However, the new class of contrast-enhanced (CE) MRA techniques is gaining importance in the head and neck area as well, because the principles of image generation provide unique advantages over the native techniques (Rofsky and Adelman 1998) (Fig. 14.4).

Unlike TOF or PC MRA methods, CE MRA does not rely on the natural flow effects, but on the shortening of the T1 relaxation time of blood after intravenous injection of a paramagnetic contrast agent bolus. By imaging with a T1-weighted sequence, angiograms can be obtained showing the cervical vessels with high contrast relative to stationary tissue.

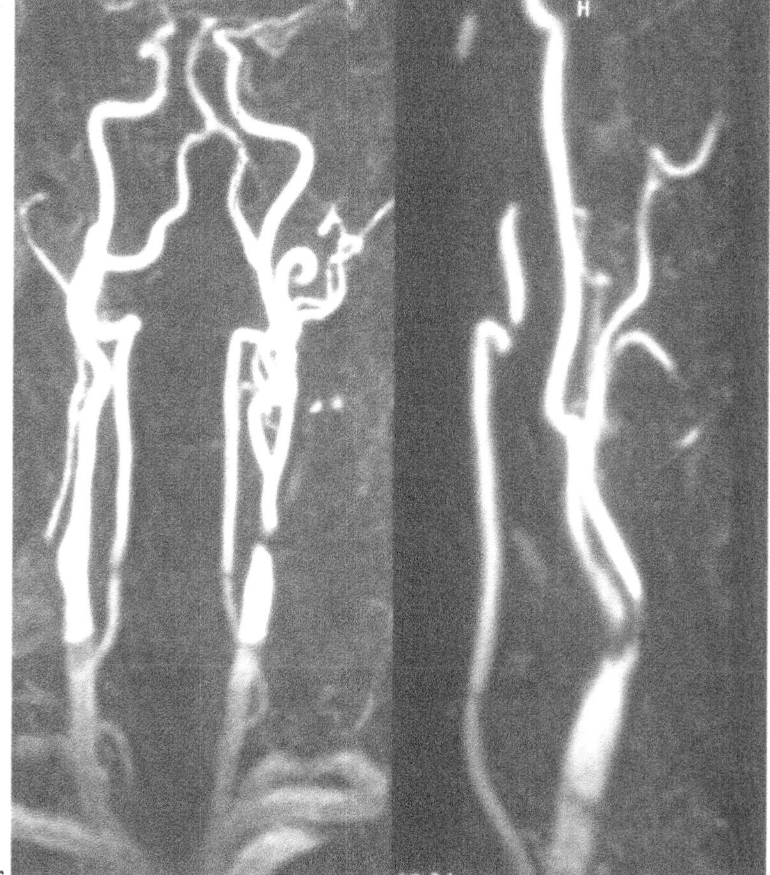

Fig. 14.4a, b. Contrast-enhanced MRA of the carotid and vertebral arteries in a patient with arteriosclerotic disease. A high-grade stenosis is readily depicted at the left carotid bifurcation in both the coronal reconstruction (**a**) and the sagittal targeted reconstruction of the left side only (**b**). The minimal residual lumen of the internal and the external carotid artery is optimally seen in the focused reconstruction

Compared with TOF techniques, saturation effects hardly occur, since the image contrast is dominated by the extremely short T1 relaxation of blood. While for TOF techniques an acquisition perpendicular to the vessel and thus in the axial plane is recommended to reduce saturation effects in carotid artery imaging, with CE MRA a 3D acquisition in the coronal plane becomes possible, covering the supra-aortic vessels in their whole extent from the aortic arch to the carotid siphon. The second advantage of the technique compared with TOF MRA is the short measurement time. Thus, artifacts from motion and swallowing play a minor role compared with TOF techniques.

Hardware prerequisites for these ultrafast imaging techniques include high-performance gradients with fast rise times and high gradient strength.

In order to standardize the intravenous administration of the contrast bolus and to ensure that the concentration of the contrast agent is kept high and constant during the image acquisition, a power injector should be used. A typical protocol represents the injection of a single dose of Gadolinium chelate at a flow rate of 2 ml/s, or the use of a double dose at a flow rate of 3 ml/s. A saline flush should be administered immediately after the contrast bolus, to obtain a "compact" bolus geometry. The image acquisition should be performed during the first pass of the contrast agent because the contrast bolus is at this moment most concentrated before it gets diluted during recirculation, and furthermore to avoid venous jugular enhancement.

This "first-pass imaging" in the head and neck area is technically the most demanding part as, compared with other regions of the body, the arteriovenous transit time is quite short (transit time from the cervical arteries to the jugular veins is below 10 s). Different technical modifications were applied to overcome this problem. With these methods, referred to as time-resolved methods, 3D data sets are acquired consecutively at relatively short intervals (usually 5–10 s) throughout the passage of the contrast agent (Korosec et al. 1996). One of the data sets should thereby solely depict the arterial phase prior to the venous return. An advantage of this method is the lack of any need for operator intervention: the scan is simply started when the injection is performed or shortly before if a mask is to be obtained. An additional benefit is that this technique allows images of late-filling vessels to be obtained in later time frames. Thus, the images provide information about flow dynamics. If 2D data sets are acquired, the temporal frame rate can be increased in the order of one projection image per second, allowing a detailed insight into the contrast agent dynamics (Wang et al. 1996; Hennig et al. 1997). The time saving in these time-resolved 2D or 3D MRA sequences, however, is at the cost of spatial resolution.

To achieve a resolution comparable to TOF MRA (e.g., voxel size of 1 mm^3), longer measurement times are required (e.g., 25 s). If these sequences are applied, the acquisition has to be synchronized with the arrival of the contrast agent such that filling of those k-space parts determining mainly the image contrast coincide with the maximal vascular signal. In the central part of k-space the low frequencies are sampled. This mainly determines the image contrast, while the higher frequencies determine the resolution and are sampled in the outer parts of the k-space. In a linear phase-encoding table (symmetrical sampling), the low frequencies are sampled at the center of the measurement time (Fig. 14.5).

If the bolus arrival time is determined with a small test bolus of contrast agent (1–2 ml) followed by a rapid and repetitive acquisition of 2D images, an exact timing of the bolus and the sequence becomes possible and images without venous overlay can be generated (Levy and Prince 1996). A drawback of

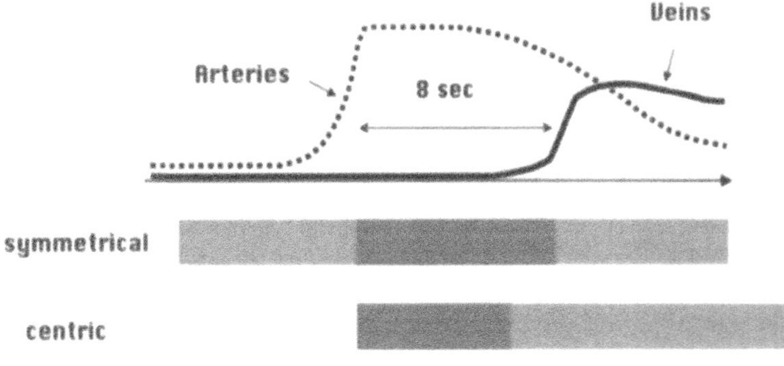

Fig. 14.5. Different methods of k-space sampling. In symmetrical sampling order, the low frequencies (*black part of the bar*), determining mainly the image contrast, are sampled at the center of the measurement time. In centric view ordering, the low frequencies are sampled initially

this method is that tracking of a separate test bolus is time consuming.

The need for a separate test bolus is overcome with a recently proposed technique: the combination of a 2D time resolved sequence with the 3D MRA sequence. The arrival of the contrast agent bolus is displayed on-line with the 2D sequence. When the arteries in the monitoring image enhance, the operator starts the angiographic 3D sequence without delay. The contrast-determining parts of k-space in this case have to be sampled initially of course, because the bolus maximum is reached at the time the 3D MRA sequence begins. This technique of k-space sampling is referred to as centric view ordering, and elliptical centric view ordering if it is centric in both phase-encoding directions (FAIN et al. 1999). This technique allows a reliable venous suppression and longer acquisition times (e.g., 40 s), whereby an improved resolution becomes possible.

Techniques to improve the image quality of CE MRA include the subtraction of a pre-contrast image set from a post-contrast angiogram. Nonenhancing stationary tissue is eliminated and fewer projection-related artifacts such as the signal loss of small vessels in regions of bright background signal are encountered.

If intensities between each point of the matrix are interpolated, the resolution improves. This technique is called zero-filling because parts of the data are filled with zero prior to the Fourier transformation (DU et al. 1994).

Typical parameter settings for a high-resolution CE MRA of the carotid artery are shown in Table 14.2.

Table 14.2. Typical parameter settings for linear/symmetric contrast-enhanced MRA of the cervical arteries (high-resolution MRA)

Parameter	
TR	<5 ms
TE	<2 ms
Flip angle	25°
Time	25 s
Contrast agent	Single dose or 20 ml
Flow	2–3 ml/s
Flush	30 ml 0.9% Nacl
Resolution	1 mm isotropy

14.3 Normal Anatomy/Variants

14.3.1 Carotid Arteries

The carotid arteries originate from the top of the aortic arch. The right artery has a common root with the right subclavian artery, called the brachiocephalic trunk, whereas the left subclavian artery originates in isolation. The most common aberrations are isolated origins of the right-sided arteries with absence of the brachiocephalic trunk, a common origin of the left carotid artery with the brachiocephalic trunk, a left-sided brachiocephalic trunk, and a variant origin of the right carotid artery from the aortic arch distal to the left subclavian artery (a. lusoria). The latter variant may cause a syndrome of dysphagia, because the misplaced right carotid crosses to the right side behind the esophagus and compresses it. The syndrome is called dysphagia lusoria.

The position of the carotid arteries' roots at the aortic arch guarantees a strong perfusion of the supra-aortic arteries, since centrifugal forces are pronounced at the outer curve of the arch. Physiologically, the flow accelerates with the diameter of the curve owing to the tendency of maintaining a straight flow direction. Therefore, a relatively large amount of the cardiac output is directly transported into the supra-aortic arteries for cerebral supply.

Depending on constitution and body size, the carotid arteries measure between 14 and 19 cm in an adult, with an average of 17 cm between the aortic arch and the siphon of the internal carotid artery. In degenerative elongation of the vessel, tremendous variation may occur. For the purpose of MRA, the distance between the aortic arch and the carotid siphon is of greater importance than the actual length of the vessel.

The area surrounding the arteries of the neck consists of soft tissue, primarily muscles and fat. Both carotid arteries are adjacent to osseous structures only at the skull base.

The carotid bifurcation projects itself onto the third or fourth cervical vertebra in conventional angiography, showing a symmetric position of both sides in about 60% of cases. A variation of more than 5 cm cephalocaudad is often found upon clinical evaluation. At the bifurcation, the external carotid artery most often shows a smaller caliber than the internal carotid and is directed 45° frontomedially. The origin of the internal carotid is larger in diameter and expanded eccentrically, forming the carotid bulb. In most cases, the carotid bulb points in the opposite direction to the external carotid artery. The carotid bulb may also include both arteries or extend solely into the external carotid artery. Evaluation of the bifurcational area can become complicated when the imaged area includes the bifurcation only, without demonstrating the peripheral vascular branches. The mainstream of the internal carotid artery preserves a straight upward direction without further truncations while the external carotid artery separates into several vessels which partially run horizontally. There is a much larger variation in the vessel's course as compared to the internal carotid (Kadir 1991).

14.3.2 Vertebral Arteries

The caliber of the vertebral arteries is small compared to the diameter of the carotid arteries. Considerable variation in symmetry exists, the extreme case comprising a unilateral vertebral artery only. The supply of the posterior cerebral circulation by the basilar artery varies to a great extent, since there is also the embryonal type of blood supply via the posterior communicating arteries. As regards the basilar pathway only, the posterior perfusion is not affected by asymmetry of the cervical vessels or even the lack of one vertebral artery as long as the other supplies sufficient blood flow.

In the case of marked asymmetry of both vertebral arteries, the smaller one often ends in a minor artery of the cerebellar vascular system like the anterior inferior cerebellar artery (AICA) or the posterior inferior cerebellar artery (PICA). Moreover, the confluence of the vertebral arteries shows variations, such as an asymmetric course of the distal vertebral arteries or a fenestration of the basilar artery, e.g., a secondary separation of the basilar artery into two parallel vessels distal to the vertebral confluence (Wentz et al. 1994).

The vertebral arteries penetrate the transverse processes of the cervical vertebrae. The close relation of bone and vessel may not only give rise to vascular stenosis but also cause problems in DSA or MRA.

In rare cases, primitive connections between the vertebral and carotid system can be found. These communicating vessels are usually unilateral, and up to four different connections are possible (Kadir 1991).

14.3.3 MRA Features in Normal Arteries of the Neck

With the TOF technique, the most important consideration in MRA of the supra-aortic vessels is the need for limitation to a certain region, e.g., to the bifurcation of the carotid arteries. Furthermore, the MRA display of the bifurcation is affected by the typical flow conditions and by the MRA parameters. In the carotid bulb, laminar flow is converted to turbulent flow or inversed flow at the outer boundary. In any case, a dephasing problem occurs at the bifurcation that may result in misdiagnoses if not properly recognized. In MRA applications which show a pronounced sensitivity to spin dephasing, a local flow void mimics stenosis or plaque of the carotid bulb, and the bulb is usually displayed too small. An advantage of CE MRA over TOF techniques is that signal voids at the carotid bifurcation are less likely as dephasing effects are diminished (Fig. 14.6). Furthermore, depending on the size of the view on the field and the size of the patient, a depiction of the entire course of the carotid arteries is possible in many cases due to the acquisition in the coronal plane. The handicap of signal saturation in TOF techniques does not occur in CE MRA. However, from a practical point of view, with the current technology the depiction of the proximal supra-aortic vessels is often impaired due to a low signal at the coil boundary. Furthermore, with CE MRA the limited coverage in the axial plane has to be taken into account for correct interpretation as parts of the vertebral arteries (especially the vertebral artery loop) are often not within the covered volume.

14.4 Pathology

14.4.1 Stenosis and Occlusion

Atheroma is the most common arterial disorder, almost universal in the elderly, and, if complicated by thrombosis or embolism, the most common cause of cerebral ischemia. The exact pathological mechanism is still unknown; however, it is quite clear that there are certain risk factors (i.e., high blood pressure, smoking, diabetes mellitus) which make the clinical consequences of atheroma more likely.

The large- (aortic arch) and medium-sized arteries, particularly at places of arterial branching such

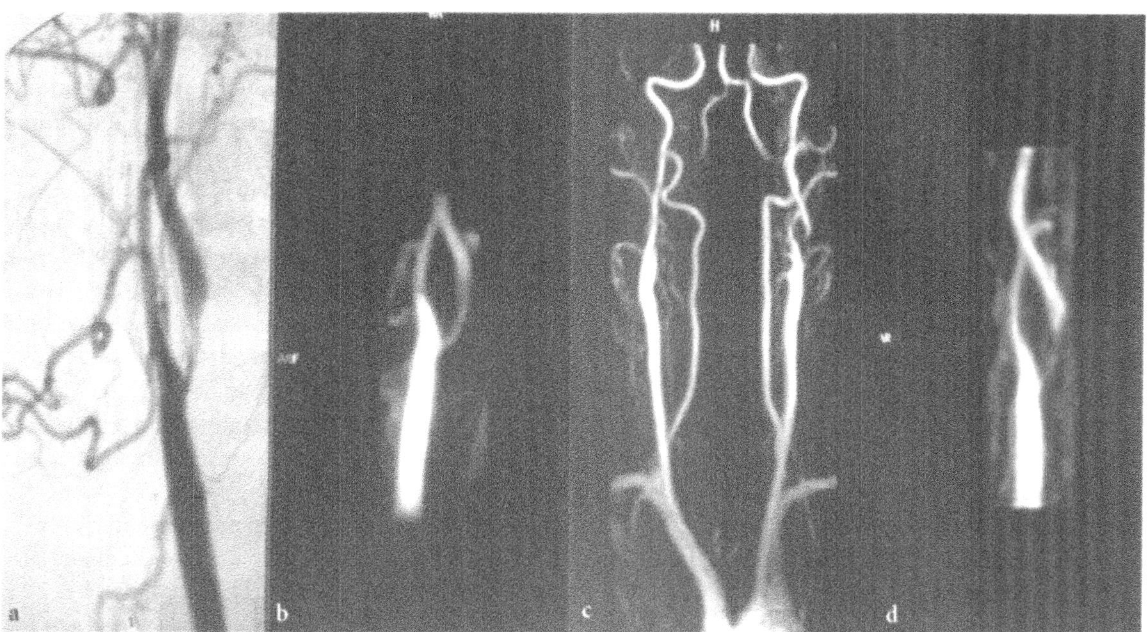

Fig. 14.6a–d. Proximal internal carotid artery stenosis at the left side. **a** DSA reveals the high-grade stenosis. **b** A targeted MIP reconstruction of a TOF MRA, the stenosis is correctly recognized with high resolution. **c** MIP reconstruction of a fluoroscopically triggered contrast-enhanced MRA with elliptical centric view ordering shows an effective venous suppression. **d** The targeted MIP reconstruction of the left carotid bifurcation shows the carotid stenosis with high accuracy

as the carotid bifurcation or of tortuosity such as the carotid siphon, are mainly affected by the atherothrombotic process. It is therefore assumed that atheroma distribution is determined by the sites of hemodynamic stress and endothelial trauma.

The atheroma formation begins as early as childhood as deposition of lipids in the arterial wall (fatty streak). Over many years, invasion of macrophages and fibrosis lead to a fibrolipid plaque that invades the media. The plaque calcifies and becomes necrotic, and platelet adhesion occurs initiating blood coagulation and thus mural thrombosis. The atherothrombotic plaque may grow to obstruct the lumen leading to a vascular stenosis or occlusion. At the carotid bifurcation, a single stenosis is the most common finding, while tandem lesions distal to the carotid bifurcation occur in approximately 6%–8% of cases (Akers 1987). Alternatively, the thrombotic part may be lysed by fibrinolytic mechanisms leading to fragmentation with the potential of obstructing a smaller distal artery.

Cerebral ischemia can therefore be due to embolic infarctions or to low flow distal to the steno-occlusive process. It is assumed that 50% of ischemic strokes, and probably also of transient ischemic attacks, are caused by atherothromboembolism, while 25% are caused by intracranial small vessel disease and 20% by cardiac embolism (Warlow et al. 1996).

To date, a single therapy does not exist that reliably prevents or cures atherothrombotic disease. From a clinical viewpoint, the distinction between symptomatic and asymptomatic manifestations is mandatory. A symptomatic stenosis leads to transient or permanent neurologic deficit due to cerebral ischemia. Symptomatic patients present with a history of at least one ischemic cerebral insult, while in asymptomatic patients the atheroma has been found by diagnostic tests only. For both groups, the treatment option depends on the severity of carotid stenosis. In the trial performed by NASCET (Collaborators North American Symptomatic Carotid Endarterectomy Trial 1991), three stages or degrees of stenosis were distinguished according to their appearance on conventional angiography:

Stage 1	Low-grade stenosis:	<30% stenosis
Stage 2	Moderate stenosis:	31%–70% stenosis
Stage 3	Severe stenosis:	71%–99% stenosis

Due to the results of this treatment study and other related studies, namely the ACAS and ECST study, the following guidelines for surgical therapy were defined: For patients with asymptomatic carotid artery disease and with a low surgical risk, carotid endarterectomy is recommended for stenotic lesions of over 60% diameter reduction, and for symptomatic patients, if the degree of carotid stenosis is above 70% (BILLER et al. 1998). Endarterectomy in symptomatic patients with stenosis of 50%–69% yielded only a moderate reduction in the risk of stroke, while patients with stenosis of less than 50% did not benefit from surgery (BARNETT et al. 1998).

Direct comparison of the results from ECST with the NASCET trial should take into account that different methods for measuring carotid artery stenosis were applied in both trials. The NASCET group used the distal internal carotid artery as its reference denominator (Fig. 14.7) and the measured stenosis as the numerator, the ECST group used an approximation of the carotid bulb diameter as the reference denominator. The relationship between the two measurement methods was found to be parabolic, a stenosis of 70%, for example, as measured by the NASCET method represents approximately a stenosis of 80% as measured by the ECST criteria (YOUNG et al. 1996).

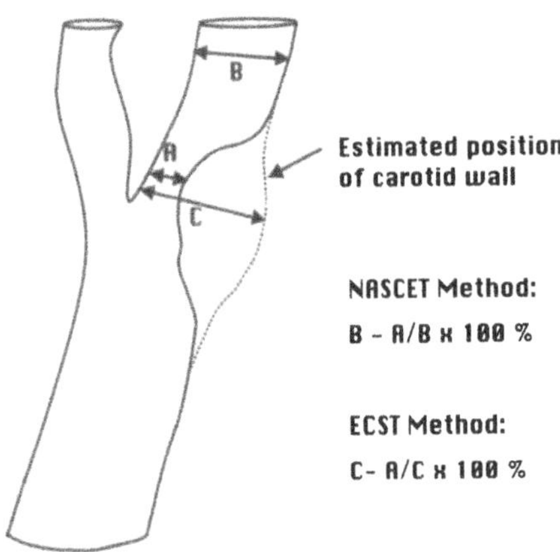

Fig. 14.7. Different grading schemes of carotid stenosis by NASCET and ECST for comparison

A major problem exists in patients with severe or subtotal stenoses: angiographic results sometimes do not enable very high-grade stenosis to be distinguished from occlusion (pseudo-occlusion) due to the slow flow and the limited resolution. On the other hand, this is an extremely important clinical question because occlusions do not require any surgical intervention while severe stenoses do. Pseudo-occlusion can be found in atherosclerotic patients or in carotid dissection.

In atherosclerotic vertebral artery stenosis, the aortic origin is the site most often affected. The intracranial portion of the vertebral arteries and the basilar artery also can be affected by atheromatous disease. Kinking or coiling due to elongation of the vessel hardly ever results in hemodynamic alterations. Osteophytes that narrow the transverse foramina and the arterial lumen are an uncommon finding (SCHILD 1994).

Surgical treatment is rarely applicable to the vertebral system. Interventional therapy in the posterior circulation focuses on acute basilar thrombosis, which represents a potentially lethal condition. Fibrinolytic therapy, in combination with conventional angiography, is regarded as the treatment of choice.

Fibromuscular dysplasia can affect all supra-aortic arteries but is most commonly found at the internal carotid arteries. The etiology remains unclear, but genetic factors are being discussed. Women are far more frequently affected than men. Secondary atheroma and stenosis are common, as are traumatic dissections of the diseased vessels (KADIR 1991).

Although it is not a disease of the vertebral arterial system, subclavian steal syndrome must be discussed within the context of diseases of the vertebral arteries. Due to an occlusion or severe stenosis of the subclavian artery proximal to the origin of the vertebral artery (right side: brachiocephalic trunk), the ipsilateral vertebral artery demonstrates an inverse flow direction for collateralization of the upper extremity. In severe cases, the steal mechanism causes relative ischemia in the posterior cerebral circulation, although the syndrome usually manifests clinically as numbness and pain in the arm and hand. For therapy planning, the length of the stenosis or occlusion must be defined by angiography or tomographic procedures. Besides atherosclerotic conditions, tumors or lymphoma can give rise to the syndrome (HENNERICI et al. 1988).

14.4.2 MRA in Carotid Atherosclerotic Disease

In previous chapters, the most useful techniques for carotid artery MRA have been described and compared with regard to advantages and artifacts. MRA is usually compared to X-ray angiography with respect to both display and results. Due to the very similar presentation of DSA and MRA MIP reconstructions, they may be regarded as identical although they are based on different phenomena. Unlike DSA, however, the original MRA data set provides a direct cross-sectional approach, and offers the chance to visualize not only the lumen but also the vascular wall (Fig. 14.2).

MRA not only delineates flow and the vascular lumen, but is also markedly affected by physical flow

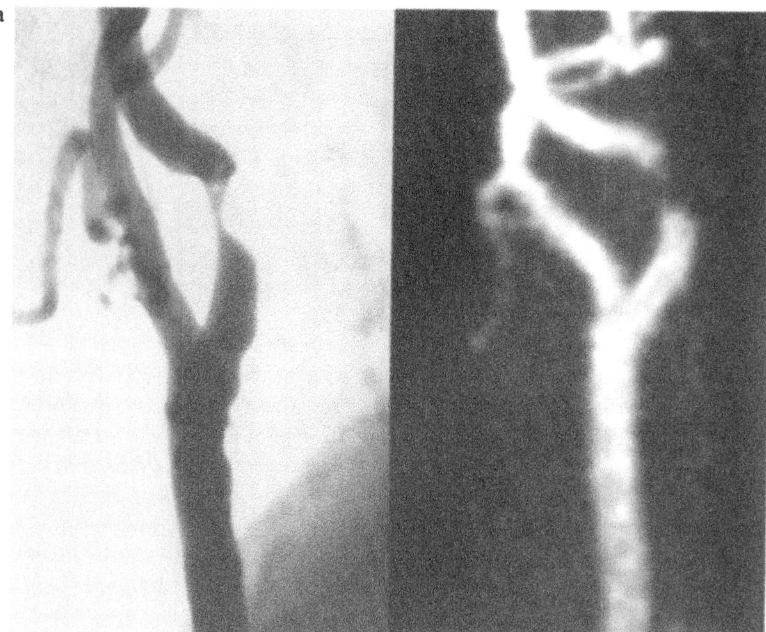

Fig. 14.8a, b. Direct comparison of a DSA and the MRA of the carotid bifurcation of a patient with severe carotid stenosis. The residual lumen is correctly seen in the conventional angiogram whereas the resolution of the MRA prevents the visualization of the vascular lumen within the stenosis. The correct diagnosis can be obtained by the high poststenotic vascular signal that proves the vessel's patency

phenomena, especially if native methods are applied. This makes interpretation more complicated and is a source of error for the inexperienced reader of MR angiograms (Fig. 14.8). Correct interpretation requires knowledge of MRA physics, flow physics, and familiarity with the applied type of MRA. The most popular flow-sensitive MRA technique, TOF MRA, is not without shortcomings.

First, due to the limited coverage of TOF MRA, the investigations focus on the bifurcation area. In most applications, the aortic origin and the distal internal carotid arteries are neglected. This is encoured by the prevalence of atherothrombotic manifestations at the carotid bifurcation. However, the presence of certain atherosclerotic plaques in the aortic arch has been identified as an independent risk factor for stroke (French Study of Aortic Plaques in Stroke Group 1996; Davila-Roman et al. 1994), and the demonstration of intracranial atherothrombosis, while not considered a contraindication to carotid endarterectomy, may influence the postoperative use of anticoagulants (Mattos et al. 1993). The limited field of view may also contribute to pitfalls regarding the interpretation of the carotid bifurcation area; for example, a branch of the external carotid artery can be misinterpreted as a continuation of the internal carotid artery when the latter is actually occluded (Litt et al. 1991).

Second, limitations include saturation and dephasing phenomena which result in, for example, a restricted capacity to distinguish a markedly narrow vessel (string sign) from occlusive disease. Concerns persist over the tendency to overestimate the grade of the lesion, and surgeons have been less accepting of carotid TOF MR imaging (Lamparello and Riles 1995).

Third, the images are often degraded by motion artifacts, especially from swallowing, due to the long measurement time.

CE MRA has markedly improved the overall acceptance of carotid MRA. Mainly due to the ultrashort echo times applied, the artificial signal loss from turbulent flow decreases, thus enabling a better depiction of the morphology of the carotid stenosis (Fig. 14.9).

A number of studies have meanwhile compared CE MRA with DSA as the standard of reference and applied the NASCET scheme for grading of stenosis. Remonda et al. (1998) used a time-resolved CE MRA technique and evaluated 44 carotid bifurcations whereby two overestimations and two underestimations by one category were reported with one overestimation of a 30%–69% stenosis and one underestimation of a 70%–99% stenosis. By use of a non-time-resolved method, 58 carotid arteries were investigated by Leclerc et al. (1998). Four overestimations and two underestimations by one category occurred, with one moderate stenosis (30%–70%) graded as severe (>70%). Sardanelli et al. (1999) who compared a breath-hold CE technique with a 2D and 3D TOF technique and DSA reported that the CE technique was significantly more accurate as compared with both TOF techniques for grading of stenoses, with only two overestimations occurring in

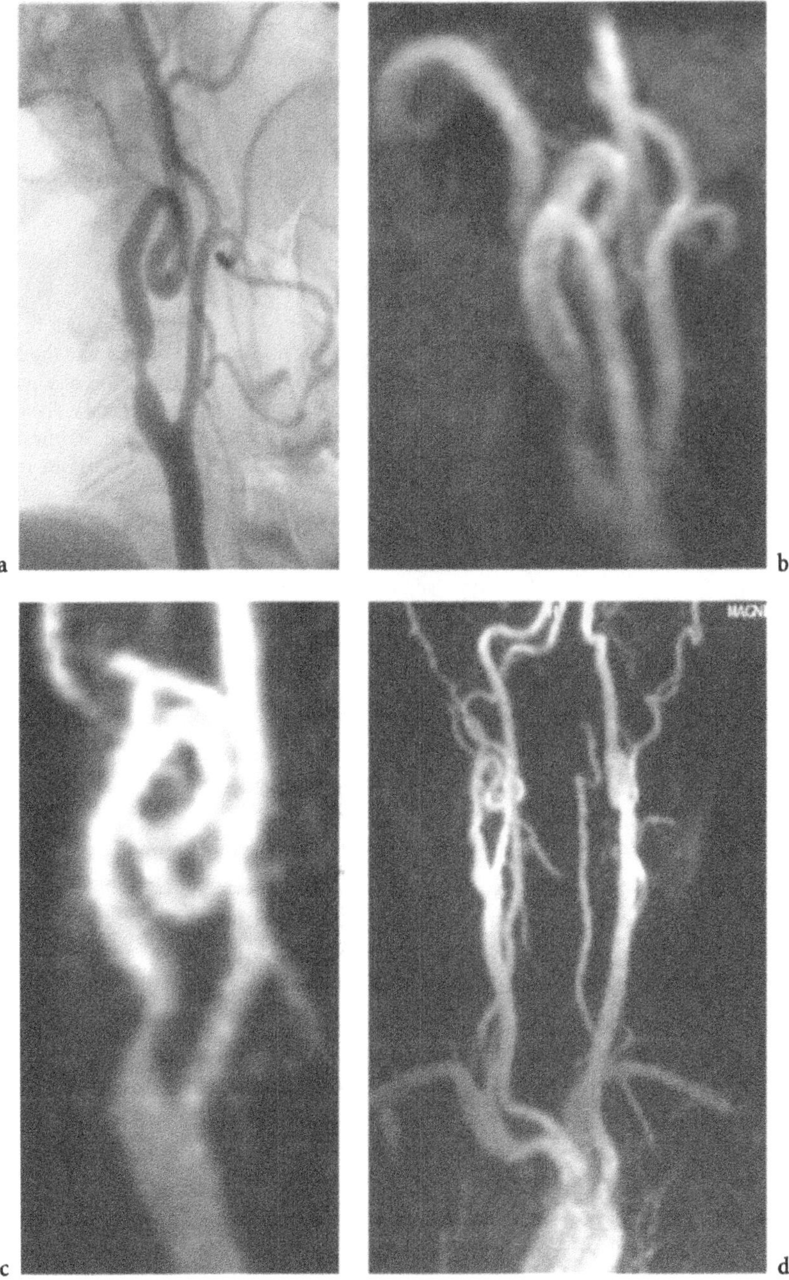

Fig. 14.9. DSA (**a**) and two different techniques of MRA (**b–d**) in a patient with atherosclerotic elongation of the internal carotid artery. The pronounced kinking of the vessel produces a remarkable signal decay in the TOF MRA (**b**) due to saturation effects while the vessel course is correctly demonstrated in CE MRA (**c**, **d**) without saturation problems

60 bifurcations investigated. In all three studies all carotid occlusions as depicted by DSA were correctly recognized by CE MRA.

Despite better accuracy for grading of carotid stenosis, the extended anatomic coverage has contributed to the improved clinical acceptance. A full coverage of the cervical arteries from the aortic arch to the intracranial part requires careful planning of the placement of the investigation volume and an appropriate coil configuration.

However, trade-offs between spatial resolution, acquisition time, and the size of the field of view are inevitable. It is likely that improved hardware configurations with higher gradient strength and rise times will enable a depiction of the entire cervical arteries at a submillimeter voxel volume resolution. However, with the current state of the technology two separate measurements of the aortic arch and the upper part of the carotid artery might be needed to obtain these very high-resolution angiograms.

14.4.3 Carotid and Vertebral Artery Dissection

Dissection of the craniocervical arteries are assumed to cause 20% of ischemic stroke in young adults (Cronqvist et al. 1986; Bogousslavsky and Regli 1987). While the dissection is frequently caused by trauma or coincides with an apparently trivial neck movement, a variety of underlying diseases are known to cause dissections such as fibromuscular dysplasia, cystic medial necrosis, or atheroma. Typical clinical findings in internal carotid artery dissection include ipsilateral pain in the face, Horner's syndrome, and lower cranial nerve palsies as a result of pressure from the expanded artery wall; vertebral artery dissection presents typically with pain in the back of the neck.

Initially, intramural hematoma develops with reactive narrowing of the vessel's lumen. The intima is elevated to a varying extent and for various lengths. The inner surface of the vascular lumen can be irregular and secondary thrombosis is known to complicate the disease. In some cases intimal flaps occur which are likely to completely obstruct the vessel (Houser et al. 1984). Carotid dissections are most often found in the midcervical portion of the internal carotid artery distal to the bifurcation with an ending proximal to the petrous part, but they may extend up to the carotid siphon. Dissections of the vertebral artery are most often localized at the level of the first and second vertebral body. Typically, diagnostic tests reveal residual flow in the narrowed vessel with distal patency - so called pseudo-occlusion. In conventional angiography, continuous narrowing of the lumen with a distally re-established flow typically correlates to pseudo-occlusion, while segmental irregularity and stenosis are regarded as the typical manifestations of carotid dissection. However, the findings on conventional angiography are nonspecific, except for the findings of a double lumen or an intimal flap, and can be mimicked by atherothrombotic disease and fibromuscular dysplasia (Provenzale 1995; Sturzenegger 1995). The hematoma and the vascular wall can be documented by ultrasonography if the dissection is close to the carotid bifurcation, but access to the distal artery and the vertebral artery is restricted.

Although there are no evidence-based guidelines for treatment of cervical artery dissection, anticoagulation is commonly initiated after diagnosis to prevent thromboembolic complications.

10.4.4 MRA in Carotid and Vertebral Artery Dissection

While atherothrombotic lesions are recognized in MRA by reference to similar criteria used in DSA, recognition of acute dissections of the cervical vessels entails use of another criterion: the direct assessment of the vessel wall. On TOF angiograms, generally the best indicator for dissection is the increase in the external diameter of the artery caused by the intramural hematoma. The chronological change of signal intensity of the hematoma follows that of an intracerebral hematoma. In the very early stage (usually up to 2 days) the hematoma is isodense to the surrounding tissue and the thickening of the vessel and narrowing of the patent lumen might be the only signs of dissection. Thereafter, due to the strong T1 effects of methemoglobin, a high signal intensity in the subacute and early chronic stage is present. In most cases it poses no problem to distinguish the high signal intensity of the intramural hematoma from the (usually slightly higher) signal of flowing blood on TOF MRA, especially if the source images are carefully studied (Fig. 14.10).

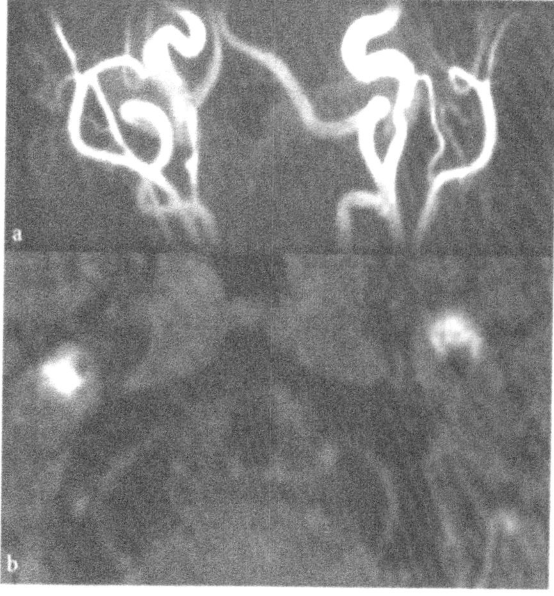

Fig. 14.10a–c. Dissection of both the left and right internal carotid artery. **a** MIP reconstruction of the 3D TOF data set shows the mural hematoma with high signal intensity and the narrowing of the perfused lumen. **b** A source image shows an eccentric hyperintense intramural hematoma on both sides

However, if problems arise, the application of an additional caudal presaturation pulse to suppress the high signal intensity from the arterial flow is useful for selective depiction of the hematoma (Kirsch et al. 1998). After about 2 months the hematomas are isointense or cannot be differentiated. Using the TOF technique, Lévy et al (Lévy et al. 1994) reported a sensitivity and specificity of 95% and 99% for the detection of carotid dissections, and in most hospitals MRA is nowadays regarded as the method of choice in suspected carotid artery dissection.

Although, the diagnosis of vertebral artery dissection is less sensitive by MRA due to the small vessel diameter and anatomic variations, the technique should be applied as it might disclose complementary information with regard to findings from selective angiography (Auer et al. 1998). Moreover, if a double lumen or a mural hematoma is depicted by MRA, there is no further indication for DSA.

The direct visualization of the hematoma is an advantage of the TOF technique over the PC technique where static tissue is entirely suppressed by subtraction. However, combination of a PC method with an axial T1-weighted spin echo sequence for depiction of the mural hematoma has been shown to be a highly accurate alternative protocol for evaluation of craniocervical dissections (Keller et al. 1997).

Contrast-enhanced MRA techniques are well suited for visualization of residual flow in narrowed vessels. However, the inherent high background suppression of these methods impairs the depiction of the arterial wall, and thus of the mural hematoma.

14.4.5 Clinical Comparison of Different Imaging Modalities for Carotid and Vertebral Artery Evaluation

Due to the inherent risk and the costs of intra-arterial DSA, there has been a search for less invasive or noninvasive tests for carotid artery disease for many years (Garrard et al. 1997). Ultrasonography represents the easiest approach to the cervical vessels covering both morphological and functional aspects. Acceptance of the method is strongly contingent upon the reputation of the investigator. Technical handicaps arise behind calcified plaques, at the intraosseous of the vertebral arteries, in severely stenosed vessels, and in tandem lesions. However, the technique has become more than a screening tool for the presence of carotid stenosis, as a high accuracy to determine a certain level of carotid stenosis is possible in most cases. MRA can be regarded as a valuable tool to confirm Doppler findings, expand the anatomical information, and identify tandem lesions (Saouf et al. 1998). Since prior to endarterectomy an a priori knowledge of the brain's status is critical, MRA can be rapidly performed in combination with an MRI examination of the brain. CTA in combination with CT has a similar potential, but the main drawbacks of that approach are the limitation in coverage of the volume to be investigated, the rather time-consuming reconstruction methods of CTA, and furthermore the lower sensitivity of CT for the detection of early stroke. The use of modern multi-array detector systems and improved postprocessing methods, however, might lead to CTA becoming an interesting and easy-to-perform alternative to MRA.

14.5 Conclusion

In the last few years, MRA has become a widely accepted clinical tool for evaluation of the cervical arteries. The introduction of contrast-enhanced MRA techniques led to a markedly improved depiction of the carotid artery and enabled a better grading of carotid stenosis than with the native techniques. The native TOF technique with its potential of displaying a mural hematoma can be considered the ideal, and in most cases sole, diagnostic tool for detection of cervical vessel dissection.

The diagnostic procedure in suspected atherothrombotic disease of the carotids still starts with ultrasonography, but inconclusive results and the diagnosis of a surgically treatable alteration demand angiographic documentation. The combination of two complementary techniques such as Doppler ultrasound and MRA is accepted in several institutions as adequate for the investigation of carotid atherosclerosis.

As to the future, technical improvements will focus on better hardware configurations to improve the resolution and coverage of CE MRA and on the optimization of data acquisition. In current clinical studies the impact of plaque morphology as displayed by ultrasound is investigated to predict which lesions are likely to rupture and cause embolism. Due to the cross-sectional approach of MRA, plaque characterization by the technique is also feasible (Luk-Pat et al. 1999). High-resolution MRA of the plaques might therefore become important in the future as an integrated part of MR examination to better define patients at risk for stroke.

To date, the rapid improvement of MRA of the cervical arteries is encouraging, and MRA can be considered as a fast, reliable, and noninvasive imaging tool for carotid and vertebral artery disease. Technical refinements are likely to improve the specificity of diagnosis, and may influence practice patterns in identifying presymptomatic patients at risk for stroke.

References

Akers D (1987) The evaluation of the aortic arch in the evaluation of cerebrovascular insufficiency. Am J Surg 154:230–236

Auer A, Felber S, Schmidauer C, et al (1998) Magnetic resonance angiographic and clinical features of extracranial vertebral artery dissection. J Neurol Neurosurg Psychiatry 64:474–481

Barnett HJM, Taylor DW, Elisaziw M, et al (1998) Benefit of carotid endarterectomy in patients with symptomatic moderate or severe stenosis. N Engl J Med 339:1415–1425

Biller J, Feinberg WM, Castaldo JE, et al (1998) Guidelines for carotid endarterectomy. A statement for healthcare professionals from a special writing group of the stroke council, American Heart Association. Stroke 29:554–562

Bogousslavsky J, Regli F (1987) Ischemic strokes in adults younger than 30 years of age: cause and prognosis. Arch Neurol 44:479–482

Bongartz G, Vestring T, Drews CI, et al (1991) Effect of slice orientation in 3D magnetic resonance angiography of the supraaortic arteries. Eur Radiol 1:158–164

Calliada F, Verga L, Pozza S, et al (1999) Selection of patients for carotid endarterectomy: the role of ultrasound. J Comput Assist Tomogr 23 [Suppl 1]:S75-S81

Cloft HJ, Joseph GJ, Dion JE (1998) Risk of cerebral angiography in patients with subarachnoid hemorrhage, cerebral aneurysm, and arteriovenous malformation. A meta-Analysis. Stroke 30:317–320

Collaborators North American Symptomatic Carotid Endarterectomy Trial (1991) Beneficial effect of carotid endarterectomy in symptomatic patients with high-grade carotid stenosis - (NASCET trial). N Engl J Med 325:445–453

Cronqvist SE, Norrving B, Nillson B (1986) Young stroke patients: an angiographic study. Acta Radiol Suppl 368:34–37

Davila-Roman VG, Barzilai B, Wareing TH, et al (1994) Atherosclerosis of the ascending aorta: prevalence and role as an independent predictor of cerebrovascular events in cardiac patients. Stroke 25:2010–2016

Du YP, Parker DL, Davis WL, et al (1994) Reduction of partial-volume artifacts with zero-filled interpolation in three-dimensional MR angiography. J Magn Reson Imaging 4:733–741

European Carotid Surgery Trialists' Collaborative Group (1998) Randomised trial of endarterectomy for recently symptomatic carotid stenosis: final results of the MRC European Carotid Surgery Trial (ECST). Lancet 351:1379–1387

Executive Committee for the Asymptomatic Carotid Atherosclerosis Study (1995) Endarterectomy for asymptomatic carotid artery stenosis. JAMA 273:1421–1428

Fain SB, Riederer SJ, Bernstein MA, et al (1999) Theoretical limits of spatial resolution in elliptical-centric contrast-enhanced 3D-MRA. Magn Reson Med 42:1106–1116

French Study of Aortic Plaques in Stroke Group (1996) Atherosclerotic disease of the aortic arch as a risk factor for recurrent ischemic stroke. N Engl J Med 334:1216–1221

Garrard CL, Manord D, Ballinger BA, et al (1997) Cost savings associated with the nonroutine use of carotid angiography. Am J Surg 174:650–654

Grant EG, Duerinckx AJ, El Saden SM, et al (2000) Ability to use Duplex US to quantify internal carotid arterial stenoses: fact or fiction? Radiology 214:247–252

Hennerici M, Klemm C, Rautenberg W (1988) The subclavian steal phenomenon: a common vascular disorder with rare neurologica deficits. Neurology 38:669–675

Hennig J, Scheffler K, Laubenberger J, et al (1997) Time-resolved projection angiography after bolus injection of contrast agent. Magn Reson Med 37:341–345

Houser O, Mokri B, Sundt T (1984) Spontaneous cervical cephalic arterial dissection and its residuum: angiographic spectrum. AJNR Am J Neuroradiol 5:27–38

Huston J, Lewis BD, Wiebers DO, et al (1993) Carotid artery: prospected blinded comparison of two-dimensional time-of-flight MR angiography with conventional angiography and duplex US. Radiology 186:339–344

Kadir S (1991) Diagnostische Radiologie. Thieme, Stuttgart

Keller E, Flacke S, Gieseke J, et al (1997) Kraniozervikale Dissektionen: Untersuchungsstrategien in der MR-Tomographie und MR-Angiographie. Fortschr Röntgensstr 167:565–571

Kido DK, Moran CJ (1994) When should third-party payers provide reimbursement for MR angiography of the carotid arteries? AJR Am J Roentgenol 162:19–20

Kirsch E, Kaim A, Engelter S, et al (1998) MR angiography in internal carotid dissection: improvement of diagnosis by selective demonstration of the intramural hematoma. Neuroradiology 40:704–709

Korosec FR, Frayne R, Grist TM, et al (1996) Time-resolved contrast-enhanced 3D MR angiography. Magn Reson Med 36:345–351

Lamparello PJ, Riles TS (1995) MR angiography in carotid stenosis: a clinical perspective. Magn Reson Imaging Clin N Am 3:455–465

Leclerc X, Martinat P, Godefroy O, et al (1998) Contrast-enhanced three-dimensional fast imaging with steady-state processing (FISP) MR angiography of supraaortic vessels: prliminary results. AJNR Am J Neuroradiol 19:1405–1413

Lévy C, Laissy JP, Raveau V, et al (1994) Carotid and vertebral artery dissections: three-dimensional time-of-flight angiography and MR imaging versus conventional angiography. Radiology 190:97–103

Levy RA, Prince MR (1996) Arterial-phase three-dimensional contrast-enhanced MR angiography of the carotid arteries. AJR Am J Roentgenol 167:11–15

Litt AW, Eidelman EM, Pinto RS, et al (1991) Diagnosis of carotid artery stenosis: comparison of 2DFT time-of-flight MR angiography with contrast angiography in 50 patients. AJNR Am J Neuroradiol 12:149–154

Liu K, Lee DH, Rutt BK (1998) Systematic assessment and evaluation of sliding interleaved ky (SLINKY) acquisition for 3D MRA. J Magn Reson Imaging 8:912–923

Luk-Pat GT, Gold GE, Olcott EW, et al (1999) High resolution three-dimensional in vivo imaging of atherosclerotic plaque. Magn Reson Med 42:762–771

Lyrer P, Bont A, Marugg A, et al (1999) Querschnittsflächenreduktion bei A.- carotis interna-Stenose. Bestimmung mit intensitätsgewichteter farbkodierter Duplexsonographie. Ultraschall Med 20:137–143

Masaryk AM, Ross JS, DiCello MC, et al (1991) 3DFT MR angiography of the carotid bifurcation: potential and limitations as a screening examination. Radiology 179:797–804

Masaryk TJ, Obuchowski NAS (1993) Noninvasive carotid imaging: caveat emptor. Radiology 186:325–331

Mattos MA, van Bemmelen PS, Hodgson KJ, et al (1993) The influence of carotid siphon stenosis on short- and long-term oucome after carotid endarterectomy. J Vasc Surg 17:902–911

Parker DL, Yuan C, Blatter D (1991) MR angiography by multiple thin slap 3D acquisition. Mag Reson Med 17:434–451

Provenzale JM (1995) Dissection of the internal carotid and vertebral arteries: imaging features. AJR Am J Roentgenol 165:1099–1104

Purdy DE, Cadena G, Laub GA (1992) The design of variable tip angle selection (TONE) pulses for improved 3D MR angiography. Society of Magnetic Resonance in Medicine, Book of Abstracts, p 882

Remonda L, Heid O, Schroth G (1998) Carotid artery stenosis, occlusion and pseudoocclusion: first-pass, gadolinium-enhanced, three-dimensional MR angiography: preliminary study. Radiology 209:95–102

Rofsky NM, Adelman MA (1998) Gadolinium-enhanced MR angiography of the carotid arteries: a small step, a giant leap? Radiology 209:31–34

Sameshima T, Futami S, Morita Y, et al (1999) Clinical usefulness of and problems with three-dimensional CT angiography for the evaluation of arteriosclerotic stenosis of the carotid artery: comparison with conventional angiography, MRA, and ultrasound sonography. Surg Neurol 51:300–309

Sardanelli F, Zandrino F, Parodi RC, et al (1999) MR angiography of internal carotid arteries: breath-hold Gd-enhanced 3D fast imaging with steady-state precession versus unenhanced 2D and 3D time-of-flight techniques. J Comput Assist Tomogr 23:208–215

Saouf R, Grassi CJ, Hartnell GG, et al (1998) Complete MR angiography and Doppler ultrasound as the sole imaging modalities prior to carotid endarterectomy. Clin Radiol 8:579–586

Schild H (1994) Angiographie – angiographische Interventionen. Thieme, Stuttgart

Sturzenegger M (1995) Spontaneous internal carotid artery dissection: early diagnosis and management in 44 patients. J Neurol 242:231–238

Urchuk SM, Plewes DB (1992) Mechanisms of flow-induced signal loss in MR angiography. J Magn Reson Imaging 2:453–462

Vanninen RL, Manninen HI, Partanen PL, Vainio PA, Soimakallio S (1995) Carotid artery stenosis: clinical efficacy of MR phase-contrast flow quantification as an adjunct to MR angiography. Radiology 194:459–1425

Wang Y, Johnston DL, Breen JF, et al (1996) Dynamic MR digital subtraction angiography using contrast enhancement, fast data acquisition, and complex subtraction. Magn Reson Med 36:551–556

Warlow CP, Dennis MS, van Gijn J, et al (1996) Stroke – a practical guide to management. Blackwell Science, Oxford

Wentz KU, Rother J, Schwartz A, et al (1994) Intracranial vertebrobasilar system: MR angiography. Radiology 190:105–110

Young GR, Humphrey PRD, Nixon TE, Smith ETS (1996) Variability in measurement of extracranial internal carotid artery stenosis as displayed by both digital subtraction angiography and magnetic resonance angiography. Stroke 27:467–473

15 The Thoracic Aorta

STEVEN DYMARKOWSKI, JAN BOGAERT

CONTENTS

15.1 Introduction

Catheter angiography, transthoracic and transoesophageal ultrasound and contrast-enhanced helical CT are generally accepted and well-established imaging modalities for detecting pathology of the thoracic aorta. The disadvantages of helical CT and X-ray angiography include the exposure of the patient to ionising radiation and the potential risk of complications of iodinated contrast agents. The known mortality and morbidity of catheter angiography, which includes iatrogenic dissection, local groin problems, pseudoaneurysm formation at the puncture site and embolisation of plaque fragments, are yet another reason to opt for a less invasive diagnostic approach. Since the advent of magnetic resonance imaging (MRI) in the field of diagnostic radiology well over a decade ago, this tendency has prevailed and is still in progress. Due to the combination of superb intrinsic contrast and spatial resolution, and the ability to acquire images in any plane, MRI is rapidly developing into the imaging modality of choice for cardiovascular pathology.

In the last few years, innovations both in hard- and software have further advanced the abilities of MRI, to the point of providing an excellent platform both for morphological and functional evaluation of the great vessels of the chest. Besides the possibility of creating high-resolution multiplanar imaging of the anatomy, MRI possesses the unique means of providing information about flow-related phenomena with bright-blood and velocity-encoded sequences.

The introduction of ultrafast gradient systems has allowed a considerable shortening of repetition times (TRs), thus effectively shortening imaging sequences. This has led to a new perspective in cardiovascular MRI: the acquisition of three-dimensional (3D) volume scans during the first pass of contrast agents. In this way, images of the thoracic aorta similar to traditional catheter angiograms can be obtained. Correlation of contrast-enhanced magnetic resonance angiography (MRA) with conventional angiography has shown that MRA is rapidly developing into a superior diagnostic procedure that may substitute vascular X-ray examination techniques in the future (MEANEY et al. 1997).

15.2 Aortic Magnetic Resonance Imaging Techniques

Like other diagnostic modalities, MRI of the vessels of the chest requires a specific imaging strategy. The thoracic cavity is intersected by vascular structures with different diameters, flow directions and flow velocities. In addition to these factors, imaging can be compromised by respiratory and cardiac blurring and pulsatile vascular flow patterns, thus constituting a situation that is not encountered in any other body part.

S. DYMARKOWSKI, M.D.
Department of Radiology, University Hospital K.U. Leuven, Herestraat 49, 3000 Leuven, Belgium
JAN BOGAERT, M.D., Ph.D.
Department of Radiology, University Hospital K.U. Leuven, Herestraat 49, 3000 Leuven, Belgium

The application of fast acquisition schemes during breath-holding and the principle of ECG-triggered segmentation of sequences have rendered the quality of MR images of the cardiovascular system sufficient for diagnosis.

15.2.1 Dark-Blood Imaging

An MRI examination of the thoracic aorta should ideally be initiated with an ECG-triggered dark-blood spin echo (SE)-based technique. The standard cardiac-gated T1-weighted spin echo sequence, which has earned much merit in the past, remains the frame of reference for great vessel imaging (LINK et al. 1993). However, recently the multislice approach has been greatly abandoned due to disadvantages such as long acquisition times, insufficient intravessel dephasing and susceptibility to respiratory artefacts (DEN BOER and ROZEBOOM 1996) in favour of more reliable single-slice sequences, which can be performed in a breath-hold period.

The problems of multislice imaging are overcome by the application of single-slice breath-hold segmented dark-blood turbo spin echo (TSE) or fast-spin echo (FSE) sequences, in which the k-space for one image is filled in 9–15 s, limiting the acquisition time to a breath-hold period.

The dark-blood effect is generated by the application of a preparation pulse pair to the sequence, which suppresses the signal from the vascular cavity. The pulse pair consists of a non-selective 180° inversion pulse, which covers the imaging slice as well as the regions below and above the imaging volume. This pulse is then immediately followed by another 180° pulse, selective for the imaging slice, thus cancelling the effects of the previous pulse on the stationary tissue in that particular slice. The result of the preparation pulse is an image with signal void in the vascular lumen, whereas the vessel walls are clearly depicted (Fig. 15.1).

In situations of slow or inverse flow, however, residual signal from the stagnant blood is detected and could be mistaken for a wall haematoma or thrombus. When in doubt, images should be acquired in a different plane (Fig. 15.2) or, alternatively, the investigator can apply bright-blood gradient echo sequences for further differentiation (SEELOS et al. 1994).

Other interesting imaging sequences include HASTE (MARCHAL and BOGAERT 1998) (Fig. 15.3) and turboFLASH (TOMIGUCHI et al. 1994), which, due to their subsecond acquisition schemes, are able to acquire images of the entire thoracic anatomy in less than 1 min. In comparison to TSE sequences, however, both HASTE and turboFLASH lack sufficient spatial resolution and signal-to-noise ratio to be of

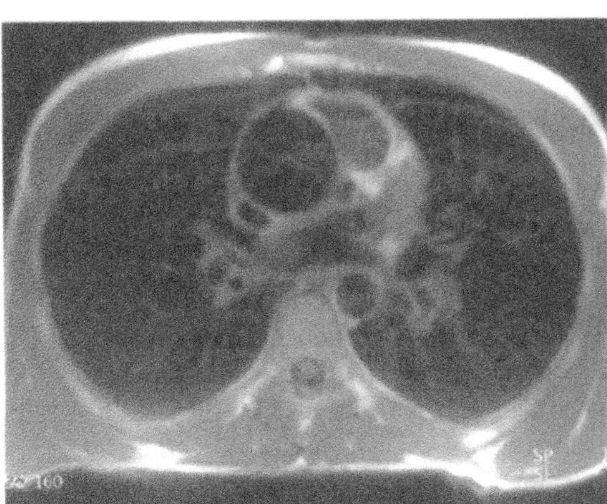

Fig. 15.1. T1-weighted turbo spin echo image at the level of the ascending aorta. There is good delineation of the vessel walls and signal void in the vascular lumen

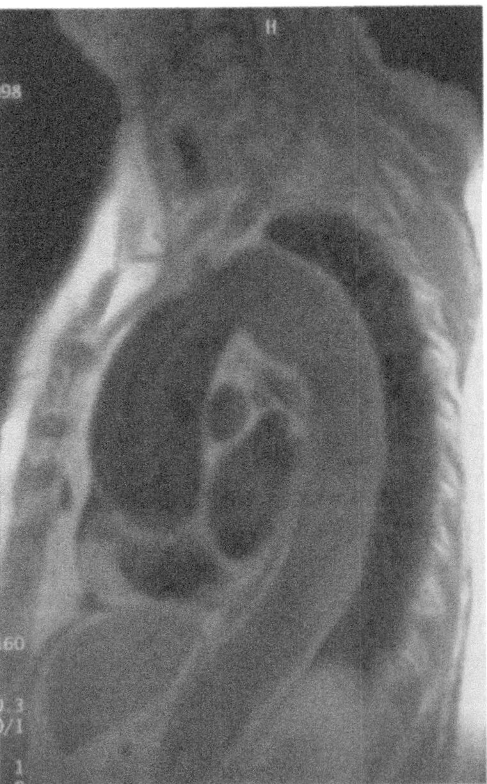

Fig. 15.2. T1-weighted turbo spin echo image in LAO incidence demonstrating residual signal from in-plane flowing blood in the descending aorta

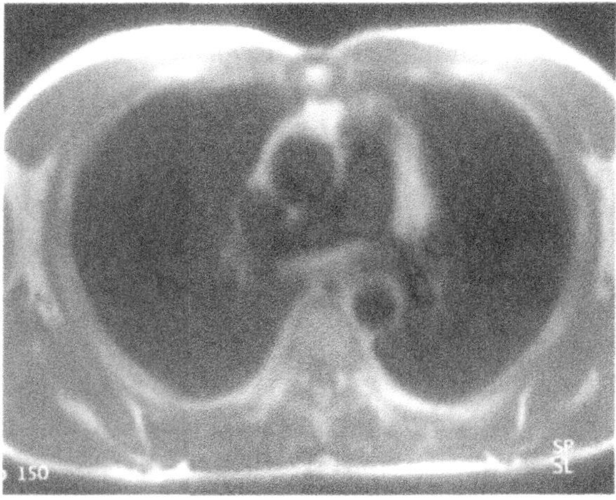

Fig. 15.3. T2-weighted HASTE image at the level of the ascending aorta. Resolution is less fine compared with turbo spin echo images

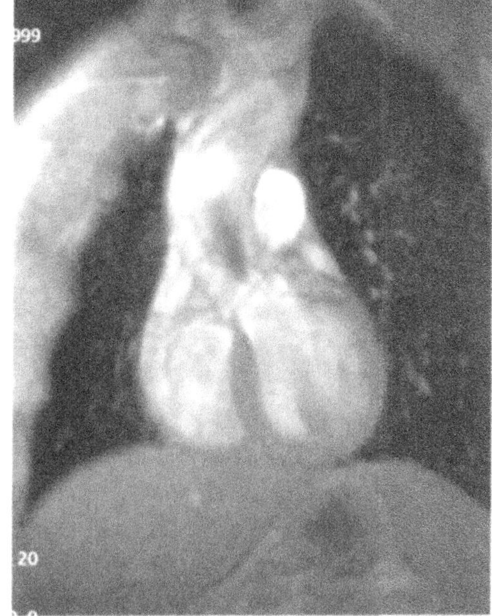

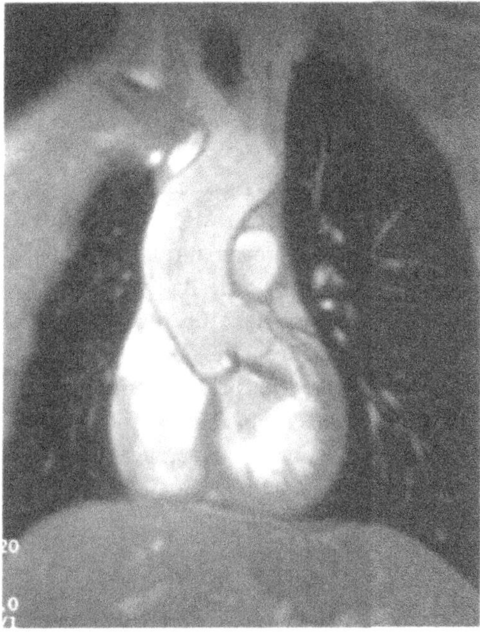

Fig. 15.4a, b. Cine MRI frames demonstrating mixed aortic valve disease. a Early systolic frame demonstrating aortic stenosis, time point, b diastolic frame with regurgitant jet from aortic insufficiency

equal diagnostic efficacy. They do offer an excellent alternative in cases where breath-holding is not possible (dyspnoea, paediatric patients).

15.2.2 Bright-Blood Imaging

15.2.2.1 Cine MRI

Unlike spin echo imaging, two-dimensional gradient echo (2D GE) cine MRI sequences display a bright signal from the vascular cavity. Because of their physical properties, these sequences possess short TRs and echo times (TEs), and thus allow for multiphase imaging. Multiphase imaging requires excitation and acquisition to occur in the same slice during different phases of the cardiac cycle (Sechtem et al. 1987). Based on this principle, fully relaxed spins enter the vascular cavity while the stationary tissue becomes progressively saturated. Maximum signal intensity will therefore be achieved when the vessels are imaged perpendicular to their longitudinal course. An interesting feature of multiphase gradient echo imaging is the possibility of displaying the consecutive images online in a continuous loop, thereby creating a dynamic overview of the different events during one cardiac cycle. Although it is not a real-time display, it permits the observer to gather additional information about the dynamic process of blood flow and to detect the presence of pathological states (Fig. 15.4a, b).

An important imaging plane for evaluation of the flow condition of the aortic arch is the left anterior oblique (LAO) incidence (Fig. 15.5) (Riquelme et al. 1999). Due to the long in-plane pathway of the aorta in this incidence, signal intensity differences derived from various in-flow patterns may be less pronounced than in a plane perpendicular to the

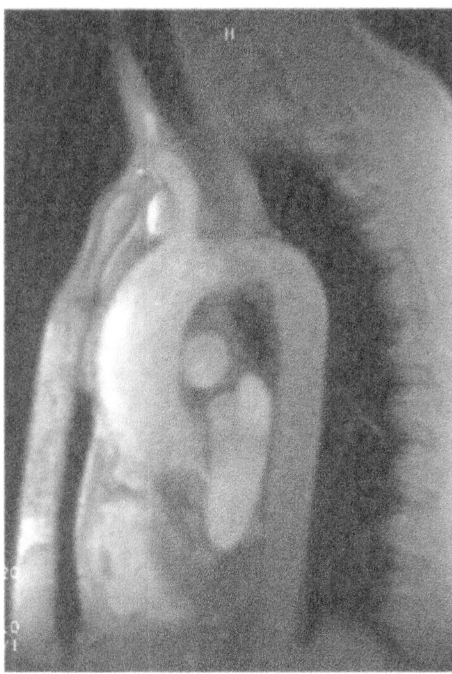

Fig. 15.5. Cine MR image of an aortic arch in LAO incidence

aorta, but nevertheless in most cases the images are of sufficient quality to be diagnostic (Kenn 1998).

The acquisition time for cine MR images depends largely on the chosen approach and the number of phases selected per cardiac cycle. Acquisition of five slices and 15 phases may take up to 10 min. The alternative strategy is to acquire single-slice data in breath-hold using faster acquisition schemes (i.e. segmented k-space approach). In these sequences, several k-space lines are acquired per heartbeat and per phase. Depending on the TR of the sequence, the amount of phase-encoding lines and the amount of k-space lines acquired per heartbeat (usually 5–9 lines) (Atkinson and Edelman 1991; Bluemke et al. 1997), the data acquisition for one slice can be completed in 15–25 heartbeats. Multiphase measurements of successive images can even share k-space data, which can further shorten acquisition time.

Although the temporal resolution of breath-hold cine MRI is usually slightly lower than the conventional multislice non-breath-hold approach, the overall image quality is better, resulting in fewer interpretational errors and respiratory artefacts.

15.2.2.2
Time-of-Flight MRA

Until recently, most MRA schemes for imaging of the thoracic aorta were based on two-dimensional time-of-flight (2D TOF) sequences. These sequences were acquired in the transverse plane, which offers the advantage of high intraluminal signal intensity due to the perpendicular course of the aorta. Total coverage of the aorta, however, remained difficult and the long acquisition times (in some cases up to 15 min) together with reconstruction difficulties proved to be of only limited clinical value.

In a similar fashion, identical problems were encountered with 3D TOF slabs of the thoracic aorta. Long acquisition times, which excluded the possibility of breath-hold imaging, and severe respiratory artefacts rendered this approach of inferior quality in evaluating aortic pathology (White et al. 1994).

To overcome these problems, specific techniques have been developed to compensate for respiratory motion by tracking the diaphragm and performing image acquisition only during specific phases of the respiratory cycle (Fig. 15.6a) (Taylor 1997, 1999; Latta et al. 1998). These techniques are being extensively used for applications which require high-resolution images, and therefore depend on long acquisition times, without the presence of motion artefacts. This so-called navigator echo technique is currently being evaluated in the field of coronary artery MRI (Fig. 15.6b) (Kessler et al. 1997).

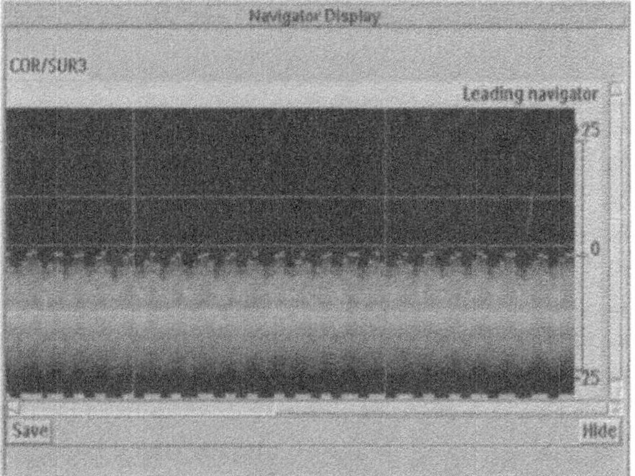

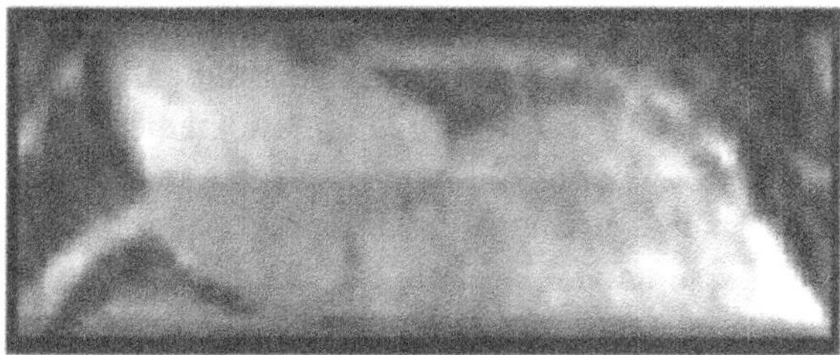

Fig. 15.6. a Excursion trace of the diaphragm obtained from a navigator echo scout sequence. **b** Example of the image quality, obtained with a cardiac-triggered, respiratory-gated 3D time-of-flight sequence, used for coronary artery imaging

15.2.2.3
Contrast-Enhanced MRA

The development of ultrafast gradient systems has led to new perspectives in MR angiography. Faster gradient rise times have allowed for TRs and TEs of 3D gradient echo sequences to be considerably shortened, thus making breath-hold 3D contrast-enhanced MRA clinically feasible. The shortening of these sequences is based on classical gradient echo time-of-flight acquisition schemes, in which the flow-compensating gradient refocusing pulses have been omitted (Krinsky and Rofsky 1998). This yields a considerable gain in time and allows the TRs and TEs to be reduced. Shorter TRs with a larger flip angle are good for optimal background suppression; however, this allows for the saturation of flowing blood, thus rendering these sequences virtually insensitive to flow effects. The principle of contrast-enhanced MRA is based on the T1-shortening of blood following a bolus injection of gadolinium chelates. The idea is to time the first pass of the bolus in the desired vessel so that it coincides with the acquisition of lower spatial frequency, i.e. contrast-rich lines of k-space of the MRA sequence (Fig. 15.7). Since the time between arterial and venous enhancement is short, timing is critical to avoid venous overlap. The total acquisition time, which mainly relies on the amount of partitions of the sequence and the matrix size, varies between 7 and 27 s in clinical practice (Revel et al. 1993).

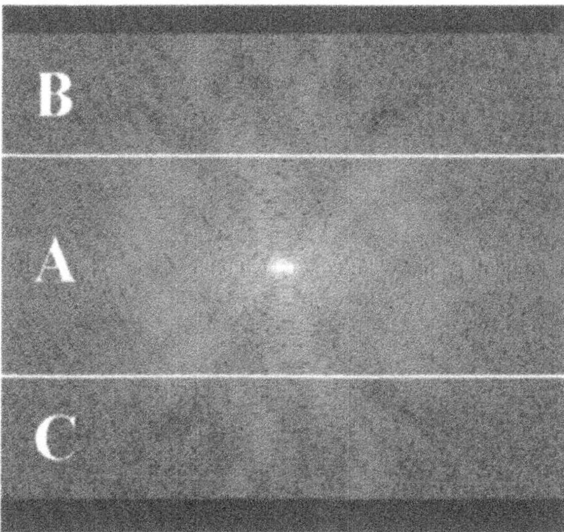

Fig. 15.7. Schematic representation of the filling of k-space. The lower spatial frequency lines, which are located in the centre of k-space, are ideally acquired during the first pass of contrast medium. The higher spatial frequency lines can be obtained before or after the first pass

Therefore, a test bolus examination (usually with 1–2 cc of contrast) should be performed in order to calculate the exact time delay before starting the MRA sequence (Fig. 15.8). Some manufacturers of MR systems have implemented a bolus-tracking algo-

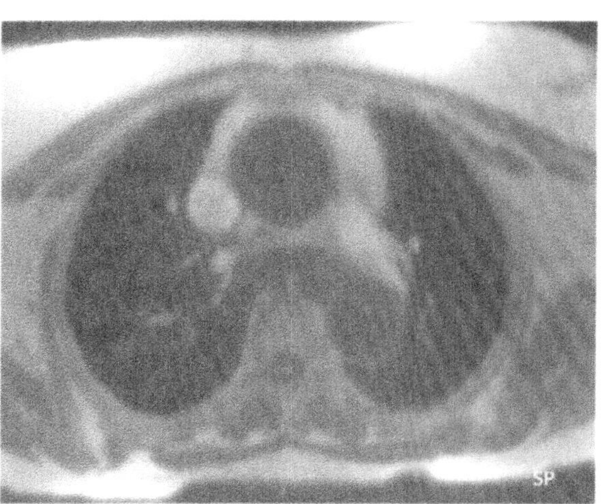

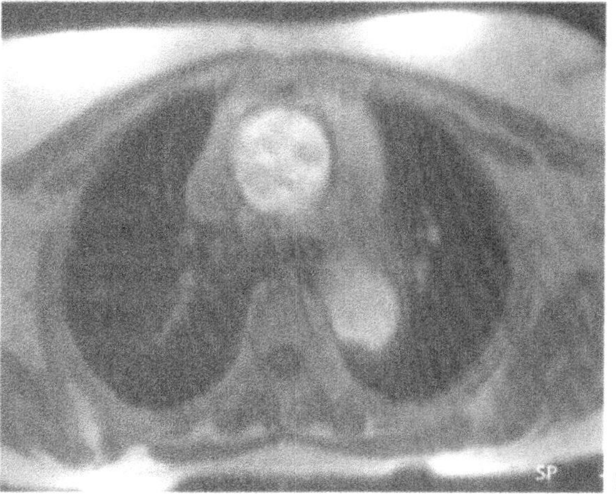

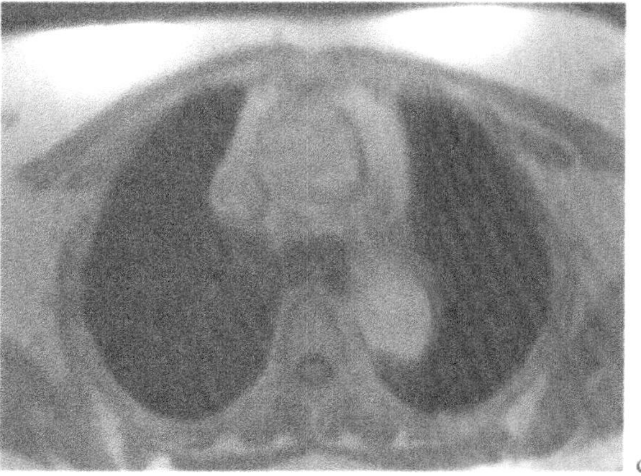

Fig. 15.8a–c. Images from a turboFLASH test bolus examination. In frame **a**, the contrast has reached the VCS and the pulmonary arteries. Frame **b** shows enhancement of the thoracic aorta. In frame **c**, contrast had divided among all vessels due to second pass effects

rithm in the MRA package. This software tool samples the signal intensity in the vessels with a 2D turboFLASH sequence and automatically initiates the 3D MRA depending on the calculated slope of the contrast arrival curve (Fig. 15.9).

Another timing approach is to keep the duration of the MRA sequence very short and perform multiple continuous measurements during breath-hold (Krinsky et al. 1998). This so-called time-resolved MRA (Van Hoe et al. 1999) allows visualisation of the passage of contrast medium in the thoracic vessels following injection in a cubital vein (superior vena cava, pulmonary artery, thoracic aorta, system venous return) without the need for proper bolus timing. This approach increases the likelihood that an arterial-only 3D image set will be obtained and allows temporal processing techniques, e.g. subtraction, to be applied to yield additional information or improve image quality (Mistretta et al. 1998). Probably the most innovative advancement to increase temporal resolution in this area is the development of "key-hole" imaging, also described as 3D-TRICKS (3D time-resolved imaging of contrast kinetics) (Korosec et al. 1996), which repeatedly acquires only partial 3D data-sets during the passage of a contrast bolus. The superior speed of this technique is generated by not collecting all of the k-space data for every reconstructed time frame. Because the lower spatial frequency lines contribute more to the image contrast, they are more regularly acquired than the higher spatial frequencies. The missing data is then estimated by interpolation between data that were collected. It is an ingenious concept which depends on a new algorithm of data reconstruction. It permits the acquisition of multiple time frames of the vascular anatomy with high temporal resolution and no significant effect on image quality. Because of its insensitivity to the shape and timing of the contrast bolus, it is a fail-safe approach to image arteries and veins of virtually any body part, producing high-quality MR angiograms, similar to conventional digital subtraction angiography.

When applied to the thoracic aorta, the time-resolved approach can be very useful in cases of aortic dissection, where there is often a difference in filling of the true and false lumen.

Post-processing of 3D MRA includes subtraction, multiplanar reformatting (MPR; Fig. 15.10), maximum intensity projections (MIP) and virtual endoscopy. Subtraction between different time frames can reveal additional information when a strictly arterial image is not obtained. MPR provides reformatted tomographic images (Leung and Debatin 1997), while MIP delivers images similar to conventional angiography (Fig. 15.11). Virtual endoscopy is a new form of virtual reality which allows the vessel walls to be viewed from the inside (Fig. 15.12). It may become important in the future for detection of atheromatous plaque; however, its precise interest in clinical imaging has yet to be defined.

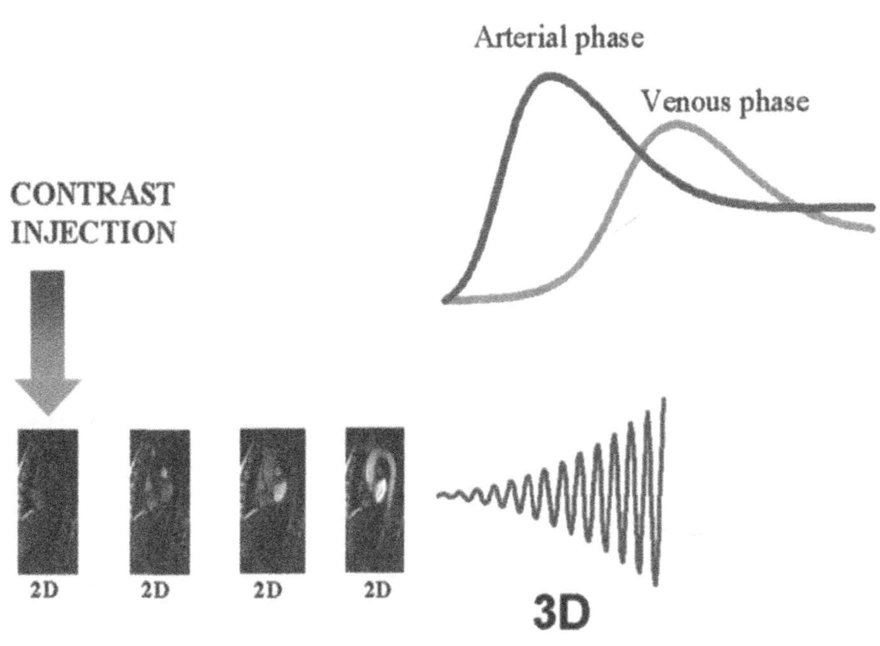

Fig. 15.9. Schematic representation of automated MRA initiation. The signal intensity in the vessel of interest is sampled at a frame rate of 1 Hz. At maximum slope of enhancement, the actual 3D gradient echo MRA sequence is started

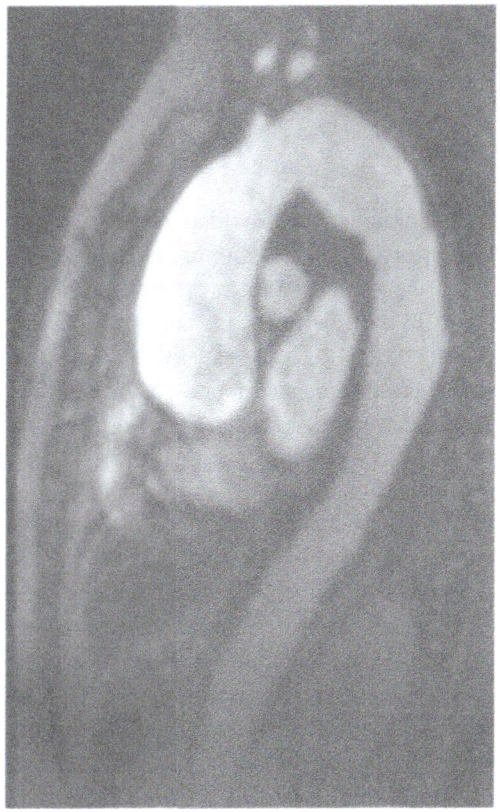

Fig. 15.10. Multiplanar reformatting (MPR) of a sagitally acquired 3D MR angiograph

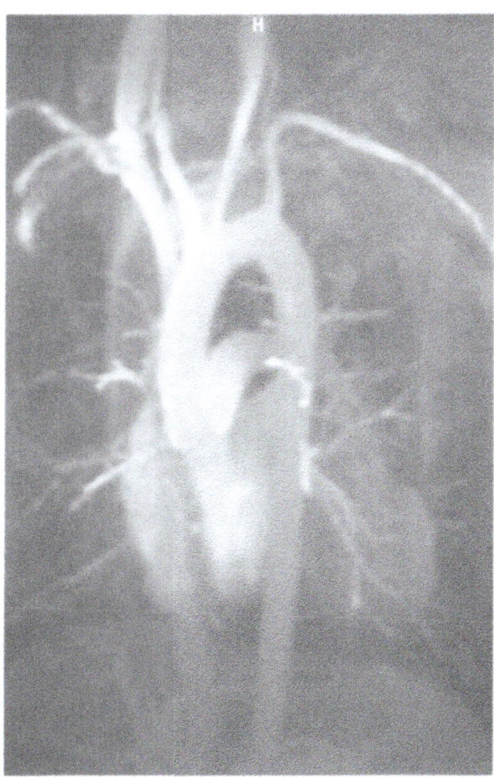

Fig. 15.11. Maximum intensity projection (MIP) of a normal aortic arch

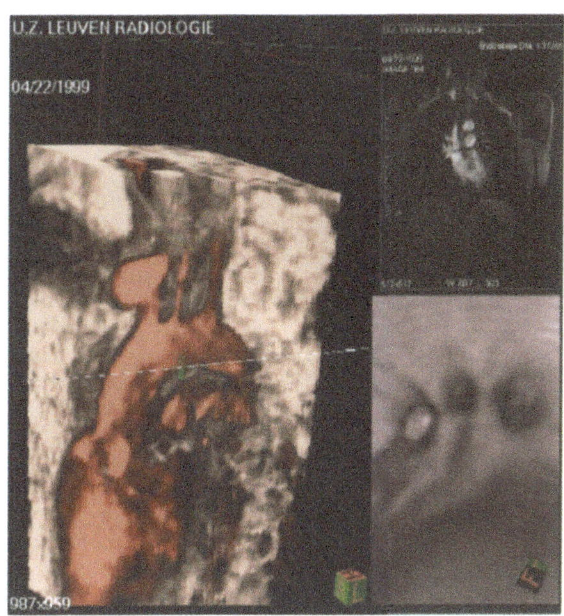

Fig. 15.12a, b. Virtual endoscopic view of the supra-aortic vessels. The *green dot* in the aortic lumen in frame **a** represents the virtual camera from which the aortic arch is viewed from the inside. The corresponding view is displayed in frame **b**. The ostia of the three supra-aortic branches can be well visualised

15.2.3 Phase Mapping

Blood flow can be quantified using differences in physical MRI properties between the spins from flowing blood and stationary tissue. By fitting a bipolar pulse to a gradient echo sequence, intravascular flowing spins will acquire a phase angle that is proportional to the gradient amplitude, to the time interval between the two pulses and, most importantly, to the velocity of the spins themselves (Peeters et al. 1995). This information can be used to quantify the absolute blood flow and to compare diseased and healthy vessels. An example of a typical flow-encoded phase image is shown in Fig. 15.13. Stationary spins are depicted as shades of grey, while flowing spins are shown in black or white, depending on the direction of flow (Hangiandreou et al. 1993). To achieve maximum accuracy in quantifying through plane flow, the imaging slice has to be positioned perpendicular to the vessel of interest. The range of velocities that can be measured is determined by the gradients and described as VENC (velocity-encoded gradient). This VENC value has to be adjusted to the expected flow velocity in the vessel of interest to avoid aliasing. For imaging of the thoracic aorta, VENC values up to 250

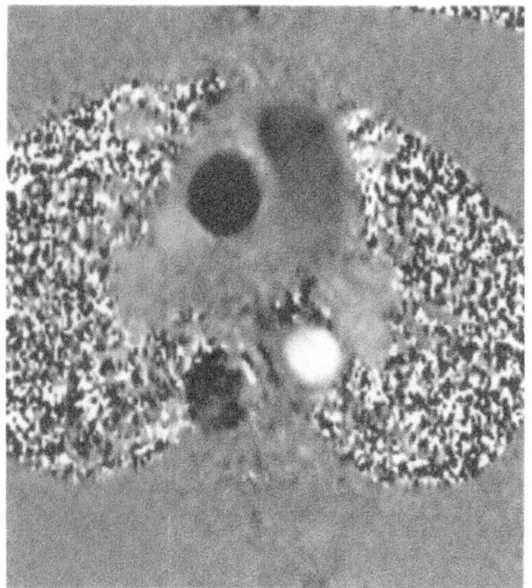

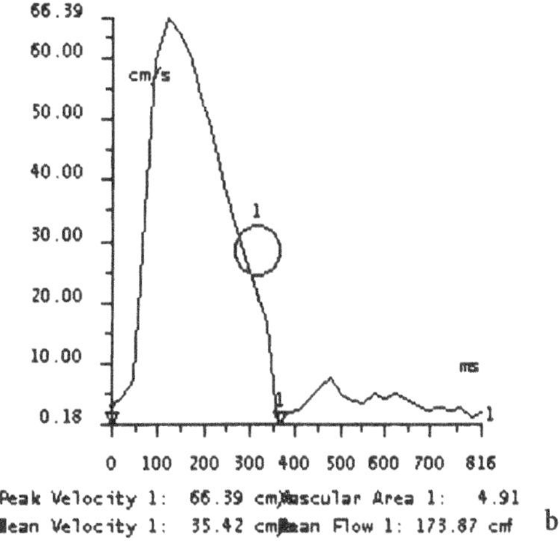

Fig. 15.13. a Typical example of a flow-encoded image through the ascending and descending aorta. Note the low intensity in the ascending aorta and the high intensity in the descending branch, due to opposite flow directions. **b** The flow curve over the cardiac cycle, obtained by integrating the instantaneous flow volume of all consecutive frames

cm/s are generally used. In cases of aortic valve stenosis, VENC values up to 400 cm/s can be required to quantify the exact grade of flow acceleration (Henk et al. 1998).

By applying cardiac-gated flow-encoded sequences about flow patterns, velocities and bulk flow volume can be obtained at any point of the cardiac cycle. The flow volume per heartbeat can be obtained by integrating the instantaneous flow volumes of all frames throughout the cardiac cycle (Wang et al.1993). This technique is very reproducible and extremely accurate and is considered to be the gold standard for in vivo flow measurements (Kondo et al. 1991).

15.3 Clinical Applications

15.3.1 Normal Anatomy

The normal thoracic aorta is divided into the ascending aorta, the aortic arch, the isthmus and descending aorta. It has the configuration of a question mark, with the aortic root arising from the centre of the cardiac base. The aortic root is usually located at the level of the eighth thoracic vertebra. The orientation of the aortic arch varies between 20° and 50° from the body's long axis. The ascending aorta rises and runs towards the right before directing itself towards the midline at the level of the brachiocephalic artery. The transverse arch, which is located at the fourth thoracic vertebra, runs further towards the left, anterior to the trachea, before joining with the descending aorta, which is located in the posterior mediastinum on the left side of the vertebral column (Fig. 15.14).

Normal vascular diameters are 33 mm at the aortic root, 30 mm in the mid-ascending aorta, 27 mm at the transverse arch and 24 mm in the descending branch (Kersting-Sommerhoff et al. 1988). Several branching patterns of the supra-aortic vessels

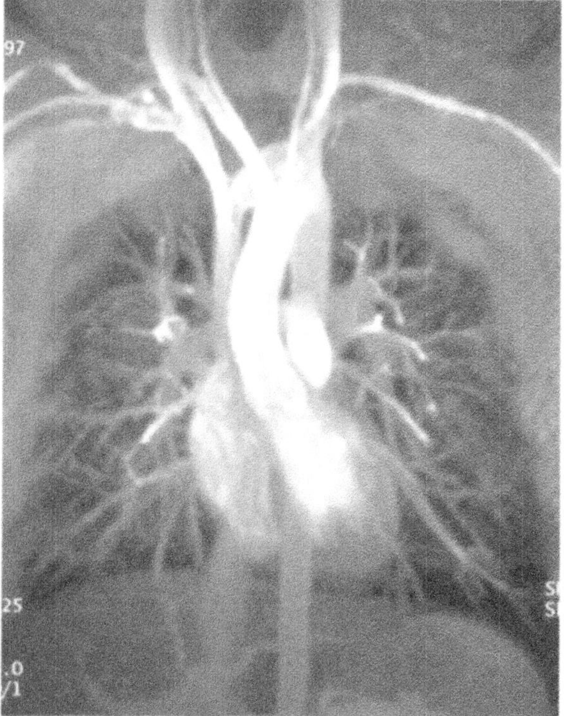

Fig. 15.14. Maximum intensity projection (MIP) of a normal aortic arch

have been described. In the most frequent pattern, which is found in 70% of the population, three vessels originate from the aortic arch from right to left: the brachiocephalic artery, the left common carotid artery and the left subclavian artery. In another 25%, a "bovine pattern" can be observed, in which the left common carotid artery has fused with the brachiocephalic artery, forming a common trunk.

Transsectional MRI and MRA are able to give a clear anatomical overview of the aorta and the supra-aortic branches in normal individuals and patients. Multiplanar breath-hold black-blood TSE sequences provide very good contrast between the dark intravascular compartment and intermediate signal from the vessel walls, while the surrounding mediastinal fat displays high signal intensities (Fig. 15.15). Although contrast-enhanced MRA is not able to clearly distinguish all small arterial branches due to its limited spatial resolution as compared to conventional aortography, the use of an interpolated 512 matrix sequence and proper contrast bolus timing permits clear visualisation of the mammarian and intercostal arteries in normal subjects and in patients.

Currently, contrast-enhanced MRA of the thoracic aorta is becoming established as the gold or reference standard for imaging of the great vessels, and it is generally accepted that the superb image quality, the reproducibility and operator-independence provide the ideal means of performing comprehensive imaging of all aspects of aortic pathology (Ruhm and Debatin 1999).

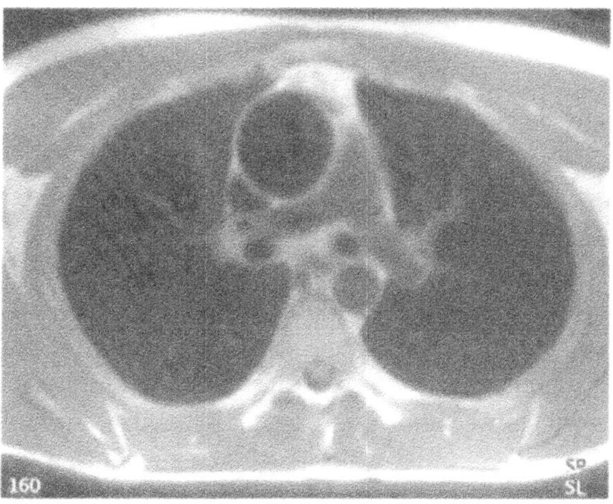

Fig. 15.15. T1-weighted turbo spin echo image transsecting the ascending and descending aorta

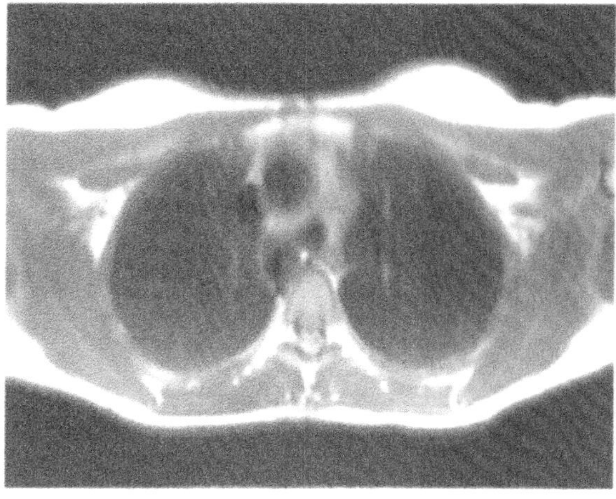

Fig. 15.16. Axial HASTE image of a right-sided aorta. The descending aorta is at the right side of the vertebral column

15.3.2 Congenital Anomalies

15.3.2.1 Right-Sided Aorta

A right-sided aortic arch forms as a result of a breach of the left branch of the Edwards hypothetical double aortic arch model distal to the ductus arteriosus (Fig. 15.16). The right-sided aortic arch passes to the right of the trachea and descends along the right side of the spine (Bogaert et al. 1992). Most cases of mirror image aortic arch occur simultaneously with other forms of congenital cardiac heart disease. Mirror image aortic arch occurs in 25% of all patients with tetralogy of Fallot and in 10%–12% of cases of open ductus of Botalli.

In some patients an aberrant left subclavian artery is found, which arises from the proximal descending aorta. Alternatively, there may be an atresia of the ostial and postostial segments and the subclavian artery may be supplied by the left vertebral artery or a patent ductus arteriosus, thereby creating a vascular ring (Fig. 15.17).

A right-sided aortic arch can be very well examined with MRI using transverse and coronal SE of breath-hold TSE sequences. They can be used in the same session to detect associated congenital intracardiac defects. Contrast-enhanced MRA acquired in the coronal plane provides a detailed overview of the aortic anatomy as well as clear insight into the branching pattern of the transverse arch. Phase mapping can be used for detection of inverse flow in case of shunting via the vertebral artery (Fig. 15.18).

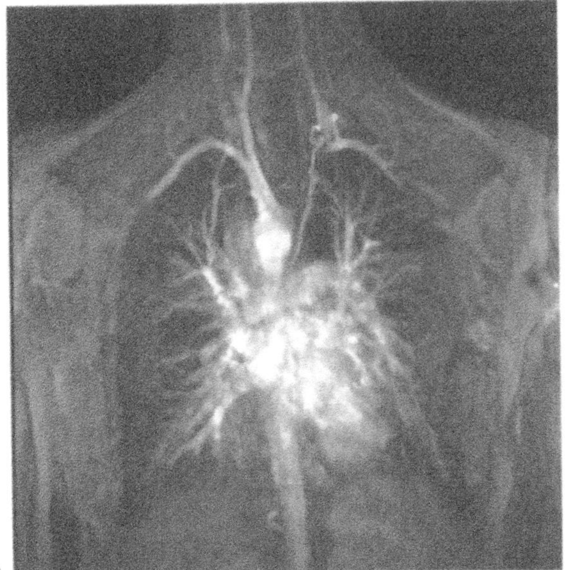

a

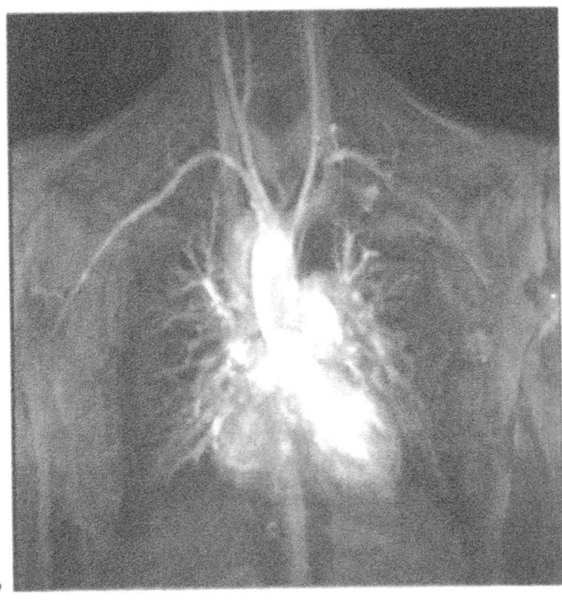

b

Fig. 15.17a, b. Maximum intensity projection of a right-sided aorta with atresia of the ostial segment of the left subclavian artery. The postostial segment is vascularised by the left vertebral artery and a collateral branch originating from the descending aorta

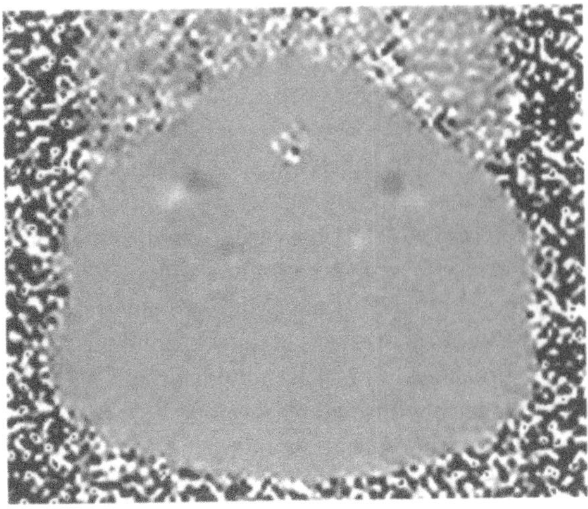

Fig. 15.18. Phase-encoded image through the vertebral arteries demonstrates reversal of flow in the presence of atresia of the ostial segment of the left subclavian artery. Same patient as in Fig. 15.19

15.3.2.2
Vascular Ring – Double Arch

A vascular ring results from a persistent double-arch model, in which the ascending aorta divides anterior to the trachea into two arches and is fused again posterior to the oesophagus and trachea to form the descending aorta (Vinstein 1990). Each arch gives rise to its own supra-aortic vessels. In this case there is no brachiocephalic trunk, but separate right and left common carotid and subclavian arteries. The descending aorta typically runs to the left side of the spinal column. Either of the arches can be dominant, although in most patients the right arch is the largest. Because of ring formation around the trachea and oesophagus, surgical intervention is warranted to relieve symptoms of dyspnea and dysphagia.

Transverse and coronal SE or TSE are well suited for detection of a double aortic arch. Due to the preceding 180° pulse in the imaging sequence, there is no apparent dephasing around the air-containing trachea as in gradient echo imaging, therefore the vascular walls can be easily detected (Roche et al. 1999). Cine MRI can be used to assess the dominance and patency of one or both arches. Contrast-enhanced MRA is generally difficult to perform in these patients due to the inherently small calibre of one of the branches of the arch. The limited ability of certain (very young) patients to perform apnoea can also be a possible compromising factor in obtaining an image with sufficient diagnostic quality.

15.3.2.3
Coarctation

Aortic coarctation is described as an infolding of the posterolateral wall of the aorta at the level of the ligamentum arteriosum, resulting in significant narrowing of the lumen. It is the most frequent form of congenital arterial stenosis, occurring in 0.7% of the general population (Simpson et al. 1988). Two clinically different forms of coarctation are differentiated. In most patients, the stenosis is located distal to

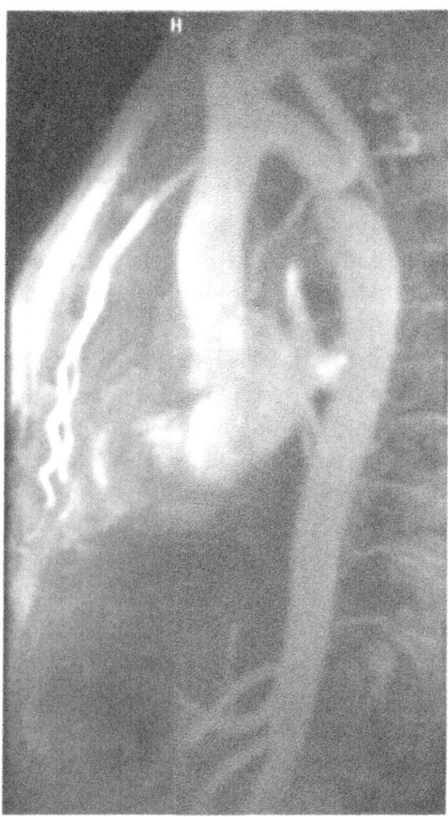

Fig. 15.19. Maximum intensity projection of a postductal coarctation. There is medium-grade narrowing which is visualised at the level of the proximal descending aorta. Note the pronounced enhancement of the mammarian arteries due to collateral flow

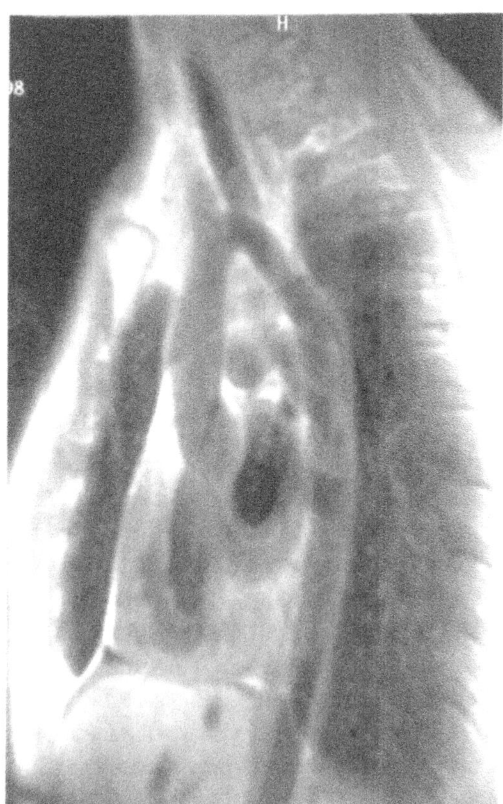

Fig. 15.20. Turbo spin echo image in LAO incidence in postductal coarctation

the ligamentum and is therefore named postductal coarctation (Fig. 15.19). It rarely gives rise to symptoms in the neonatal period or early childhood, hence it is also called adult coarctation (HARTNELL and MEIER 1995; HARTNELL et al. 1996).

The second type occurs proximal to the ligamentum and is named infantile coarctation, due to its manifestation in cardiovascular symptoms and growth disorders on the left side of the body and lower limbs (WIMPFHEIMER and BOXT 1999).

The length of the stenosis is usually short, and therefore accessible to surgery or balloon dilation. Complications of treatment include fusiform aneurysm formation in cases of patch graft surgery (BOGAERT et al. 1995), restenosis (SIBLINI et al. 1998) and dissection of the descending aorta (PHADKE et al. 1993; HUBBARD et al. 1998).

The main MRI features of coarctation are dilation of the ascending aorta, associated bicuspid aortic valve, the stenosis itself and forming of collateral circulation. Usually the mammarian arteries and the intercostal arteries, which display a corkscrew appearance, are markedly pronounced on contrast-enhanced MRA images (Fig. 15.19). TSE images in the LAO plane can very accurately demonstrate the site of stenosis (Fig. 15.20). The use of thin slices is strongly recommended, as the partial volume effect and differences in breath-hold depth can obscure clear visualisation of the grade of stenosis. Cine MRI is very effective in demonstrating post-stenotic jet-phenomena, since accelerated flow will result in signal void in the intravascular compartment.

Pressure gradients over the coarctation determined by velocity-encoded sequences above and beneath the level of stenosis are very accurate and agree well with findings of Doppler-ultrasound measurements (SOLER et al. 1998).

Contrast-enhanced MRA is best performed in the sagittal plane. Both MIR and MPR reconstructions are very adequate in demonstrating the severity of vessel stenosis as well as the relation of the stenosis to the rest of the thoracic aorta and allow the precise measurement of dilation of the ascending aorta, if present (TANEJA et al. 1998). In this patient population, MRA constitutes a comfortable and completely non-invasive approach towards diagnosis and post-therapeutic follow-up, virtually eliminating the need for invasive diagnostic procedures (Godart et al. 1998).

15.3.3 Acquired Disease

15.3.3.1 Aneurysm

Dilation of the thoracic aorta, or aneurysm formation, can be grossly divided into two categories. When the entire vascular wall is involved in the expansion, the pathology is described as a true aneurysm. The wall of the aneurysm contains all the components of a normal arterial vessel wall (endothelium, intima, media, adventitia). Conversely, in false aneurysms – also called pseudoaneurysms – there is a limited perforation of the intima and the media, while the adventitia forms the barrier of containment against exsanguination.

True aneurysms form the vast majority, of which most are caused by atherosclerotic degeneration and loss of elasticity of the inner vessel walls. This is a diffuse process, which only very rarely presents itself as a focal phenomenon. The form of an aneurysm is determined by the degree and stage of involvement and is described as saccular, cylindrical or fusiform. Other coinciding findings in atherosclerotic disease of the thoracic aorta include kinking, apparent lengthening and tortuosity (Fig. 15.21).

Accurate imaging of thoracic aorta aneurysms is very important in order to establish the cause, the need for surgery and the prognosis of the patient. It may also be necessary to look for associated complications of aortic aneurysms such as rupture, periaortic haematoma and aortic valve insufficiency (Fig. 15.22) (Carpenter et al. 1997; Murray et al. 1997].

Multiplanar breath-hold TSE MRI is very effective in providing information about the extent of dilation, the location of the aneurysm and also supplies relevant information regarding the vessel wall, e.g. whether there is an intramural haematoma or atherosclerotic plaque formation (Dowd et al. 1996; Bon-

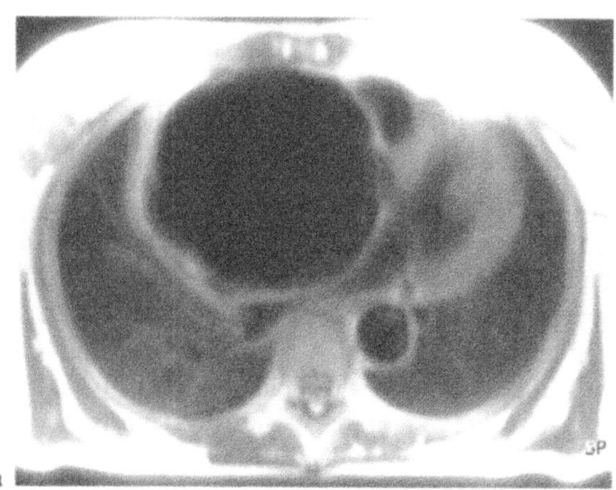

a

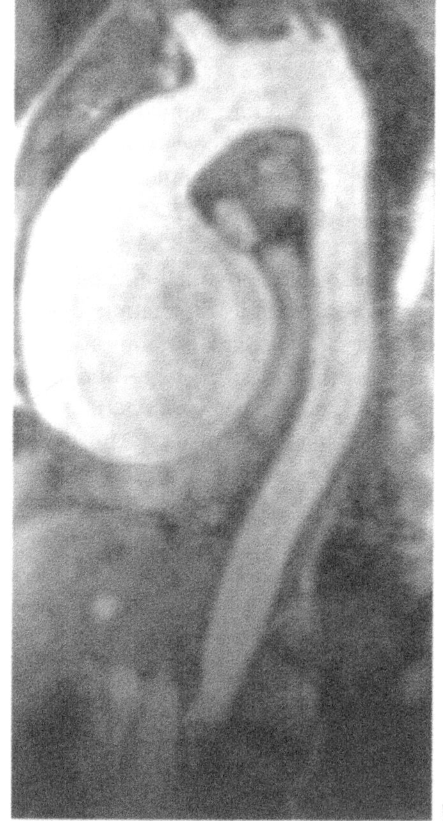

b

Fig. 15.21a, b. Giant aortic aneurysm. **a** Axial T2-weighted TSE image clearly demonstrates an aneurysm of the ascending aorta measuring 11 cm. **b** Multiplanar reconstruction of a 3D MRA in LAO incidence

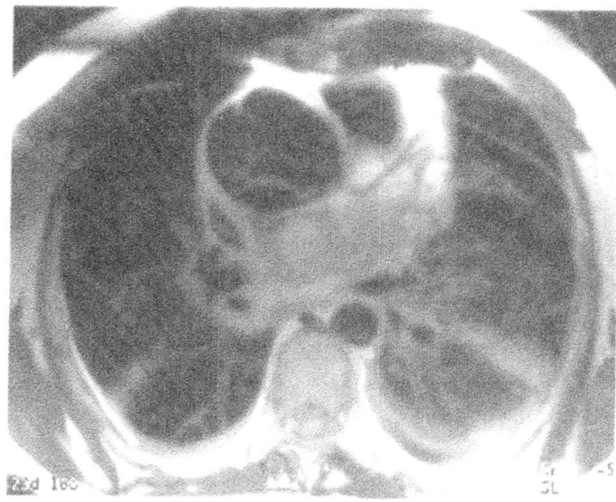

Fig. 15.22. T2-weighted image in axial incidence of a rupture of an ascending aorta aneurysm towards the aortic anulus and the coronary sinuses. Note the different signal intensities in the forming pseudoaneurysm, indicating both bleeding and slow flow

GARTZ et al. 1997). The advantage of spiral CT is definitely constituted by the ability to differentiate acute intramural haemorrhage from thrombotic material or plaques, since an acute haematoma will display increased signal intensity on T1-weighted images, whereas thrombus has a low signal intensity (HARTNELL 1997).

Functional studies of saccular aneurysms of the ascending aorta, which are predominantly caused by degenerative annuloaortic ectasia and Marfan's syndrome (RAMMOHAN et al. 1998), display a varying degree of aortic regurgitation, depending on the severity of involvement (Fig. 15.23). On the other hand, a bicuspid or heavily calcified aortic valve can lead to an asymmetric systolic jet directed towards the anterior wall of the thoracic aorta, which in the long run leads to aneurysm formation (FRAYNE and RUTT 1995; BONGARTZ et al. 1997).

Both entities can be accurately demonstrated using GE cine MRI (Fig. 15.4). The jet of regurgitation from aortic valve stenosis appears as an area of signal void on these bright-blood images, whereas the vascular lumen remains clearly visible (BOGREN et al. 1995).

Quantification of valve function by velocity mapping may aid in pretherapeutic decision making regarding medical or surgical treatment of aortic aneurysms.

Contrast-enhanced MRA acquired in the sagittal plane, particularly due to the possibility of multiplanar reformatting, is the ideal approach to describe the precise extent of an aortic aneurysm and the possible involvement of the supra-aortic vessels in one single field of view (BONGARTZ et al. 1994). Reformattings in the LAO plane, in particular, are very useful in determining the severity of involvement.

15.3.3.2 Dissection

Dissection of the thoracic aorta is - similar to the pathogenesis of aneurysms - the result of intimal degeneration and subsequent subintimal haemorrhage and tear formation, or repetitive media trauma. Promoting factors are coexisting hypertension, atherosclerotic aneurysm or aortic trauma. Hypertension, in particular, is a causal agent in the propagation of a small rent into a tear that may extend into the entire thoracic and abdominal aorta (HEKALI et al. 1986).

Thoracic aorta dissection is classified according to the Debakey classification independent of the origin of the intimal flap. Type I dissections involve the ascending aorta, the aortic arch and the descending aorta (Fig. 15.24). Type II dissections are confined to the ascending aorta, whereas type III dissections begin distal to the left subclavian artery. Alternatively, thoracic artery dissections can be specified by the Stanford classification, where a type A dissection

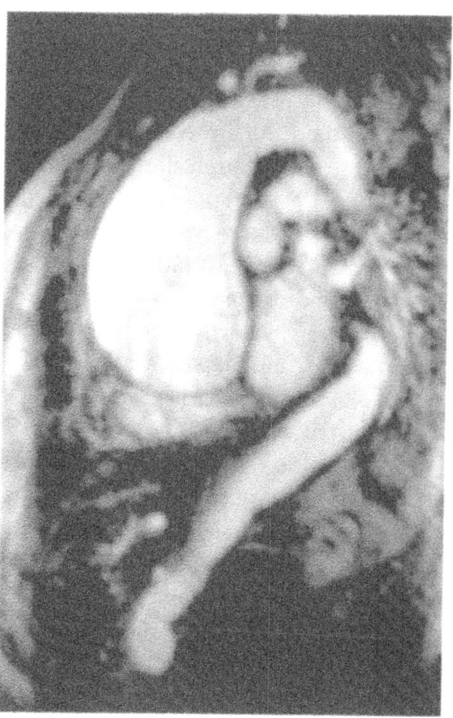

Fig. 15.23. Marfan syndrome. Annuloaortic ectasia demonstrated by 3D MRA. There is marked fusiform dilatation of the ascending aorta and proximal aortic arch. MPR view in LAO incidence

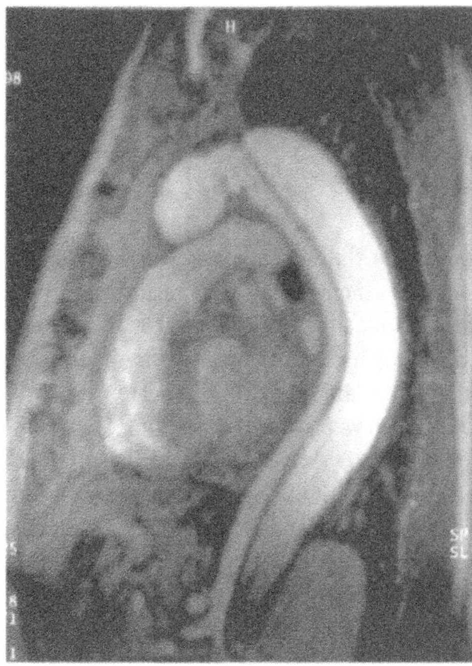

Fig. 15.24. Type III dissection in the Debakey classification. The intimal flap originates distal to the left subclavian artery and is propagated into the abdominal aorta

corresponds with types II and I. Type B is the analogous term for a Debakey type III dissection.

The determination of the extent of a dissection is of crucial importance for the management and the prognosis of the patient (Hartnell 1995). Dissections of the ascending aorta are considered as life threatening and are treated surgically by replacing the ascending aorta by a graft, possibly with incorporation of a prosthetic aortic valve and reimplantation of the coronary arteries (Robbins et al. 1993). Complications of ascending aorta dissection include intrapericardial haemorrhage with tamponade and propagation of the tear into the supra-aortic vessel with occlusion of the carotid artery (Veyssier-Belot et al. 1993; Cherington et al. 1995).

Dissections confined to the descending aorta are treated medically, in which control of blood pressure and hyperlipidaemia are key elements. Descending aorta aneurysms very often extend into the abdominal aorta and past the iliac bifurcation, possibly compromising the patency of one or more intra-abdominal side branches (Bogaert et al. 1997).

The typical appearance of an aortic dissection on MR images is the "double-barrel" aorta, in which two lumina can be clearly delineated. SE or TSE sequences display a dark signal from the cavities, whereas the intimal flap is characterised by an intermediate signal intensity (Ho and Prince 1998). In the false lumen, flow deceleration may be present, thus compromising the efficacy of the dark-blood preparation pulses. This can lead to a heterogeneous signal from the cavity of the false lumen and may be mistaken for thrombus or an intramural haematoma. It is the virtue of bright-blood sequences to demonstrate the presence of slow flow. On cine MRI images, there is a distinct difference in signal intensities between the two lumina, especially in the systolic phase of the cardiac cycle, where the false channel is markedly less bright than the true lumen, due to reduced inflow effects (Fig. 15.25).

In the majority of aortic dissections (up to 89%), re-entry is experienced further downstream and most of these have multiple re-entry sites (Chung et al. 1994). On T1-weighted TSE images, these fenestrations in the intimal flap can be visualised. Because these fenestrations are very small, they are more

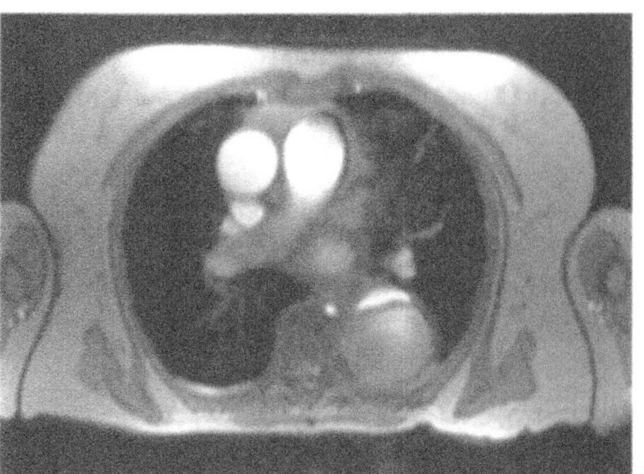

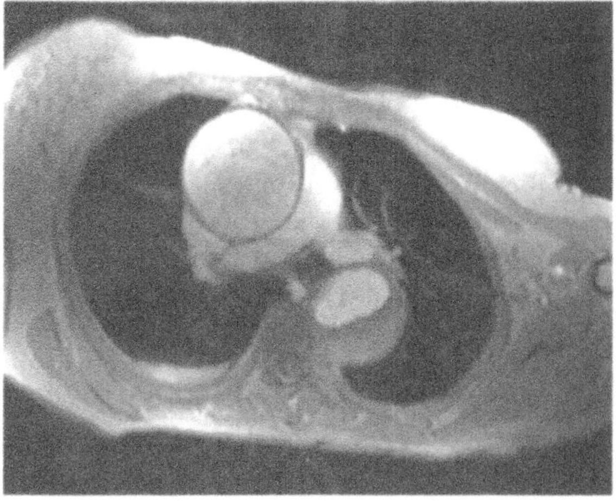

Fig. 15.25a, b. Cine MRI in aortic dissection. In image **a**, the false (posterior) lumen is markedly less bright than the smaller true lumen, due to reduced inflow effects. Frame **b** shows complete thrombosis of the false lumen. No inflow signal is detected in the false lumen

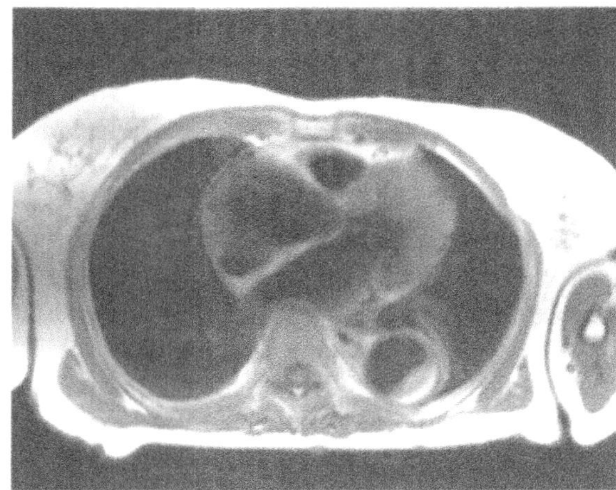

Fig. 15.26. Axial HASTE image of type III aortic dissection. The slower flow in the false lumen at the level of the descending aorta causes decreased efficiency of the preceding dark-blood pulse, resulting in bright signal from the blood

effectively demonstrated on contrast-enhanced 3D MRA scans due to the absence of slice misregistration and the possibility of reformatting to get in a plane exactly perpendicular to the intimal flap (Fig. 15.26).

Although the general approach of contrast-enhanced MRA towards dissection is similar to that of aneurysm, specific attention should be paid to visualise both lumina properly to avoid misinterpretation. Since flow in the false lumen is slower, the contrast arrival time following a bolus injection will also be delayed by several seconds. Acquisition of a single slab may thus reveal only enhancement of the true lumen, since contrast accumulation in the false lumen has not yet occurred at the time point which is ideal to image the true channel. It is therefore recommended to acquire multiple contiguous timeframes, i.e. time resolved 3D MRA or even faster, to use the 3D TRICKS technique. In Fig. 15.27, two consecutive time frames are shown. Note the enhancement only of the true lumen, which gives the impression that no dissection is present. The second time point, acquired 10 s later, clearly shows both "barrels" of the dissected descending aorta.

For the correct preoperative work-up of a patient with thoracic aorta dissection, the combination of these formerly discussed techniques results in an MR examination with high sensitivity and specificity, which is able to replace the need for an invasive vascular X-ray exam. Indeed, in patients with acute dissection, renal and cardiac function may be impaired and injection of large quantities of iodinated contrast media should be avoided.

Currently, MRA is progressively being accepted as a new gold standard for imaging of dissection of the thoracic aorta. However, the relatively long examination time and limited availability still prevent MRA from being the examination of choice in emergency department patients, a role which is currently reserved for transoesophageal ultrasound and spiral CT (Laissy et al. 1995; Sarasin et al. 1996).

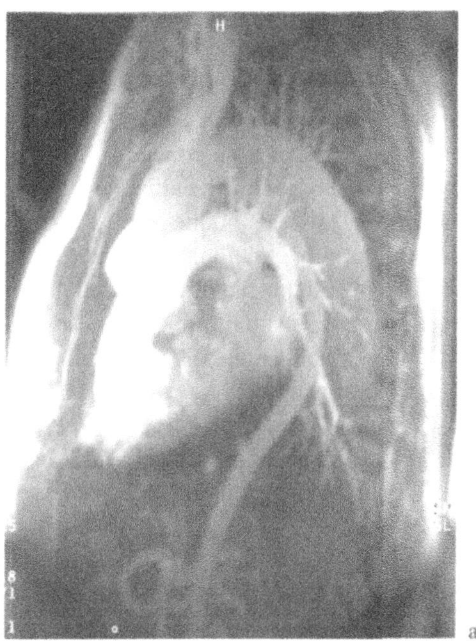

a

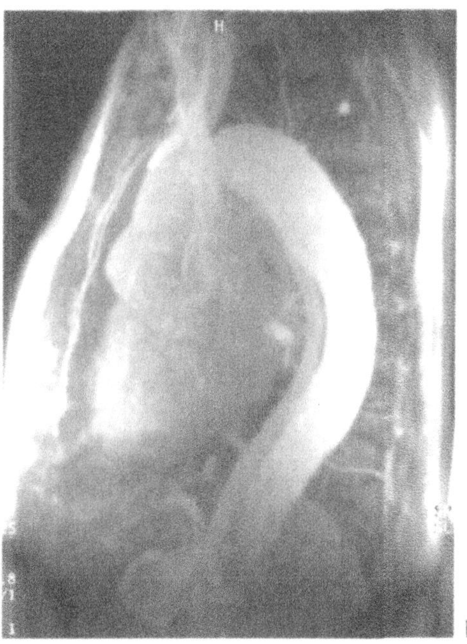

b

Fig. 15.27a, b. Two consecutive time frames of a contrast-enhanced MR angiograph of aortic dissection. Note the differential enhancement of the false and true lumen due to delayed contrast arrival in the false lumen

15.3.3.3
Inflammatory Disease

Among the many causes of aortitis, the one most eligible for MRI is Takayasu's arteritis. This disease causes multiple, diffuse stenoses in the aorta, creating a most precarious situation for catheterisation. Other causes of aortic inflammation include bacterial endocarditis, sepsis, the presence of prosthetic heart valves and a history of aortic surgery (Fig. 15.28).

Although MRI is not commonly considered as the examination of choice in cases of infectious or inflammatory diseases of the aorta, it can be valuable by providing information which cannot be detected by echocardiography, including the presence of a mediastinal abscess and the involvement of the branch vessels in any inflammatory state (HATA and NUMANO 1995). TSE imaging provides a detailed overview of the vascular anatomy and besides vascular wall thickening it can demonstrate infiltration of the mediastinal or paravalvular tissues (FLAMM et al. 1998), while GE cine MRI is very useful and accurate in detecting any aortic valve abnormalities. Additionally, valvular function can be quantified using velocity-encoded techniques.

Infectious diseases can also lead to the formation of aneurysms, albeit less frequently than those caused by atherosclerosis. In particular, saccular aneurysms caused by syphilis or infective endocarditis are very well known. In some cases pseudoaneurysms are found, of which the lumen may contain infectious material, subject to haematogenous spread and mycotic aneurysm formation (BERKMEN 1998). As previously described, MRA can be considered an investigation of choice in the non-acute patient to further differentiate the origin and extent of thoracic aorta aneurysms.

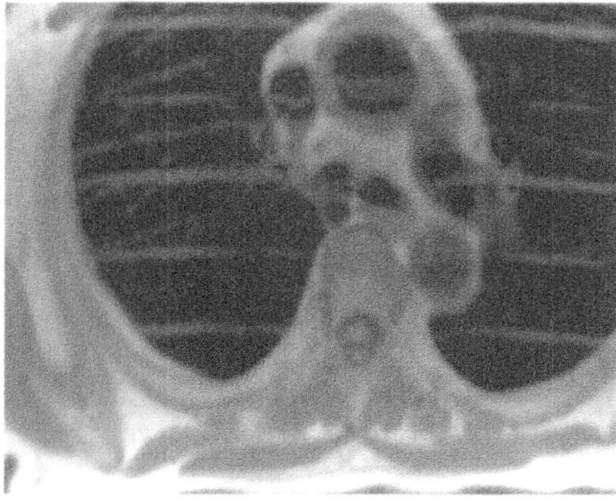

Fig. 15.28. Axial T1-weighted TSE image in a patient with staphylococcal aortitis. Note the pronounced thickening of the wall of the ascending aorta

15.3.3.4
Aortic Trauma

Aortic trauma is in the majority of cases the result of blunt trauma to the chest, and even more specifically, the consequence of a deceleration injury. Most patients have suffered a fall from a great height or were involved in a motor vehicle accident in which they had impact of the chest on the steering wheel.

Traumatic lacerations of the thoracic aorta occur at the level of the proximal ascending aorta or at the insertion of the ligamentum arteriosum.

The aftermath of an aortic rupture is critical, to say the least. Sudden death occurs in 85%–90% of cases (DAVIES 1998). Of those fortunate to survive the initial hours, 90% will die if not properly treated. Therefore, fast and accurate diagnosis is imperative. A thorough study of the literature fails to reveal any experience with MRI on aortic trauma, which is logically explained by the impracticality of MRI in this class of patients, who most likely have other life-threatening injuries (HUGHES et al. 1994).

However, MRI and MRA are frequently used in the diagnosis of small aortic tears that are initially missed, which appear in the form of chronic pseudoaneurysms. These pseudoaneurysms are located in the vicinity of the ligamentum arteriosum, on the internal border of the distal aortic arch. They often display heterogeneous signal intensity on SE and TSE images, due to the presence of intraluminal slow flow and haematoma in different stages of organisation (Fig. 15.29). Contrast-enhanced MRA is able to demonstrate a residual lumen, if present, but often underestimates the actual size of the aneurysm itself. This can be explained by the presence of susceptibility artefacts, owing to the high association with calcification at the site of injury.

15.3.4
Imaging of the Side Branches

As previously discussed, the branching pattern of the supra-aortic vessels can be efficiently described in normal individuals and patients using transsectional MRI and MRA. Clinical applications which may necessitate imaging of these vessels include, among others, propagation of aortic dissection into

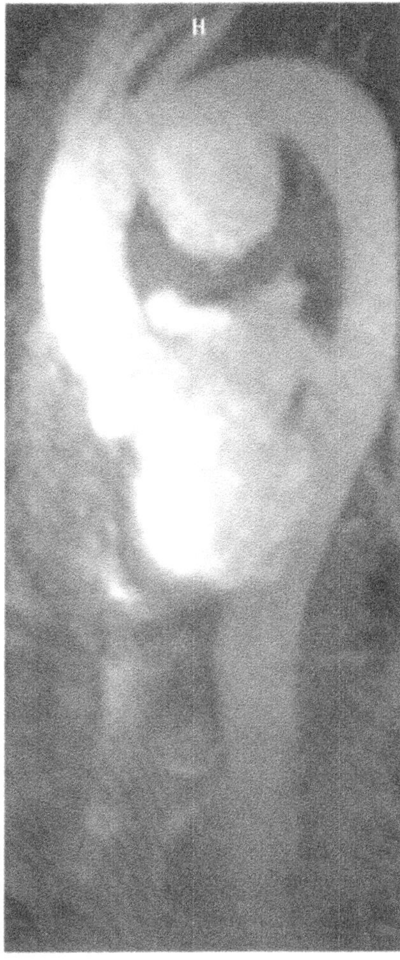

Fig. 15.29. Post-traumatic aneurysm of the aortic arch. MIP view

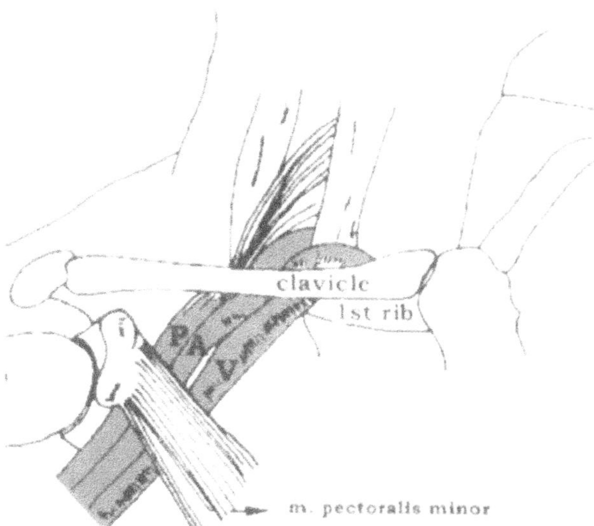

Fig. 15.30. Schematic representation of the anatomy of the thoracic outlet. *P*, brachial plexus; *A*, subclavian artery; *V*, subclavian vein; *SA*, scalenus anterior muscle; *SM*, scalenus medius muscle

the carotid or subclavian arteries, aneurysm formation at the origin on the aorta, subclavian steal syndromes and the thoracic outlet syndrome.

15.3.4.1 Thoracic Outlet Syndrome

The thoracic outlet is the anatomical region where the subclavian vessels and the brachial plexus structures exit the thoracic cavity in their path to the upper extremity through the axilla (Fig. 15.30). The subclavian artery curves over the upper margin of the first rib, posterior to the insertion of the scalenus anterior muscle, and continues as the axillary artery under the clavicle though the crevice formed by the coracoid process of the scapula and the tendinous insertion of the pectoralis minor muscle on this process. The brachial plexus is found immediately posterior to the artery, anterior to the scalenus medius muscle. The 'interscalene triangle' is thus defined as the anatomical space between the scalenus anterior and medius muscle, with the first rib as its inferior boundary. The subclavian vein follows the artery, but runs anterior to the scalenus anterior muscle. Thoracic outlet syndrome refers to neurovascular complaints attributable to compression of either the brachial plexus or the subclavian vessels. Pressure on or elongation of the vascular or neural structures, or both, in this area can occur at various locations. The most critical point appears to be the costoclavicular area (i.e. between the first rib and the clavicle). Anatomical variants of these bones can narrow this space, thereby obstructing the normal course of the interposed structures. Second, obstruction can exist when a broad insertion of the scalenus anterior muscle on the clavicle or the presence of a cervical rib narrows the interscalene triangle. Finally, the wedge formed by the coracoid process and the tendon of the pectoralis minor muscle can cause an impingement of the vascular and neural structures during abduction of the arm.

In patients with chronic and acute ischemia of the arm, clinical signs of stenosis or occlusion of the subclavian artery can be found: a palpable thrill over the artery, diminished radial pulsations and lowered brachial blood pressure. Several examination manoeuvres have been described to diagnose thoracic outlet syndrome, including the Adson, costoclavicular and hyperabduction tests. Many diagnostic procedures have been described to confirm neurovascular compression or to differentiate it from other diseases (Cherington et al. 1995). These examinations include conventional angiography, peripheral nerve conduction measurements, brachial plexus neurography, Duplex scanning [5] and, more recently, two-dimensional time-of-flight (TOF) MRA (Esposito et al. 1997). Of these examinations, most procedures, including conventional angiography, are fairly non-specific, whereas neurography, electromyography and somatosensory-evoked potentials are found to be more specific. One should note that complaints related to thoracic outlet syndrome can be caused by brachial plexus compression without vascular abnormalities, and in fact, nerve-related problems are much more common than vascular compression syndromes, in some studies even reported up to 98%. However, patients with a thoracic outlet syndrome without evidence suggesting vascular elongation or compression are deemed not eligible for surgery, due to the high degree of postoperative recurrences of complaints and the risk of definitive damage to the brachial plexus by an unwarranted resection of the first rib. Therefore it is interesting to include an MR investigation in the preoperative work-up to evaluate the vascular status.

To evaluate the effect of arm position on vessel patency, the patients are positioned with the arms in hyperabduction after which time-resolved contrast-enhanced 3D MRA is performed in the coronal plane (Fig. 15.31). An example of typical imaging parameters of the MRA sequence is: TR 3.8 ms, TE 1.3 ms, flip angle 250, 1 acquisition, matrix 134+160, slab thickness 60 mm, number of partitions 30, with a rectangular field of view of 306+350 mm. Interpolation along the k_z-direction in k-space is used to obtain 60 slices with an effective thickness of 1.0 mm. This results in an acquisition time of 15 s per slab. Three consecutive measurements are recorded, of which the first was performed during the first pass of the contrast agent through the subclavian arteries. Timing is calculated based on a test bolus injection of 1 ml of contrast medium to ensure that the first scan coincides with the arterial first pass. The second and third acquisition both generally showed mixed arterial and venous images.

The patients are then repositioned with arms in adduction, after which T1-weighted breath-hold TSE sequences are performed in the coronal and the sagittal planes. A second session of MRA is then performed, again acquiring three time-resolved sets. The average total imaging time is about 25 min. The time interval between the two MRA sessions should be no less than 10 min, allowing signal intensities in the vessels to return to their pre-injection values.

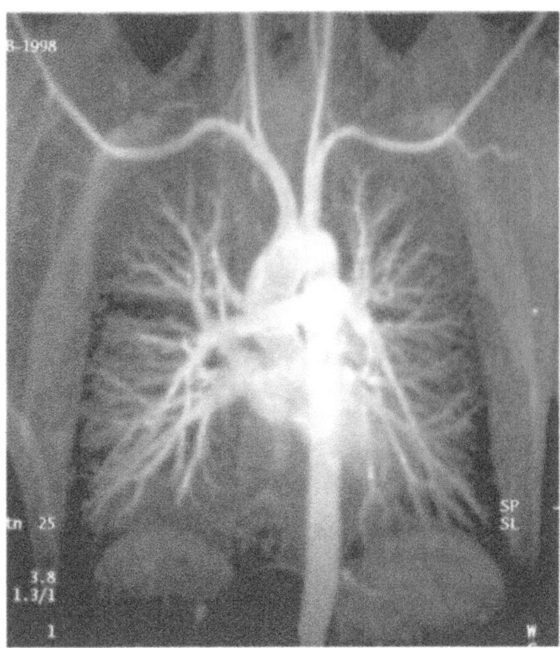

Fig. 15.31. First-pass MR angiogram obtained with arms in hyperabduction in a patient with pain in both arms. Intermediate-grade stenosis of the left subclavian artery becomes apparent

In this patient group, the combination of T1-weighted TSE image acquisition and 3D MRA is able to identify the anatomical structures responsible for vessel compression during hyperabduction of the arms as well as to demonstrate the grade of vessel patency itself, whereas the angiograms during adduction show regular vessel patency (Fig. 15.32). Maximum intensity projections of MR angiograms allow a clear diagnosis of the site of stenosis, whereas multiplanar reformatting of the 3D data sets is more useful in determining the grade of vessel compression (Dymarkowski et al. 1999). It is a non-invasive approach, and requires neither ionising radiation nor the administration of iodinated contrast agents. The ultrafast contrast-enhanced 3D contrast-enhanced MRA approach holds many advantages over the two-dimensional sequences formerly used, such as speed, lack of dephasing, and an improved signal-to-noise ratio. These advantages clearly compensate for i.v. injection of a contrast agent. Although the imaging itself is fast, the need for an interval between the two series of MR angiograms is time consuming. This is a drawback in the current approach. However, blood pool agents will soon become available for clinical use that can counteract this disadvantage, as only one injection will be required. In the future, larger comparative studies are required to confirm whether this

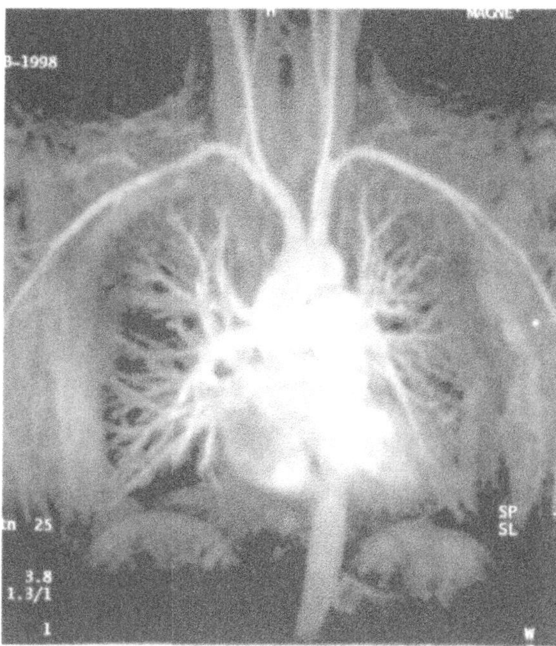

Fig. 15.32. Same patient as in Fig. 15.31. First-pass MR angiogram obtained with arms in adduction show subclavian vessels as normal

procedure deserves a place among other more established diagnostic techniques.

15.4 Conclusion

Due to recent high-end technological improvements, MRI and MRA have evolved to highly sensitive and accurate imaging techniques to evaluate congenital or acquired pathology of the thoracic aorta. In the era where availability of MR systems is increasing and radiologists are systematically trained in understanding how to use these modalities to their fullest extent to thoroughly evaluate the pathology under investigation, the acceptance of MRI for diagnosing diseases of the great vessels is no longer a future perspective but a fact. By combining different concepts of MRI - ranging from dark-blood pulses in spin echo sequences, inflow enhancement on cine MR images, velocity measurements derived from flow-encoded sequences and the ability of contrast-enhanced MRA to selectively image the arterial vessels - a comprehensive anatomical and functional evaluation of the thoracic aorta can be provided in a single examination. Further technical improvements may in the future lead to the acceleration of scan speed, higher resolution and possibly the efficient incorporation of interventional procedures.

Such combined non-invasive MR examinations may some day become the ultimate cost-effective screening tool for diseases of the great vessels of the chest.

References

Atkinson DJ, Edelman RR (1991) Cineangiography of the heart in a single breath hold with a segmented turboFLASH sequence. Radiology 178:357-360

Berkmen T (1998) MR angiography of aneurysms in Behcet disease: a report of four cases. J Comput Assist Tomogr 22:202-206

Bluemke DA, Boxerman JL, Mosher T, Lima JA (1997) Segmented K-space cine breath-hold cardiovascular MR imaging. II. Evaluation of aortic vasculopathy. AJR Am J Roentgenol 169:401-407

Bogaert J, Verschakelen JA, Smet MH, Baert AL (1992) Pictorial essay: right aortic arch. J Belge Radiol 75:406-409

Bogaert J, Gewillig M, Rademakers F, Bosmans H, Verschakelen J, Daenen W, Baert AL (1995) Transverse arch hypoplasia predisposes to aneurysm formation at the repair site after patch angioplasty for coarctation of the aorta. J Am Coll Cardiol 26:521-527

Bogaert J, Meyns B, Rademakers FE, Bosmans H, Verschakelen J, Flameng W, Marchal G, Baert AL (1997) Follow-up of aortic dissection: contribution of MR angiography for evaluation of the abdominal aorta and its branches. Eur Radiol 7:695-702

Bogren HG, Mohiaddin RH, Yang GZ, Kilner PJ, Firmin DN (1995) Magnetic resonance velocity vector mapping of blood flow in thoracic aortic aneurysms and grafts. J Thorac Cardiovasc Surg 110:704-714

Bongartz G, Behrendt J, Schuierer G, Reimer P, Peters PE (1994) Magnetic resonance angiography of supra-aortic arteries. Radiologe 34:430-436

Bongartz G, Boos M, Winter K, Brandli M, Scheffler K (1997) MR angiography of thoracic blood vessels. Radiologe 37:529-538

Bongartz GM, Boos M, Winter K, Ott H, Scheffler K, Steinbrich W (1997) Clinical utility of contrast-enhanced MR angiography. Eur Radiol 7 [Suppl 5]:178-186

Carpenter JP, Holland GA, Golden MA, Barker CF, Lexa FJ, Gilfeather M, Schnall MD (1997) Magnetic resonance angiography of the aortic arch. Vasc Surg 25:145-151

Cherington M, Wilbourn AJ, Schils J, Whitaker J (1995) Thoracic outlet syndromes and MRI. Brain118:819-821

Chung JW, Park JH, Kim HC, Han MC (1994) Entry tears of thoracic aortic dissections: MR appearance on gated SE imaging. J Comput Assist Tomogr 18:250-255

Davies RH (1998) Imaging the thoracic aorta in the injured patient. Heart 79:631

Den Boer JA, Rozeboom AR (1996) Artifact in SE phase images can mimic aortic dissection. J Magn Reson Imaging 6:964-965

Dowd SB, Wilson BG, Hall JD, Steves A, Benson T (1996)

Review of techniques used to image aortic dissection. Radiol Technol 67:223–230; quiz 231–232
Dymarkowski S, Bosmans H, Marchal G, Bogaert J (1999) Three-dimensional MR angiography in the evaluation of thoracic outlet syndrome AJR Am J Roentgenol 173:1005–1008
Earls JP, DeSena S, Bluemke DA (1998) Gadolinium-enhanced three-dimensional MR angiography of the entire aorta and iliac arteries with dynamic manual table translation. Radiology 209:844–849
Esposito MD, Arrington JA, Blackshear MN, Murtagh FR, Silbiger ML (1997) Thoracic outlet syndrome in a throwing athlete diagnosed with MRI and MRA. J Magn Reson Imaging 7:598–599
Flamm SD, White RD, Hoffman GS (1998) The clinical application of 'edema-weighted' magnetic resonance imaging in the assessment of Takayasu's arteritis. Int J Cardiol 66 [Suppl 1]:S151–159; discussion S161
Frayne R, Rutt BK (1995) Understanding acceleration-induced displacement artifacts in phase-contrast MR velocity measurements. J Magn Reson Imaging 5:207–215
Godart F, Beregi JP, Rey C, Louvegny S, Desmoucelles F, Nicol L, Vaksmann G, Breviere GM, Francart C (1998) Does NMR provide information complementary to cardiac catheterization in aortic coarctation? Arch Mal Coeur Vaiss 91:587–592
Hangiandreou NJ, Rossman PJ, Riederer SJ (1993) Analysis of MR phase-contrast measurements of pulsatile velocity waveforms. J Magn Reson Imaging 3:387–394
Hartnell GG (1995) MR imaging in the diagnosis of aortic dissection. Radiology 197:314–315
Hartnell GG (1997) Disease of the supraaortic branches: spiral CT versus MR imaging. Radiology 202:285
Hartnell GG, Meier RA (1995) MR angiography of congenital heart disease in adults. Radiographics 15:781–794
Hartnell GG, Cohen MC, Meier RA, Finn JP (1996) Magnetic resonance angiography demonstration of congenital heart disease in adults. Clin Radiol 51:851–857
Hata A, Numano F (1995) Magnetic resonance imaging of vascular changes in Takayasu arteritis. Int J Cardiol 52:45–52
Hekali P, Velt P, Gutierrez O, Tottemann S, Mare K (1996) Radiology of aortic dissection: pitfalls in diagnosis. Eur J Radiol 6:314–318
Henk CB, Schlechta B, Grampp S, Gomischek G, Klepetko W, Mostbeck GH (1998) Pulmonary and aortic blood flow measurements in normal subjects and patients after single lung transplantation at 0.5 T using velocity encoded cine MRI. Chest 114:771–779
Ho VB, Prince MR (1998) Thoracic MR aortography: imaging techniques and strategies. Radiographics 18:287–309
Hubbard AM, Fellows KE, Weinberg PM, Fogel MA (1998) Preoperative and postoperative MRI of congenital heart disease. Semin Roentgenol 33:218–227
Hughes JP, Ruttley MS, Musumeci F (1994) Case report: traumatic aortic rupture: demonstration by magnetic resonance imaging. Br J Radiol 67:1264–1267
Kenn W (1998) Cardiac anatomy, mass and function-great vessels. MAGMA 6:88–90
Kersting-Sommerhoff BA, Higgins CB, White RD, Sommerhoff CP, Lipton MJ (1988) Aortic dissection: sensitivity and specificity of MR imaging. Radiology 166:651–655
Kessler W, Achenbach S, Moshage W, Zink D, Kroeker R, Nitz W, Laub G, Bachmann K (1997) Usefulness of respiratory gated magnetic resonance coronary angiography in assessing narrowings >or = 50% in diameter in native coronary arteries and in aortocoronary bypass conduits. Am J Cardiol 80:989–993
Kondo C, Caputo GR, Semelka R, Foster E, Shimakawa A, Higging CB (1991) Right and left ventricular stroke volume measurements with velocity-encoded cine MR imaging : in vitro and in vivo validation. AJR Am J Roentgenol 157:9–16
Korosec FR, Frayne R, Grist TM, Mistretta CA (1996) Time-resolved contrast-enhanced 3D MR angiography. Magn Reson Med 36:345–351
Krinsky G, Rofsky NM (1998) MR angiography of the aortic arch vessels and upper extremities. Magn Reson Imaging Clin N Am 6:269–292
Krinsky GA, Kaminer E, Lee VS, Rofsky NM, Weinreb JC (1998) The effects of apnea on timing examinations for optimization of gadolinium-enhanced MRA of the thoracic aorta and arch vessels. J Comput Assist Tomogr 22:677–681
Laissy JP, Blanc F, Soyer P, Assayag P, Sibert A, Tebboune D, Arrive L, Brochet E, Hvass U, Langlois J, et al (1995) Thoracic aortic dissection: diagnosis with transesophageal echocardiography versus MR imaging. Radiology 194:331–336
Latta P, Jellus V, Budinsky L, Mlynarik V, Tkac I, Luypaert R (1998) Motion artifacts reduction in DWI using navigator echoes: a robust and simple correction scheme. MAGMA 7:21–27
Leung DA, Debatin JF (1997) Three-dimensional contrast-enhanced magnetic resonance angiography of the thoracic vasculature. Eur Radiol 7:981–989
Link KM, Loehr SP, Baker DM, Lesko NM (1993) Magnetic resonance imaging of the thoracic aorta. Semin Ultrasound CT MR 14:91–105
Marchal G, Bogaert J (1998) Non-invasive imaging of the great vessels of the chest. Eur Radiol 8:1099–1105
Meaney JF, Weg JG, Chenevert TL, Stafford-Johnson D, Hamilton BH, Prince MR (1997) Diagnosis of pulmonary embolism with magnetic resonance angiography. N Engl J Med 336:1422–1427
Mistretta CA, Grist TM, Korosec FR, Frayne R, Peters DC, Mazaheri Y, Carrol TJ (1998) 3D time-resolved contrast-enhanced MR DSA: advantages and tradeoffs. Magn Reson Med 40:571–581
Murray JG, Manisali M, Flamm SD, VanDyke CW, Lieber ML, Lytle BW, White RD (1997) Intramural hematoma of the thoracic aorta: MR image findings and their prognostic implications. Radiology 204:349–355
Peeters F, Luypaert R, Eisendrath H, Osteaux M (1995) Time resolved flow quantification with MRI using phase methods: a linear systems approach. Magn Reson Med 33:337–354
Phadke K, Dyet JF, Aber CP, Hartley W (1993) Balloon angioplasty of adult aortic coarctation. Br Heart J 69:36–40
Rammohan M, Milind U, Karuna T, Kumar AS (1998) Management of annuloaortic ectasia in association with aortic regurgitation. Tex Heart Inst J 25:68–71
Revel D, Loubeyre P, Delignette A, Douek P, Amiel M (1993) Contrast-enhanced magnetic resonance tomoangiography: a new imaging technique for studying thoracic great vessels. Magn Reson Imaging 11:1101–1105
Riquelme C, Laissy JP, Menegazzo D, Debray MP, Cinqualbre A, Langlois J, Schouman-Claeys E (1999) MR imaging of

coarctation of the aorta and its postoperative complications in adults: assessment with spin-echo and cine-MR imaging. Magn Reson Imaging 17:37–46

Robbins RC, McManus RP, Mitchell RS, Latter DR, Moon MR, Olinger GN, Miller DC (1993) Management of patients with intramural hematoma of the thoracic aorta. Circulation 88:1–10

Roche KJ, Krinsky G, Lee VS, Rofsky N, Genieser NB (1999) Interrupted aortic arch: diagnosis with gadolinium-enhanced 3D MRA. J Comput Assist Tomogr 23:197–202

Ruhm SG, Debatin JF (1999) Contrast-enhanced 3D MR-angiography of the thorax, abdomen and lower extremities. Radiologe 39:100–109

Sarasin FP, Louis-Simonet M, Gaspoz JM, Junod AF (1996) Detecting acute thoracic aortic dissection in the emergency department: time constraints and choice of the optimal diagnostic test. Ann Emerg Med 28:278–288

Sechtem U, Pflugfelder P, Higgins CB (1987) Quantification of cardiac function by conventional and cine magnetic resonance imaging. Cardiovasc Intervent Radiol 10:365–373

Seelos KC, von Smekal A, Steinborn M, Gieseke J, Kaas P, Urban J, Redel DA, Reiser M (1994) MR angiography of the heart and thoracic blood vessels. Use of rapid ECG-triggered techniques with multiplanar reconstruction capability. Radiologe 34:454–461

Siblini G, Rao PS, Nouri S, Ferdman B, Jureidini SB, Wilson AD (1998) Long-term follow-up results of balloon angioplasty of postoperative aortic recoarctation. Am J Cardiol 81:61–67

Simpson IA, Chung KJ, Glass RF, Sahn DJ, Sherman FS, Hesselink J (1988) Cine magnetic resonance imaging for evaluation of anatomy and flow relations in infants and children with coarctation of the aorta. Circulation 78:142–148

Soler R, Rodriguez E, Requejo I, Fernandez R, Raposo I (1998) Magnetic resonance imaging of congenital abnormalities of the thoracic aorta. Eur Radiol 8:540–546

Taneja K, Kawlra S, Sharma S, Rajani M (1998) Pseudocoarctation of the aorta: complementary findings on plain film radiography, CT, DSA, and MRA. Cardiovasc Intervent Radiol 21:439–441

Taylor AM, Jhooti P, Wiesmann F, Keegan J, Firmin DN, Pennell DJ (1997) MR navigator-echo monitoring of temporal changes in diaphragm position: implications for MR coronary angiography. J Magn Reson Imaging 7:629–636

Taylor AM, Jhooti P, Firmin DN, Pennell DJ (1999) Automated monitoring of diaphragm end-expiratory position for real-time navigator echo MR coronary angiography. J Magn Reson Imaging 9:395–401

Tomiguchi S, Morishita S, Nakashima R, Hara M, Oyama Y, Kojima A, Takahashi M (1994) Usefulness of turbo-FLASH dynamic MR imaging of dissecting aneurysms of the thoracic aorta. Cardiovasc Intervent Radiol 17:17–21

Van Hoe L, De Jaegere T, Bosmans H, Bogaert J, Oyen R, Marchal G (1999) Time-resolved MR angiography of the upper abdomen: initial clinical experience. Eur Radiol 9:418–421

Veyssier-Belot C, Cohen A, Rougemont D, Levy C, Amarenco P, Bousser MG (1993) Cerebral infarction due to painless thoracic aortic and common carotid artery dissections. Stroke 24:2111–2113

Vinstein AL (1990) Neonatal radiology casebook. Double aortic arch. J Perinatol 10:209–210

Wang Y, Weber DM, Korosec FR, Mistretta CA, Grist TM, Swan JS, Turski PA (1993) Generalized matched filtering for time-resolved MR angiography of pulsatile flow. Magn Reson Med 30:600–608

White RD, Obuchowski NA, VanDyke CW, Tkach JA, Geisinger MA, Link KM, Ruggieri PM, Dillinger JJ, Lytle BW (1994) Thoracic aortic disease: evaluation using a single MRA volume series. J Comput Assist Tomogr 18:843–854

Wimpfheimer O, Boxt LM (1999) MR imaging of adult patients with congenital heart disease. Radiol Clin North Am 37:421–438

16 The Coronary Arteries

André J. Duerinckx

CONTENTS

16.1 Introduction

Magnetic resonance angiography (MRA) of the coronary arteries became possible in 1991 with the development of a new group of fast MR imaging sequences (Duerinckx 1995, 1996, 1997, 1999, 2001a, b; Wielopolski et al. 1998, 2000; Woodard et al. 1999; Danias et al. 1998; Manning and Edelman 1993). Coronary MRA has since been used with great success in key clinical applications, such as the detection of coronary artery variants and the imaging of coronary stents and bypass grafts. The new magnetic resonance imaging (MRI) techniques also allow quantification of velocity and flow in coronary arteries. Most promising is the potential role of coronary MR angiography in screening for coronary artery lesions, which is actively being investigated.

Coronary artery disease remains the leading cause of death in the United States and is responsible for an estimated 900,000 deaths per year. The estimated cost of these deaths and the additional 1.5 million heart attacks annually exceeds $60 billion in the United States alone (American Heart Association 1996). X-ray contrast angiography is widely accepted as the definitive method to define coronary anatomy. However, given that currently more than 1 million diagnostic cardiac catheterizations are performed annually in the USA (Johnson et al. 1989) and the relative high procedural cost of $3000 to $5000, any less-expensive noninvasive alternative test would be welcome. Coronary MRA offers the potential to replace diagnostic and screening X-ray coronary angiography in the near future in selected population groups. The impact of cardiac MRI on the global cost of healthcare and the use of diagnostic tests for myocardial ischemia will be enormous. This review introduces the novice to these new cardiac MRI technologies and their proven and future applications. More advanced readers will find extensive discussions of the research and preclinical work done by many investigators since 1991.

16.1.1 What Is Coronary MRA?

Unlike other blood vessels, coronary arteries are small tortuous vessels subjected to significant physiological motion, both cardiac and respiratory, which present a tremendous challenge to conventional MRI

A.J. Duerinckx, MD, PhD (e-mail: andrejd@earthlink.net)
VA North Texas Healthcare System, 4500 South Lancaster Road, Dallas, Texas 75216, USA

and MRA techniques. With the development in 1991 of a new group of fast MRI pulse sequences "reliable and reproducible" MRA of the coronary arteries has become possible and was described in the first preclinical studies published in 1993 and 1994 (Manning et al. 1993a, b; Duerinckx and Urman 1994a). The term "reliable" means simply that images of good quality can routinely and reproducibly be obtained in the majority of patients. Prior to the development of these newer techniques coronary artery MRI was possible, but was much less reliable and not considered a clinical application of cardiac MRI.

Several generations of coronary MRA techniques have since been described (see Table 16.1). All techniques use ECG triggering. First-generation breath-hold techniques, as described in 1991, acquire one two-dimensional (2D) image per breath-hold and are commercially available on almost all new MRI scanners. They are robust and have been successfully used for specific clinical applications. All imagers should become familiar with their use.

Table 16.1. Coronary MR Angiography technique classification, as proposed by Duerinckx (2001) (Modified from: Duerinckx AJ (1999) (Clinics) Coronary magnetic resonance angiography. Radiol Clin North Am 37:273–318, with permission)

Coronary MR angiography techniques Generation	Principle	Pros and cons
First	One slice per breath-hold	2D; spatial registration problems; available on all commercial scanners
Second	Free-breathing	3D and high resolution; but long acquisition times (up to 15 min)
Third	3-D volume in a single breath-hold	3D and low spatial resolution; short acquisition times

The second generation techniques use navigator pulses for respiratory gating or triggering and are referred to as "non-breath-holding" or "free-breathing" techniques, as they do not require breath-holding. Although the initial implementations were somewhat unreliable, dramatic improvements have since been made. Third generation techniques allow three-dimensional (3D) volume acquisitions (multiple 2D images) in a single breath-hold, which in combination with real-time interactive slice positioning, appears very promising. MR contrast agents, real-time slice positioning, and higher-resolution acquisition schemes, such as spiral MRA, can further improve and facilitate the use of these coronary MRA techniques.

Technical progress and changes in this subfield of cardiac MRI have been so rapid that large-scale preclinical trials have not been (and probably never will be) conducted with the majority of the first and second generation coronary MRA pulse sequences as known today. In this chapter we review the development of these new cardiac MRI techniques and the initial successes with clinical applications using commercial MR scanners.

16.1.2 Clinical Indications for Coronary MRA

Coronary MRA is a cardiac MRI technique used to visualize the proximal and middle portion of most coronary arteries and some coronary artery branches. The techniques and practice of coronary MRA can easily be learned. Even though it is not equivalent to conventional X-ray-based coronary angiography, coronary MRA can and should be used for noninvasive imaging in a variety of clinical situations. We will discuss the evaluation of congenital coronary artery anomalies and the noninvasive determination of the patency of bypass grafts and coronary stents. Coronary MRA can also be used in the follow-up of known proximal coronary lesions, such as after angioplasty. However, the use of coronary MRA for blind prospective detection of unknown coronary lesions is still being evaluated. Coronary MRA techniques may become an integral part of the clinical evaluation and screening of patients with ischemic heart disease. Coronary MRI techniques appear very promising in the quantification of coronary flow and flow reserve.

16.2 Coronary MRA Techniques

Conventional cardiac-triggered MRI has provided reliable, clinically useful, diagnostic images of cardiac structures and large vessels within the thorax for many years (Higgins et al. 1990; Higgins 1992; Blackwell et al. 1992; Duerinckx et al. 1994; Bogaert et al. 1999). With conventional cardiac MRI it has been possible to visualize coronary bypass grafts, evaluate bypass graft patency, and quantitate flow in bypass grafts. Bypass grafts in general are easier to image than native coronary vessels because they are larger in size and because they are usually located further away from the heart and therefore undergo less cardiac motion. It is well known that traditional cardiac-triggered spin echo (SE) and gradient recalled echo (GRE) images can occasionally show small portions of the native coronary artery tree (LIEBERMAN et al. 1984; PAULIN et al. 1987; CASSIDY et al. 1989) and they have been used to visualize congenital coronary artery variants (BISSET et al. 1989; DOOREY et al. 1994). However, these techniques have significant limitations: motion artifacts and pulsatile flow artifacts preclude visualization of all except the very proximal or abnormally dilated vessel anatomy; it is difficult to distinguish between coronary arteries and veins; and the pericardial space can easily be mistaken for portions of a vessel or bypass graft. In contrast to this, the new coronary MRA techniques allow much more reliable and consistent visualization of the proximal native coronary tree (DUERINCKX 1995, 1996, 1999; WIELOPOLSKI et al. 2000; MANNING and EDELMAN 1993; PENNELL et al. 1993; BOGAERT et al. 1994).

Conventional MRA techniques depict and characterize blood vessels and blood flow and are relatively well established in clinical practice (ARLART et al. 1996; ANDERSON et al. 1993; POTCHEN et al. 1995; ATKINSON and TERESI 1995; BRANT-ZAWADZKI et al. 1993; PRINCE et al. 1999). However, when it comes to imaging small tortuous vessels in the chest or abdomen or even any large vessel in the thorax, none of the traditional MRA techniques (such as time-of-flight, TOF, and phase contrast, PC) have been able to perform consistently or adequately. The newer contrast-enhanced 3D MRA techniques now reliably image not only the abdomen and periphery, but also the chest. MRA of pulmonary arteries, the aortic arch, and even coronary bypass grafts using these new CE 3D MRA techniques is performed in daily clinical practice at many centers. However, these newest MRA techniques are not routinely cardiac-gated and are thus inadequate for imaging of native coronary vessels or the distant anastomoses of coronary bypass grafts.

16.2.1 History of Coronary MRA Pulse Sequences

Advances in MR pulse sequence design (with the first described cardiac applications in 1991) have resulted in a significant reduction in both respiratory motion artifacts (by eliminating, correcting, or compensating for respiratory motion) and pulsatile flow artifacts (by always using cardiac triggering and mid-diastolic acquisitions), while maintaining a reasonably short image acquisition time (by segmenting the data acquisition in k-space) (PEARLMAN and EDELMAN 1994; LAUZON and RUTT 1993; MEZRICH 1995). Coronary MRA does significantly differ from conventional MRA in that it incorporates mechanisms to compensate for both cardiac and respiratory motion. Even though some of the techniques are variants of 2-D MRI sequences, and not really MRA techniques, we will always refer to these MR techniques as "coronary MRA," because they are used to visualize coronary vessels. Most of the new coronary MRA techniques can also be applied to image larger thoracic vessels (HARTNELL et al. 1994; HERNANDEZ et al. 1993) and improved cardiac imaging in general (BOGAERT et al. 1999; BLUEMKE et al. 1997a, b). Knowledge of coronary MR imaging is relevant to any imager (radiologist, cardiologist, or other physicians) interested in improving the quality of vascular imaging using MRI or MRA.

The new MRI sequences which allow reliable and reproducible MRA of the coronary arteries can be classified in many ways. In this review we opted for a classification based partially on historical developments, but also on the amount of information obtained (single 2D images versus 3D slabs) for a given level of patient comfort (breath-holding versus non-breath-holding) and the total duration of the data acquisition. The first generation of coronary MRA techniques was first described in 1991 and are now commercially available on most clinical MRI scanners. These techniques rely upon a combination of segmental acquisition in k-space of the data to minimize cardiac motion and the use of a single breath-hold to minimize respiratory motion artifacts. They require sequential single breath-holds, with a total examination time from 30 to 60 min. The typical coronary MRI quality obtained is illustrated in Figs. 16.1 and 16.2. A second generation of techniques described in 1993–1994 allows image acquisition during repeated breath-holding or during "free breathing" and opens the way for higher resolution coronary MRA with increased patient comfort. These techniques are referred to as the "navigator" techniques and are based on concepts developed for abdominal imaging many years ago. They are still undergoing extensive fine-tuning. They typically require 5–12 min per 3D slab acquisition, with three slabs being adequate to cover most of the heart. The coronary MR image quality that can be obtained is illustrated in Fig. 16.3. Improvements to these tech-

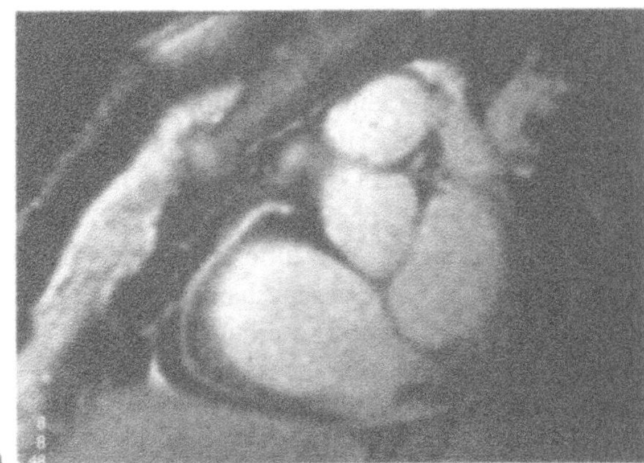

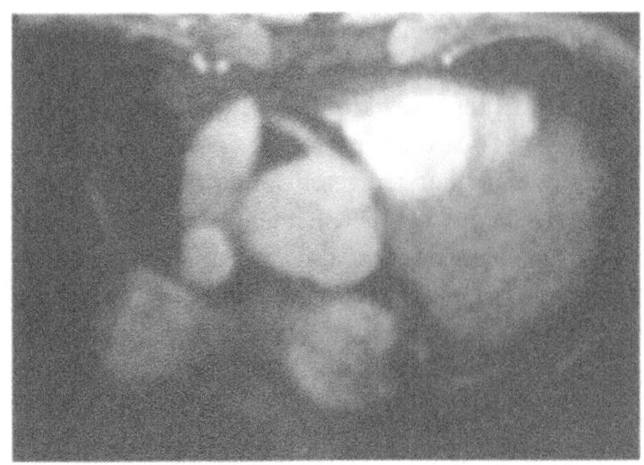

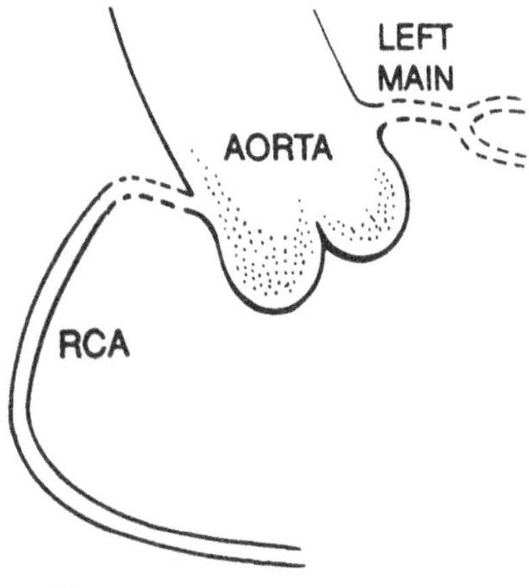

Fig. 16.1a–c. The right coronary artery (RCA) imaged with a first generation coronary MR angiographic technique. Each image was obtained within a breath-hold. The RCA lies in the anterior atrioventricular groove. A large portion of the RCA can usually be visualized with a single imaging plane through the anterior atrioventricular groove (**a**). Often one additional transaxial plane is needed to clearly show the ostium of the RCA (**b**). A schematic drawing of the typical appearance of the RCA on coronary MR angiograms is shown (**c**). **a** The proximal and middle RCA are shown; the distal RCA is slightly out-of-plane and better seen in an image obtained in a parallel imaging plane. The origin of the RCA is out-of-plane. **b** Origin of the RCA best seen on oblique transaxial plane. **c** Schematic drawing of a typical appearance of the proximal and mid-RCA on coronary angiograms. The origin is shown in *dashed (thin) lines* to emphasize the point that often the origin is better seen in an additional plane. Also shown are: the pericardial sac. (Fig. 1 a, c from: Duerinckx AJ (1995) MR angiography of the coronary arteries. Top Magn Reson Imaging 7:267–285; with permission) (Fig. 1b from: Duerinckx AJ (1996) Coronary MR angiography. Magn Reson Imaging Clin North Am 4:361–418, with permission)

niques have made them into very robust and clinically useful techniques which are now available on several commercial scanners (Stuber et al. 1999a, b). Exciting and promising third generation techniques have been under development since 1995. The combination of second and third generation techniques provides the ultimate compromise between user-friendliness, high spatial resolution, and acquisition speeds. The best approach may indeed be to use both techniques at all times, as needed. They require one or several breath-holds for a full survey of the heart and coronary vessels. The coronary MRI quality that can be obtained is illustrated in Fig. 16.4. The combination of MR contrast agents (and in the near future also MR blood pool agents) with any of these coronary MRA techniques seems very promising, according to initial results in animals (Johansson et al. 1999; Li et al. 1998a; Sakuma et al. 1999; Taylor et al. 1999; Zheng et al. 2000a) and in humans (Li et al. 1998b; Lorenz and Johansson 1999). The use of new MR blood pool contrast agents may open up a whole new world for coronary MRA, similar to what happened after Martin Prince introduced the concept of contrast-enhanced 3D MRA for body, peripheral, and chest MRA applications.

Because only the first and second generation coronary MRA techniques are now universally available on most commercial MRI equipment, the bulk of the published preclinical literature on this topic has been limited to these techniques. We refer the reader to more detailed reviews of the coronary MRA techniques (Duerinckx 1995, 1996, 1997, 1999; Wielopolski et al. 1998; Danias et al. 1998; Manning and Edelman 1993; Pennell et al. 1993; Bogaert et al. 1994; Duerinckx and Lipton 1998). Other technical developments such as SMASH (Sodickson and Manning 1997; Sodickson et al. 1999), SENSE (Pruessmann et al. 1999; Weiger et al. 1999), segmented echo planar MR, the use of True FISP (Deshpande et al. 2000; Chung et al. 2000; Duerk et al. 1998; Wendt et al. 1999), spiral imaging (Taylor et al. 2000a), keyhole imaging, and hybrid techniques (Foo et al. 2000) are all very promising, but beyond the scope of this clinically oriented review. Prone

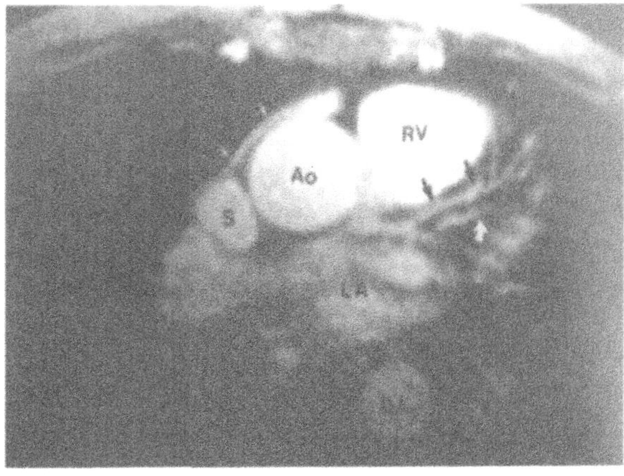

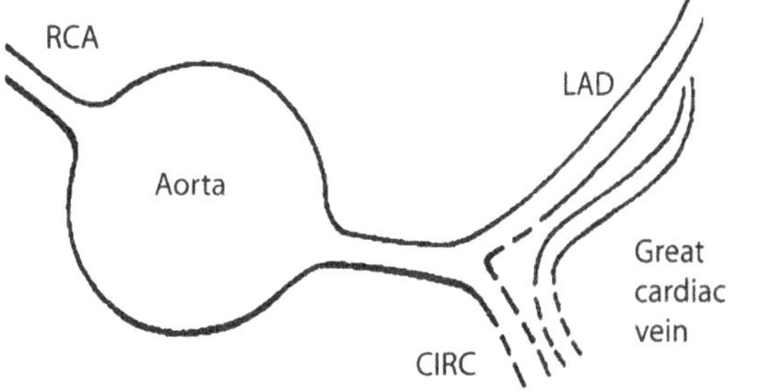

Fig. 16.2a, b. Left coronary artery system imaged with a first generation coronary MRA technique. The left coronary artery system is relatively complex and requires multiple imaging planes to visualize its proximal course. **a** Oblique transaxial plane showing the proximal and middle left anterior descending coronary artery (LAD; *arrows*) and the great cardiac vein (*curved arrows*). **b** Schematic drawing of a typical appearance of the left main, LAD, proximal circumflex and great cardiac vein on oblique transaxial planes. The origin of the LAD and circumflex are shown in *dashed (thin) lines* to emphasize the point that often these origins are better seen in another plane. Also shown are: the pericardial sac (*thin arrows*). (*Ao*, ascending aorta; *RV*, right ventricle; *LV*, left ventricle; *LA*, left atrium; *DA*, descending aorta; S, superior vena cava) (From: Duerinckx AJ (1995) MR angiography of the coronary arteries. Top Magn Reson Imaging 7:267–285, with permission)

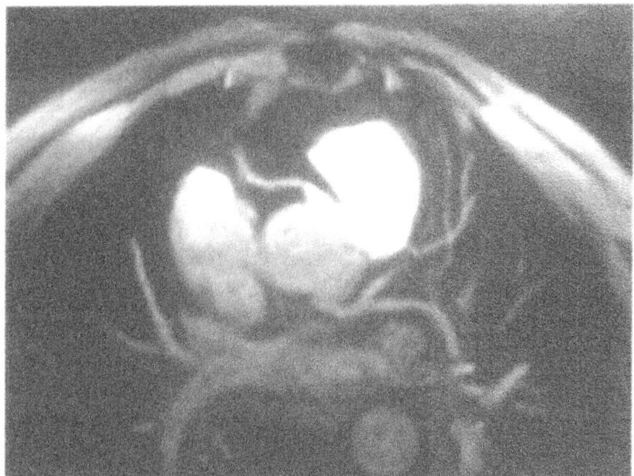

Fig. 16.3. Proximal right and left coronary arteries imaged with an early version of a second generation coronary MR angiographic technique and intensive postprocessing of the data. and A maximum intensity projection (MIP) of a 3D coronary MR angiogram acquired in a patient without breath-holding but with retrospective respiratory gating. A maximum intensity projection (MIP) image derived from a 3D MR angiographic data set with 16 partitions, $1.2\times2\times2$ mm^3 resolution and five averages. Overlapping blood pool signal was removed prior to the MIP reconstruction. An edge-preserving filter was applied to improve the signal-to-noise ratio. Note the excellent delineation of the RCA, circumflex, and a 50%–75% stenosis of the proximal LAD. (From: Haacke EM, Li D, et al (1995) Cardiac MR imaging: principles and techniques. Top Magn Reson Imaging 7:200–217, with permission)

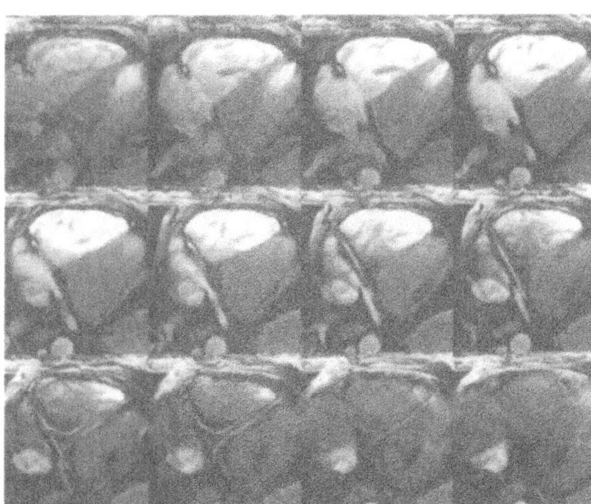

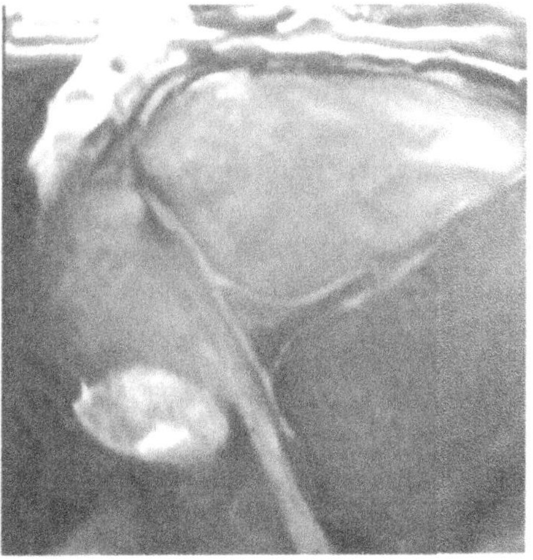

Fig. 16.4a, b. Distal right coronary artery (RCA) and posterior descending artery (PDA) imaged with a third generation technique. **a** The center nine sections (from the 16 reconstructed for VCATS) are displayed. **b** Volume rendering integrates the entire course of the distal RCA. Acquisition parameters: 16 1.5-mm-thick sections were reconstructed for VCATS by using 21 heartbeats, a 126×256 matrix with partial Fourier encoding, and a FOV of 240×320 mm. (From: Wielopolski, et al (1998) Breath-hold coronary MRA with volume-targeted imaging. Radiology 209:209–219, with permission)

imaging, used almost exclusively in the early days of first generation techniques, is being reevaluated again (Ms et al. 2001).

16.2.2 Other Techniques for Noninvasive Imaging of the Coronary Arteries

Many imaging tools exist to directly evaluate the coronary artery anatomy: electron-beam computed tomography (EB-CT), multi-slice helical CT, coronary MRA, echocardiography (both transthoracic and transesophageal), intravascular ultrasound, and invasive X-ray coronary angiography, today's gold standard. EB-CT, multi-slice CT, and MRI appear to be very close competitors for the same market. However, unlike CT, coronary MRA does not require iodinated contrast agents or X-ray radiation and has the potential to become a more widespread and easy to use cardiac screening tool. Since the year 2000, cardiac-gated multi-slice CT has emerged as a very serious competitor for both EB-CT and MRI/MRA-based coronary imaging (Van Geuns et al. 2000a; Ohnesorge et al. 2000).

16.2.3 How To Perform Coronary MRA

It is extremely important that all cardiac imagers (radiologists, cardiologists, and others) keep up with the latest advances in this subfield of cardiac MRI so that we can offer these new cardiac MRI studies to our patients. In order to do this, however, we need to be knowledgeable about the coronary MRA sequences available today on commercial MRI scanners. Radiologists need to be prepared to work with cardiologists when using these new cardiac MRI applications, and vice versa. The two groups need each other to fully utilize the potential of cardiac MRI and make this available to patients. The coronary MRA techniques that have been developed and tested in preclinical trials are well described (Duerinckx 2001a). The imager who is not yet a specialist in cardiac MR imaging and coronary MRA should focus on those MR techniques which seem most likely to provide good results in the hands of the majority of users. Very promising future developments such as a combination of second and third generation approaches to coronary MRA and the use of MR blood pool contrast agents have also been described.

There are differences from country to country and from continent to continent as to what are realistic clinical applications of and expectations for coronary MRA. In the November 1999 special issue on Cardiovascular MRI of the *Journal of Magnetic Resonance Imaging*, clinical experience with coronary MRA in Japan, the US, and Europe were described (Nitatori et al. 1999; Danias et al. 1999; Bunce and Pennell 1999). In general, the future of coronary MRA appears very promising (Duerinckx 1999; Wielopolski et al. 2000; Polak 2000).

We refer the readers to the specialized literature, conference proceedings, and web sites for further information on these topics beyond February 2001. Specifically, there is a textbook (Duerinckx 2001a) and the program, abstracts, and proceedings of the First International Workshop on Coronary MR and CT angiography, held 1–3 October 2000, in Lyon, France, and organized by the North American Society for Cardiac Imaging (NASCI), provide added information (Duerinckx 2000). More recent information can be found in the Proceedings and Abstracts of the Second International Workshop on Coronary MR and CT Angiography, 1–2 October 2001, in Chicago, Ill. (Duerinckx 2001c). Other good sources of additional information are the North American Society for Cardiovascular Imaging (NASCI) (www.nasci.org), the Society for Cardiovascular Magnetic Resonance (www.scmr.org) and the International Society for Magnetic Resonance in Medicine (www.ismrm.org). Other web sites provide direct links to information on cardiac MRI in general (www.cardiac-mri.com) and coronary MRA specifically (for example: www.bidmc.harvard.edu/cmr/cmr-network.html and www.nasci.org). Results of multicenter industry-sponsored trials to test new coronary MRA techniques and contrast agents are underway and will undoubtedly further increase our confidence in coronary MRA.

16.3 Clinical Applications of Coronary MRA Today

Most of the clinical applications of coronary MRA have been validated using first generation techniques with breath-holding. For a clinician thinking about ordering a coronary MR angiogram, it is important to know when such a study can add value to the patient work up and what the confidence level is for obtaining a definitive clinical diagnosis and answer.

It is equally important to know when coronary MRA is the only modality that can provide the answer, such as in certain cases of congenital coronary anatomy. This chapter provides a brief review of the existing literature of proven clinical applications of coronary MRA. We will point out along the way which applications are easy to perform, which are more difficult, and which are still somewhat experimental.

Clinical applications of 2D coronary MRA include: coronary lesion detection (MANNING et al. 1993a; DUERINCKX and URMAN 1994a; POST et al. 1996, 1997; HUNDLEY et al. 1995; PENNELL et al. 1996); the delineation of congenital coronary artery anomalies (VANCAMPEN et al. 1995; DUERINCKX et al. 1995a, 1997a, 1999a; MANNING et al. 1995; MCCONNELL et al. 1995; POST et al. 1995a); the characterization of previously known coronary lesions (PENNELL et al. 1996; BRIFFA et al. 1996); coronary bypass graft patency (BUSER and HIGGINS 1994; GALJEE et al. 1996; SCHMIDT et al. 1996; VRACHLIOTIS et al. 1997; WINTERSPERGER et al. 1997, 1998) and complications of coronary bypass surgery (DUERINCKX et al. 1996); vessel patency and evaluation after coronary stent placement (DUERINCKX et al. 1995b; DE COBELLI et al. 1997, 1998); coronary anatomy after heart transplantation (MOHIADDIN et al. 1996a; DAVIS et al. 1996); and coronary flow reserve quantification (CLARKE et al. 1995; SAKUMA et al. 1996a; HOFMAN et al. 1996; HUNDLEY et al. 1996).

16.3.1 Imaging Congenital Anomalies of the Coronary Arteries

Until a few years ago there were only isolated reports on the use of MRI to determine the origin or proximal course of an anomalous coronary artery. For example, DOOREY et al. (1994) reported on five patients with anomalous coronary artery. In all five patients, MRI definitively confirmed the courses of the anomalous left and right coronary arteries. This study was performed using T1-weighted SE sequences in multiple planes on the 1.5T GE signal scanner. No coronary MRA technique was used. More recently, several new case reports appeared which describe the use of coronary MRA to evaluate such anomalous vessels (VANCAMPEN et al. 1995; DUERINCKX et al. 1995; MANNING et al. 1995). Then, in the 1 December 1995 issue of *Circulation*, two major articles were published which established coronary MRA as the technique of choice for the delineation of the origin and proximal course of anomalous coronary arteries (MCCONNELL et al. 1995; POST et al. 1995a). Each one of these publications will be discussed in more detail later. Since then, the use of MRI and/or coronary MRA for the detection of coronary artery aneurysms or arteriovenous (AV) fistulas has also been well documented (BISSET et al. 1989; DUERINCKX et al. 1997, 1999a; DUERINCKX and TAKAHASHI 1996; HWANG et al. 1997). All of these studies are easy to perform. Most radiologists should be able to reproduce the results shown in the literature with the existing first generation coronary MRA techniques.

In the first 1995 article in *Circulation* by MCCONNELL et al. (1995) from the Cardiovascular Divisions, Beth Israel Hospital and Brigham and Women's Hospital, a total of 16 patients (nine men, seven women; age 44–81 years) with anomalous aortic origins of the coronary arteries according to conventional X-ray angiography were studied with coronary MRA. Multiple images of the major epicardial coronary arteries were obtained by use of a first generation breath-hold technique (a fat-suppressed, segmented k-space GE pulse sequence) in a blinded fashion by the investigators who were blinded to previous X-ray angiography data. The anomalous coronary pathology as determined by the X-ray coronary angiography included: right-sided left main coronary artery (n=3), right-sided left circumflex artery (n=6), separate left-sided left anterior descending and left circumflex arteries (n=2), left-sided right coronary artery (n=4), and an anteriorly displaced right coronary artery (n=1). Coronary MRA correctly identified the anomalous coronary vessels in 14 of 15 patients. In only one patient was the anomalous vessel incorrectly identified, and in two patients the course of the anomalous vessel was not clearly seen; one of these was a nondominant anomalous right coronary artery. The authors of this publication conclude that coronary MRA is a useful technique for the noninvasive identification of anomalous coronary arteries and their anatomic course.

In a second article POST et al. (1995a), from the Free University Hospital and the Institute for Cardiovascular Research of the Free University, Amsterdam/InterUniversity Cardiology Institute of the Netherlands, Utrecht, reported on a study of 38 patients, of which 19 had an anomalously originating coronary artery. The question specifically asked was: is coronary MRA of the anomalous coronary arteries the new gold standard for delineating the proximal course of these vessels? Both the origin and the proximal course of the coronary arteries were defined. After separate analysis of the MRI and conventional X-ray angiography studies, a final consensus result was defined for each patient. Coronary MRA was successfully performed in 37 or 38 patients. An X-ray coronary angiogram was available in 36 of the 38 patients. Sensitivity and specificity for detecting anomalous coronary arteries and delineating the proximal course in this second study were 100%. The data in this study suggest that coronary MRA is highly accurate in determining the origin and in delineating the proximal course of anomalous coronary arteries, even in those cases in which X-ray coronary angiographic diagnosis was difficult or even erroneous. In three patients, differences of opinion existed about the proximal course (but not the origin) of the anomalous artery. However, after a joint review of three cases, it was unanimously decided that MRA unambiguously delineated the proximal course of these anomalous arteries, whereas conventional X-ray angiography interpretation of this course had been erroneous or at least difficult.

16.3.2 Coronary MRA in Patients with Adult Congenital Heart Disease (Grown Up Congenital Heart Disease)

Taylor et al. described coronary artery imaging in grown up congenital heart disease and the complementary role of MRA and X-ray coronary angiography (Taylor et al. 2000b). There is a high incidence of anomalous coronary arteries in subjects with congenital heart disease. These abnormalities can be responsible for myocardial ischemia and sudden death or be damaged during surgical intervention. It can be difficult to define the proximal course of anomalous coronary arteries with the use of conventional X-ray coronary angiography. Magnetic resonance coronary angiography (MRCA) has been shown to be useful in the assessment of the 3D relationship between the coronary arteries and the great vessels in subjects with normal cardiac morphology but has not been used in patients with congenital heart disease. Taylor et al. studied 25 adults with various congenital heart abnormalities (Taylor et al. 2000b). X-ray coronary angiography and respiratory-gated MRCA were performed in all subjects. Coronary artery origin and proximal course were assessed for each imaging modality by separate, blinded investigators. Images were then compared, and a consensus diagnosis was reached. With the consensus readings for both magnetic resonance and X-ray coronary angiography, it was possible to identify the origin and course of the proximal coronary arteries in all 25 subjects: 16 with coronary anomalies and nine with normal coronary arteries. Respiratory-gated MRCA had an accuracy of 92%, a sensitivity of 88%, and a specificity of 100% for the detection of abnormal coronary arteries. The MRCA results were more likely to agree with the consensus for definition of the proximal course of the coronary arteries (p=0.02). Taylor et al. concluded that, for the assessment of anomalous coronary artery anatomy in patients with congenital heart disease, the use of the combination of MRCA with X-ray coronary angiography improves the definition of the proximal coronary artery course. MRCA provides correct spatial relationships, whereas X-ray angiography provides a view of the entire coronary length and its peripheral run-off. Furthermore, respiratory-gated MRCA can be performed without breath-holding and with only limited subject cooperation.

16.3.3 AV Fistulas and Other Congenital Variants

The use of MRI and coronary MRA for the detection of coronary artery aneurysms or AV fistulas has also been well documented (Bisset et al. 1989; Duerinckx et al. 1997a, 1999a, 2000; Duerinckx and Takahashi 1996, Hwang et al. 1997). Kawasaki disease, a generalized vasculitis of unknown etiology, is a leading cause of acquired heart disease in children in the US and has widespread cardiovascular involvement, including coronary arterial aneurysms (Chung and Stein 1998). Coronary aneurysms in patients with Kawasaki disease can easily be visualized by MR (Fig. 16.5). Coronary AV fistulas are malformations of the coronary circulation. Prior to surgical or interventional therapy, the anatomy of these complex vascular structures needs to be imaged. Coronary MRA offers a noninvasive imaging approach to these coronary anomalies. Sequential transaxial 2D breath-hold coronary MR angiograms can be obtained. 3D volume renderings can then be obtained from these 2D transaxial images. The 3D reconstructions visualize all abnormally enlarged coronary arteries and the proximal portions of the normal coronary artery anatomy in most cases. All of these applications of coronary MRA are easy to perform. Most radiologists should be able to reproduce the results with existing first generation coronary MRA techniques.

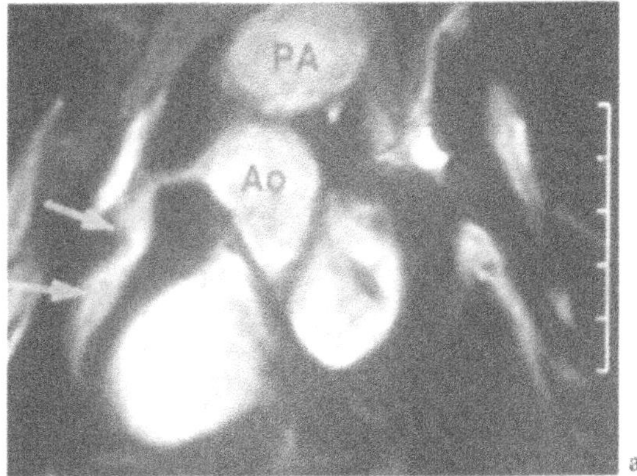

a

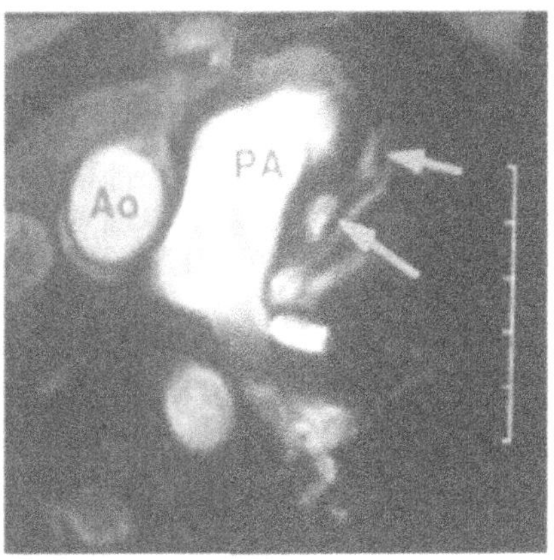

b

Fig. 16.5a, b. An 11-year-old boy with a 3-year history of clinically stable Kawasaki disease. **a** Coronary MR angiogram of right coronary artery (RCA) with the imaging plane in right atrioventricular groove reveals ostium and proximal RCA within normal limits. Note that the proximal RCA then widens into fusiform and segmented aneurysm. The more distal RCA, which is partially revealed, appears of normal caliber. (*Ao*, ascending aorta; *PA*, pulmonary artery). **b** Coronary MR angiograms in two oblique transaxial planes with slightly different angulation show normal left main coronary artery and proximal left anterior descending artery that has two smaller aneurysms. (*Ao*, ascending aorta; *PA*, pulmonary artery; *D*, descending aorta; *S*, superior vena cava). (Reproduced with permission from: Duerinckx AJ, et al (1997) Coronary MR angiography in Kawasaki disease. A case report. AJR Am J Roentgenol 168:114–116)

16.3.4 Imaging of Coronary Artery Bypass Grafts

Patients having one or more coronary artery bypass graft operations constitute an important part of the practice of cardiac radiology. Because coronary artery bypass grafts (CABG) are performed in a very large number of Americans annually, and follow-up studies have shown a rather significant number of postoperative occlusions, there is a great interest in providing imaging techniques for CABG occlusion. It has been shown that 10%–30% of grafts are occluded 1–2 years and 45%–55% are occluded 10–12 years after grafting. There are major differences in occlusion rates between the saphenous vein and internal mammary artery graft, with occlusion rates in the first postoperative year of 20% and 5%. To date, the gold standard for evaluating graft patency in CABG patients is still coronary angiography, an invasive and costly procedure that is not risk free. There are other direct methods such as ultrasound, CT, EB-CT, MRI and Doppler sonography. Indirect imaging methods include radionuclide ventriculopathy, Thallium-201 scintigraphy, and position imaging tomography.

Besides the gold standard of X-ray-based coronary angiography, the other direct imaging modalities such as transthoracic echocardiography, Doppler sonography, and CT have some limitations. The great disadvantage of transthoracic echocardiography is that it requires considerable expertise and it is difficult to differentiate the graft flow signal from that generated by the aorta and pulmonary arteries. The technique is also less applicable for circumflex grafts that are located more posteriorly. Published sensitivities and specificities for the technique run from 83% to 92% and 56% to 100%, respectively (Stanford et al. 1991). Conventional and ultrafast CT offer another alternative. Ultrafast CT has shown considerable promise in imaging bypass graft. A multicenter study by Stanford et al. (1988) has shown a sensitivity of 93% for detecting angiographically patent grafts and a specificity of 89% for determining angiographically closed grafts. The overall accuracy was 92%. The number of technically adequate studies was more than 94%. Many other published studies have reported results from the use of ultrafast CT for determining CABG patency (Stanford et al. 1991). An example of CABG imaged with ultrafast CT is shown in Fig. 16.6.

MRI offers an important alternative approach to imaging of CABG. Bypass grafts are relatively stationary when compared to native coronary arteries. This explains why cardiac-gated spin-echo (dark blood) and GRE (bright blood) MRI techniques to evaluate graft patency have shown relatively good success rates. It also explains the relative success of the other noninvasive imaging techniques. Figure 16.7 shows the typical locations of saphenous vein bypass grafts. The more proximal portions of the grafts are subjected to less cardiac motion than the distal anastomosis to the native vessels. In the early days, the MRI technique focused on determining graft patency by

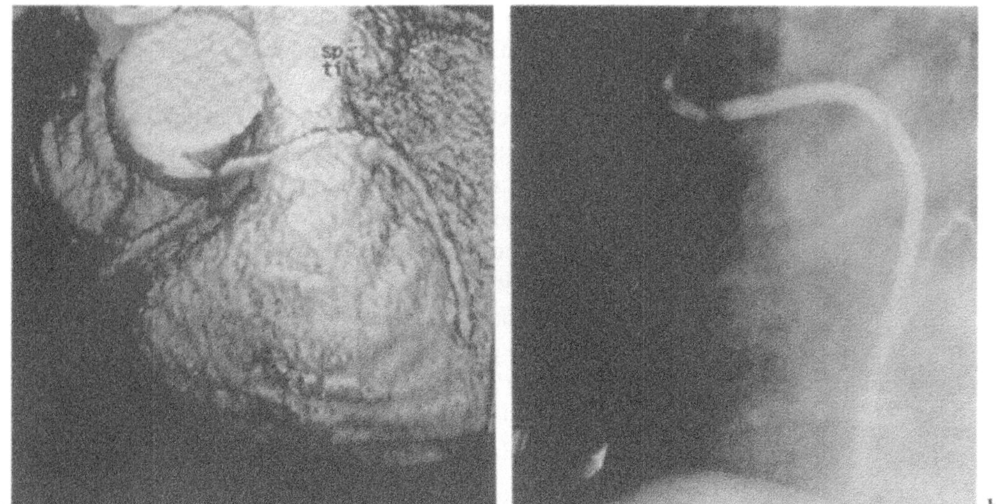

Fig. 16.6. Coronary artery bypass graft is imaged with electron-beam CT (EB-CT). A (*left*). Volume-rendered EB-CT angiogram of a bypass graft to the LAD. 1. (*right*) Corresponding selective coronary X-ray angiogram. (From: Achenbach S, et al (1998) Non-invasive coronary angiography by contrast-enhanced electron-beam computer tomography. Clin Cardiol 21:323–330, with permission)

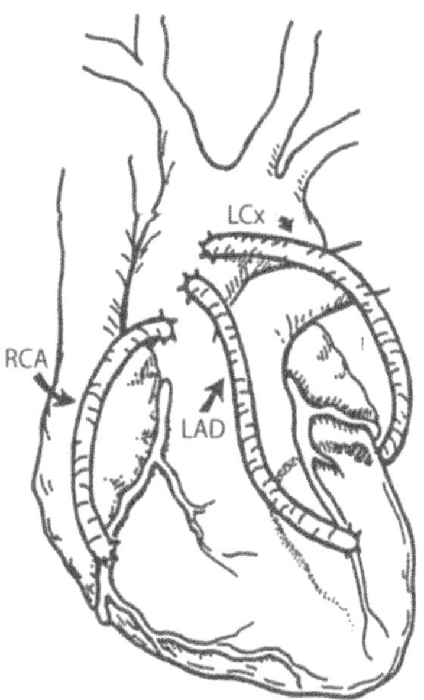

Fig. 16.7. Typical location of saphenous vein bypass grafts coming off the proximal ascending aorta and anastomosing the native coronary arteries (artist's drawing)

imaging a small portion of the bypass graft. In fact, a single cross-section of the graft in one or two transaxial planes was all that was usually imaged. These techniques used traditional ECG-gated MR pulse sequences: cardiac gated T1-weighted SE imaging where patent grafts appeared as flow void (dark blood), and cine MR where a patent graft shows up as a high signal area (bright blood). We refer the reader to several excellent reviews of the literature on this early use of MRI for assessing graft patency (Danias et al. 1998; Buser and Higgins 1994; Stanford et al. 1991). Although one might have hoped that coronary MRA would be very helpful for such applications, this has not been the case. The first generation coronary MRA techniques require pre-test knowledge of the position of the blood vessels. The location of native coronary vessels with respect to the heart is relatively well known, thus allowing easy selection of appropriate imaging planes. However, following the course of bypass grafts, without clear landmarks inside the chest cavity, can be more difficult. This explains why no extensive studies using a first generation coronary MRA technique to image large sections of a bypass grafts have been performed. Studies to image internal mammary artery grafts have been performed (Duerinckx et al. 1997b), as the course of these vessels is more predictable, as shown in Fig. 16.8. Also somewhat easier to image with coronary MRA is the distal graft anastomosis, as it is located close to an easy to visualize cardiac surface (see later discussions).

Given the great challenges of interactively tracking the course of a bypass graft though the chest cavity with no clear landmarks, the advent of new 3D MRA techniques with short acquisitions times (within a single breath-hold, thus eliminating breathing motion) has dramatically changed our ability to image these vessels. These new non-cardiac-gated 3D MRA techniques are adequate to image the proxi-

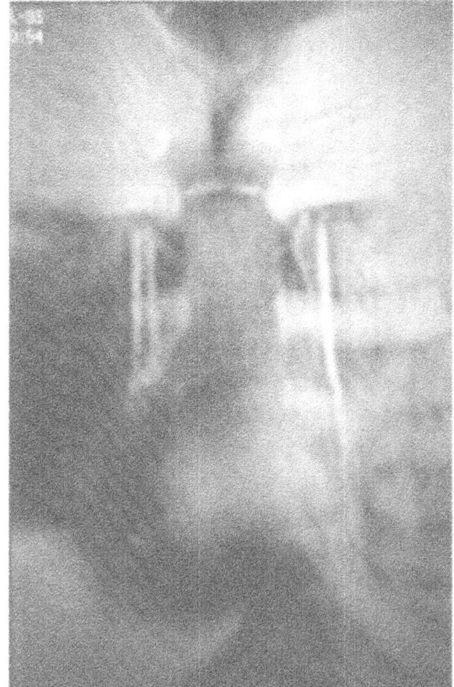
a

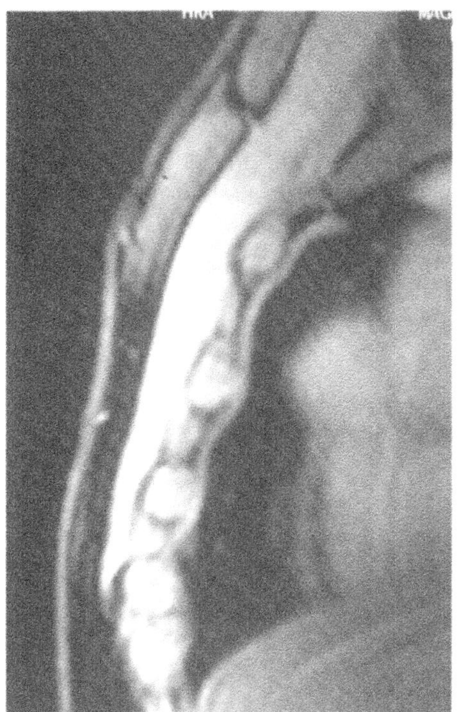
b

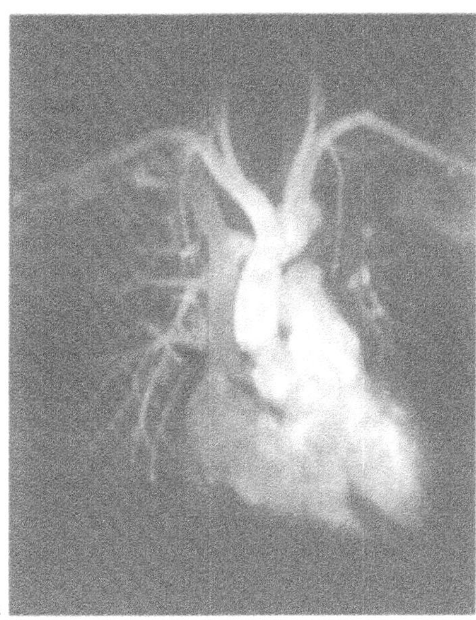
c

Fig. 16.8a–c. Typical appearance of the internal mammary vessels (arteries and veins) as seen on first generation coronary MR angiograms. **a** Coronal image obtained along the anterior chest wall, with the patient prone on a standard a spine coil. **b** Sagittal image of the right/left mammary vessels. Unlike saphenous vein grafts these vessels are easy to track and follow (see text). **c** Coronal image of the mammary vessel during a dynamic contrast-enhanced MRA.

mal and middle portion of grafts, but not the distal anastomosis where cardiac motion is still a problem. Since they were first described in 1993 by Prince et al. (1993), enormous progress has been made with these 3D dynamic gadolinium-enhanced MRA techniques (Prince et al. 1995a, b, 1996). The duration of 3D slab acquisitions has decreased from several minutes in 1993 to time periods under 8 s for carotid MRA in 1998. These contrast-enhanced 3D non-cardiac-gated MRA approaches are now being routinely used to image the thoracic aorta, the renal arteries, and the abdominal aorta and are starting to be used for imaging of the carotid arteries (Cloft et al. 1996; Kim et al. 1998) and the pulmonary arteries (Meaney et al. 1997; Duerinckx et al. 1998a). Most recently it has been applied in use for CABG imaging (Vrachliotis et al. 1997; Wintersperger et al. 1997, 1998). These techniques nicely complement the cardiac-gated coronary MRA techniques which offer direct visualization of native coronary arteries, small segments, and the distal anastomosis of a CABG and internal mammary arteries and veins (Galjee et al. 1996; Duerinckx et al. 1997b), as illustrated in Fig. 16.8. Moreover, the capability for 3D visualization and 3D reconstruction from MRA data has tremendously improved the visualization of much longer portions of coronary bypass grafts. It should be noted that metal artifacts from sternal sutures, surgical clips, or stents do not usually interfere with visualization of a graft. They only obscure the graft in very small focal areas and still allow clear visualization of the majority of the largest portion of the graft.

We will now review the more promising recently published approaches to CABG imaging. Most of these should be easily reproducible on any clinical MRI scanner.

In a first study, published in the April 1997 issue of the *American Journal of Roentgenology* by VRACHLIOTIS et al. (1997), a total of 45 grafts (29 saphenous vein bypass grafts, 12 left internal mammary artery grafts, and four right internal mammary artery grafts) were evaluated in 15 patients. These 15 patients underwent 3D breath-hold ECG-triggered contrast-enhanced MRA on a 1.5T commercial scanner (Magnetom Vision Scanner, Siemens Medical Systems, Iselin, NJ) with 25 mT/m gradients and 600-ms rise time. These MRA studies were performed within 24 h of the conventional coronary angiography studies. MRA was in agreement with the coronary angiography in 42 of the 44 grafts, after exclusion of one saphenous vein graft which was revealed as occluded by X-ray coronary angiography but was patent by MRA.

In a second study by WINTERSBERGER et al. (1997, 1998) breath-hold contrast-enhanced MRA was also evaluated as a tool to assess CABG patency. These authors set out to demonstrate the feasibility and reliability of the contrast-enhanced MRA technique in the assessment of venous and internal mammary artery graft patency after CABG surgery, using X-ray coronary angiography as a reference. The study included 27 patients with a total of 76 (48 venous/28 IMA) coronary bypass grafts. These patients were examined 26.5±5.8 months after surgery with both MRA and X-ray angiogram within 12.6±10.5 h. MRA was performed on a 1.5T whole-body scanner (Magnetom Vision Scanner, Siemens Medical Systems, Germany) using the same contrast-enhanced 3D GE sequence, i.e., a 3D FLASH sequence without ECG triggering with the following parameters: TR=4.4 ms, TE=1.8 ms, and 40° flip angle; matrix size of 512 with field of view (FOV) of 500 mm. The rectangular FOV was used as needed. The 3-D volume slab had a thickness of 96 mm subdivided into 26–40 partitions with an acquisition time of about 30 s. The typical slice thickness was 3 mm. A single bolus of 20 cc gadopentetate dimeglumine (Magnevist, Schering AG, Germany) followed by a saline flush was used. Arrival time of the bolus was also calculated using a test bolus. These authors found that coronary MRA and traditional X-ray coronary angiography were in agreement in 70 of 76 grafts. Sensitivity was 95% for venous grafts, 96% for internal mammary artery graft, and 95% overall. Specificity was 85% for venous graft and 67% for internal mammary artery grafts. These authors concluded that with contrast-enhanced MRA, a reliable assessment of CABG patency is possible.

In the above studies, the following definitions of sensitivity, specificity and predicted values were used. An occluded (by coronary angiography) graft was defined as true positive (occluded, diseased). Conversely, a patent (by coronary angiography) graft was defined as true negative. In these studies, no specific attempt was made to identify focal lesions, focal stenosis, or anastomotic problems. Although these newer studies visualize larger portions of the graft, they still only look at patency. Thus, no attempt is ever made to evaluate underlying stenosis or partial thrombus. As the high sensitivity in most of the studies illustrates, MRI is a relatively good tool for detecting a totally occluded graft. However, the relatively lower specificity also means that a significant proportion of patent grafts (by X-ray coronary angiography) are erroneously labeled as being occluded by MRI. This is because MRI failed to visualize the graft or failed to visualize flow in the patent portion of the graft. Calcifications, metal clips, thickened pericardium, and small pericardial collections of fluid can mimic the signal void of flowing blood on SE images. Flowing blood on GE images is depicted as a bright signal. Because of this it has been suggested that the specificity of MR imaging for graft patency will be improved with GRE techniques.

As mentioned before, these non-cardiac-gated 3D contrast-enhanced MRA techniques cannot visualize the distal CABG anastomosis. For visualization of distal anastomosis, ECG-triggered techniques are needed. Preliminary success with an ECG-triggered approach has been described by VRACHLIOTIS et al. (1997) and also in two case reports (DUERINCKX et al. 1996; WARNER et al. 1996). An example of the use of a first generation coronary MRA technique to visualize a bypass graft is shown in Fig. 16.9. WARNER et al. (1996) describes how MRI of the coronary artery was useful when planning a re-do of a CABG operation. Specifically, this was the case of a 57-year-old man who had undergone triple vessel CABG surgery. Because the previous saphenous vein graft to the left anterior descending coronary artery (LAD) was aneurysmal, there was very poor opacification of the distal LAD during a repeat X-ray coronary angio-

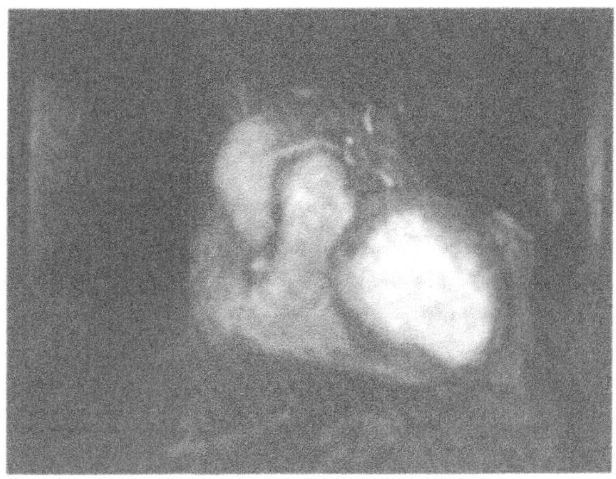

Fig. 16.9. Coronal projection image of a bypass graft, extracted from a 3D contrast-enhanced MRA, usind a small subset of the data to create a maximum intensity projection (MIP)

gram. In this particular case, the coronary MRA technique clearly showed the distal LAD to be of sufficient quality to be able to re-do the bypass surgery. In another case report by DUERINCKX et al. (1996) an area of aneurysmal dilatation was also found in the saphenous vein graft to the LAD in a 74-year-old man. Although the major problems after CABG surgery are graft stenoses, pseudoaneurysms do occur and MRI represents a good modality to visualize these grafts. This case report is another example of how MRI can significantly help the cardiologist when the amount of contrast available via conventional contrast-enhanced coronary X-ray angiography is insufficient and further clarification is required. It also illustrates how these coronary MRA sequences can occasionally be used without breath-holding and still produce relatively good results.

Another and very different approach to bypass graft evaluation is the combination of traditional imaging of patency of the graft with flow profile analysis. Several recent papers have addressed this. GALJEE et al. studied 47 patients with a previous history of CABG who underwent angiography and both SE and cine phase velocity imaging (GALJEE et al. 1996). Twenty-three grafts were patent; 25 were occluded. The typical flow pattern was a balance biphasic for a floor pattern. The ultimate role of adding flow measurement is unknown, but appears very promising (SCHREIBER et al. 1999; SAKUMA et al. 1996b; VAN ROSSUM et al. 1999; VOIGTLANDER 1998; WALPOTH et al. 1999).

MRA and flow quantification of the internal mammary artery graft after minimally invasive direct coronary artery bypass have also been successfully performed (MILLER et al. 1999). Six patients who had undergone minimally invasive direct coronary artery bypass surgery were examined to evaluate an MRI protocol that provided information about cardiac function, bypass graft patency, and flow characteristics with a single examination. Preliminary results by MILLER et al. suggest that the imaging protocol allows accurate follow-up of patients after minimally invasive direct coronary artery bypass surgery (MILLER et al. 1999). Bypass graft patency was correctly determined in all patients. In four patients, anastomoses were visualized by MRA, and flow measurements revealed a volume range of 28–84 ml/min (native and grafted internal mammary arteries) and a trend for the flow values of bypass grafts to be lower than those of native vessels. Interobserver reproducibility was good (r=.99; slope, .98).

Cardiac-gated coronary MRA for imaging of bypass grafts has also been described. As stated earlier, first generation techniques require lengthy interactive search patterns, with one 2D image per breath-hold, to locate the grafts and can thus be time consuming (VAN ROSSUM et al. 1997). The third generation techniques, with thin-slab 3D breath-hold scans, are easier to use for this purpose because the 3D slabs cover larger volumes (see Fig. 22 in WIELOPOLSKI et al. 2000). The second generation, navigator-based techniques offer an even easier approach as they cover larger 3D slabs (WIELOPOLSKI et al. 2000; KESSLER et al. 1997; MOLINARI et al. 1999). Using a retrospective, navigator-based second generation coronary MRA technique, KESSLER et al. reported the results on seven patients with CABGs within a large study on coronary artery stenosis detection, correctly classifying four occluded and 13 of 15 patent grafts (KESSLER et al. 1997).

Another approach for CABG imaging uses cardiac-gated breath-hold black-blood fast SE (HASTE) (KALDEN et al. 1999a, b; WITTLINGER et al. 1999). KALDEN et al. evaluated the patency of CABG with a 2D T2-weighted breath-hold turbo-spin-echo sequence (HASTE). The HASTE technique has been well described elsewhere (REGAN 1999; LAUB et al. 1995; DUERINCKX et al. 1999b; AERTS et al. 1996). KALDEN et al. studied 38 patients with 97 grafts (19 internal mammary artery and 78 saphenous vein grafts) and a total of 120 distal anastomoses at 1.5 T in supine position using a phased-array body coil (KALDEN et al. 1999a). An ECG gated 2D T2-weighted HASTE study was performed. The reference method was selective coronary angiography. The image material was evaluated independently by two radiologists (observer one, a radiological fellow, and observer two, a staff radiologist). Observer 1 reached a sensitivity of 96% (72/75) and a specificity of 91% (20/22); positive predictive value was 97%, and negative predictive value 87%. Of the 97 (81%) patent distal anastomoses, 79 were correctly identified. Observer 2 achieved a sensitivity of 92% (69/75) and a specificity of 82% (18/22); positive and negative predictive values were 95% and 75%, respectively. From 97 patent distal anastomoses, 59 (61%) were recognized. The interobserver agreement was good (Cohen's kappa=68%, *p*-value; McNemar=58%). KALDEN et al. concluded that the HASTE sequence makes a reliable assessment of graft patency possible and that this sequence is a helpful tool for planning flow measurements and 3-D MRA (KALDEN et al. 1999a). In addition, HASTE can be a great compliment to non-cardiac-gated 3D MRA (described earlier) because its shorter acquisition times allows better imaging of distal graft anastomoses.

16.3.5 Imaging of Coronary Artery Stents

Another potentially important application of coronary MRA is determining the patency of coronary vessels after stent placement. Because stents are metallic objects and cause a major image artifact on the MR images, they are very easy to localize. Coronary MRA can then be used to determine flow in the vessels proximal and distal to the stent and thus determine vessel patency. Lesion severity or partial thrombosis cannot be assessed at the present time, only total occlusion versus (total or partial) patency (DUERINCKX et al. 1995b, 1998b; DE COBELLI et al. 1997, 1998). The clinical implications of this are that conventional X-ray angiography techniques are still better than MRI, depending on what the clinical question is. However, when clinical suspicion is low and the clinician prefers an initial noninvasive imaging study, coronary MRA could provide a very good initial imaging step.

Newer stents made of nickel-titanium, tantalum, and other new materials in which the metal stent artifact may no longer be a problem have already been tested in humans (TEITELBAUM et al. 1989; LAISSY et al. 1995). Preliminary reports suggest that these newer stents may offer great potential for the imaging of partial thrombosis stenosis within the stent.

Patients are routinely given anticoagulants for 30 days after stent deployment. During this 30-day window, cardiologists are reluctant to perform angiography because anticoagulation must first be reversed. Thus, when patients present acutely after stent placement with signs and/or symptoms suggestive of stent thrombosis but a clinical picture that is not clear, they would benefit from a noninvasive imaging technique to evaluate stent patency. A self-imposed 8-week waiting period for MRI after stent placement has been suggested by the stent manufacturers (KOTSAKI et al. 1997). Until MRI can be recommended for imaging during the immediate post-stent placement period, a repeat coronary angiogram is still the only alternative . These conventional contrast coronary angiograms can definitively establish patency of the stent, but are invasive and represent somewhat of a risk in the acute stage. Furthermore, the location of the stents cannot always easily be established by angiography, as stainless steel stents are radiolucent, and one widely used version of stent (the Palmaz-Schatz stent) is barely visible by fluoroscopy (YAMOAKA et al. 1995). Therefore, there is a great interest in newer noninvasive imaging methods, such as CT and MRI, which could offer additional insight under those circumstances.

Coronary MRA of stents is a safe and noninvasive imaging procedure. Coronary artery stents are not significantly influenced by the magnetic fields that are used for imaging in clinical MR imaging systems at 1.5 T (SCOTT and PETTIGREW 1994) and, thus, routine MR imaging of patients with coronary or saphenous vein graft stents should not cause significant motion of the prosthesis (DUERINCKX et al. 1995b; KOTSAKIS et al. 1997; FRIEDRICH et al. 1999). A possible explanation is the relatively low ferromagnetic nature of the metals used for the manufacture of coronary stents. SHELLOCK and SHELLOCK (1999) evaluated safety during MR imaging (i.e., magnetic field interactions, heating, and artifacts) for metallic stents. Different types of metallic stents were tested for magnetic field interactions, heating, and artifacts using a 1.5T MR system. Magnetic field-related translational attraction and torque were assessed using previously described techniques. Heating was evaluated using an infrared thermometer to record temperatures immediately before and after performing MR imaging using a whole-body-averaged specific absorption rate of 1.3 W/kg. Artifacts were assessed by placing the stents inside a fluid-filled phantom and performing MRI using fast spoiled GE and T1-weighted SE pulse sequences. For the ten different stents evaluated, SHELLOCK and SHELLOCK (1999) found no magnetic field interactions, and any artifacts involved signal voids that would not create diagnostic problems as long as the area of interest was not positioned exactly where a particular stent was located. STROHM et al. (1999) examined 14 different coronary stents from seven manufacturers in 1.0T and 1.5T systems (STROHM et al. 1999). They demonstrated no evidence of stent motion or measurable change in temperature in explanted pig hearts. KRAMER et al. (1999, 2000) have also assessed safety of stents during MRI early after stent placement for acute myocardial infarction. They reported no significant safety problems. SCHROEDER et al. (2000) also confirmed that MRI seems safe in patients with intracoronary stents.

A case report described how ultrafast CT enabled the clear detection of a Palmaz-Schatz stent without artifacts and was valuable in confirming its location (YAMOAKA et al. 1995). Another report discussed the use of ultrafast CT to evaluate a stent after a patient developed chest pain following bypass grafting and after later implementation of a Gianturco-Roubin stent (NYMAN et al. 1993). SCHMERMUND et al. (1995, 1996) have described the use of EB-CT to assess coronary vessel patency after stent imaging in 22 patients. Quantitative analysis of densitometric curves in a region of interest distal to the stented vessel segment was performed to establish patency or occlusion. Another case report described how MR imaging localized a Palmaz-Schatz stent in the right coronary artery (RCA) and showed vessel patency distal to the stent (DUERINCKX et al. 1995b).

The first study on the assessment of coronary artery patency following stent placement using coronary MRA was published by DUERINCKX et al. (1998b). In this study, the authors studied 16 patients with 26 stents. The study was performed on a 1.5T Siemens scanner. The distribution of stent locations was: ten in the RCA, ten in the LAD, two in the circumflex coronary artery (Circ), and four in the saphenous vein graft (SVG) to RCA. One patient had two RCA and two LAD stents, one had three RCA and one LAD stent, and one had three saphenous vein graft (SVG) stents and two had double RCA stents. The authors concluded that coronary MRA is safe for noninvasive imaging of coronary artery stents and that in the proper clinical setting it can be used to help suggest patency. However, it cannot exclude partial occlusion of partial thrombosis. Representative examples of such coronary stent images are shown in Figs. 16.6–16.8.

A follow-up report by DE COBELLI et al. (1997–1999) confirmed similar findings about stent patency assessment by MRI in 13 stented coronary vessels with 18 stents 1 day to 8 months after stent placement. Different types of stents were evaluated: Palmaz-Schatz (n=6), Multilink (n=6), Crossflex (n=5), and Wiktor (n=1). The study was performed on a 1.5T GE scanner. Both studies (DE COBELLI et al. 1997; DUERINCKX et al. 1998b) confirmed the safety of the MRI studies.

AMANO et al. have described artifacts of coronary stents (AMANO et al. 1999; BAUM et al. 2000; LENHART et al. 2000; MANKE et al. 2000). MR flow measurements after stent placement are also possible (NAGEL et al. 1998).

16.3.6 Imaging in Postsurgical Patients

The use of coronary MRA in postsurgical patients or after interventional procedures is increasing. Rapid heart rates, sternal wires, and altered cardiac orientation do not prevent coronary MRA in heart transplant recipients (DAVIS et al. 1996; MOHIADDIN et al. 1996b). Artifacts from bypass graft markers or clips can interfere with complete visualization of a graft and could simulate stenosis in a graft. Sternal wires do not interfere with imaging of the majority of native coronary arteries and bypass grafts.

16.3.7 Post- and Preangioplasty Follow-up

Although existing coronary MR angiographic pulse sequences may not be adequate to replace conventional coronary angiography for screening and detecting of coronary arterial lesions, they can play a significant role in the evaluation and follow-up of known proximal coronary artery lesions. If and when a proximal coronary arterial lesion can be detected with coronary angiography, it is relatively easy and totally noninvasive to study the anatomy of this lesion periodically with MRI as needed, for example, after interventional procedures such as angioplasty (PENNELL et al. 1994a).

DUERINCKX et al. (1999c) have also described the usefulness of coronary MRA prior to angioplasty. The range of indications for percutaneous transluminal coronary angioplasty (PTCA) has increased greatly since the procedure was initially introduced. The success rate depends on the anatomy and length of the occlusion and on the state of the distal vessel. DUERINCKX et al. (1999c) present a case in which MRA was used to evaluate the length of a subtotal occlusion prior to PTCA, and thus could have had an impact on therapeutic decisions. This capability may further expand the clinical use of MR technology in the practice of cardiology.

16.3.8
Coronary Blood Flow and Flow Reserve

Being able to measure blood flow as well is a major advantage of coronary MRA over coronary X-ray angiography. The clinical significance of determining coronary flow reserve and changes in velocity and flow in coronary vessels cannot be emphasized enough. Early work – before the advent of breath-hold velocity-encoded cine MRI – concentrated on flow measurements in mammary arteries, as they are subjected to much less respiratory motion than the native vessels (Debatin et al. 1992, 1993; Duerinckx 1993). More recent work using the breath-hold velocity-encoded cine MRI has shown promising initial results in native vessels (Clarke et al. 1995; Sakuma et al. 1996b; Hofman et al. 1996; Hundley et al. 1996), bypass grafts, and mammary arteries (Sakuma et al. 1996). The results obtained so far have been limited to small portions of the proximal coronary artery territory and the coronary sinus. The reproducibility has not been good at some laboratories (Nitz et al. 1996); nevertheless, the preliminary results are extremely encouraging and are pointing us in the right direction. More basic and applied clinical work will be needed to validate these techniques. Many theoretical reasons could be suggested as to why none of the MRI based techniques used to quantitate coronary flow could possibly work (Frayne et al. 1997). Nevertheless, most experimental data seem to suggest otherwise. The techniques are still being refined (Langerak et al. 2001).

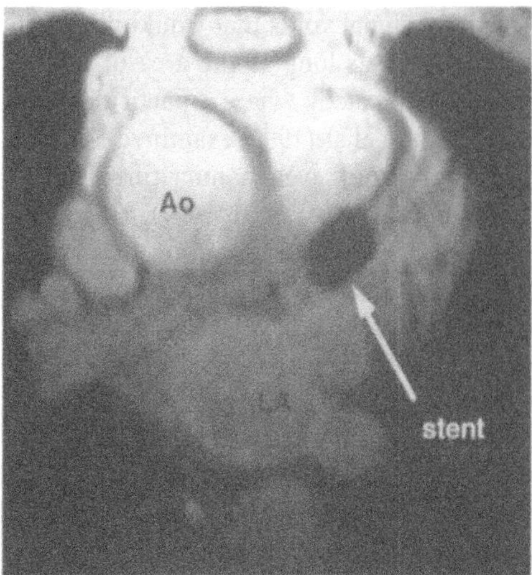

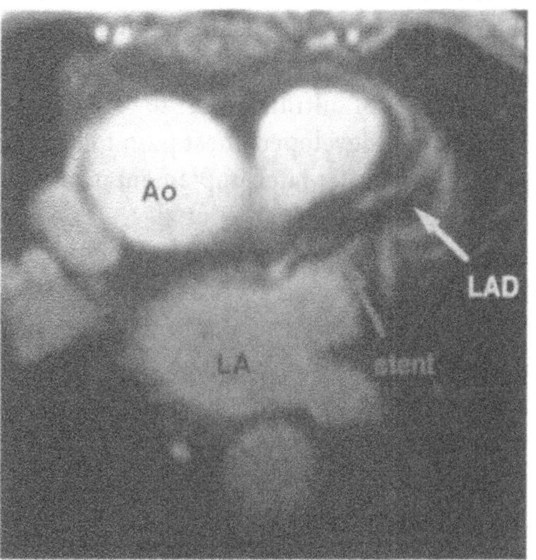

Fig. 16.10a, b. A 55 -year-old man with a single stent in the proximal left anterior descending artery (LAD). **a** Oblique transaxial images with fat-suppression. The proximal LAD, mid-LAD (*white arrow*) and great cardiac vein are shown. An area of signal void due to the susceptibility artifact of the stent is visualized. Also shown are the ascending aorta (*Ao*) and the descending aorta (*D*). **b** Oblique transaxial images without fat-suppression. The area of signal void due to the susceptibility artifact of the stent is better visualized. The mid LAD is only faintly seen. Also shown are the ascending aorta (*Ao*) and the descending aorta. (With permission from: Duerinckx AJ, et al (1998) Assessment of coronary artery patency after stent placement using magnetic resonance angiography. J Magn Reson Imaging 8:896–902)

16.4
Coronary Artery Lesion Detection

The use of coronary MRA for blind prospective detection of coronary lesions is still being evaluated, and improved coronary MR angiographic techniques may become an integral part of the clinical evaluation and screening of patients with ischemic heart disease. It is still premature to judge the ultimate capability of coronary MRA in screening for coronary artery disease.

16.4.1 Imaging Coronary Artery Lesions by MR

The detection of coronary artery lesions by MR is probably the most talked about and investigated future application of coronary MRA. Interestingly enough, it is still the least mature and most experimental application. Coronary lesion detection represents the "Holy Grail" of cardiac MR imaging (CAPUTO 1991, 1994; ROGERS 1998; DINSMORE 1995; GOLDSMITH 1994). From the beginning it was hoped that coronary MRA could become a noninvasive screening tool for the detection of all (or most) coronary artery lesions. This is still our hope today, at least for proximal lesions in the main coronary arteries and their larger side branches. The fact that after 7 years of preclinical trials of coronary MRA techniques their sensitivity and specificity for coronary lesion detection still does not compare with traditional contrast coronary angiography (DUERINCKX 1999; WIELOPOLSKI et al. 1998; DANIAS et al. 1998; DINSMORE 1995) should not discourage us. There are many reasons why we have not yet seen "perfect" results, such as 99% sensitivity for detection of all coronary lesions. First, the MRI technology and coronary MRA pulse sequences changed and improved so quickly over the last 5 years that few large preclinical trials were ever performed with any of them. Secondly, because the first and second generation coronary MRA techniques required respectively great skill or less skill but much longer acquisition times, few investigators were willing to take on the challenge. Thirdly, many people wanted coronary MRA to perform like the established invasive gold standard contrast X-ray coronary angiography, even though this was never the case for other noninvasive techniques such as nuclear cardiology or exercise stress testing. There is a need to reassess unrealistic expectations about what coronary MRA should be able to do. Being able to detect 70%–90% of all significant proximal coronary artery lesions is already a very worthwhile goal. It is not necessary for a noninvasive imaging technique for patients with ischemic heart disease to detect every single minor lesion in small coronary side branches. In addition, with the advent of the third generation coronary MR angiographic techniques, improved post-processing, more interest on the part of clinical users, the availability of new dedicated "cardiac" MR scanners, and new MR blood pool agents (both indicating industry's interest in this issue), the use of coronary MRA in daily clinical practice will soon become reality. Coronary MRA for lesion detection is now available to clinical users and not just investigators at major academic centers or clinics. Coronary MRA will have an important role in the work-up of patients with ischemic heart disease in the very near future.

16.4.2 Coronary Artery Lesion Detection by MRI: How Does It Differ from Imaging in Other Vascular Territories?

The physiology of blood flow in coronary arteries is very different from the physiology of blood flow in large vessels such as the carotid arteries and the abdominal aorta. In the coronary arteries flow velocities are lower than in other large vessels; there is less or no turbulent flow; and there is potential for collateral blood flow. Normal coronary arteries and veins appear as high-signal linear structures on coronary MR angiograms. Distal to a total occlusion, vessels with no collateral flow have decreased signal intensity or background (fat-suppressed) signal intensity. However, occasionally a vessel shadow is visible, possibly corresponding to the wall of the occluded vessel, and this could be misconstrued as representing reduced flow beyond a subtotal occlusion. Reverse flow distal to a total occlusion cannot be distinguished from forward flow past a subtotal occlusion without determining direction of flow.

16.4.3 Coronary Wall and Plaque Imaging

Coronary MRA can be performed using bright blood or black blood sequences (STUBER and MANNING 2000). With some of the bright blood sequences, the wall and arterial blood inside the vessel wall may have very similar signal characteristics. The use of black blood imaging or MR contrast agents may be needed to distinguish between wall and blood content. T2-weighted preparation pulses may also improve the distinction between coronary vessel wall and blood content.

Imaging of the coronary wall and plaque inside the wall has been described by several groups (MEYER, unpublished; WORTHLEY et al. 1999, 2000a–d; BOTNAR et al. 1999, 2000; FAYAD et al. 2000a, b; ZHENG et al. 2000b; FAYAD and FUSTER 2000). This an extension to coronary MRA of very exciting work on the use of MRI for atherosclerotic plaque characterization (YUAN et al. 1997; TROUARD et al. 1997; TOUSSAINT et al. 1998; HATSUKAMI et al. 1997; BONN 1999; LUK-PAT et al. 1999; SHINNAR et al. 1999; ZIMMERMANN-PAUL et al. 1999).

16.4.4 Lesion Detection Using First, Second and Third Generation Coronary MRA: the 1993–2001 period

It was originally hoped that coronary MRA could become a noninvasive screening tool for the detection of coronary artery lesions. The results with first generation coronary MRA in the 1993–1994 period were very promising but somewhat variable. The first generation 2D breath-hold MR imaging technique was tested by several investigators on a total of approximately 224 patients and was able to detect significant coronary artery lesions (greater than 50% diameter narrowing) with a sensitivity ranging from 33% to 100%. The reported sensitivity also varied depending upon the vessel examined. Because all the early studies were done with a surface coil positioned on the anterior chest wall, the more posteriorly located circumflex coronary artery was the more difficult one to visualize. Later studies used phased-array thoracic coils, with better visualization of the circumflex coronary artery. The early 3D techniques did not make a significant difference. The initial clinical results were very disappointing, with a sensitivity of 0%–38%. Then in 1994–1995 came the second generation 3D coronary MRA trials using navigator-pulse feedback. With the original implementation of these techniques a few investigators were able to demonstrate a sensitivity from 65% to 87% for lesion detection. Many modifications and improvements in this second generation coronary MRA approach have since been proposed and implemented, with better results for lesion detection (Huber et al. 1999; Sardanelli et al. 2000). These improved second generation coronary MRA show great promise. However, even these improved navigator techniques still require long acquisition times with all the inherent risks of erratic breathing or motion. Thus, the interest has grown in developing newer techniques which allow multiple slice acquisition in one breath-hold, referred to as the third generation coronary MRA techniques. Only preliminary clinical results are available for the third generation coronary MRA techniques (Van Geuns et al. 2000b), as illustrated in Fig. 16.11. After 7 years of preclinical trials of many different coronary MRA techniques, none has yet emerged as a clear winner that can provide a sensitivity and specificity for coronary lesion detection that compares with traditional contrast coronary angiography (Duerinckx 2001a, b). Table 16.2 summarizes the results from published reports on coronary artery lesion detection using MRI and MRA.

16.4.5 Coronary Lesion Detection by MRI in the Future

Coronary MRA technique development has been proceeding at a very fast pace, indeed so fast that most techniques never even have a chance of being evaluated by more than one or two investigators before everybody moves on to the next technique. Clinical users should not be disappointed by this or view this as an indication that these techniques are not working. First generation coronary MRA techniques are more than adequate for a large number of specific clinical applications. They are even capable of detecting significant coronary lesions, with a 65%–80% sen-

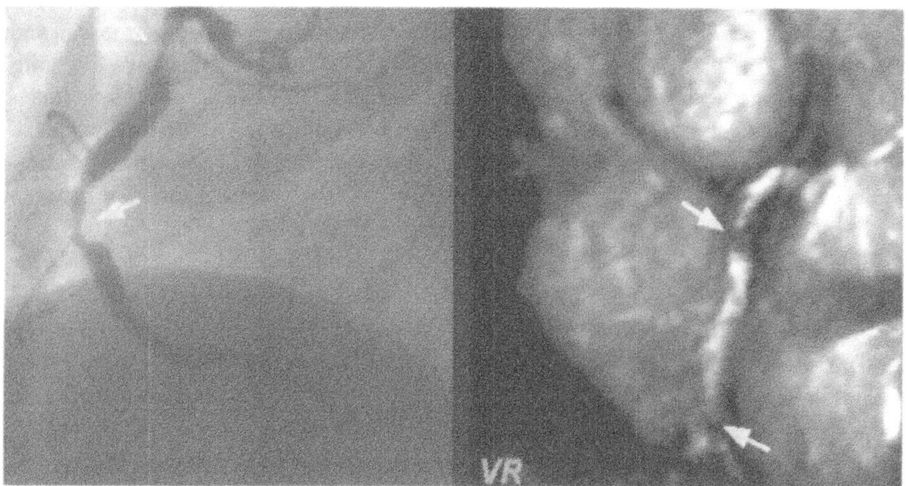

Fig. 16.11a, b. Detection of a RCA lesion using the VCATS technique. **a** Conventional X-ray coronary angiogram. **b** 3D rendering of the RCA using VCATS data (from Van Geuns and Wielopolski, with permission)

Table 16.2. Sensitivity and specificity for coronary lesion detection by coronary magnetic resonance angiography: a literature survey (1993–2000)

First generation techniques (2D) (*one slice; one breath-hold*)	*n*	# les	Sensitivity (%)	Specificity (%)
Manning et al. 1993	39	52a	90	92
Manning et al. 1994	72	81	90	
Duerinckx et al. 1993, Duerinckx and Urman 1994b, Duerinckx and Urman 1994a	20	27	63 (0 75)b	n/a
Post et al. 1994a	14	14	36	
Post et al. 1995b	35	35	33b 75b	
Pennell et al. 1994a	17	23	65	
Pennell et al. 1994b	31	41	88c	
Nitatori et al. 1995a, Nitatori et al. 1995b	50	n/a	83100	
Pennell et al. 1996	39	n/a	85 (75–100)	
Mohiaddin et al. 1996a, Mohiaddin et al. 1996b	16	9	56	82
Yoshino et al. 1997	36	31	83 LAD 100 RCA	98 LAD 100 RCA
Post et al. 1997	35		53 LAD 71 RCA	73 LAD n/a RCA
Total number of patients[d]	224			
Transition from first to second generation: Multi-slice acquisitions				
Post et al. 1994b	22	17	0	
Post et al. 1996	20	21	38	95
Second generation techniques (3D) (navigator pulses; no breath-holding) (retrospective navigator approach)				
Müller et al. 1996	33	n/a	87	97
Müller et al. 1997	35	54	83	94
Kessler et al. 1997	73	43	65	n/a
Woodard et al. 1996, Woodard et al. 1998	10	10	80	
Huber et al., 1999	20	53 53e	73 79	50 54
Sandstede et al. 1999	30	37	81	89
Van Geuns et al. 1999	29	26	50	91
Sardanelli et al. 2000	42	n/a	82	89
Second generation techniques (3D) (navigator pulses; no breath-holding) (prospective navigator approach)				
Lethimonnier et al. 1999	20	17	65	93
Total number of patients[d]	118			
Third generation techniques (3D) (multiple slices; one breath-hold)				
Hu et al. 1996	23	27	63	
Van Geuns et al. 1998	13	9	66	n/a
Regenfus et al. 1999	30	31	77	94

Results of clinical trials using coronary magnetic resonance angiography (sensitivity and specificity), as compared with conventional angiography, to identify individual vessels with = 50% angiographic stenoses. Results are expressed in percent (%).All results published as peer-reviewed journal articles are indicated in italic lettering.
n number of subjects; # *les* number of lesions with significant disease)
[a] Number of vessels instead of lesions.
[b] Variable sensitivities depending upon detection threshold used to interpret images (see Duerinckx 1996).
[c] Study interpretation not fully blinded.
[d] Total number of patients; this total does not reflect numbers reported at meetings in partial or preliminary oral or poster reports.
[e] Sensitivity and specificity for subset of images with higher image quality.

sitivity in many centers. The early implementations of the second generation coronary MR angiographic techniques (using retrospective respiratory gating) required long acquisition times, which explains their unpredictable behavior. When images were good they were very good, but equally often they were very bad and not interpretable. The improved second generation coronary MR angiographic techniques using navigator pulse feedback and adaptive prospective (or retrospective or interactive) correction of slice position or signal averaging dramatically improve the reliability and image quality and thus have increased the sensitivity of the technique (DANIAS et al. 2000). The newer third generation techniques appear very promising and easy to use (VAN GEUNS et al. 2000b). The advent of blood pool agents will also impact our capability to detect lesions better (JOHANSSON et al. 1999; TAYLOR et al. 1999; HOFMAN et al. 1999). Hopefully, we will soon have a useful array of complementary noninvasive MRA approaches for evaluating coronary lesions which will be easy to use and will provide reproducible results. In the year 2000 cardiac-gated multi-slice CT emerged as a very serious competitor for both EB-CT and MRI/MRA-based coronary imaging (VAN GEUNS et al. 2000a; OHNESORGE et al. 2000). The jury is still out as to which imaging modality will ultimately prevail, and this topic continues to be hotly debated at many cardiac imaging meetings.

References

Aerts P, VanHoe L, Bosmans H, Oyen R, Marchal G, Baert AL (1996) Breath-hold MR urography using the HASTE technique. AJR Am J Roentgenol 166:543–545

Amano Y, Ishihara M, Hayashi H, et al (1999) Metallic artifacts of coronary and iliac arteries stents in MR angiography and contrast-enhanced CT. Clin Imaging 23:85–89

American Heart Association (1996) Heart and stroke facts: 1996 statistical supplement. American Heart Association, Dallas, Texas

Anderson CM, Edelman RR, Turski PA (1993) Clinical magnetic resonance angiography. Raven Press, New York

Arlart IP, Bongartz GM, Marchall G (1996) Magnetic resonance angiography. Springer, Berlin Heidelberg New York

Atkinson D, Teresi L (1995) Magnetic resonance angiography (review article). Magn Reson Q 10:149–172

Baum F, Vosshenrich R, Fischer U, Castillo E, Grabbe E (2000) [Stent artifacts in 3D MR angiography: experimental studies]. Rofo Fortschr Geb Röntgenstr Neuen Bildgeb Verfahr 172:278–281

Bisset GS, Strife JL, McCloskey J (1989) MR imaging of coronary artery aneurysms in a child with Kawasaki disease. AJR Am J Roentgenol 152:805–807

Blackwell GG, Cranney GB, Pohost GM (1992) MRI: cardiovascular system. Gower Medical Publishing, New York

Bluemke DA, Boxerman JL, Mosher T, Lima JA (1997a) Segmented K-space cine breath-hold cardiovascular MR imaging. II. Evaluation of aortic vasculopathy. AJR Am J Roentgenol 169:401–407

Bluemke DA, Boxerman JL, Atalar E, McVeigh ER (1997b) Segmented k-space cine breath-hold cardiovascular MR imaging. I. Principles and technique. AJR Am J Roentgenol 169:395–400

Bogaert J, Duerinckx AJ, Baert AL (1994) Coronary MR angiography: a review. J Belge Radiol 77:255–261

Bogaert J, Duerinckx AJ, Rademakers FE (1999) Magnetic resonance of the heart and great vessels: clinical applications. Springer, Berlin Heidelberg New York

Bonn D (1999) Plaque detection: the key to tackling atherosclerosis? [news]. Lancet 354:656

Botnar RM, Matthias Stuber, Kraig V Kissinger, Manning WJ (1999) Real-time navigator gated and corrected coronary vessel wall imaging [abstract]. In: Cardiovascular Imaging 1999. The 27 th Annual Meeting of the North American Society for Cardiac Imaging (NASCI), 6 November 1999, Atlanta, Georgia

Botnar RM, Stuber M, Kissinger KV, Manning WJ (2000) In-vivo imaging of coronary artery wall in humans using navigator and free-breathing [abstract]. In: Book of abstracts and Proceedings of the 8th Meeting of the International Society of Magnetic Resonance in Medicine (ISMRM 2000 Proceedings available on CD-ROM). Denver, Colorado, 1–7 April 2000

Brant-Zawadzki M, Boyko OB, Jensen MC, Gillan GD (1993) MR angiography: a teaching file. Raven, New York

Briffa NP, Clarke S, Kugan G, Coulden R, Wallwork J, Nashef SA (1996) Surgical angioplasty of the left main coronary artery: follow-up with magnetic resonance imaging. Ann Thorac Surg 62:550–552

Bunce NH, Pennell DJ (1999) Coronary MRA – a clinical experience in Europe. J Magn Reson Imaging 10:721–727

Buser PT, Higgins CB (1994) Coronary artery graft disease: diagnosis of graft failure by magnetic resonance imaging. In: Lüscher TF, Turina M, Braunwald E (eds) Coronary artery graft disease: mechanisms and prevention. Springer, Berlin Heidelberg New York, pp 99–112

Caputo GC (1991) Coronary arteries: potential for MR imaging [editorial]. Radiology 181:629–630

Caputo RC (1994) Coronary MR angiography: a clinical perspective [editorial]. Radiology 193:596–598

Cassidy M, Schiller N, Botvinick E, et al (1989) Assessment of coronary artery imaging by gated magnetic resonance; an evaluation of the utility and potential of the currently available imaging methods. Am J Card Imaging 3:100–107

Chung CJ, Stein L (1998) Kawasaki disease: a review. Radiology 208:25–33

Chung HW, Chen CY, Zimmerman RA, Lee KW, Lee CC, Chin SC (2000) T2-weighted fast MR imaging with true FISP versus HASTE: comparative efficacy in the evaluation of normal fetal brain maturation. AJR Am J Roentgenol 175:1375–1380

Clarke GD, Eckels R, Chaney C, et al (1995) Measurement of absolute epicardial coronary artery flow and flow reserve with breathhold cine phase-contrast magnetic resonance imaging. Circulation 91:2627–2634

Cloft HJ, Murphy KJ, Prince MR, Brunberg JA (1996) 3D gad-

olinium-enhanced MR angiography of the carotid arteries. Magn Reson Imaging 14:593–600
Danias PG, Edelman RR, Manning WJ (1998) Coronary MR angiography. Cardiol Clin 16:207–225
Danias PG, Stuber M, Edelman RR, Manning WJ (1999) Coronary MRA: a clinical experience in the United States. J Magn Reson Imaging 10:713–720
Danias P, Kissinger K, Stuber M, Botnar R, Manning W, et al (2000) MR coronary artery multi-center study with the Boston Cookbook protocol [abstract]. In: Book of abstracts of the First International Workshop on Coronary MR and CT Angiography, Lyon, France, 1–3 Oct 2000. Organized and published by the North American Society for Cardiac Imaging. Reprinted in: Int J Card Imaging
Davis SF, Kannam JP, Wielopolski P, Edelman RR, et al (1996) Magnetic resonance coronary angiography in heart transplant recipients. J Heart Lung Transplant 15:580–586
Debatin J, Strong J, Negro-Vilar R, Sostman H, Pelc N, Herfkens R (1992) MR characterization of blood flow in native and grafted internal mammary arteries [abstract]. In: Proceedings of the RSNA 78th Scientific Assembly and Annual Meeting. Chicago. 185:102
Debatin JF, Strong JA, Sostman HD, et al (1993) MR characterization of blood flow in native and grafted internal mammary arteries. J Magn Reson Imaging 3:443–451
De Cobelli F, Rosanio S, Vanzulli A, Mellone R, Chierchia S, Del-Maschio A (1997) Breathhold cine coronary MR angiography: patency assessment after stent placement. [abstract]. In: 1997 Scientific program of the 83rd Scientific Assembly and Annual Meeting of the Radiological Society of North America (RSNA). 30 November–5 December 1997, Chicago, Illinois. Radiology 205:154
De Cobelli F, Guidetti D, Vanzulli A, Mellone R, Chierchia S, Del Maschio A (1998) [Magnetic resonance angiography of coronary arteries: assessment in patients with coronary stenosis and control after stent positioning]. Radiol Med 95:54–61
De Cobelli F, Cappio S, Vanzulli A, Del Maschio A (1999) MRI assessment of coronary stents. Rays 24:140–148
Deshpande V, Gerhard Laub, Orlando Simonetti, et al (2000) 3D MR coronary artery imaging using magnetization-prepared TrueFISP [abstract]. In: Book of abstracts of the First International Workshop on Coronary MR and CT Angiography, Lyon, France, 1–3 Oct 2000. Organized and published by the North American Society for Cardiac Imaging. Reprinted in: Int J Card Imaging. 16:z
Dinsmore RE (1995) Noninvasive coronary arteriography – here at last? [comment]. Circulation 91:1607–1608
Doorey AJ, Wills JS, Blasetto J, Goldenberg EM (1994) Usefulness of magnetic resonance imaging for diagnosing an anomalous coronary artery coursing between aorta and pulmonary trunk. Am J Cardiol 74:198–199
Duerinckx AJ (1993) Coronary hemodynamics in patients with artery bypass grafts using phase contrast MRI [abstract]. In: 16th Annual Meeting of Society for Cardiac Angiography and Interventions. San Antonio, Texas, 18–22 May 1993
Duerinckx AJ (1995) Review: MR angiography of the coronary arteries. Top Magn Reson Imaging 7:267–285
Duerinckx AJ (1996) Coronary MR angiography. In: Boxt LM (ed) Cardiac MR imaging. Saunders, Philadelphia, pp 361–418 (MRI clinics of North America, vol 3).
Duerinckx AJ (1997) MRI of coronary arteries. Int J Card Imaging 13:191–197
Duerinckx AJ (1999a) Coronary MR angiography. Radiol Clin North Am 37:273–318
Duerinckx AJ (1999b) Coronary MR angiography [invited article]. In: Boxt LM (ed) Cardiac radiology. Saunders, Philadelphia, pp 273-318 (The radiological clinics of North America, vol 37)
Duerinckx AJ (2000) Abstracts, program and proceedings of the First International Workshop on Coronary MR and CT Angiography, 1–3 October 2000, Lyon, France. Organized by the North American Society for Cardiac Imaging (NASCI). Int J Card Imaging 16:185–212
Duerinckx AJ (2001a) Coronary MR Angiography (a textbook). Springer, New York Berlin Heidelberg
Duerinckx AJ (2001b) Imaging of coronary artery disease – MR. J Thorac Imaging 16:25–34
Duerinckx AJ (2001c) Abstracts, program and proceedings of the Second International Workshop on Coronary MR and CT Angiography, 1–2 October 2001, Chicago, Illinois. Organized by the North American Society for Cardiac Imaging (NASCI). [In press] International Journal of Cardiovascular Imaging 17:
Duerinckx AJ, Urman M (1994a) Two-dimensional coronary MR angiography: analysis of initial clinical results. Radiology 193:731–738
Duerinckx AJ, Urman MK (1994b) Hemodynamically significant coronary artery lesions missed with MR coronary angiography [abstract]. In: Printed program of the First Meeting of the Society of Magnetic Resonance (SMR). Dallas, Texas, 5–9 March 1994. J Magn Reson Imaging 4:80
Duerinckx AJ, Takahashi M (1996) Coronary MR angiography in Kawasaki disease [abstract]. Radiology 201:274
Duerinckx AJ, Lipton MJ (1998) Noninvasive coronary artery imaging using CT and MR imaging [comment]. AJR Am J Roentgenol 170:900–902
Duerinckx AJ, Urman M, Sinha U, Atkinson D, Simonetti O (1993) Evaluation of gadolinium-enhanced MR coronary angiography [abstract]. In: 79th Scientific Assembly and Annual Meeting of the Radiological Society of North America (RSNA). Chicago, 28 November –3 December 1993. Radiology 189:278
Duerinckx A, Higgins C, Pettigrew R (1994) MRI of the cardiovascular system (The Raven Press MRI Teaching File). Raven, New York
Duerinckx AJ, Bogaert J, Jiang H, Lewis BS (1995a) Anomalous origin of the left coronary artery: diagnosis by coronary MR angiography [case report]. AJR Am J Roentgenol 164:1095–1097
Duerinckx AJ, Atkinson D, Hurwitz R, Mintorovitch J, Whitney W (1995b) Coronary MR angiography after coronary stent placement [case report]. AJR Am J Roentgenol 165:662–664
Duerinckx AJ, Lewis BS, Louie HW, Urman MK (1996) MRI of pseudoaneurysm of a brachial venous coronary bypass graft. Cathet Cardiovasc Diagn 37:281–286
Duerinckx AJ, Troutman B, Allada V, Kim D (1997a) Coronary MR angiography in Kawasaki disease. A case report. AJR Am J Roentgenol 168:114–116
Duerinckx AJ, Grieten M, Atkinson D, Altamirano J (1997b) Breathhold MR angiography of the internal mammary arteries [abstract]. In: Book of abstracts and Proceedings of the 5th Meeting of the International Society of Magnetic Resonance in Medicine (ISMRM). Vancouver, B.C., Canada, April 12–18, 1997 2:840 (Abstract 840)

Duerinckx AJ, Grant EG, Bakhda RK, To SY, Peters G, Shaaban A (1998a) A phase II study of the use of a new blood pool agent (NC100150) for pulmonary angiography [abstract]. Radiology 209:494

Duerinckx AJ, Atkinson D, Hurwitz R (1998b) Assessment of coronary artery patency after stent placement using magnetic resonance angiography. J Magn Reson Imaging 8:896–902

Duerinckx AJ, Perloff JK, Currier JW (1999a) Arteriovenous fistulae of the circumflex and right coronary arteries with drainage into an aneurysmal coronary sinus. Circulation (11 May 1999):

Duerinckx AJ, Yu WD, El-Saden S, Kim D, Wang JC, Sandhu HS (1999b) MR imaging of cervical spine motion with HASTE. Magn Reson Imaging 17:371–381

Duerinckx AJ, Laughrun D, Lewis BS (1999c) Usefulness of coronary MR angiography prior to angioplasty [in process citation]. Int J Card Imaging 15:533–540

Duerinckx AJ, Shaaban A, Lewis A, Perloff J, Laks H (2000) 3D MR imaging of coronary arteriovenous fistulas. Eur Radiol 10:1459–1463

Duerk JL, Lewin JS, Wendt M, Petersilge C (1998) Remember true FISP? A high SNR, near 1-second imaging method for T2- like contrast in interventional MRI at .2 T. J Magn Reson Imaging 8:203–208

Fayad ZA, Fuster V (2000) Characterization of atherosclerotic plaques by magnetic resonance imaging. Ann N Y Acad Sci 902:173–186

Fayad ZA, Fuster V, Fallon JT, et al (2000a) Noninvasive in vivo human coronary artery lumen and wall imaging using black blood MR [abstract]. In: Book of abstracts and Proceedings of the 8 th Meeting of the International Society of Magnetic Resonance in Medicine (ISMRM 2000 Proceedings available on CD-ROM). Denver, Colorado, 1–7 April 2000; Vol .. of 3: ...

Fayad ZA, Fuster V, Fallon JT, et al (2000b) Noninvasive in vivo human coronary artery lumen and wall imaging using black-blood magnetic resonance imaging. Circulation 102:506–510

Foo TK, Ho VB, Hood MN (2000) Vessel tracking: prospective adjustment of section-selective MR angiographic locations for improved coronary artery visualization over the cardiac cycle. Radiology 214:283–289

Frayne R, Polzin JA, Mazaheri Y, Grist TM, Mistretta CA (1997) Effect of and correction for in-plane myocardial motion on estimates of coronary-volume flow rates. J Magn Reson Imaging 7:815–828

Friedrich MG, Kivelitz D, Strohm O, et al (1999) Intracoronary stents are safe during MR imaging of the heart [abstract]. In: Society for Cardiovascular Magnetic Resonance, Second Meeting, 22–24 January 1999. Atlanta, Georgia, p 36

Galjee MA, vanRossum AC, Doesburg T, vanEenige MJ, Visser CA (1996) Value of magnetic resonance imaging in assessing patency and function of coronary artery bypass grafts. An angiographically controlled study. Circulation 93:660–666

Goldsmith MF (1994) Realizing potential of MR coronary angiography may ease patients' test load and diagnosis costs [editorial]. JAMA 271:256

Hartnell GG, Finn JP, Zenni M, et al (1994) MR imaging of the thoracic aorta: comparison of spin-echo, angiographic and breath-hold techniques. Radiology 191:697–704

Hatsukami TS, Ferguson MS, Beach KW, et al (1997) Carotid plaque morphology and clinical events. Stroke 28:95–100

Hernandez RJ, Aisen AM, Foo TK, Beekman RH (1993) Thoracic cardiovascular anomalies in children: evaluation with a fast gradient-recalled-echo sequence with cardiac-triggered segmented acquisition. Radiology 188:775–780

Higgins CB (1992) Essentials of cardiac radiology and imaging. Lippincott, Philadelphia

Higgins CB, Silverman NH, Kersting-Sommerhoff VA, Schmidt K (1990) Congenital heart disease: echocardiography and magnetic resonance imaging. Raven, New York

Hofman MB, Henson RE, Kovacs SJ, et al (1999) Blood pool agent strongly improves 3D magnetic resonance coronary angiography using an inversion pre-pulse. Magn Reson Med 41:360–367

Hofman MBM, van Rossum AC, Sprenger M, Westerhof N (1996) Assessment of flow in the right human coronary artery by magnetic resonance phase contrast velocity measurements: effects of cardiac and respiratory motion. Magn Reson Med 35:521–531

Hu BS, Meyer CH, Macovski A, Nishimura DG (1996) Multislice spiral magnetic resonance coronary angiography [abstract]. In: Book of abstracts of the 4th Meeting of the International Society of Magnetic Resonance in Medicine (ISMRM). New York, NY, 27 April–3 May 1996, vol 1, p 671 (Abstract 176)

Huber A, Nikolaou K, Gonschior P, Knez A, Stehling M, Reiser M (1999) Navigator echo-based respiratory gating for three-dimensional MR coronary angiography: results from healthy volunteers and patients with proximal coronary artery stenoses. AJR Am J Roentgenol 173:95–101

Hundley WG, Clarke GD, Landau C, et al (1995) Noninvasive determination of infarct artery patency by cine magnetic resonance angiography. Circulation 91:1347–1353

Hundley WG, Lange RA, Clarke GD, et al (1996) Assessment of coronary arterial flow and flow reserve in humans with magnetic resonance imaging. Circulation 93:1502–1508

Hwang SW, Yucel EK, Bernard S (1997) Aortic root abscess with fistula formation. Chest 111:1436–1438

Johansson LO, Nolan NM, Taniuchi M, Fischer SE, Wickline SA, Lorenz CH (1999) High resolution magnetic resonance coronary angiography of the entire heart using a new blood-pool agent, NC100150 injection: comparison with invasive X-ray angiography in pigs. J Cardiovasc Magn Reson 2:139–144

Johnson LW, Lozner EC, Johnson S, et al (1989) Coronary arteriography 1984–1987: a report of the registry of the society for cardiac angiography and interventions. Cathet Cardiovasc Diagn 17:5–10

Kalden P, Kreitner KF, Wittlinger T, et al (1999a) [The assessment of the patency of coronary bypass vessels with a 2D T2- weighted turbo-spin-echo sequence (HASTE) in the breath-hold technic]. Rofo Fortschr Geb Röntgenstr Neuen Bildgeb Verfahr 170:442–448

Kalden P, Kreitner KF, Wittlinger T, et al (1999b) Assessment of coronary artery bypass grafts: value of different breath-hold MR imaging techniques. AJR Am J Roentgenol 172:1359–1364

Kessler W, Achenbach S, Moshage W, et al (1997) Usefulness of respiratory gated magnetic resonance coronary angiography in assessing narrowings > or = 50% in diameter in native coronary arteries and in aortocoronary bypass conduits. Am J Cardiol 80:989–993

Kim JK, Farb RI, Wright GA (1998) Test bolus examination

in the carotid artery at dynamic gadolinium-enhanced MR angiography. Radiology 206:283–289

Kotsakis A, Tan KH, Jackson G (1997) Is MRI a safe procedure in patients with coronary stents in situ? [editorial]. Int J Clin Prac 51:349

Kramer CM, Rogers WJ, Mankad SV, Pakstis DL, Vido D, Reichek N (1999) Short and long-term safety of magnetic resonance imaging soon after stenting for acute myocardial infarction [abstract]. In: Society for Cardiovascular Magnetic Resonance, Second Meeting, 22–24 January 1999. Atlanta, Georgia, p 99

Kramer CM, Rogers WJ, Pakstis DI (2000) Absence of adverse outcomes after magnetic resonance imaging early after stent placement for acute myocardial infarction: a preliminary study. J Cardiovasc Magn Reson 2:257–262

Laissy JP, Grand C, Mator C, Struyven J, Berger JF, Schounan-Claeys E (1995) Magnetic resonance angiography of intravascular endoprosthesis: investigation of three devices. Cardiovasc Intervent Radiol 18:360–366

Langerak SE, Kunz P, Vliegen HW, et al (2001) Improved MR Flow mapping in coronary artery bypass grafts during adenosine-induced stress. Radiology 218:540–547

Laub G, Simonetti O, Nitz W (1995) Single-shot imaging of the heart with HASTE [abstract]. In: Book of abstracts of the 3rd Meeting of the Society of Magnetic Resonance (SMR) and the 12th Annual Scientific Meeting of the European Society for Magnetic Resonance in Medicine and Biology (ESMRMB). Nice, France, 20–25 August 1995 1:246 (Abstract 246)

Lauzon ML, Rutt BK (1993) Generalized k-space analysis and correction of motion effects in MR imaging. Magn Reson Med 30:438–446

Lenhart M, Volk M, Manke C, et al (2000) Stent appearance at contrast-enhanced MR angiography: in vitro examination with 14 stents. Radiology 217:173–178

Lethimonnier F, Furber A, Morel O, et al (1999) Three-dimensional coronary artery MR imaging using prospective real-time respiratory navigator and linear phase shift processing: comparison with conventional coronary angiography. Magn Reson Imaging 17:1111–1120

Li D, Dolan RP, Walovitch RC, Lauffer RB (1998a) Three-dimensional MRI of coronary arteries using an intravascular contrast agent. Magn Reson Med 39:1014–1018

Li D, Zheng J, Bae KT, Woodard PK, Haacke EM (1998b) Contrast-enhanced magnetic resonance imaging of the coronary arteries. A review. Invest Radiol 33:578–586

Lieberman LM, Botti RE, Nelson AD (1984) Magnetic resonance of the heart. Radiol Clin North Am 22:847–858

Lorenz CH, Johansson LO (1999) Contrast-enhanced coronary MRA. J Magn Reson Imaging 10:703–708

Luk-Pat GT, Gold GE, Olcott EW, Hu BS, Nishimura DG (1999) High-resolution three-dimensional in vivo imaging of atherosclerotic plaque. Magn Reson Med 42:762–771

Manke C, Nitz WR, Lenhart M, et al (2000) Magnetic resonance monitoring of stent deployment: in vitro evaluation of different stent designs and stent delivery systems. Invest Radiol 35:343–351

Manning W, Edelman R (1993) Magnetic resonance coronary angiography. Magn Reson Q 9:131–151

Manning WJ, Li W, Edelman RR (1993a) A preliminary report comparing magnetic resonance coronary angiography with conventional angiography. N Engl J Med 328:828–832

Manning WJ, Li W, Boyle NG, Edelman RE (1993b) Fat-suppressed breath-hold magnetic resonance coronary angiography. Circulation 87:94–104

Manning WJ, Li W, Wielopolski P, Gaa J, Kannam JP, Edelman RR (1994) Magnetic resonance coronary angiography: comparison with contrast angiography [abstract]. In: Book of abstracts and Proceedings of the 2nd Meeting of the the Society of Magnetic Resonance (SMR). San Francisco, California, 6–12 August 1994, vol 1, p 368 (Abstract 368)

Manning WJ, Li W, Cohen SI, Johnson RG, Edelman RR (1995) Improved definition of anomalous left coronary artery by magnetic resonance coronary angiography. Am Heart J 130:615–617

McConnell MV, Ganz P, Selwyn AP, Li W, Edelman RR, Manning WJ (1995) Identification of anomalous coronary arteries and their anatomic course by magnetic resonance coronary angiography. Circulation 92:3158–3162

Meaney JF, Prince MR, Nostrant TT, Stanley JC (1997) Gadolinium-enhanced MR angiography of visceral arteries in patients with suspected chronic mesenteric ischemia. J Magn Reson Imaging 7:171–176

Mezrich R (1995) A perspective on k-space. Radiology 195:297–315

Miller S, Scheule AM, Hahn U, et al (1999) MR angiography and flow quantification of the internal mammary artery graft after minimally invasive direct coronary artery bypass. AJR Am J Roentgenol 172:1365–1369

Mohiaddin RH, Bogren HG, Lazim F, et al (1996a) Magnetic resonance coronary angiography in heart transplant recipients [abstract]. In: Book of abstracts of the 4th Meeting of the International Society of Magnetic Resonance in Medicine (ISMRM). New York, NY, 27 April–3 May 1996. 2:671 (Abstract 671)

Mohiaddin RH, Bogren HG, Lazim F, et al (1996b) Magnetic resonance coronary angiography in heart transplant recipients. Coron Artery Dis 7:591–597

Molinari G, Sardanelli F, Zandrino F, Balzan C, Masperone MA (1999) Magnetic resonance assessment of coronary artery bypass grafts. Rays 24:131–139

Ms M, Danias PG, Rm R, Sodickson DK, Kissinger KV, Manning WJ (2001) Superiority of prone position in free-breathing 3D coronary MRA in patients with coronary disease. J Magn Reson Imaging 13:185–191

Müller MF, Fleisch M, Kroeker R (1996) Coronary arteries: three-dimensional MR imaging with fat saturation and navigator echo [abstract]. Radiology 201:274

Müller MF, Fleisch M, Kroeker R, Chatterjee T, Meier B, Vock P (1997) Proximal coronary artery stenosis: three-dimensional MRI with fat saturation and navigator echo. J Magn Reson Imaging 7:644–651

Nagel E, Hug J, Bunger S, et al (1998) Coronary flow measurements for evaluation of patients after stent implantation. Magma 6:184–185

Nitatori T, Hachiya J, Korenaga T, Hanaoka H, Yoshino A (1995a) Clinical application of coronary MR angiography. Studies on shortening of time for examination [abstract]. In: Book of abstracts of the 3rd Meeting of the Society of Magnetic Resonance (SMR) and the 12th Annual Scientific Meeting of the European Society for Magnetic Resonance in Medicine and Biology (ESMRMB). Nice, France, 20–25 August 1995 (Abstract 1390)

Nitatori T, Hanaoka H, Yoshino A, Tominaga M, et al (1995b) Clinical application of magnetic resonance angiography for coronary arteries: correlation with conventional angiography and evaluation of imaging time. Nippon Acta Radiol 55:670–676

Nitatori T, Yoshino H, Yokoyama K, Hachiya J, Ishikawa K (1999) Coronary MR angiography-a clinical experience in Japan. J Magn Reson Imaging 10:709–712

Nitz WR, Kessler W, Stingl D, Moshage W, Laub G (1996) Can we trust breath-hold MR velocity measurements of coronary blood flow? [abstract]. Radiology 201:166

Nyman MA, Schwartz RS, Breen JF, Garratt KN, Holmes DR (1993) Ultrafast computed tomographic scanning to assess patency of coronary artery stents in bypass grafts. Mayo Clin Proc 68:1021–1023

Ohnesorge B, Flohr T, Becker CR, Knez A, Reiser MF (2000) ECG-gated multi-slice cardiac volume CT for coronary CT angiography – initial experience [abstract]. In: Book of abstracts of the First International Workshop on Coronary MR and CT Angiography, Lyon, France, 1–3 Oct 2000. Organized and published by the North American Society for Cardiac Imaging. Reprinted in: Int J Card Imaging

Paulin S, vonSchulthess GK, Fossel E, Krayenbuehl HP (1987) MR imaging of the aortic root and proximal coronary arteries. AJR Am J Roentgenol 148:665–670

Pearlman JD, Edelman RE (1994) Ultrafast magnetic resonance imaging: segmented TurboFLASH, echo-planar, and real-time nuclear magnetic resonance. Radiol Clin North Am 32:593–612

Pennell DJ, Keegan J, Firmin DN, Gatehouse PD, Underwood SR, Longmore DB (1993) Magnetic resonance imaging of coronary arteries: technique and preliminary results. Br Heart J 70:315–326

Pennell DJ, Bogren HG, Keegan J, Firmin DN, Underwood SR (1994) Detection, localization and assessment of coronary artery stenosis by magnetic resonance imaging [abstract]. In: Book of abstracts and proceedings of the 2nd Meeting of the the Society of Magnetic Resonance (SMR). San Francisco, California, 6–12 August 1994. 1:369 (Abstract 369)

Pennell DJ, Bogren HG, Keegan J, Firmin DW, Underwood SR (1994) Coronary artery stenosis: assessment by magnetic resonance imaging [abstract]. In: Book of abstracts of the 11th Annual Scientific Meeting of the European Society for Magnetic Resonance in Medicine and Biology. Vienna, Austria, 20–24 April 1994, p 374 (Abstract 374)

Pennell DJ, Bogren HG, Keegan J, Firmin DN, Underwood SR (1996) Assessment of coronary artery stenosis by magnetic resonance imaging. Heart 75:127–133

Polak JF (2000) MR coronary angiography: are we there yet? [editorial; comment]. Radiology 214:649–650

Post JC, van Rossum AC, Hofman MBM, Valk J, Visser CA (1994a) Current limitations of two dimensional breathhold MR angiography in coronary artery disease [abstract]. In: Book of Abstracts and Proceedings of the 2nd Meeting of the the Society of Magnetic Resonance (SMR). San Francisco, California, 7–12 August 1994; Vol I (Abstract 508)

Post JC, van Rossum AC, Hofman MBM, Valk J, Visser CA (1994b) Respiratory-gated three dimensional MR angiography of coronary arteries and comparison with X-ray contrast angiography [abstract]. In: Book of abstracts and Proceedings of the 2nd Meeting of the the Society of Magnetic Resonance (SMR). San Francisco, California, 7–12 August 1994, (Abstract 509)

Post JC, van Rossum AC, Bronzwaer JGF, et al (1995a) Magnetic resonance angiography of anomalous coronary arteries. A new gold standard for delineating the proximal course? Circulation 92:3163–3171

Post JC, van Rossum AC, Hofman MBM, Valk J, Visser CA (1995b) Clinical utility of two dimensional breathhold MR angiography in coronary artery disease. [abstract]. In: Book of abstracts of the 3rd Meeting of the Society of Magnetic Resonance (SMR) and the 12th Annual Scientific Meeting of the European Society for Magnetic Resonance in Medicine and Biology (ESMRMB). Nice, France, 20–25 August 1995 (Abstract 1394)

Post JC, van Rossum AC, Hofman MB, Valk J, Visser CA (1996) Three-dimensional repiratory-gated MR angiography of coronary arteries: comparison with conventional coronary angiography. AJR Am J Roentgenol 166:1399–1404

Post JC, van Rossum AC, Hofman MB, de Cock CC, Valk J, Visser CA (1997) Clinical utility of two-dimensional magnetic resonance angiography in detecting coronary artery disease. Eur Heart J 18:426–433

Potchen EJ, Haacke EM, Siebert JE, Gottschalk A (1995) Magnetic resonance angiography: concepts and applications. Mosby, St Louis

Prince MR, Yucel EK, Kaufman JA, Harrison DC, Geller SC (1993) Dynamic Gadolinium-enhanced three-dimensional abdominal MR arteriography. J Magn Reson Imaging 3:877–881

Prince MR, Narisimham DL, Stanley JC, et al (1995a) Breath-hold Gadolinium- enhanced MR angiography of the abdominal aorta and its major branches. Radiology 197:785–792

Prince MR, Narasimham DL, Stanley JC, et al (1995b) Gadolinium-enhanced magnetic resonance angiography of abdominal aortic aneurysms. J Vasc Surg 21:656–669

Prince MR, Narasimham DL, Jacoby WT, et al (1996) Three-dimensional Gadolinium-enhanced MR angiography of the thoracic aorta. AJR Am J Roentgenol 166:1387–1397

Prince MR, Grist TM, Debatin JF (1999) 3D contrast MR angiography, 2nd edn. Springer, Berlin Heidelberg New York

Pruessmann KP, Weiger M, Scheidegger MB, Boesiger P (1999) SENSE: sensitivity encoding for fast MRI. Magn Reson Med 42:952–962

Regan F (1999) Clinical applications of half-Fourier (HASTE) MR sequences in abdominal imaging. Magn Reson Imaging Clin North Am 7:275–288

Regenfus M, Ropers D, Achenbach S, et al (1999) Gadolinium enhanced 3D breathhold magnetic resonance angiography for detection of coronary artery stenosis in oblique projection angiograms [abstract]. In: Book of abstracts and Proceedings of the 7th Meeting of the International Society of Magnetic Resonance in Medicine (ISMRM). Philadelphia, 22–28 May 1999, vol 2, p 1262

Rogers LF (1998) The heart of the matter: noninvasive coronary artery imaging [editorial]. AJR Am J Roentgenol 170:841–841

Sakuma H, Blake LM, Amidon TM, et al (1996a) Coronary flow reserve: noninvasive measurement in humans with breath-hold velocity-encoded cine MR imaging. Radiology 198:745–750

Sakuma H, Globits S, O'Sullivan M, et al (1996b) Breath-hold MR measurements of blood flow velocity in internal mammary arteries and coronary artery bypass grafts. J Magn Reson Imaging 6:219–222

Sakuma H, Goto M, Nomura Y, Kato N, Takeda K, Higgins CB (1999) Three-dimensional coronary magnetic resonance angiography with injection of extracellular contrast medium [in process citation]. Invest Radiol 34:503-508

Sandstede JJ, Pabst T, Beer M, et al (1999) Three-dimensional MR coronary angiography using the navigator technique compared with conventional coronary angiography. AJR Am J Roentgenol 172:135-139

Sardanelli F, Molinari G, Zandrino F, Balbi M (2000) Three-dimensional, navigator-echo MR coronary angiography in detecting stenoses of the major epicardial vessels, with conventional coronary angiography as the standard of reference [see comments]. Radiology 214:808-814

Schmermund A, Haude M, Sehnert C, et al (1995) [Noninvasive evaluation of the patency of coronary vessel stents using electron beam tomography segment images with administration of contrast media]. Z Kardiol 84:892-897

Schmermund A, Haude M, Baumgart D, et al (1996) Non-invasive assessment of coronary Palmaz-Schatz stents by contrast enhanced electron beam computed tomography. Eur Heart J 17:1546-1553

Schmidt HC, Voigtlaender T, Kreitner KF, Wittlinger T, Meyer J, Thelen M (1996) Assessment of patency of bypass grafts to the left anterior descending coronary artery: correlation of MR imaging with coronary angiography [abstract]. Radiology 201:273

Schreiber WG, Voigtländer T, Kreitner K-F, et al (1999) Measurement of flow reserve in coronary bypass grafts [abstract]. In: Book of abstracts and proceedings of the 7th Meeting of the International Society of Magnetic Resonance in Medicine (ISMRM). Philadelphia, 22-28 May 1999, vol 1

Schroeder AP, Houlind K, Pederson EM, Thuesen L, Nielsen TT, Egleblad H (2000) Magnetic resonance imaging seems safe in patiens with intracoronary stents. J Cardiovasc Magn Reson 2:43-49

Scott NA, Pettigrew RI (1994) Absence of movement of coronary stents after placement in a magnetic resonance imaging field. Am J Cardiol 73:900-901

Shellock FG, Shellock VJ (1999) Metallic stents: evaluation of MR imaging safety. AJR Am J Roentgenol 173:543-547

Shinnar M, Fallon JT, Wehrli S, et al (1999) The diagnostic accuracy of ex vivo MRI for human atherosclerotic plaque characterization [in process citation]. Arterioscler Thromb Vasc Biol 19:2756-2761

Sodickson DK, Manning WJ (1997) Simultaneous acquisition of spatial harmonics (SMASH): fast imaging with radiofrequency coil arrays. Magn Reson Med 38:591-603

Sodickson DK, Griswold MA, Jakob PM (1999) SMASH imaging. Magn Reson Imaging Clin North Am 7:237-254

Stanford W, Brundage B, MacMillan R, et al (1988) Sensitivity and specificity of assessing coronary bypass graft patency with ultrafast computed tomography: results of a multicenter study. J Am Coll Cardiol 12:1-7

Stanford W, Galvin JR, Skorton DJ, Marcus ML (1991) The evaluation of coronary bypass graft patency: direct and indirect techniques other than coronary arteriography [review article]. AJR Am J Roentgenol 156:15-22

Strohm O, Kivelitz D, Gross W, et al (1999) Safety of implantable coronary stents during 1H-magentic resonance imaging at 1.0 and 1.5 T. J Cardiovasc Magn Reson 1:239-245

Stuber M, Botnar RM, Danias PG, et al (1999a) Double-oblique free-breathing high resolution three-dimensional coronary magnetic resonance angiography. J Am Coll Cardiol 34:524-531

Stuber M, Botnar RM, Danias PG, Kissinger KV, Manning WJ (1999b) Submillimeter three-dimensional coronary MR angiography with real-time navigator correction: comparison of navigator locations. Radiology 212:579-587

Stuber M, Manning WJ (2000) Black-blood coronary MRA [abstract]. In: Book of abstracts of the First International Workshop on Coronary MR and CT Angiography, Lyon, France, 1-3 Oct 2000. Organized and Published by the North American Society for Cardiac Imaging. Reprinted in: Int J Card Imaging

Taylor AM, Panting JR, Keegan J, et al (1999) Safety and preliminary findings with the intravascular contrast agent NC100150 injection for MR coronary angiography. J Magn Reson Imaging 9:220-227

Taylor AM, Keegan J, Jhooti P, Gatehouse PD, Firmin DN, Pennell DJ (2000a) A comparison between segmented k-space FLASH and interleaved spiral MR coronary angiography sequences. J Magn Reson Imaging 11:394-400

Taylor AM, Thorne SA, Rubens MB, et al (2000b) Coronary artery imaging in grown up congenital heart disease: complementary role of magnetic resonance and X-ray coronary angiography. Circulation 101:1670-1678

Teitelbaum GP, Raney M, Carvlin MJ, Matsumoto AH, Barth KH (1989) Evaluation of ferromagnetism and magnetic resonance imaging artifacts of the tantalum vascular stent. Cardiovasc Intervent Radiol 12:125-127

Toussaint JF, Southern JF, Kantor HL, Jang IK, Fuster V (1998) Behavior of atherosclerotic plaque components after in vitro angioplasty and atherectomy studied by high field MR imaging. Magn Reson Imaging 16:175-183

Trouard TP, Altbach MI, Hunter GC, Eskelson CD, Gmitro AF (1997) MRI and NMR spectroscopy of the lipids of atherosclerotic plaque in rabbits and humans. Magn Reson Med 38:19-26

VanCampen LC, deCock C, Bronzwaer JG, vanRossum AC (1995) Single coronary artery: morphological and functional evaluation by MRI [letter]. Eur Heart J 16:2003-2004

Van Geuns RJM, Wielopolski PA, Rensing B, Debruin HG, Defeyter PJ, Oudkerk M (1998) Clinical evaluation of breath-hold MR coronary angiography using targeted volumes [abstract]. In: Proceedings of the Sixth Scientific Meeting of the International Society for Magnetic Resonance in Medicine (ISMRM), 18-24 April 1998. Sydney, Australia, vol 1, p 324 (Abstract #324)

Van Geuns RJ, de Bruin HG, Rensing BJ, et al (1999) Magnetic resonance imaging of the coronary arteries: clinical results from three dimensional evaluation of a respiratory gated technique. Heart 82:515-519

Van Geuns RJ, vanOoijen PMA, Nieman K, Rensing BJ, Oudkerk M, deFeyter PJ (2000a) Initial results with retrospective ECG gated quarter second multi-slice spiral CT [abstract]. In: Book of abstracts of the First International Workshop on Coronary MR and CT Angiography, Lyon, France, 1-3 Oct 2000. Organized and published by the North American Society for Cardiac Imaging. Reprinted in : Int J Card Imaging

Van Geuns RJ, Wielopolski PA, de Bruin HG, et al (2000b) MR coronary angiography with breath-hold targeted volumes: preliminary clinical results. Radiology 217:270-277

VanRossum AC, Galjee MA, Post JC, Visser CA (1997) A practical approach to MRI of coronary artery bypass graft patency and flow. Int J Card Imaging 13:199-204

VanRossum AC, Bedaux WL, Hofman MB (1999) Morphologic and functional evaluation of coronary artery bypass conduits. J Magn Reson Imaging 10:734–740

Voigtlander T (1998) Coronary artery and bypass flow measurement–basic methodology and current status. Magma 6:96–97

Vrachliotis TG, Bis KG, Aliabadi D, Shetty AN, Safian R, Simonetti O (1997) Contrast-enhanced breath-hold MR angiography for evaluating patency of coronary artery bypass grafts. AJR Am J Roentgenol 168:1073–1080

Walpoth BH, Muller MF, Genyk I, et al (1999) Evaluation of coronary bypass flow with color-Doppler and magnetic resonance imaging techniques: comparison with intraoperative flow measurements. Eur J Cardiothorac Surg 15:795–802

Warner OJ, Ohri SK, Pennell DJ, Smith PLC (1996) Magnetic resonance coronary artery imaging for redo coronary operations [case report]. Ann Thorac Surg 62:1513–1516

Weiger M, Pruessmann KP, Boesiger P (1999) High performance cardiac real-time imaging using SENSE [abstract]. In: Book of abstracts and proceedings of the 7th Meeting of the International Society of Magnetic Resonance in Medicine (ISMRM), Philadelphia, PA, 22–23 May 1999, vol 1

Wendt M, Wacker F, Wolf KJ, Lewin JS, Duerk JL (1999) [Keyhole-true FISP: fast T2-weighted imaging for interventional MRT at 0.2 T]. Rofo Fortschr Geb Röntgenstr Neuen Bildgeb Verfahr 170:391–393

Wielopolski PA, van Geuns RJ, de Feyter PJ, Oudkerk M (1998) Coronary arteries. Eur Radiol 8:873–885

Wielopolski PA, van Geuns RJ, de Feyter PJ, Oudkerk M (2000) Coronary arteries. Eur Radiol 10:12–35

Wintersperger BJ, von Smekal A, Engelmann MG, et al (1997) [Contrast media enhanced magnetic resonance angiography for determining patency of a coronary bypass. A comparison with coronary angiography]. Rofo Fortschr Geb Röntgenstr Neuen Bildgeb Verfahr 167:572–578

Wintersperger BJ, Engelmann MG, von Smekal A, et al (1998) Patency of coronary bypass grafts: assessment with breath-hold contrast-enhanced MR angiography – value of a non-electrocardiographically triggered technique. Radiology 208:345–351

Wittlinger T, Voigtlander T, Grauvogel K, et al (1999) [Noninvasive evaluation of coronary bypass grafts by magnetic resonance imaging. Comparison of the Haste and Fisp-3-D sequences with the conventional coronary angiography]. Z Kardiol 89:7–14

Woodard PK, Li D, Dhawale P, et al (1996) Identification of coronary artery stenosis with 3D retrospective respiratory gating [abstract]. In: 96th Annual Meeting of the American Roentgen Ray Society, Supplement to AJR. San Diego, May 5–10, 1996. AJR Am J Roentgenol 166 [Suppl]

Woodard PK, Li D, Haacke EM, et al (1998) Detection of coronary stenosis on source and projection images using three-dimensional MR angiography with retrospective respiratory gating: preliminary experience. AJR Am J Roentgenol 170:883–888

Woodard PK, Li D, Zheng J, Haacke EM, Gropler RJ (1999) Coronary MR angiography. Magn Reson Imaging Clin North Am 7:365–378

Worthley SG, Helft G, Fayad Z, et al (1999) MR imaging documents coronary artery atherosclerotic severity and composition:ex vivo and in vivo studies in a porcine model [abstract]. In: Cardiovascular imaging 1999. The 27 th Annual Meeting of the North American Society for Cardiac Imaging (NASCI), 6 November 1999, Atlanta, Georgia

Worthley SG, Helft G, Fuster V, et al (2000a) Serial in vivo MRI documents arterial remodeling in experimental atherosclerosis. Circulation 101:586–589

Worthley SG, Helft G, Fuster V, et al (2000b) Noninvasive in vivo magnetic resonance imaging of experimental coronary artery lesions in a porcine model. Circulation 101:2956–2961

Worthley SG, Helft G, Fuster V, et al (2000c) High resolution ex vivo magnetic resonance imaging of in situ coronary and aortic atherosclerotic plaque in a porcine model. Atherosclerosis 150:321–329

Worthley SG, Helft G, Fayad ZA, et al (2000d) Images in cardiovascular medicine. Magnetic resonance imaging and asymptomatic aortic dissection. Circulation 101:2771

Yamaoka O, Ikeno K, Fujioka H, et al (1995) Detection of Palmaz-Schatz stent by ultrafast CT. J Comput Assist Tomogr 19:128–130

Yoshino H, Nitatori T, Kachi E, et al (1997) Directed proximal magnetic resonance coronary angiography compared with conventional contrast coronary angiography. Am J Cardiol 80:514–518

Yuan C, Petty C, O'Brien KD, Hatsukami TS, Eary JF, Brown BG (1997) In vitro and in situ magnetic resonance imaging signal features of atherosclerotic plaque-associated lipids. Thromb Arteriosc1 17:1496–1503

Zheng J, Finn JP, Li D (2000a) Contrast-enhanced MR coronary artery imaging on a porcine model: in vivo experience [abstract]. In: Book of abstracts of the First International Workshop on Coronary MR and CT Angiography, Lyon, France, 1–3 Oct 2000. Organized and Published by the North American Society for Cardiac Imaging. Reprinted in: Int J Card Imaging

Zheng J, Li D, Finn JP, Simonetti O, Cavagna FM (2000b) Coronary vessel wall MR imaging: initial experience [abstract]. In: Book of abstracts and Proceedings of the 8th Meeting of the International Society of Magnetic Resonance in Medicine (ISMRM 2000 Proceedings available on CD-ROM). Denver, Colorado, 1–7 April 2000

Zimmermann-Paul GG, Quick HH, Vogt P, von Schulthess GK, Kling D, Debatin JF (1999) High-resolution intravascular magnetic resonance imaging: monitoring of plaque formation in heritable hyperlipidemic rabbits. Circulation 99:1054–1061

17 Pulmonary Vessels

STEFAN SONNET and GEORG M. BONGARTZ

CONTENTS

17.1 Normal Anatomy

The total weight of the lung is about 300–400 g: only about 10% of the lung consists of solid tissue, whereas the rest is composed of airways (dead air space, gas exchange portions) and blood. The supporting structures must be strong enough to maintain architectural integrity and delicate to allow gas exchange. The lungs have a pulmonary and systemic vascular supply.

17.1.1 Anatomy of the Pulmonary Vessels

The pulmonary arteries originate at the pulmonic valve and divide within the pericardium into right and left branches. The right ramus divides into an anterior trunk (to the right upper lobe) and a larger inferior trunk that supplies both, the middle and lower lobes. The portion of the inferior right artery between the lower and middle lobes in the major fissure is called the interlobar artery, in accordance with the bronchial tree. The left ramus is a continuation of the main truncus and divides into an upper and lower lobe artery that supply the upper and lower lobe (including the lingular lobe). The lobar arteries further divide into segmental and subsegmental arteries. Pulmonary arteries take their course in the center of the lobules along the bronchial tree (GREENE 1989). Pulmonary veins run separately from the arteries and can be distinguished by the fact that they are unaccompanied by bronchi and that they extend toward the left atrium. Therefore, lower lobe veins take a more horizontal course and upper lobe veins a more vertical one than the arteries. Arteries that run parallel to veins are difficult to distinguish in magnetic resonance angiography (MRA). Arteriovenous shunts can physiologically be found to various extend in the normal lung, depending on the actual situation and oxygen utilization. The diameter of the thorax in an anterior–posterior orientation often reaches 20 cm, which is important for determining the MRA acquisition volume (Fig. 17.1).

S. SONNET, MD
Department of Radiology, University Hospital, Kantonsspital Basel, Petersgraben 4, 4031 Basel, Switzerland
G.M. BONGARTZ, PhD, MD
Department of Radiology, University Hospital, Kantonspital, Petersgraben 4, 4031 Basel, Switzerland

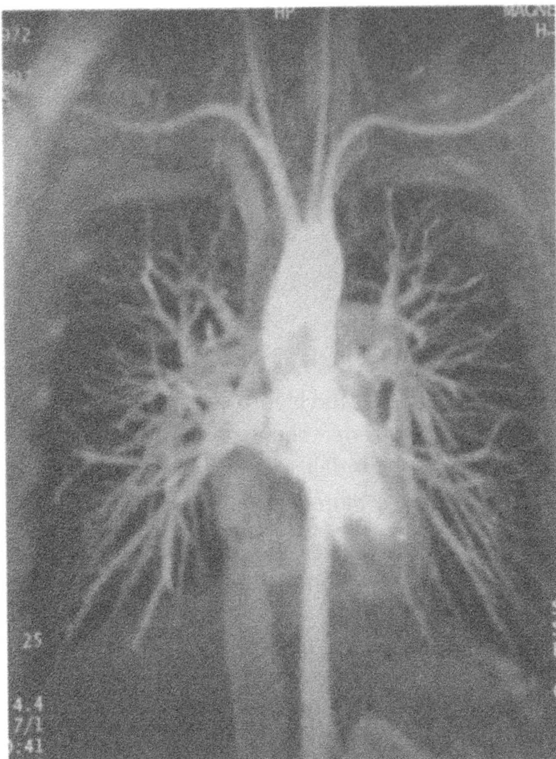

Fig. 17.1. MRA in a healthy volunteer. Pulmonary arteries and veins are both contrasted. Detailed information on the lung's vascular geometry was gained in a single volume measurement of 30 s. For differentiation of venous and arterial vessels, secondary reconstruction of the data is necessary

17.1.2 Pulmonary Blood Supply

The systemic bronchial circulation arises from the thoracic aorta to supply the airways, pulmonary arteries, and veins to the level of the terminal bronchioles. The bronchial arteries originate from the thoracic aorta between the T3 and T7 vertebrae. Up to 35% of individuals have aberrant bronchial arteries which arise from intercostal arteries, internal mammary arteries, the thyrocervical or costocervical trunk, or from the inferior aspect of the aortic arch (Najarian and Morris 1998). The normal bronchial artery is less than 2 mm in size (Song et al. 1998).

The bronchial circulation drains via systemic and pulmonary veins. Drainage through the pulmonary veins produces a small left to right shunt in all individuals.

17.2 Pulmonary Embolism

The role of MRA in different pulmonary vascular diseases is strongly dependent on the relation of vessel size and spatial resolution. Pathological conditions of the pulmonary vasculature comprise occlusion or stenosis of the pulmonary arteries, caused by thromboembolism or external compression (neoplastic disease), congenital cardiovascular anomalies, arteriovenous malformations, and pulmonary hypertension. Diagnosis and exclusion of pulmonary embolism is the central and most crucial indication for pulmonary angiography – therefore, it must be discussed with greater detail than other vascular pathologies.

17.2.1 Etiology and Pathogenesis

It is estimated that in the US 650,000 cases of pulmonary embolism occur each year (Bell and Simon 1982). It accounts for approximately 100,000 deaths per year as the sole cause and is a major contributing cause of death in another 100,000 patients. Pulmonary embolism is the third most frequent cause of death overall (Dalen et al. 1975). Although early detection is very important, the diagnosis is missed in 60%–70% of fatal cases, as shown by autopsy studies.

Pulmonary thromboembolism is characterized by the transport of a fragment of thrombus to the pulmonary circulation and its impaction in the lung. This process is preceded by the formation of a thrombus somewhere in the peripheral venous system.

In most cases the pulmonary emboli derive from the deep veins of the legs. Other relatively common sites are the pelvic veins and the inferior vena cava. Though rare, emboli may also arise from the right ventricle, right-sided heart valves, the superior vena cava, veins of the neck and arms, or hepatic and renal veins. The pathogenesis of cardiac or venous thrombosis is related to one or more of the following factors:

1. Alteration of blood flow caused by stasis or local turbulence
2. Damage to the vessel wall
3. Changes in the coagulability of the blood

Stasis is a quite common cause, resulting from bed rest, for example, in the postoperative period, left-sided heart-failure and shock (decreased arterial output), or prolonged periods of sitting such as during air or ground travel.

Furthermore, in up to 50% of the cases of fatal pulmonary embolism, the source could not be found during life and was not even identified at autopsy (Greenberg 1965; Sevitt 1962).

17.2.2 Symptoms and Signs

In a series of 327 patients a variety of symptoms were observed: chest pain (88%), pleuritis (74%), dyspnea (84%), apprehension (59%), and cough (53%). Symptoms such as hemoptysis (30%), diaphoresis (27%), and syncope (13%) were present only in a minority of the patients.

The most common clinical sign was tachypnea (92%) followed by rales (58%), increased pulmonic secondary sound (53%), tachycardia (44%), and fever (43%). Gallop rhythms (34%), phlebitis (32%), edema (24%), murmur (23%), and cyanosis (19%) were less common signs (Bell et al. 1977).

17.2.3 Ultrasonography and D-Dimer Assay

The deep venous system of the legs is the most frequent origin of pulmonary embolism. Diagnosis of deep venous thrombosis by ultrasonography relies on lack of compressibility rather than on visualization of the thrombus itself. Duplex and color Doppler ultrasound examinations are often used to verify the findings obtained by the compression technique. In areas in which compression may be difficult, such as the adductor canal or the inguinal ligament, Duplex and color Doppler ultrasound can confirm venous patency.

The compression ultrasound examination has several limitations: deep venous thrombi in the calf usually remain undetected, even with color Doppler ultrasonography. Compression abnormalities are sometimes indistinguishable from the original findings of deep venous thrombosis. Thus, it may not be possible to differentiate between a new acute deep venous thrombosis and a previous episode. Furthermore, the ultrasound results are strongly dependent on the operator and on the tissue echo characteristics of the patient.

In about one-third of patients with pulmonary embolism there is no imaging evidence of deep venous thrombosis. In these cases, the thrombus might derive from the pelvic veins, where ultrasonography is usually unreliable, or the thrombus may have already embolized into the lung. Even in normal ultrasound examinations, the work-up for pulmonary embolism must be continued if there is high clinical suspicion of pulmonary embolism. Among symptomatic out-patients suspected of having deep venous thrombosis of the thigh, the reliability of venous ultrasonography is well established. The combination of this noninvasive test with ventilation–perfusion scintigraphy has increased the rate of positive identification of patients who would profit from therapeutic anticoagulation to 71% (Mayo et al. 1997).

The quantitative plasma D-dimer enzyme-linked immunosorbent assay (ELISA), indicating endogenous thrombolysis, is a noninvasive test to rule out pulmonary embolism. It has a high sensitivity and negates the need for further diagnostic work-up. No patient with pulmonary embolism or deep venous thrombosis had a negative D-dimer assay as shown in a study by Owings et al. (2000). The specificity of this assay is low, however, since D-dimer levels increase in patients after surgical interventions, myocardial infarction, sepsis, and some other systemic disorders.

17.2.4 Conventional Pulmonary Angiography and Scintigraphy

Conventional pulmonary angiography with its exquisite resolution still serves as the gold standard for the diagnosis of pulmonary embolism, showing a high sensitivity and specificity and offering the option of introducing therapeutic local fibrinolysis or mechanical disintegration of central emboli (Stock et al. 1997).

The need to search for a noninvasive method of detecting pulmonary embolism was prompted by the known morbidity and mortality of invasive pulmonary angiography (6% and 0.5%, respectively) (Mayo et al. 1997). The most frequently applied noninvasive test is ventilation–perfusion scintigraphy if pulmonary embolism is suspected. According to the outcome of the PIOPED study (Prospective Investigation Of Pulmonary Embolism Diagnosis; PIOPED Investigators 1990) the reliability of this test is under debate: A normal result of pulmonary scintigraphy and a low-probability scan in combination with low clinical suspicion can rule out the diagnosis of a pulmonary embolism. In those patients in whom a high-probability scan is associated with a strong clinical suspicion of pulmonary embolism, the positive predictive value reaches 96%. In-between this margins, all other combinations give equivocal results. In the population investigated by the PIOPED study, about 66% of the cases could not be diagnosed definitively by scintigraphy and clinical investigation alone (Kelley et al. 1991; Gefter et al. 1995; Bergin et al. 1997).

17.2.5 Computed Tomographic Angiography

Spiral computed tomographic (CT) angiography is an excellent technique for imaging the pulmonary arteries up to a segmental level with a high sensitivity and specificity. Helical CT is easy to implement and gives quick results and additional information about other thoracic pathologies. The low invasiveness and the fast scanning procedure make CT angiography the number one clinical diagnostic evaluation of pulmonary embolism today. Several protocols have been suggested, with emphasis on thin-slice acquisition techniques with optimized contrast within the pulmonary arteries (Rémy-Jardin et al. 2000). With the recent development of multislice scanning technology, even faster data acquisition is possible and the improved image resolution provides excellent depiction of subsegmental emboli.

17.2.6 Diagnostic Work-up of Pulmonary Embolism

When pulmonary embolism is suspected clinically, a fixed protocol should be initiated which includes different tests in a defined order, starting with the blood D-dimer assay as a noninvasive and effective method to rule out pulmonary embolism. If the result of this test is negative, no further diagnostic studies are needed because a thromboembolic event is excluded with very high probability and, therefore, expensive or invasive diagnostic tests can be avoided (Owings et al. 2000). Of course, in rare cases false-negative results may occur, namely, in small emboli or metabolic disorders.

If the results of the D-dimer test are positive, evaluation of the deep venous system of the legs by ultrasonography is the second step in the diagnostic hierarchy. If a deep venous thrombosis is found in the legs, no further diagnostic steps are required and therapy for PE is indicated. If there is no evidence of deep venous thrombosis by ultrasonography, diagnostic work-up must be continued.

The next step is spiral CT angiography of the pulmonary arteries, which can visualize the embolus directly as a partial or complete intravascular obliteration of the contrast media bolus. Exclusion of emboli is possible up to the segmental arteries whereas detection and exclusion in the subsegmental vessels is less certain. CT angiography, to date, is regarded as the method of choice in the evaluation of pulmonary embolism; it is even considered superior to digital subtraction angiography (DSA) because of the cross-sectional and three-dimensional access to the image information.

The reliability of ventilation–perfusion scintigraphy is under debate since the PIOPED study presented only successful and reliable results in only one third of the cases. Scintigraphy can primarily be regarded as insufficient when coexisting pulmonary diseases such as emphysema are present.

17.2.7 Possible Role of MRA

MRA is known to have a superior contrast resolution and optimal suppression of background tissue. Initial studies demonstrated the ability of MRA to visualize subsegmental pulmonary arteries with fine detail and to profit from the well-tolerated non-nephrotoxic contrast medium. With further improvement in acquisition speed and with more skill in monitoring the patients in the magnet, MRA may offer an alternative or even compete with CT angiography in patients suspected of having pulmonary embolism.

17.3 MRA of Pulmonary Vessels: Imaging Techniques

17.3.1 Two- and Three-dimensional Time-of-Flight Techniques

Time-of-flight angiography (inflow angiography) was successfully applied to image the pulmonary arteries (Wielopolski et al. 1993) in the early 1990s. This technique is based on saturation of the stationary tissue, which is optimal in the lung, and on the strong signal enhancement from in-flowing blood. The saturation of stationary tissue can be further improved by fast repetition of the radio frequency pulses. The signal enhancement of the flowing blood depends on several factors, including the velocity of the flowing blood, the flow profile, and unsaturated blood in volume of interest. It has been proven that three-dimensional time-of-flight techniques are superior to two-dimensional techniques for imaging of segmental pulmonary arteries (Scialpi et al. 1998) due to the low resolution of the two-dimensional technique. By using three-dimensional applications both the signal-to-noise ratio and resolution are improved. Furthermore, flow void due to intravoxel dephasing is reduced by the smaller voxel size of three-dimensional data sets, and multiplanar reprojection and maximum intensity projection reconstructions are possible. All time-of-flight techniques are associated with artifacts due to slow flow, field distortion artifacts and motion from cardiac pulsation and breathing. Therefore, tremendous misregistration may occur and slow-flowing blood in segmental pulmonary arteries can be misinterpreted as embolus.

Scanning time is long and varies from around 5 to 13 min. Breath-holding is therefore not feasible for three-dimensional time-of-flight imaging. Two different techniques, pseudogating and respiratory gating, have been developed to suppress motion artifacts from breathing (Wielopolski et al. 1992).

Time-of-flight techniques without the use of contrast agents for the detection of pulmonary emboli are time consuming and hampered by motion artifacts, insufficient resolution, and saturation (Hoffmann et al. 1999).

17.3.2 Contrast-Enhanced MRA

Because of the close proximity to the heart very fast flow velocities are found in the thoracic vessels. To reduce motion artifacts caused by breathing and pulsation, faster imaging concepts and new data acquisition techniques are required. With the recent generations of scanners, new strong and ultrafast gradient echo sequences were also developed to perform ultrafast MRA. The fundamentals of pulmonary contrast-enhanced MRA are extremely fast gradient switching times and sufficiently short duty cycles of the powerful gradient systems. Still, residual artifacts, especially at the cardiac border are inevitable since standard data acquisition times for ultrafast MRA vary from around 10 to 30 s. Measuring times have to be kept as short as possible because patients with pulmonary embolism are usually short of breath and the arteriovenous circulation time is very short. Patients can often tolerate breath-hold periods even up to 30 s, whereas most times breath-hold periods as short as 20 s are already too long. It is sensible to practice the actual breath-hold period prior to the examination and to supply oxygen via a nasal tube.

17.3.3 Acquisition Volume

The vascular tree of the lung is larger in the cephalocaudad direction than in the anterior–posterior direction. Therefore, in order to restrict the number of slices required to cover the entire vasculature of the lung to the smallest possible number, a frontal (coronal) imaging plane is beneficial. It covers both lungs simultaneously. Anteroposteriorly, it can even be restricted to a volume slightly smaller than the entire lung. The acquisition plane is usually tilted along the vertebral axis into an oblique frontal-axial orientation. By doing so, some vessels of the lung base are missed, but the overlying signals from the heart are also cut off (Fig. 17.2).

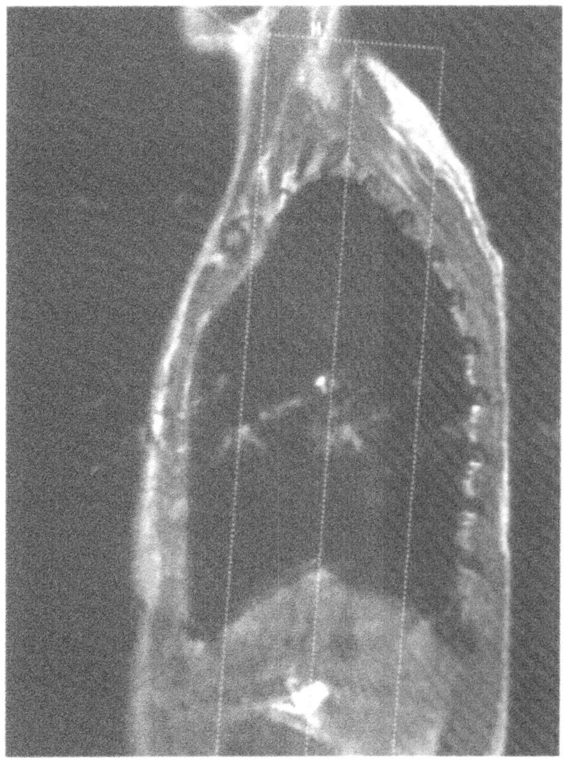

Fig. 17.2. The three-dimensional acquisition volume is tilted along the vertebral axis into an oblique frontal-axial orientation. Some vessels of the lung base are missed, but also the overlying signals from the heart are cut off

Another approach for visualizing the pulmonary vessels by MRA is to separately measure each lung in a sagittal orientation. There are two main advantages: first, improved resolution, and second, cut off of the cardiac signals. The disadvantage of sequential imaging is the doubled amount of contrast medium required and the prolonged imaging time. By a simultaneous, double-slab acquisition, contrast medium can be saved, but at the cost of resolution.

Three-dimensional contrast-enhanced MRA is related to the maximal intravascular T1 shortening during the data acquisition period. For pulmonary MRA, body phased-array coils should be used to improve the signal-to-noise ratio and to reduce the active imaging field to a minimum to prevent aliasing of structures from outside the thorax. Positioning patients with the arms elevated is optimal, but they cannot always tolerate this position throughout the entire imaging procedure. When the arms are positioned along the thorax, aliasing must be prevented by applying a larger field of view. Alternatively, the arms can be placed anteriorly outside the coil.

17.3.4 Flip Angle

Background saturation can be improved by using a higher flip angle (Bosmans and Marchal 1996; Stehling et al. 1996). Thus, if the T1 values of the contrasted blood are reduced to 20–80 ms, which is readily achieved by a dilution of up to 1/200, the optimal flip angle can be calculated to 20–40° (for TR=5 ms). The slice profile varies with different flip angles, since for lower flip angles the entire profile is more homogeneous because the edges are less pronounced than with higher flip angles. At higher flip angles, short T1 tissues such as fat at the outer contour of the imaging volume can cause signal overlay, resulting in diagnostic problems.

17.3.5 Contrast Media Administration

For ultrafast MRA a fast contrast medium bolus and the data acquisition period must be coordinated to achieve optimal image quality. In thoracic MRA the entire pulmonary circulation should be covered, separately for arteries and veins. MRA must be able to clearly define vascular occlusions. The most important issues are sufficient covering of the volume to be investigated within the given time frame, sufficient image resolution and reconstructability, as well as timing problems concerning the patient's compliance and bolus timing. During the data acquisition period, 3D MRA requires a stable maximum of intravascular T1 shortening, which is achieved by an adequately timed and configured intravenous gadolinium bolus. The contrast provided by the contrast medium does not need to persist at a maximum level during the entire measurement, but must be maximized during acquisition of the central part of the k - space (Bongartz et al. 1997). During this period, the contrast of the entire MR angiogram is defined owing to the holographic nature of signal determination in MRI (see Chap. 4, this volume). Pulmonary arteries and veins can only be distinguished by the exact timing of the contrast bolus injection and coordination to the center of the k-space acquisition.

To obtain optimal results, the individual pulmonary circulation time should be tested by peripherally injecting a contrast media test bolus of 1–2 ml. Simultaneous to the injection of the test bolus, a time-resolved, single slice sequence is started to evaluate the bolus arrival time (BAT) at the vessel of interest. To reduce in-flow phenomena, the image orientation has to be adjusted to the main in-flowing artery (coronal or sagittal). Alternatively, presaturation pulses can be applied. For acceptable image quality, a single dose of a standard gadolinium compound (0.1 mmol per kg BW) has been shown to be sufficient using a flip angle of 25° (Bongartz et al. 1997); a double dose (0.2 mmol/kg BW) added only little information, whereas a half dose (0.05 mmol/kg BW) gave lower image quality. The quality of these three dosages was described according to the signal to noise ratio at the main pulmonary arteries and the number of visible vascular generations at the mediobasal lower lobe.

Another alternative is to perform a high resolution three-dimensional angiography during the contrast steady state by using blood pool agents (such as USPIO, Nycomed Amersham). Consequently, longer acquisition times are possible, whereby the signal to noise ratio and therefore resolution are improved. However, longer acquisition times require compensation mechanisms for respiratory motion such as navigator techniques (Ahlstrøm et al. 1998): Every time a new line of the k-space is acquired, data on the position of the diaphragm are recorded simultaneously. Data are only accepted for image processing if the diaphragm is within a preset threshold. Therefore a breath-hold period is not necessary, which is an advantage in patients who suffer from severe dyspnea.

The above mentioned contrast media are non-nephrotoxic and low-allergenic.

17.3.6 Sequences

Acceptable image quality can be achieved in patients who can hold their breath only for 5–10 s by interactive triggering of the data acquisition (Riederer et al. 1998). With fluoroscopic triggering single two-dimensional slices at the main pulmonary artery are acquired in 1 s time resolution and displayed in real-time. When the contrast agent reaches the vessel of interest, the operator immediately starts a centrically reordered three-dimensional angiography (Wilman and Riederer 1997). Optimally, an elliptical, centric view order of data sampling in both phase-encoding directions is applied in this type of interactive sequence to optimize contrast within the arteries under investigation. The centrically reordered acquisition is mandatory since the contrast medium has already reached the vascular area of interest when the sequence is started. Suppression of the venous signal by individually suited fluoroscopic timing is superior to symmetric k-space data order.

Subtraction technique (DS-MRA) can be applied to pulmonary MRA in order to improve vascular contrast, mainly by suppression of high-signal areas such as fatty tissue of the thoracic wall or at the mediastinum. Prior to the original data acquisition, an identical three-dimensional data set is acquired. It serves as background subtraction of the contrast-enhanced data set on a pixel-by-pixel basis. A minor mismatch of the vascular geometry can be neglected, because the vessels are dark during the first (native) sequence and the direct surrounding pulmonary tissue is free of signal in both acquisitions. In direct comparison of a subtracted and a nonsubtracted MR angiogram, the gain in peripheral detail detectability is readily apparent (Fig. 17.3a, b).

Repetition of several measurements of 20 s acquisition time each, separated by a short breathing interval of 5–10 s, makes it possible to observe several perfusion phases, e.g., arterial and venous phases of the pulmonary vascular perfusion. Especially in cases of vascular anomalies, arteriovenous malformations or venous obstructions, the delayed images are very important clinically. Subtraction techniques can also be used for improvement of vascular contrast; the different phases of arterial, arteriovenous, and venous signals can be subtracted in order to provide venous angiograms or arterial angiograms separately.

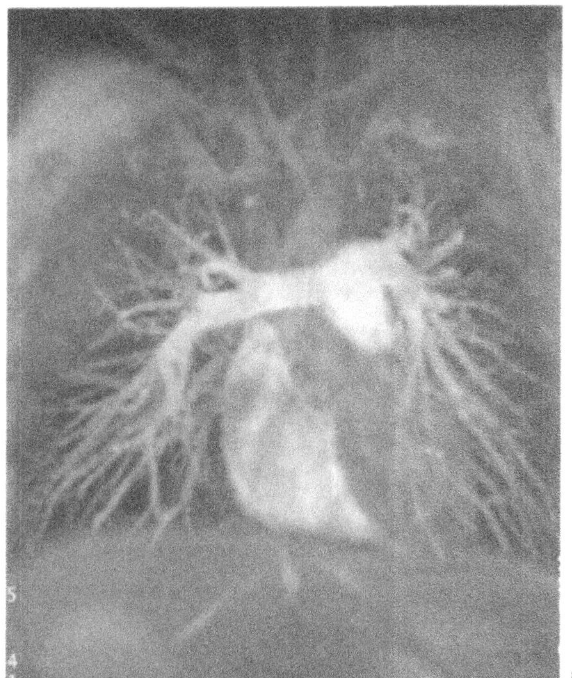

a

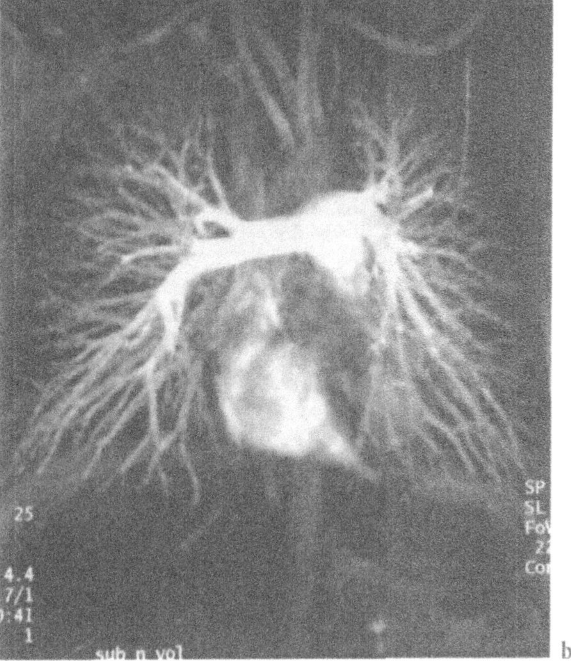

b

Fig. 17.3a, b. Example of the value of subtraction technique (DS-MRA). Before contrast media injection, an identical three-dimensional native data set is acquired, which is subtracted from the contrast enhanced MRA (**a**). The direct comparison of a subtracted (**b**) and a non-subtracted MR angiogram (**a**) demonstrates better peripheral detail in (**b**)

Technically, the acquisition of the huge amount of data can cause problems if the computer does not have sufficient random access memory (RAM). Postponing data processing until after the measurement facilitates the sequential MRA approach.

In order to assess not only perfusion of the major vessels but also of the lung parenchyma (small interstitial vessels), the data acquisition must be accelerated, i.e., to the order of seconds. Of course, three-dimensional data sets as usually used for pulmonary MRA are too long to achieve this information.

Fast projective MRA is a valuable alternative: the technique recently has been introduced for cerebral projection MRA (WETZEL et al. 2001) but can be applied to the pulmonary vasculature accordingly.

An ultrafast gradient echo sequence based two-dimensional MRA with a slab thickness of 8–10 cm and a high in-plane resolution is applied in coronal direction to cover the entire lung (Fig. 17.4).

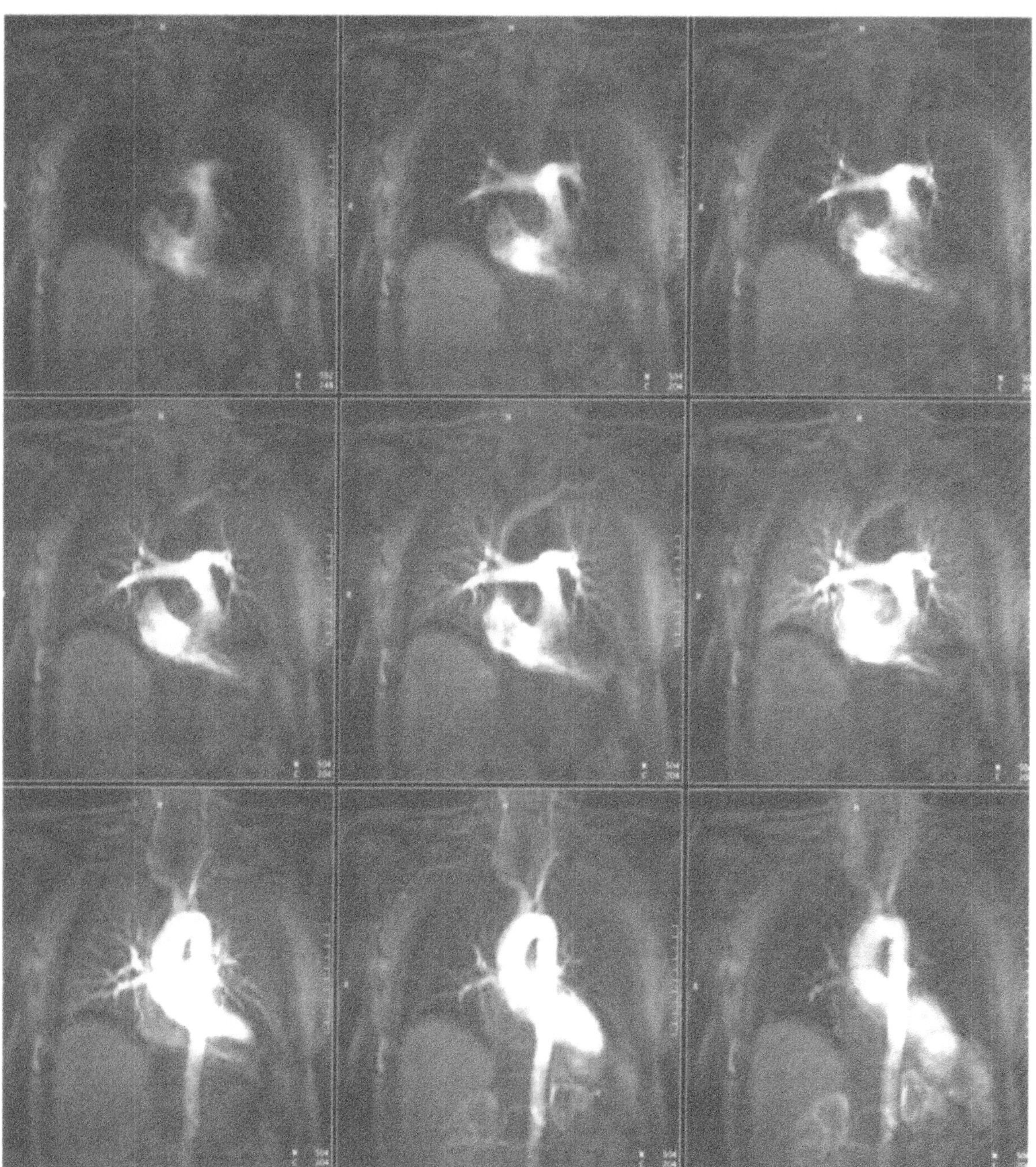

Fig. 17.4. Two-dimensional contrast-enhanced projection angiography allowing high time resolution to depict the pulmonary vessels in a single projection. Parenchymal perfusion is demonstrated by selected sequential images

17.3.7 Postprocessing

In pulmonary MRA source image review and image postprocessing are mandatory. Frequently, pathological conditions are easily demonstrated on the standard maximum intensity projection (MIP) images. Sometimes, however, conditions such as pulmonary emboli are hidden at locations where an abrupt change in vessel size occurs, e.g., at vascular branches. In these cases dedicated MIP reconstructions are useful: subvolume targeting on MR angiograms with smaller, 1- to 2-cm volumes are supposed to be ideal to show all components of a branching vessel and give an optimal image perspective. Larger subvolumes often show an overlap of vessels within the chosen volume and are therefore less useful, but good overall demonstration of the pulmonary vessels can be obtained.

Other techniques such as multiplanar reconstruction (MPR) or volume rendering (VR) help to increase confidence in determining the presence or absence of a pathologic condition (Fig. 17.5a,b). Of course correct windowing is of major importance, because suboptimal window settings may obscure pulmonary vascular pathologies (Gupta et al. 1999).

For blood pool contrast MRA, complicated and time consuming postprocessing is required for the differentiation between arteries and veins and is still under evaluation.

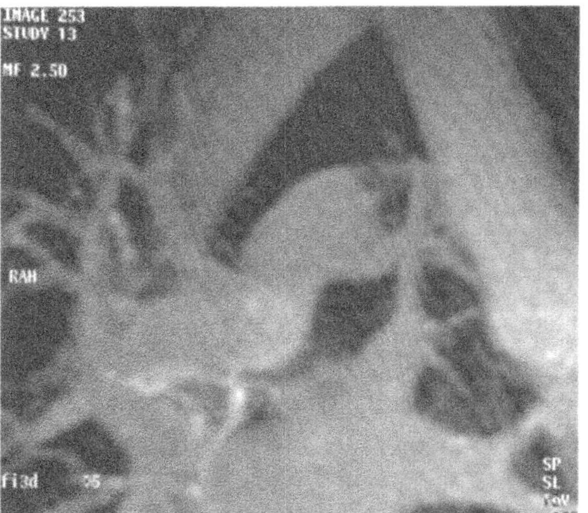

a

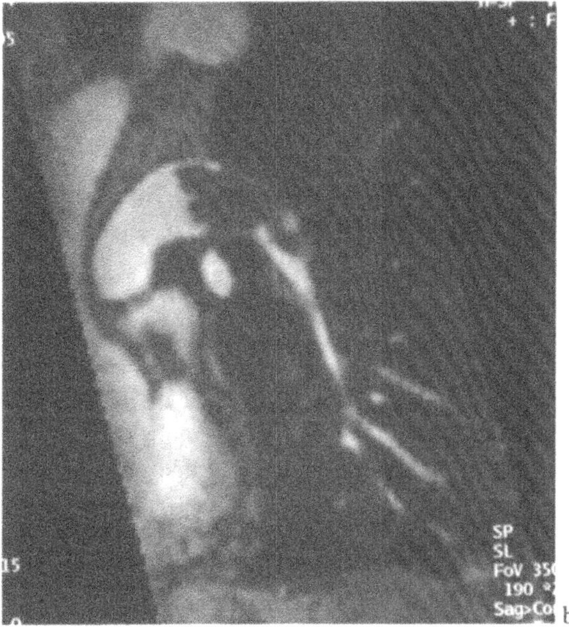

b

Fig. 17.5. MRA is displayed as a semi-coronal MIP reconstruction in (**a**), in which the dark thromboembolism is partially covered by the descending thoracic aorta and as a multiplanar reconstruction along the course of the left main pulmonary artery in (**b**), where the same pathology is perfectly separated. The subtotal occlusion has led to prestenotic enlargement of the vessel and narrowing of the lumen distally

17.4 Clinical MRA

Besides pulmonary embolism the main indications for performing pulmonary MRA are congenital heart anomalies, pulmonary arteriovenous malformation or fistulas, vascular anomalies, pulmonary hypertension, and obstruction of the pulmonary arteries by a tumorous mass.

17.4.1 Usefulness and Advantages of Pulmonary MRA

The advantages of MRA are the lack of radiation, the non-nephrotoxic and low-allergenic contrast media, and the three-dimensional access to the vessels with the possibility of reconstructing the data individually. Pulmonary MRA may be preferred to CT angiography in patients who are allergic to CT contrast agents containing iodine or during pregnancy.

MRA, like CT angiography, provides cross-sectional and thus three-dimensional information on the pathology and enables dedicated image reconstruction which is focussed on the pathology. It can offer simultaneous access to the vascular lumen, the vessel wall, and surrounding tissues.

17.4.2 Indications for Pulmonary Angiography

17.4.2.1 *Pulmonary Embolism*

Segmental and subsegmental arteries can be displayed by MRA, which supports its use in patients with pulmonary embolism. The thromboembolic material usually consists of older clots, fibrous tissue, and fresh thrombotic material, which together often give a heterogeneous signal intensity. The embolus should be delineated because the contrasted blood has a significantly shorter T1. Demonstration and exact localization of central and peripheral emboli have been shown in several publications (Bongartz et al. 1997; Gupta et al. 1999; Meaney et al. 1997) and the use of MRA in the clinical work-up of the disease has been foreseen. The superiority of this technique in demonstrating subsegmental pathologies is encouraging.

The simultaneous demonstration of the direct effects on the pulmonary tissue by means of perfusion MRA underline the potential usefulness of MR investigations in patients suffering from pulmonary embolism.

Pulmonary angiography often fails in patients with pulmonary embolism because they are usually very short of breath and need to be monitored throughout the investigation. All secondary instrumentation such as control monitors, ECG leads, pulse oxygenation control, and others add problems to the MR investigation. The required breath-hold periods of 15–20 s for optimal MRA results are most times too long for these patients, who, moreover, frequently present with claustrophobia. Further problems are given by the limited access to suitable MR technology in many clinics. For correct interpretation of the image highly experienced radiologists are needed who are familiar with postprocessing procedures.

17.4.2.2 *Anomalies and Chronic Disorders*

Pulmonary MRA is an excellent imaging modality in patients with chronic disease who present without acute clinical symptoms and can easily tolerate the imaging procedure. In congenital pulmonary vascular malformations such as pulmonary sequestration, anomalous venous return (PAPVR), or other anomalies, pulmonary MRA is an excellent method for demonstrating the aberrant vessel course in a three-dimensional display (Fig. 17.6). Therefore, MRA is often superior to projective DSA. Time-resolved, sequential MRA is helpful in the evaluation of anomalous vessels, especially when clinically relevant shunts occur. Some vessels may be hidden in the static three-dimensional MIP display of the entire vascular tree and only become visible during a short period of time and, thus, in sequential acquisition.

In patients with pulmonary arteriovenous malformation MRA images may provide information about the number and size of feeding and draining vessels prior to surgery or radiological embolization therapy.

Hemangiomas may be able to be visualized, depending on their perfusion rate and the size of the vascular supply (Fig. 17.7a, b).

17.4.2.3 *Vascular Compression*

Furthermore, MRA is used to show the relationship between malignant central neoplasms and contiguous vessels. The degree of vascular compression is demonstrated in multiple views and the effect on the lung parenchyma in severe stenoses can be

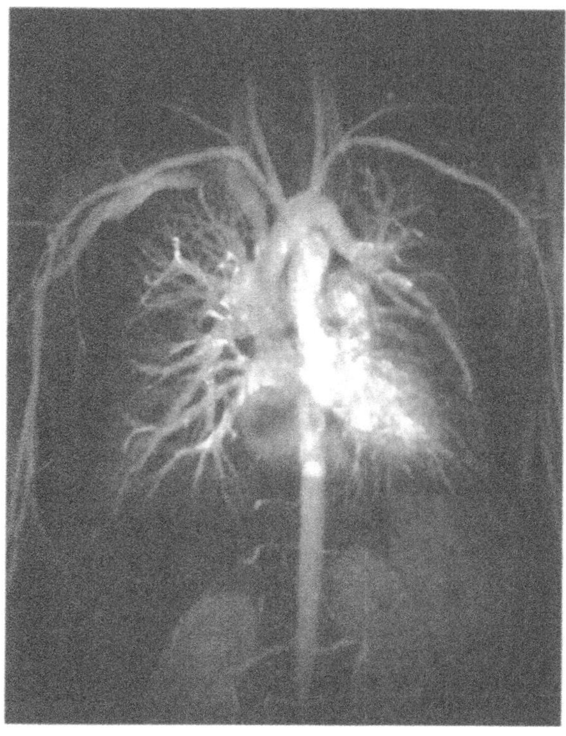

Fig. 17.6. Partial anomalous pulmonary venous return in which the anomalous vein of the left upper lobe drains into the high portion of superior vena cava. The pathological details are clearly shown by three-dimensional contrast-enhanced MRA

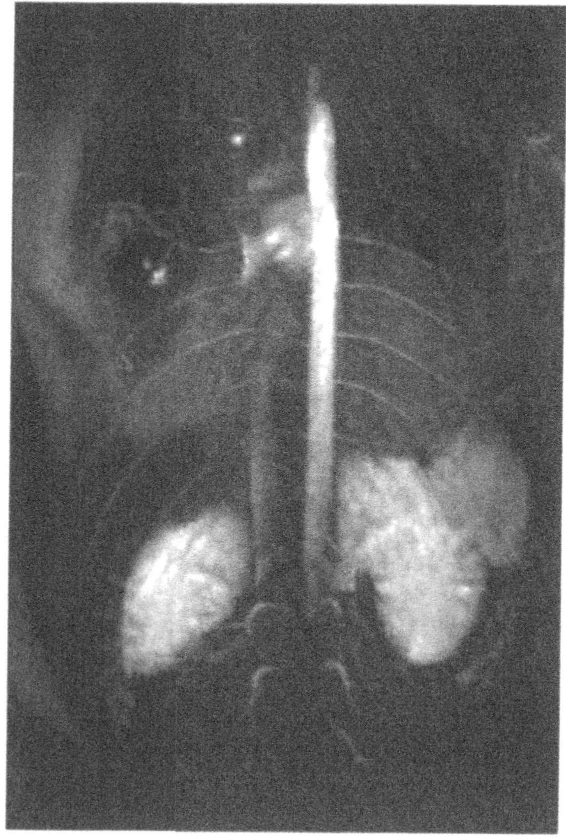

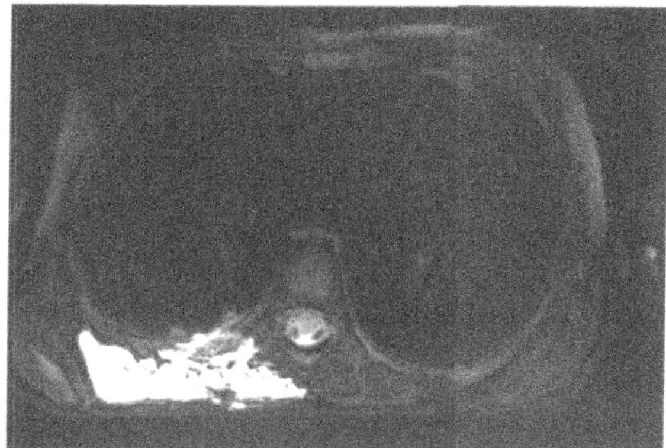

Fig. 17.7a, b. A huge hemangioma of the dorsal thoracic wall in a 18-year-old patient. The presurgical diagnostic work-up included MRI to demonstrate the depth and invasiveness of the tumor (**b**). The high-resolution MRA of the region displayed a small feeding vessel deriving from the 8th intercostal artery directly pointing at an aneurysmatic vascular dilatation within the hemangioma. Another aneurysmatic alteration is visible three segments further in cephalad direction (**a**)

documented simultaneously. The direct access to the tumor and the vessel by combining MRI and MRA is clinically significant for treatment planning (Fig. 17.8).

17.4.3 Results and Comparison with other Imaging Modalities

Of course, the spatial resolution of CT and MRA is worse than that of conventional pulmonary angiography, but imaging of the pulmonary arteries and exclusion or proof of pulmonary embolism is possible to the level of segmental arteries: In several articles the diagnosis of pulmonary embolism with spiral CT has been described. Since RÉMY-JARDIN et al. published the first prospective study comparing conventional pulmonary angiography and helical CT in 1992, several subsequent studies have also confirmed the high competence of helical CT in the diagnosis of pulmonary embolism, with approximately 90% specificity and 90% sensitivity at the segmental level and above (RÉMY-JARDIN et al. 1992, 1996).

In a prospective study comparing MRA to conventional pulmonary angiography in 30 patients clinically suspected of having pulmonary embolism,

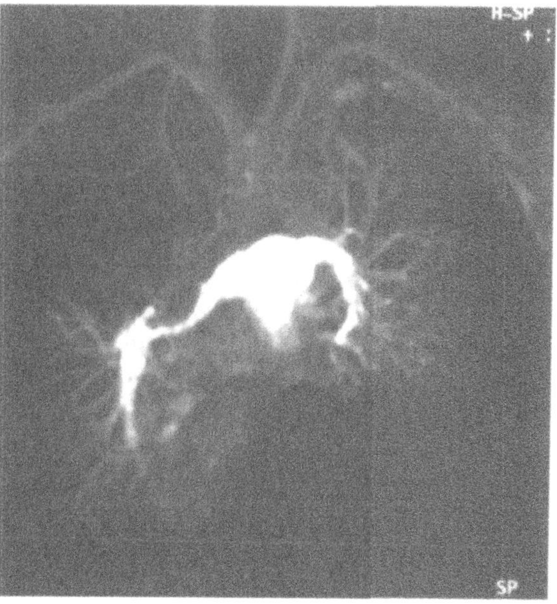

Fig. 17.8. Three-dimensional contrast enhanced MRA (maximum intensity projection reconstruction) demonstrating an osteogenic sarcoma of the pulmonary artery in the lumen of the right pulmonary artery. The artery of the right upper lobe is not contrasted due to tumor occlusion

Meaney et al. (1997) described a sensitivity of 87.3% and a specificity of 96.6%. With conventional angiography, 22 sites of pulmonary embolism were detected: five emboli were identified as lobar disease and 17 emboli in the segmental arterial branches. Overall, 21 of these 22 sites of embolism were equally detected with MRA: one segmental embolus identified by conventional angiography was not detected by MRA and only one false-positive finding in MRA was found by two of the three readers.

Another prospective evaluation of pulmonary MRA compared to conventional pulmonary angiography in 36 consecutive patients by Gupta et al. (1999) reached a sensitivity of 87% and a specificity of 100% when subsegmental emboli were ignored. A total of 19 acute pulmonary emboli were depicted in 13 patients by conventional pulmonary angiography whereas 13 of these emboli were prospectively found by pulmonary MRA. Six emboli were missed by MRA, of which four were localized subsegmentally and only two were on a segmental level. Therefore, MRA demonstrated a high accuracy for detecting acute emboli on a lobar or segmental level.

In another study, three-dimensional contrast-enhanced MRA was compared with selective intraarterial DSA in 20 patients with chronic thromboembolic hypertension by Kreitner et al. (2000). MRA depicted the pulmonary vessels up to a segmental level in all patients and demonstrated a sensitivity of 87% and a specificity of 100% in delineation of the subsegmental arteries (371/424 patent subsegmental arteries).

17.5 Conclusion

The niche for noninvasive angiographic imaging of pulmonary embolic disease is defined by the known diagnostic problems caused by the results of ventilation–perfusion scintigraphy. In about two thirds of the cases, the combined diagnostic results of clinical investigation and scintigraphy are not sufficient to submit the patient to a defined therapeutic regimen. Among the two methods CT angiography and MRA, only CT angiography is currently used in clinical routine and is an approved method for diagnosis of pulmonary thromboembolic disease. CT angiography will be improved by fast multislice scanners in the future.

Three-dimensional contrast-enhanced MRA is a excellent noninvasive imaging technique for the pulmonary arteries and an accurate technique for depicting central, lobar, and segmental emboli. It is still an unreliable method for detecting small subsegmental emboli. Moreover, MRA is performed with non-nephrotoxic and low-allergenic contrast media and does not require ionizing radiation. In comparison to pulmonary angiography it is less expensive and does not require hospitalization. Faster data acquisition with even shorter TE and TR will lead to shorter breath-hold periods, fewer artifacts caused by motion, and improved resolution. Furthermore, ultrasmall superparamagnetic iron oxide particles as a blood pool contrast agent have already been developed and will improve imaging quality in the future, in combination with navigator gating without breath-hold and with intelligent postprocessing. MRA still is under technical development and is steadily being improved.

Nevertheless, the role of MRA for the diagnosis of pulmonary embolism is uncertain. Among the two methods CT angiography and MRA, only CT is used today in the clinical routines for diagnosis of pulmonary thromboembolic disease. The clinical use of MRA is hampered by problems in patient monitoring, the limited access to suitable MR technology, patient claustrophobia, and the still relatively long measurement time which necessitates a relatively long breath-hold period. Furthermore, correct image interpretation is difficult and requires complicated postprocessing procedures and highly experienced radiologists. MR perfusion imaging is a new technique for the detection of perfusion defects distal to pulmonary emboli (Haraldseth et al. 1999) and might be promising in the future in combination with MRA.

References

Ahlstrøm H, Johansson L, Ragnarsson A, Borseth A (1998) Pulmonary MRA during continuous breathing using a blood pool agent and navigator echo. In: Proceedings of the International Society of Magnetic Resonance Medicine, Sixth Scientific Meeting, Abstract 170

Bell WR, Simon TL (1982) Current status of pulmonary thromboembolic disease: pathophysiology, diagnosis, prevention, and treatment. Am Heart J 103:239–262

Bell WR, Simon TL, DeMets DL (1977) The clinical features of submassive and massive pulmonary emboli. Am J Med 62:355–360

Bergin CJ, Sirlin CB, Hauschildt JP, Huynh TV, Auger WR, Fedullo PF, Kapelanski DP (1997) Chronic thromboembolism: diagnosis with helical CT and MR imaging with angiographic and surgical correlation. Radiology 204:695

Bongartz G, Boos M, Winter K, Brändli M, Scheffler K (1997) MR Angiographie der Thorakalgefässe. Radiologe 37:529

Bongartz G, Boos M, Scheffler K, Steinbrich W (1998) Pulmonary circulation. Eur Radiol 8:698–706

Bosmans H, Marchal G (1996) Contrast enhanced MR angiography. Radiologe 36:115

Gefter WB, Hatabu H, Holland GA, Gupta KB, Henschke CI, Palevsky HI (1995) Pulmonary thromboembolism: recent developments in diagnosis with CT and MR imaging. Radiology 197:561

Greenberg H (1965) Refractory dyspnea and orthopnea. Evidence of recurrent pulmonary embolism and infarction. Am Rev Respir Dis 92:215

Greene RE (1989) Anatomical and functional basis of imaging of the respiratory system. In: Taveras JM, Ferrucci JT (eds) Radiology: diagnosis-imaging-intervention, vol 1. Lippincott, Philadelphia, chapter 39

Gupta A, Frazer CK, Ferguson JM, Kumar AB, Davis SJ, Fallon MJ, Morris IT, Drury PJ, Cala LA (1999) Acute pulmonary embolism: diagnosis with MR angiography. Radiology 210:353–359

Haraldseth O, Amundsen T, Rinck PA (1999) Contrast-enhanced pulmonary MR imaging. MAGMA 8:146–153

Hoffmann U, Schima W, Herold C (1999) Pulmonary magnetic resonance angiography. Eur Radiol 9:1745–1754

Indik JH, Alpert JS (2000) Detection of pulmonary embolism by D-dimer assay, spiral computed tomography, and magnetic resonance imaging. Prog Cardiovasc Dis 42:261–272

Kelley MA, Carson JL, Palevsky HI, Schwartz JS (1991) Diagnosing pulmonary embolism: new facts and strategies. Ann Intern Med 114:300

Kreitner KF, Ley S, Kauczor HU, Kalden P, Pitton MB, Mayer E, Laub G, Thelen M (2000) Contrast media enhanced three-dimensional MR angiography of the pulmonary arteries in patients with chronic recurrent pulmonary embolism – comparison with selective intra-arterial DSA. Rofo Fortschr Geb Röntgenstr Neuen Bildgeb Verfahr 172:122–128

Mayo JR, Remy-Jardin M, Müller NL, Remy J, Worsley DF, Hossein-Foucher C, Kwong JS, Brown MJ (1997) Pulmonary embolism: prospective comparison of spiral CT with ventilation-perfusion scintigraphy. Radiology 205:447

Meaney JMF, Weg JG, Chenevert TL, Stafford-Johnson D, Hamilton BH, Prince MR (1997) Diagnosis of pulmonary embolism with magnetic resonance angiography. N Engl J Med 336:1422

Najarian KE, Morris CS (1998) Arterial embolization in the chest. J Thorac Imaging 13:93–104

Owings JT, Gosselin RC, Battistella FD, Anderson JT, Petrich M, Larkin EC (2000) Whole blood D-dimer assay: an effective noninvasive method to rule out pulmonary embolism. J Trauma 48:795–799; discussion 799–800

Rémy-Jardin M, Rémy J, Wattinne L, Giraud F (1992) Central pulmonary thromboembolism: diagnosis with spiral volumetric CT with the single-breath-hold technique – comparison with pulmonary angiography. Radiology 185:381–387

Rémy-Jardin M, Rémy J, Deschildre F, Artaud D, Beregi JP, Hossein-Foucher C, Marchandise X, Duhamel A (1996) Diagnosis of pulmonary embolism with spiral CT: comparison with pulmonary angiography and scintigraphy. Radiology 200:699–706

Rémy-Jardin M, Baghaie F, Bonnel F, Masson P, Duhamel A, Rémy J (2000) Thoracic helical CT: influence of subsecond scan time and thin collimation on evaluation of peripheral pulmonary arteries. Eur Radiol 10:1297–1303

Riederer SJ, Kruger DG, Wilman AH, Rossman PJ, Huston J, Ehrman RL, Breen JF, LaPlante CL (1998) Contrast-enhanced 3D MR angiography using fluoroscopic triggering: technical reliability and applicability in 250 patients. In: Proceedings of the International Society of Magnetic Resonance Medicine, Sixth Scientific Meeting, Abstract 169

Scialpi M, Scapati C, Carriero A, Bonomo L, Rotondo A (1998) Segmental pulmonary arteries: two-dimensional and three-dimensional time of flight magnetic resonance angiography. J Thorac Imaging 13:123–127

Sevitt S (1962) Venous thrombosis and pulmonary embolism. Their prevention by oral anticoagulation. Am J Med 33:703

Song JW, Im JG, Shim YS, Park JH, Yeon KM, Han MC (1998) Hypertrophied bronchial artery at thin-section CT in patients with bronchiectasis: correlation with CT angiographic findings. Radiology 208:187–191

Stehling MK, Holzknecht N, Gauger J, Luboldt W, Smekal A von, Laub G, Reiser M (1996) Gadolinium enhanced magnetic resonance angiography with ultra-short echo-times. Initial experiences. Radiologe 36:670

Stock EW, Jacob AL, Schnabel KJ, Bongartz G, Steinbrich W (1997) Massive pulmonary embolism: treatment with thrombus fragmentation and local fibrinolysis with recombinant tissue plasminogen activator. Cardiovasc Intervent Radiol 20:364

Wetzel SG, Haselhorst R, Bilecen D, Lyrer PA, Seifritz E, Bongartz GM, Radue EW, Scheffler K (2001) Preliminary experience with dynamic MR projection angiography in the evaluation of cervicocranial steno-occlusive disease. Eur Radiol 11(2):295–302

Wielopolski PA, Haacke EM, Adler LP (1992) Three-dimensional MR pulmonary vascular imaging: preliminary experience. Radiology 183:465–472

Wielopolski PA, Haacke EM, Adler LP (1993) Evaluation of the pulmonary vasculature with three-dimensional magnetic resonance imaging techniques. MAGMA 1:21–34

Wilman AH, Riederer SJ (1997) Performance of an elliptical centric view order for signal enhancement and motion artifact suppression in breath-hold three-dimensional gradient echo imaging. Magn Reson Med 38:793–802

18 Abdominal Aorta and Its Branches

INGOLF P. ARLART and ANNA GERLACH

CONTENTS

18.1 Introduction

The abdominal aorta is responsible for transporting blood into the arteries of the intra- and retroperitoneal parenchymal organs as well as into the pelvis and lower extremities. The main branches of the abdominal aorta are the splanchnic and renal arteries. Splanchnic vessels supply the liver, spleen, pancreas, duodenum, and the stomach via the celiac artery, and the intestinal tract via the superior mesenteric artery (SMA) and the inferior mesenteric artery (IMA). Through the renal arteries approximately 20% of the cardiac output volume is transported into the kidneys.

Both splanchnic and renal arteries are responsible for maintaining parenchymal nutrition and the different functions, which are very specific for each organ.

Diagnostic imaging of the abdominal aorta and its branches is mainly necessary in acute and chronic occlusive disease, aneurysmal disease, and in dissection. Each of these lesions normally presents typical symptoms with respect to its site, which indicates angiographic evaluation. The diagnostic tools include conventional angiography, ultrasonography (US), computed tomographic (CT) angiography, and magnetic resonance (MR) angiography. A large number of publications is available in the current literature concerning the usefulness and value of the different diagnostic methods.

Conventional Angiography. Conventional angiography or digital subtraction angiography (DSA) each visualize in a highly specific way not only the course, location, perfused lumen, and the inner wall condition of the abdominal aorta but also the different branches arising from the aortic lumen (ABRAMS 1983a, b; BAUM 1983; BOIJSEN 1983; LIPCHIK and ROGOFF 1983a, b). Major advantages of conventional angiography are its high spatial and temporal resolution. Due to the peripheral location of important vascular pathologies, selective catheter angiography of the splanchnic arterial system and the renal parenchyma is regarded as the method of first choice. In addition, conventional angiography plays a prominent role as a highly accurate imaging procedure in selected patients, providing the possibility of measuring intraluminal distances for vascular therapy with calibrated catheters and of performing percutaneous endovascular interventions immediately after the diagnostic visualization of a pathological condition within the same procedure.

The drawbacks of conventional angiography are the invasive character of the examination with potential risks for the patient caused by arterial puncture, catheter manipulations, and the use of contrast material that has shown to be nephrotoxic, particularly in patients with diabetes mellitus, multiple myeloma, impaired kidney function, and in combination with drugs containing metformin (MORCOS et al. 1999). Additionally, conventional angiography is associated with high examination costs and the necessity of hospitalizing the majority of patients, and diagnostic information about the intravascular space is limited. As a result of these drawbacks, technically highly developed noninvasive color-coded duplex Doppler US and contrast-enhanced CT angiography, which is

I.P. ARLART, MD; A. GERLACH, MD
Radiologisches Institut Stuttgart, Katharinenhospital, Kriegsbergstrasse 60, 70174 Stuttgart, Germany

considered a minimally invasive technique due to the necessity of intravenous administration of iodinated contrast material, became of interest and were introduced successfully into the armamentarium for evaluating vascular abnormalities of the abdominal aorta and its branches. In addition to intravascular information, all these methods are able to supply information about the para-aortic space and adjacent soft tissue structures.

Ultrasonography. In recent years US has been improved significantly by combining morphologic imaging and dynamic color-coded functional Doppler flow measurements (MERRITT 1992) and was optimized by high-resolution tissue harmonic imaging, power Doppler technology, three-dimensional (3D) imaging, and the use of specifically developed contrast agents. Using this approach, experienced examiners are able to depict the aorta, the aortic wall structures, and main aortic branches directly. The initial limitations of US, including a low depiction rate of smaller branches when older equipment was used, have been partially overcome. In addition to the direct depiction of angiomorphologic disease, functional disorders can be determined routinely in different vascular areas by analyzing Doppler spectra. However, this method is not able to provide objective images similar to those obtained by angiography which clearly visualize the complete morphologic information of aortic, splanchnic, and renovascular structures. Abdominal vessel structures of interest can be partially or completely masked by obesity and overlying calcifications, bone structures, or air-filled areas, also obscuring the Doppler signal. Doppler dynamic flow measurements can be potentially falsified by examination failures, and the reliability of factors that, for instance, cause intrarenal flow abnormalities in stenotic disease are still being critically discussed. These limitations of US made it apparent that alternative noninvasive imaging techniques are needed which are based on a standardized imaging protocol, cover large areas of the abdominal vasculature, and are able to present information similar to that provided by conventional angiography.

CT Angiography. As a minimally invasive approach, single- or multislice helical acquisition CT angiographic techniques have been developed and replaced conventional CT completely in vascular imaging (RUBIN 1998; RUBIN et al. 2000). Biphasic CT angiographic image acquisition using a single i.v. contrast bolus injection can be performed during two repetitive breath-holds. In the early arterial phase, abnormalities of the aorta and the aortic wall can be visualized, and the depiction of main central splanchnic and renal branches as well as accessory renal arteries is possible. In a delayed phase, venous structures of the splanchnic and renal circulation can be evaluated, and lesions of the renal, splenic, pancreatic or hepatic parenchyma can be detected.

Following contrast enhancement, CT angiograms with a large field of view can be postprocessed directly using techniques such as two-dimensional (2D) and 3D multiplanar reformatting (MPR) in any desired plane, 3D shaded surface display (SSD), 3D volume-rendering techniques (VR), and maximum intensity projection (MIP) imaging. With the introduction of helical CT angiography, the indications for conventional angiography of the abdominal aorta and its branches have been reduced and changed. However, compared with conventional angiography, CT angiography shows a lower spatial resolution, there is no temporal resolution within the arterial or venous phase acquisition, and side effects due to the iodinated contrast material may occur. Furthermore, the high radiation exposure of the patient is a critical issue, particularly when multislice technique is used and functional imaging – with which quantitative flow measurement is comparable to that of Doppler US or radionuclide studies – is not available.

MR Angiography. Noninvasive MR angiographic techniques, in principle, have been regarded as the ideal alternative to conventional angiography, US, and CT due to their potential of combining angiomorphologic and functional information. When MR angiography was first introduced, this method was able to visualize the abdominal aorta and its proximal branches on the basis of flow-sensitive 2D or 3D GRE-sequences, including time-of-flight (TOF) (EDELMAN et al. 1989; ARLART et al. 1992; LEWIN et al. 1991) and phase-contrast (PC) (DUMOULIN et al. 1990; AMANUMA et al. 1992) techniques. Using these approaches, intraluminal aortic flow could be visualized with a bright signal and the perivascular space could be evaluated as with US and CT. In pre-existing morphologic vascular lesions the 2D and 3D PC MR techniques could be used to yield information on the functional effect on blood flow (BASS et al. 1997; DONG et al. 1999) and quantification of flow velocities and flow volumes (DEBATIN et al. 1994, SCHOENBERG et al. 1997). However, it could be observed that the quality of flow-sensitive MR angiograms was limited by a variety of factors. The vascular signal became obscured, particularly under slow or turbulent flow conditions, reducing spatial resolution and signal inhomogeneities or signal voids due to phase dispersion, in-plane saturation, susceptibility artifacts, respiratory artifacts, and ghosting artifacts. Thus, the imaging of aortic branches, in particular, achieved only limited acceptance; its application was not considered clinically satisfactory, nor was it regarded as a method with the potential of replacing conventional angiography. However, problems of flow-sensitive MR angiography could be widely solved by intravenously administered paramagnetic contrast material, introduced by Prince et al. (1993, 1994), and optimized by ultrafast image acquisition (Holland et al. 1996; Alley et al. 1998; Shirkhoda et al. 1997; Dong et al. 1999) and time-resolved multiphase imaging within a single breath-hold (Schoenberg et al. 1999; Van Hoe et al. 2000). The contrast material used in MR angiography showed no relevant side effects; in particular, it was not nephrotoxic (Prince et al. 1996). Arterial 3D data acquisition during the early phase of intravenously administered paramagnetic extracellular contrast agents most recently has proven to be superior to acquiring data during the equilibrium phase when colloidal superparamagnetic contrast material was used, because attendant venous overlap limited the assessment of arterial structures (Weishaupt et al. 2000).

18.2 Technical Considerations

In a large number of patients with abdominal aortic diseases, intraluminal disorders may be associated with abnormalities of vessel wall structures, the perivascular space, and the parenchymal organs supplied by aortic branches. In addition, knowledge of blood flow alteration and reduction, respectively, that may occur particularly in occlusive disease is important for planning suitable therapeutic strategies. For this reason, the aim of abdominal vascular MR imaging is to create the new diagnostic gold standard by combining modalities which are able to provide morphologic information of the vascular lumen, vessel wall structures, and perivascular space as well as functional quantitative blood flow information within different vascular areas. Depending on the individual diagnostic problem, standardized examination protocols are available today which include either a single MR angiographic sequence or complementary MR sequences. The goal of abdominal MR angiography, the modality of major interest, is to provide temporally and spatially resolved vascular information similar to that of DSA. Since optimized gadolinium-enhanced 3D MR angiography using ultrafast spoiled 3D GRE-sequences has been developed and successfully introduced into clinical practice, this technique presently seems to be the most promising modality to replace invasive conventional angiography. In the following sections of this chapter, technical considerations of gadolinium-enhanced 3D MR angiography, sequence designs, postprocessing techniques, and examination protocols of different vascular structures are presented, including complementary sequences useful to complete morphologic and functional vascular imaging of the abdominal aorta and its branches.

18.2.1 General Aspects

MR angiography of the abdominal aorta and its branches requires data to be acquired during a breath-hold in order to avoid motion artifacts that may significantly reduce image quality. Thus, the examination time of a 3D data acquisition is limited to approximately 30 s. Moreover, if the image acquisition time is short the concentration of paramagnetic contrast material is optimized in the arterial system if a short bolus administration time is used. Current MR angiography protocols for imaging the abdominal aorta have incorporated these prerequisites and are based on different capabilities of the presently available high-performance MR equipment which operate at 1.0 to 1.5 Tesla, a gradient field strength of more than 20 mT/m, and a rise time shorter than 500 µs. In optimized high-performance equipment, the gradient field strength is higher than 30 mT/m and rise time is shorter than 200 µs. Image acquisition with a four-channel phased-array body coil significantly improves the signal-to-noise ratio, and a high image quality can be achieved with adequate postprocessing. As a general recommendation, patients should be prepared for the examination. Because breath-holding periods for acquisition of abdominal gadolinium-enhanced 3D MR angiographic images normally are longer than 20 s, in older patients or patients with cardiopulmonary disease, hyperventilation exercises should be performed or oxygen administered before the study in order to prolong the breath-hold period (Marks et al. 1997). Intravenous administration of glucagon may be useful when artifacts are expected due to bowel motion.

18.2.2 Contrast-Enhanced 3D MR Angiography

18.2.2.1 Sequence Design

In an early and preliminary study of PRINCE et al. (1993) preferential arterial enhancement of the abdominal aorta was achieved with 3D TOF dynamic MR imaging during manual intravenous injection of an extracellular-compartment paramagnetic contrast agent (gadolinium-DTPA) over an infusion time of 5 min, corresponding to a total acquisition time of 5:10 min. Already at that time it was suggested that newer, rapid imaging techniques, a mechanical injection technique of the contrast agent, a variable injection rate such that the center of the k-space is covered during the period of maximum injection, and the use of image subtraction and fat saturation techniques might offer potentials for improving the quality of arterial imaging. Today these perspectives have been widely become reality. Rapid 3D data acquisition is the prerequisite for imaging multiple temporal phases or multiple locations. Temporal resolution is important because the arterial phase typically only lasts a few seconds before venous enhancement begins. Therefore, the shortest possible sequence repetition time (TR) is desired. Ultrashort TR can be achieved by optimization of the gradient configuration, the reduced-power selective radio frequency pulses, and the receiver bandwidth for data acquisition. Radiofrequency spoiling can be used to improve the suppression of static tissue. With this configuration it is possible to achieve a TR/TE of less than 5/2.5 ms for a 3D data set with 2- to 3-mm-thick sections and a resolution of 256 points in the frequency-encoding direction. The acquisition time can be further reduced by fractional symmetric k-space collection in either the frequency- or phase-encoding direction, and by using interpolation schemes. By collecting 63% of the echo (fractional echo) in the readout direction, it is possible to reduce the TR/TE to 4.0/1.0 ms. Fractional coverage in the phase-encoding direction allows a greater reduction in overall acquisition time because fewer sequence repetitions are needed. The ability to zero fill the acquired data in the section-encoding direction can be used to produce finer sampling in the section direction at no cost to the imaging time. This technique is useful for reducing partial-volume artifacts, which can lead to a loss of signal in smaller vessels (ALLEY et al. 1998). The acquisition of a single 3D data set within seconds is possible by using asymmetric centric data sampling in the k-space and half-Fourier analysis with 63% of the phase-encoding steps, allowing the acquisition of several 3D data sets during a single breath-hold. However, when this time-resolved multiphase technique is used, voxel size increases compared with the single-phase acquisition and, consequently, spatial resolution of the angiographic images decreases. The flip angle should be tuned for optimum T1 contrast according to TR and the expected blood gadolinium concentration, i.e., it could be larger for higher doses of gadolinium and longer TR or lower doses of gadolinium and shorter TR. The extravascular signal can be reduced by subtracting a nonenhanced 3D data set from the enhanced data set. Background adipose tissue signal around aortic branches can be eliminated by fat-suppression techniques. Fat can be suppressed by applying a frequency-selected pulse or spectral technique and an inversion pulse and may improve the visualization of small vessels of the splanchnic artery system. A rectangular field-of-view prevents aliasing in the phase-encoding direction, improves spatial resolution, and shortens acquisition time. For correct planning of the 3D volume, a nonenhanced localizer sequence has to be applied in three planes (transverse, coronal, and sagittal) before acquisition of the enhanced data sets.

The state-of-the-art concept of time-resolved ultrafast contrast-enhanced (CE) GRE MR angiography of the abdominal aorta and its branches can focus on two different techniques available at the moment. One technique includes the high spatially resolved acquisition of a single coronal 3D data set within a breath-hold with two or three contiguous acquisitions for late arterial and venous information during repetitive breath-holds (ALLEY et al. 1998). Useful sequence parameters are recommended in Table 18.1.

Table 18.1. Sequence parameters of contrast-enhanced 3D MR angiography

Parameters	Single-phase	Multiphase
Plane	Coronal	Coronal
Field of view (cm)	30–48	30–35
Number of frequency-encoded steps	256–512	256
Number of phase-encoded steps	128–512	140–180
Repetition time (ms)	4.5–7.0	3.2
Echo time (ms)	1.0–2.1	1.1
Flip angle (degrees)	25–45	30
Slab (mm)	80–140	80–90
No. of sections	28–44	16–22/44–50
Section thickness (zero filled) (mm)	1.8–4.0	1.8–2.5
Bandwidth	31.25 kHz	650 Hz/pixel
No. of excitations	0.5–1	1
Acquisition time (s)	15–58	28 (4×7)

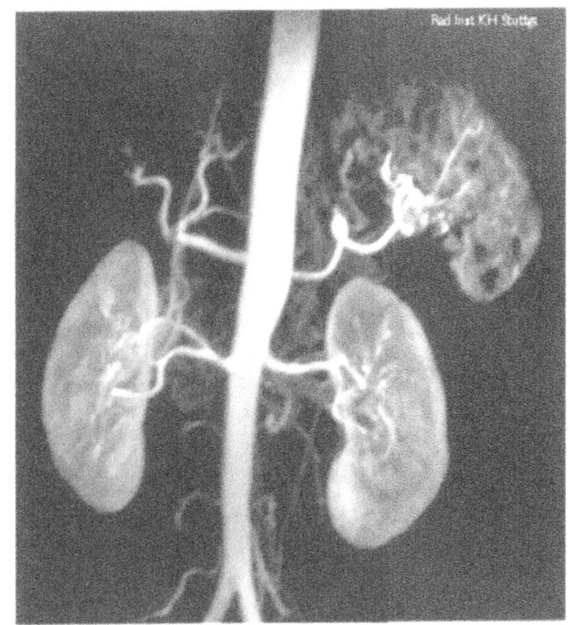

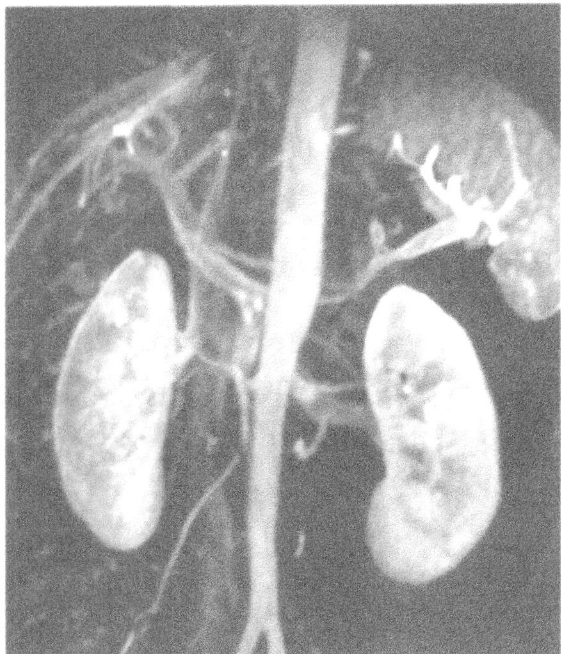

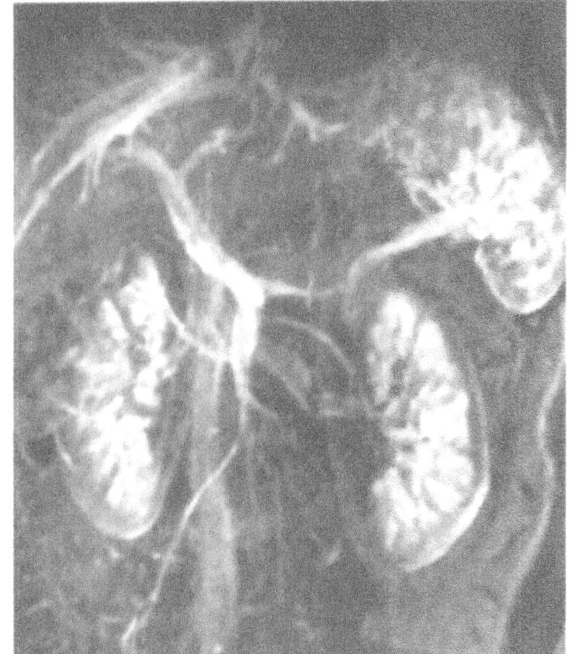

Fig. 18.1. Dynamic CE 3D GRE MR angiograms (maximum intensity projection images) of the normal abdominal aorta in the early arterial (**a**), late arterial (**b**), and venous phase after image subtraction (**c**). Coronal data acquisition was performed during three repetitive breath-holds (each data set within a breath-hold) using the following sequence parameters (1.5 T, body coil): 40 cm field-of-view, 41.7 kHz bandwidth, 5.3/1.7 ms TE/TR, 35°flip angle, 256×192 matrix, 36 sections, 1.6-mm section thickness after zero-filling, 0.5 nex (number of excitations), fat saturation, 22 s acquisition time, 25 ml gadolinium-DTPA (1.5 ml/s flow rate)

This technique requires appropriate timing of the acquisition and the contrast bolus (Fig. 18.1a–c).

The other technique, which presumably will become the leading technique when optimized, is based on dynamic multiphase acquisition of four to five repetitive measurements of 6–7 s with an intermittent delay of 150 ms between the 3D data sets within a single breath-hold (Fig. 18.2a–f). Ultrashort sequence TR and TE can be obtained by a self-refocusing radiofrequency pulse for excitation of the 3D volume and the use of an asymmetric k-space sampling (140–160 data points) in the read-out, phase-encoding, and partition direction. Filtering of raw data and zero filling in the k-space may reconstruct the voxel size such that it is nearly identical to that obtained with a standard 3D MR angiographic sequence (Schoenberg et al. 1999; Van Hoe et al. 2000). Useful sequence parameters are demonstrated in Table 18.1. The acquisition can be started 8 s after beginning of the bolus injection of contrast material. A bolus timing has proven not to be necessary due to the multiphase acquisition, which guarantees a maximum arterial phase. The dose and flow rate per second which are selected can be identical to those

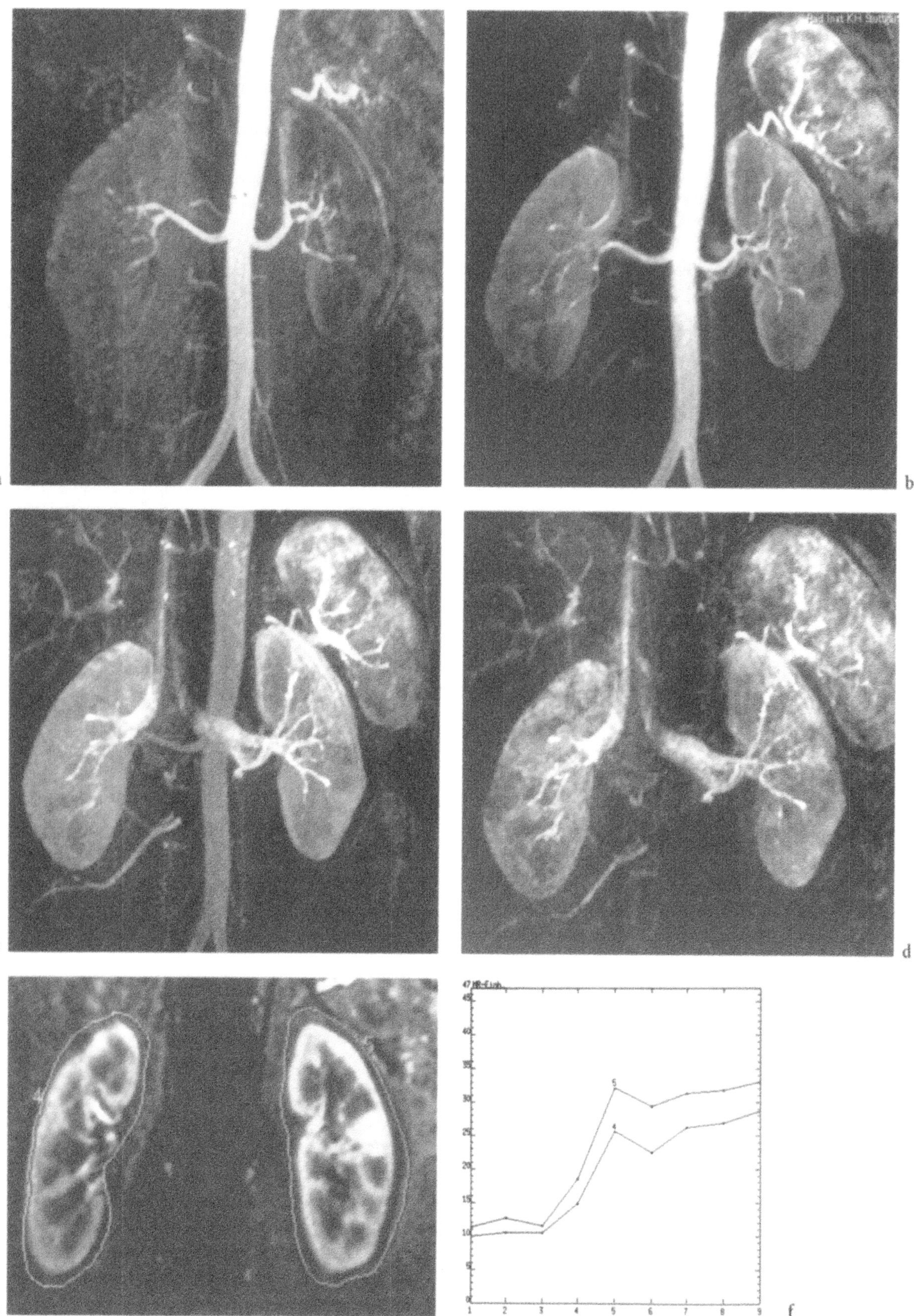

Fig. 18.2a–f. Dynamic multiphase CE 3D MR angiograms of normal kidneys. Six coronal data sets were acquired during two repetitive breath-holds, i.e., three data sets during a single breath-hold. Representative images of the early (**a**) and late (**b**) arterial phase, the parenchymal (**c**) and venous phase after subtraction of arterial information (**d**) are shown. Dynamic parenchymal gadolinium enhancement (**e**) is demonstrated on time-dependent signal intensity curves (**f**) over both kidneys. Sequence parameters for this renal study (1.5 T, 4 channel phased-array coil) include a 32×40 cm field-of-view, 83.3 kHz bandwidth, 3.9/1.3 ms TR/TE, 25°flip angle, 256×160 matrix, 26 sections, 1.6 mm section thickness after zero filling, 0.5 nex, 28 s acquisition time for three data sets, 25 ml of gadolinium-DTPA (1.5 ml/s flow rate)

used in a standard 3D MR angiography sequence. The consecutive 3D data sets cover early and late arterial enhancement, perfusion of the abdominal viscera, and enhancement of venous structures.

18.2.2.2
Features of Aortic MR Angiography

In abdominal aortic disorders MR angiographic information should primarily include the perfused vascular lumen of the aorta and the aortic bifurcation, the iliac arteries, and the proximal visceral arteries with their ostia. Thus, a large field-of-view of 45–48 cm has to be planned to cover all vascular areas of interest. Multiphase imaging is useful for depicting arterial lesions under normal and low-flow conditions, to evaluate the parenchyma of abdominal viscera, and to visualize abdominal venous structures. In patients with complex thoracoabdominal aortic disease, a particular examination technique has been described in which two contiguous 3D data sets are acquired during a single administration of contrast bolus using dynamic table translation (EARLS et al. 1998). The 3D volume can be tailored to each patient, depending on his/her size and anatomy and according to coronal and transverse localizing sections and should prescribe the extent, posteriorly, to include the descending thoracic aorta and, anteriorly, to include the common femoral arteries.

In a variety of vascular lesions sequences complementary to MR angiography are of particular interest to provide secondary morphologic imaging of aortic wall structures and the para-aortic space. T1- and T2-weighted SE images have been shown to be useful in the detection and analysis of mural thrombi (CASTRUCCI et al. 1995). Post-contrast, T1-weighted, fat-saturated GRE imaging in the transverse and/or coronal acquisition plane (52 transverse sections within four repetitive breath-holds) immediately following the CE 3D MR angiographic study is able to cover the entire abdominal aorta, the iliac arteries, and the perivascular space. On the basis of these images vascular distances can be measured, and aortic atheromatous material, thrombotic intimal layers, mural thrombi, inflammatory aortic wall thickening, and productive periaortic fibrosis can be visualized and quantified.

18.2.2.3
Features of Splanchnic MR Angiography

In patients with splanchnic artery disease, the acquisition volume has to be localized mainly in the region of the mesenteric, celiac, or hepatic vasculature. A field-of-view of 35–40 cm has been shown to be useful. The CE 3D data should be acquired in coronal or oblique coronal plane with a slab positioned parallel to the aorta and which includes the anterior portion of the aorta (SHIRKHODA et al. 1998; KOPKA et al. 1999). This placement appears to be most beneficial in terms of the mesenteric orientation and for covering the origin of the SMA. The quality of MR angiographic imaging of the mesenteric branches can be significantly improved by a variety of procedures such as subtraction of 3D data sets performed once before and again during administration of contrast material, fat saturation, intravenous administration of glucagon, and a standard caloric meal before the examination (HANY et al. 1998a; KOPKA et al. 1999), which stimulates an increase in flow volume in the mesenteric vasculature. For the mesenteric and hepatic arterial phase, it is extremely important to tailor the contrast material bolus to the contrast-sensitive low-frequency lines of the k-space. Three repetitive 3D data acquisitions should be performed in order to obtain different phases of the mesenteric and hepatic vasculature, including the arterial (Fig. 18.3a–c), venous, and portal venous phase. By systematic subtraction of the arterial phase image (second acquisition) from the delayed venous phase image, a pure MR venogram can be obtained. The data from each of the CE measurements can be subjected to a MIP or MPR algorithm for postprocessing in three planes. Using transverse reformatting as a guide, a sagittal oblique subvolume lined up with the celiac artery and SMA can be selected. This subvolume of sagittal data can be displayed as a MIP, which will show the celiac, SMA, and IMA, as well as the anterior and posterior margins of the aorta. In this way, the delineation of ostial mesenteric occlusive disease can be improved. Similarly, using reformatting and subvolume MIP technique, it is possible to depict hepatic lesions and the visualize feeding or draining vessels.

CE 3D MR angiography in conjunction with 2D cine PC imaging (BURKART et al. 1993) provides a comprehensive morphologic and functional analysis of the splanchnic vasculature. The imaging protocol can be completed in less than 20 min and requires only short periods of breath-holding. Using thin-section MR angiograms, quantitative velocity images

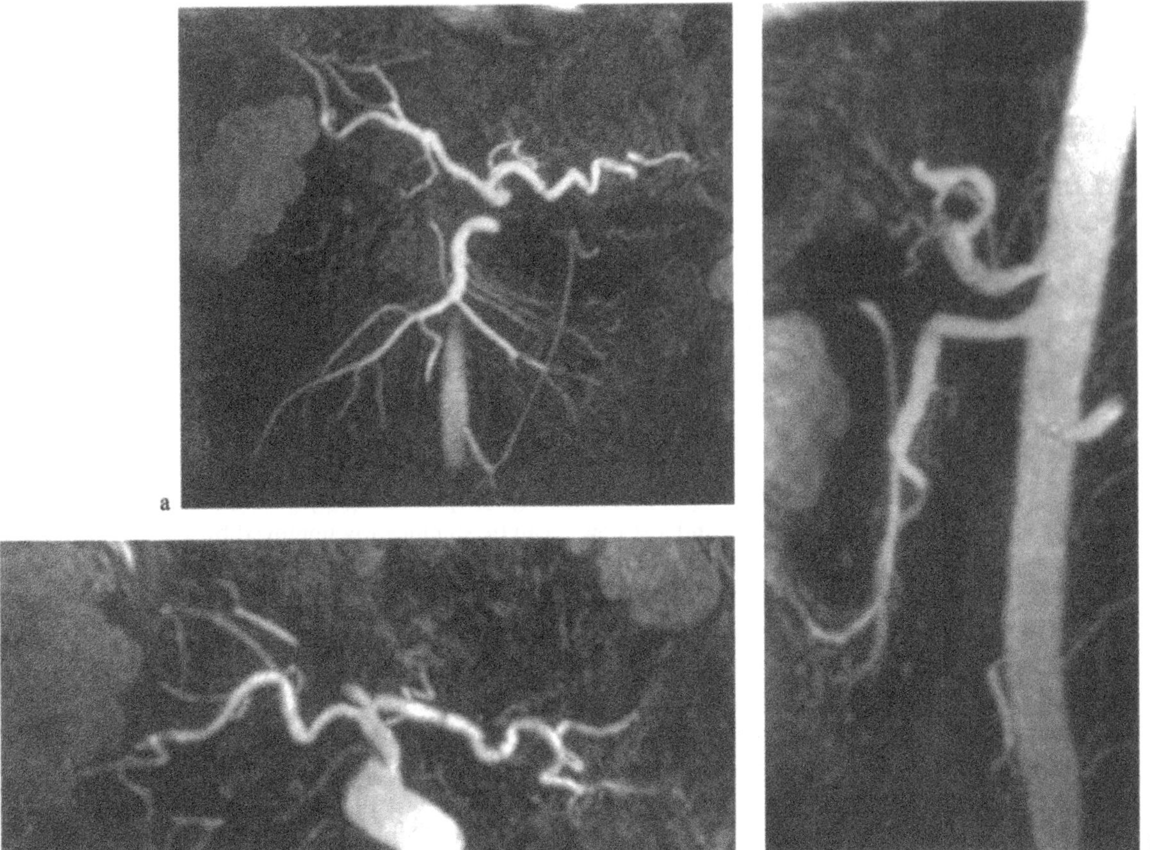

Fig. 18.3a–c. Normal anatomy of splanchnic vessels. Single-phase CE 3D MR maximum intensity projection (MIP) angiogram of the celiac, superior and inferior mesenteric artery in coronal (**a**, MIP), sagittal (**b**, reformatted image) and transverse (**c**, reformatted image) plane

perpendicular to the celiac axis or the SMA and SMV can be obtained to calculate flow with 2D PC mapping (see Chap. 10). MR oximetry, a functional MR imaging technique in suspected cases of reduced perfusion of the superior mesenteric vasculature, has been successfully applied in animal studies (Chan et al. 1999). This approach seems to be promising in the evaluation of mesenteric ischemia and may find its way into clinical routine. MR oximetry is based on a sequence which is designed to produce fat-suppressed T2-weighted multiecho images with minimum T2* and flow-related signal loss (Wright et al. 1991). The T2 values of blood in the SMV and the IVC are measured on images taken at four different echo times: 30, 78, 126, and 222 ms. Images for all four echoes are obtained in less than 5 min. Using an empirically established formula, relating T2 of the blood to oxygen saturation (% $Hb0_2$), the oxygen saturation can be calculated by estimation from their corresponding T2 blood values measured on the images according to the formula:

$$1/T2\ blood = 1/T2o + k(1 - \%Hb0_2/100)^2$$

where T2o is T2 blood at 100% oxygen saturation and k is the calibration coefficient.

18.2.2.4 Features of Renal MR Angiography

In renovascular MR imaging both angiomorphologic imaging of the renal arteries and functional determination of blood flow in occlusive disease are of particular interest. A standardized imaging protocol has been established which includes a combination of ultrafast CE 3D MR angiography with a functional imaging modality, i.e., 2D or 3D PC technique, respectively (Dong et al. 1999; Schoenberg et al. 1997, 1999). The multiphase dynamic renal CE 3D MR angiography is able to provide not only angiograms of the arterial and venous vasculature but also information about kidney perfusion and renal function. With multiphase acquisition the nonenhanced phase can be distinguished from an early arterial phase with minor parenchymal enhancement, a main arterial phase with maximum enhancement of the main renovascular tree, and major enhancement of the renal parenchyma and minor enhancement of distal veins, an early venous phase with complete depiction of the proximal veins and the IVC, and a late venous phase with maximum enhancement of the venous system (SCHOENBERG et al. 1999) (Fig. 18.2a–d). The visualization of dynamic contrast flow during the different phases in dynamic multislice CE 3D MR angiography makes it possible to evaluate unilateral morphologic and functional parenchymal disorders, particularly when comparing the two kidneys (Fig. 18.2e, f). Useful parameters are kidney size, temporal enhancement of renal parenchyma (Ros et al. 1995), thickness of renal cortex and differentiation of corticomedullary anatomy (PRINCE et al. 1997b), effects of converting-enzyme inhibition on renal enhancement pattern (GRENIER et al. 1996), and the excretory function of gadolinium (WALSH et al. 1996). In their study Ros et al. (1995) described the technique of MR renography and the gadolinium-based measurement of glomerular filtration rate. In MR renography intrarenal kinetics are studied, which is based on gadolinium-enhancement curves that show signal intensity in both kidneys over time by measuring the time of arrival of gadolinium in the renal cortex and outer medulla. Measurements of the glomerular filtration rate are based on the disappearance of gadolinium in the plasma as determined by MR relaxometry. A postcontrast, multislice spoiled GRE sequence with fat-saturated T1-weighted imaging in the coronal and transverse planes should be included in the protocol, which allows the accurate evaluation of the renal parenchyma and the perirenovascular space.

After 3D data acquisition, postprocessing is required to obtain reliable information about the renal arteries, including the segmental, accessory, and pole arteries. In order to avoid false interpretations of the renal arterial lumen, it is extremely important that each renal artery will be analyzed and documented in two perpendicular planes using source images, multiplanar reformatted imaging, and subvolume MIP imaging in the coronal oblique and transverse oblique planes. The renal artery ostia and eccentric atherosclerotic plaques can then be identified accurately. Moreover, on subvolume MIP images from the early arterial phase, vessel-to-background contrast of the segmental arteries is higher than on standard 3D angiograms, allowing a continuous analysis of the course of the vessel – including the segmental arteries. Using this technique, arterial branches are free from vascular overlap, and distal stenotic disease, found particularly in fibromuscular dysplasia (FMD), can be excluded. Septum-like artifacts of the main renal artery that may appear in 3D reformatted projection angiograms due to the stack of source images used for image reconstruction can mimic FMD. In order to avoid this phenomenon, the section thickness should not be more than 2 mm (1 mm zero-filled) in patients with suspected FMD.

For renal transplant examination the field-of-view has to be localized so as to encompass the lower abdominal aorta and extending down to the femoral bifurcation. Multiphase CE 3D MR angiography is able to evaluate the arterial and venous vasculature as occlusive disease can develop in both arteries and veins. Since both anastomosis and the course of renal transplant artery may vary, depending on different operative techniques and anatomic conditions, the sagittal plane, in addition to the coronal plane, has also been shown to be useful for data acquisition to optimize spatial resolution of reformatted images. Because the anastomotic region is the main location of stenotic disease, it is important to visualize this area in two perpendicular views. The transplanted renal vein can also be analyzed by a similar procedure on the late enhanced images.

18.2.3 Use of Contrast Material

Degradation of image quality and flow signal due to turbulent flow, in-plane saturation and motion artifacts, which is known from inflow TOF MR angiography, can be widely avoided by using 3D GRE techniques with a short acquisition time. The prerequisite for short acquisition within a breath-hold is a very short sequence TR. However, when the TR is short, a lack of contrast between blood and tissue will be evident, causing blood to appear nearly isointense with background tissue. With paramagnetic contrast agents the vascular signal can be improved due to a relative reduction in the T1 of blood compared with that of fat, muscle, and other background tissue (see Chap. 6). Imaging during the first transit time of the contrast material, i.e., depiction of the arterial phase, is essential for short TR CE 3D MR angiography because sufficiently short T1 of blood is only achieved during the peak vascular concentration of paramagnetic contrast material. Thus, an individually planned correct timing of the contrast material bolus relative to the start of data acquisition has a significant effect on image quality and diagnostic utility. In a breath-hold 3D GRE sequence, the central lines of the k-space are responsible for image contrast, whereas peripheral lines determine spatial resolution (Prince et al. 1997b). The time delay of the contrast bolus should be short enough to ensure appropriate detection of the arterial phase in patients with short acquisition times and long enough to maximize the monitoring period in patients with delayed bolus passage. In order to reduce blurring of contrast-enhanced vascular structures, a contrast bolus injection should cover not only the central parts but also the peripheral lines of k-space responsible for spatial resolution. Depending on the mode of k-space filling, different bolus timing techniques have been shown to be useful. When k-space is filled sequentially, the peak contrast bolus should appear during data acquisition after approximately the first third and be finished after the second third of the total acquisition period. When the k-space is filled centric or centric–elliptic, peak contrast of the bolus should appear when the acquisition is started and should cover approximately half of the total acquisition period. Because estimation of the optimum delay time from the beginning of contrast material administration to the beginning of data acquisition is difficult, a number of techniques for monitoring the arterial arrival of maximum concentration of contrast material have been described in the literature. By injection of a small test bolus (Earls et al. 1998) on the basis of sequential fast GRE imaging or interactive scanning of one frame per second, the appearance of the contrast bolus can be determined in the region of interest. Moreover, automated contrast material detection sequences (Prince et al. 1997a), i.e., "smart prep" (GE Med.System), "bolus track" (Philips Med.System), and "care bolus" (Siemens Med.System), have been introduced, and direct monitoring of the arrival of the contrast bolus in a sequence of real time "MR fluoroscopy" with a means of immediately triggering the 3D MR angiographic sequence (Wilman et al. 1997) has been described. Although automatic contrast material detection is most commonly used for aortic MR angiography, administration of a test bolus is recommended when two channels with different velocities exist in an aortic dissection that may distort the accuracy of the automated detection sequence. If a multiphase time-resolved 3D acquisition technique is used within a single breath-hold (Schoenberg et al. 1999; Van Hoe et al. 2000), contrast bolus timing is basically unnecessary due to the fact that at least one k-space will be filled during peak arterial enhancement. In aortic MR angiography the injection of the contrast bolus should be performed mechanically by using a power injector, a standard dose of 0.2 mmol/kg and a flow rate of 1.5–2.0 ml/s, followed by a flush of 20 ml of normal saline.

18.2.4 Image Analysis and Postprocessing

A separate workstation and suitable software are necessary to perform the different postprocessing techniques available today in vascular imaging. Standardized image evaluation should include the analysis of individual source images, MIP images, images established by thin MPR of the underlying 3D data set, and digital subtraction of the precontrast image from the dynamic arterial, or venous phase image data. In addition, volume rendering (VR) imaging, and surface rendering (SR) imaging can be considered if necessary (see Chap. 7). MIP images are produced with a ray-tracing algorithm by collecting maximum intensity values of displayed pixels along each selected ray. The appearance of MIP images resembles that of conventional angiograms. Since total volume MIP images may be corrupted by venous overlap, arterial vessels can be distinguished from venous vessels using subvolume MIP and MPR techniques. VR technique has shown to be useful for imaging aortic structures. VR is a 3D postprocessing algorithm based on a selection of the voxels of the image and adjusting the signal intensity for each selected material to allow change in the transparency. SR technique is based on a ray-casting algorithm that selects visible voxels by tracing rays from an instantaneous viewing position and exoscopically and endoscopically reconstructing the images (Davis et al. 1997). With exoscopic viewing, the virtual light source and the observer are positioned outside the vessel; with endoscopic viewing they are positioned inside the vessel. By endoscopic "virtual" SR, the examiner is allowed to navigate interactively through the inside of a vessel with a 3D view of the interior vessel wall. For reformatting the coronally acquired 3D image data in a sagittal or transverse plane, it is important to use the thinnest section possible. This consideration must be balanced with the volume that needs to be covered and the duration of breath-hold required.

18.2.5 2D/3D PC Techniques

Several MR-based imaging techniques have been proposed for evaluating the hemodynamics in vascular structures (see Chap. 8). Particularly in stenotic disease, reports include 2D cine PC techniques for measurement of renal blood flow (Debatin et al. 1994; Schoenberg et al. 1997; De Haan et al. 2000), and 3D PC imaging for the identification of the turbulence-induced spin dephasing at a significant lesion (Prince et al. 1997b, Bass et al. 1997, Wasser et al. 1997).

18.2.5.1
2D Cine PC MR Flow Mapping

Using a cardiac-gated 2D cine PC sequence functional disorders can be reliably quantified by measuring blood flow velocities. The most experience has been gained in the determination of mesenteric (Burkart et al. 1993) and renal blood flow (Debatin et al. 1994; Schoenberg et al. 1997; De Haan et al. 2000). By quantifying flow dynamics hemodynamically significant arterial stenosis can be evaluated. When the examination is planned in renal arteries, an oblique section is positioned on the transverse course of each of the vessels visualized on the MR angiogram to obtain an in-plane view. Measurements should be obtained 1–2 cm downstream from a stenosis. A block of transverse sections is positioned at the level of the vascular pedicles, and freely obtained slabs are positioned along the axial course of the renal arteries. On the in-plane image, the section for flow measurement is projected perpendicular to the vessel axis. Cine PC flow measurements in cross-sectional vessel areas are performed with a fast spoiled GRE sequence (see Chap. 10). The measurement necessitates acquisition of two corresponding phase images. One image has no flow information (flow-compensated image); the other image is subjected to a phase shift which linearly depends on the flow velocity (flow-sensitive image). Velocity information is extracted by subtracting the two-phase images. Suitable velocity encoding (VENC) has to be calculated individually, varying between 20 and up to 150 cm/s; for normal cases 50 cm/s has been recommended , for patients with heart failure, aortic aneurysm, or reduced intrarenal flow or aged over 70 years down to 20 cm/s, and for young healthy individuals up to 60 cm/s and more (Prince et al. 1997b). To obtain flow data for the different phases of the cardiac cycle, the PC images should be recorded with standard cardiac gating. Respiration-controlled examination (breath-hold technique, respiratory-gated technique) is recommended to eliminate respiratory motion as a source of error in the measurement (de Haan et al. 2000). Flow analysis on a separate workstation using software-based postprocessing of the image data includes

1. Definition of the region of interest
2. Calculation of flow velocity (minimum, maximum, mean; cm/s) and mean arterial blood flow (ml/min)
3. Quantification of flow at stenoses to estimate pressure gradient according to the modified Bernoulli's equation

18.2.5.2
3D PC MR Angiography

The image quality of 3D PC MR angiography has been shown to be substantially improved after the administration of gadolinium, so that the 3D PC technique is qualified as a complementary sequence to contrast-enhanced 3D MR angiography in depicting stenotic disease (Dong et al. 1999). Transverse 3D PC images can be acquired within approximately 15 min and are reconstructed with the phase-difference method, illustrating maximum velocity in all directions as well as right-to-left flow to evaluate the retrocaval course of the right renal artery. Subvolume MIP images and single-voxel-thick reformatting should be performed through the origins of each of the major aortic branch vessels. For tortuous vessels, individual, curved reformations can be established along the course of the arteries. Depending on the degree of signal void distal to the lesion, stenotic grading can be calculated. In patients with slow flow or renal failure or when VENC does not closely match the renal flow velocity, 3D PC MR imaging is limited. Spin dephasing and, as a result, artifacts, may occur at the renal origins.

18.3
Applications of MR Angiography

18.3.1
Normal Anatomy and Variants

18.3.1.1
Abdominal Aorta

The abdominal aorta extends from the diaphragmal hiatus (Th12–L1) to the aortic bifurcation at L4 or L5. Its course is in the left prevertebal retroperitoneum; its diameter varies and ranges from 1.5 to 3.0 cm depending on habitus and age. The space adjacent to the outer aortic wall normally contains fat and less fibrous tissue. The aortic bifurcation is frequently lower in older individuals and those with arterial tortuosity, ectasia, and axial rotation, which may displace the orifices of the aortic branches (Kadir 1991).

MR Angiography. The abdominal aorta can be morphologically visualized in the transverse and coronal planes using T1-weighted SE sequences (Higgins 1992). Commonly, intravascular flow signal appears black when this technique is applied, and both aortic wall structures and the periaortic space can be evaluated. However, alterations in the flow signal may occur due to turbulent or inverse flow that cannot be differentiated reliably from pathologic states. Vascular dimensions and distinct wall-adherent atheromatous plaques or aortic wall thickening due to different causes can be evaluated by using a CE fat-saturated T1-weighted fast GRE sequence. The combination of MR imaging with MR angiography makes it possible to depict both morphologic and blood flow information. CE 3D MR aortography is an accurate modality for visualizing the perfused aortic lumen and the aortic branch ostia (Prince 1994; Alley et al. 1998). Time-resolved early and late arterial phase images and venous phase images can be acquired either within separate consecutive breath-holds or within a single breath-hold when multiphase technique is used (Fig. 18.1a–c and Fig. 18.2a–d).

18.3.1.2 Splanchnic Arteries

The main sources of blood supply of the gastrointestinal tract are the celiac artery, SMA, and IMA. In approximately 65% of individuals, the celiac artery divides into three branches: the splenic, left gastric, and hepatic arteries. In about 10% the right hepatic artery is replaced by a branch of the SMA. The splanchnic circulation has two major sources of arterial flow, that is, the celiac artery and the SMA. There are minor, collateral, communicating vessels between the celiac artery and SMA as well as the SMA and the IMA (Kadir 1991). The visualization of a normal splanchnic vasculature and, in particular, the hepatic vessels is required due to the increasing number of patients being treated for liver cirrhosis and malignant liver disease, or in whom liver transplantation is being planned.

MR Angiography. In depicting the main splanchnic arteries, flow-sensitive MR angiography plays only a limited role compared with other imaging modalities, such as color-coded duplex US (Moneta et al. 1993) and CE CT angiography (Kanematsu et al. 1995; Johnson et al. 1996; Hong and Freeny 1999), which demonstrate a high accuracy in visualizing main branches. Compared with 3D PC MR angiography (Wasser et al. 1996), CE 3D MR angiographic examination is superior in visualizing the main splanchnic arteries in the coronal and sagittal planes and has been reported to agree with conventional angiography in 79% of cases (Prince et al. 1995). Breath-hold imaging results in a 25%–50% greater signal-to-noise (S/N) ratio and a 60%–120% greater contrast-to-noise (C/N) ratio than non-breath-hold imaging. Sequence optimization, including fat saturation, high-resolution technique, and a short examination time, provides a good to excellent angiographic quality of the SMA trunk in 85%, of the celiac arteries in 75%, and of the IMA in 25% of cases (Shirkhoda et al. 1997) (Fig. 18.3a–c). Moreover, visualization of first-order branching is reported in 75%, second-order branching in 60%, and third-order branching in 50% (Shirkoda et al. 1997); arterial variations appeared identical to those in DSA (Ernst et al. 2000). While the most relevant proximal vessel segments of the SMA usually become visible even under fasting conditions, caloric stimulation increases flow volumes and improves the visualization of smaller vessels (Hany et al. 1998a).

Using optimized multiphase CE 3D MR angiography, the hepatic supply, including the arterial, hepatovenous, and portal venous vasculature, can be visualized in a quality comparable to CT angiography (Chambers et al. 1995; Kraus et al. 1995; Winter et al. 1995) and mostly superior to color-coded duplex US (Roobottom et al. 1993; Lomas et al. 1994). Compared with DSA, the results of MR angiography are similar for evaluating the main arterial system and better for demonstrating the portal vein and its intrahepatic branches up to second-order branching (Misri et al. 1998; Hawighorst et al. 1999; Kopka et al. 1999). Compared with single-phase CE 3D MR angiography, the current multiphase time-resolved imaging technique still shows limitations in depicting smaller hepatic arterial branches due to reduced spatial resolution (Van Hoe et al. 2000).

18.3.1.3 Renal Arteries

As regards the arterial supply of the kidneys, a single right and left renal artery can be found in about two thirds of individuals. Multiple renal arteries occur unilaterally in 32% and bilaterally in 12%. An independent superior renal pole artery can be observed in 7%, and an inferior pole artery in about 5%. An aberrant renal vascular supply can be expected in renal malformations or horseshoe kidneys. An atypical accessory supply via collaterals is seen in proximal renovascular occlusion or hypervascularized renal tumors (Kadir 1991). A variety of non- or minimally invasive and cost-saving methods have been established for imaging of the renal vasculature, such as color-coded duplex Doppler US, CT angiography, and MR angiography in order to replace invasive diagnostic arteriography.

MR Angiography. Flow-sensitive MR angiographic techniques are able to satisfactorily depict the proximal parts of main renal arteries, whereas the visualization of segmental arteries is usually not possible and the identification of accessory renal arteries is limited, ranging from 0% to 61% (Loubeyre et al. 1996a; de cobelli et al. 1997; Hahn et al. 1999). Administration of contrast material can achieve a 2.2-fold improvement in the S/N ratio in the distal renal arteries, reflecting improved visualization of segmental arteries particularly in conditions of slow blood flow along the arterial wall (Bass et al. 1997). Multiphase CE 3D MR angiography within a single or three repetitive breath-holds as the state-of-the-art technique achieves an accuracy of 100% in the visualization of main and segmental renal arteries, renal parenchyma, and renal vein structures in different phases (Prince et al. 1997; Wilman et al. 1997; Dong et al. 1999; Thornton et al. 1999), an accuracy ranging from 63% to 94% in the depiction of accessory renal arteries (Holland et al. 1996; Prince et al. 1995; Hahn et al. 1998; De Cobelli et al. 1997, 2000) (see Fig. 18.22), and a sensitivity of 90% and specificity of 100%, respectively, in the detection of renovascular anatomic variants (Van Hoe et al. 2000). In living renal allograft donors, this technique has shown to be 100% accurate and as reliable as conventional angiography in the determination of the renal vascular anatomy, which suggests that invasive conventional angiography can be replaced at a 31% cost savings (Buzzas et al. 1997). Generally, MR angiographic results are similar to those reported with CT angiography (Beregi et al. 1996; Kaatee et al. 1997; Johnson et al. 1999), and better than those reported with color-coded duplex Doppler US (Berland et al. 1990; Desberg et al. 1990, Hansen et al. 1990, House et al. 1999, De Cobelli et al. 2000). Comparing single-phase and multiphase time-resolved imaging within a breath-hold, it has been demonstrated that multiphase technique is more robust and easier to perform, imaging is less disturbed by artifacts, shows an improved contrast enhancement, and allows simultaneous evaluation of arterial and venous disease (Van Hoe et al. 2000). However, multiphase CE MR angiography has a larger voxel size, resulting, at the moment, in a lower spatial resolution. Abnormalities of renal veins can be depicted more clearly when arterial phase images are subtracted from images which showed adequate venous enhancement.

In addition to morphologic imaging of the renal vasculature, CE 3D MR angiography provides functional information about the kidney. In combination with MR renography, the measurement of the glomerular filtration rate based on plasma clearance of gadopentate-dimeglumine correlates well with 99mTc-DTPA clearance (Ros et al. 1995). Renal blood flow can be determined with cardiac-gated 2D cine PC flow mapping techniques, which correlate well with flow values measured by para-amino-hippurate-clearance (Debatin et al. 1994). The validity and reproducibility of breath-hold and respiratory-triggered PC MR imaging techniques in the measurement of renal blood flow have been demonstrated by De Haan et al. (2000).

18.3.2 Pathological Conditions

18.3.2.1 Abdominal Aorta

18.3.2.1.1 Occlusive Disease

Abdominal aortic occlusive disease is mainly caused by atherosclerosis, and the most common site is the infrarenal distal portion of the vessel, including the aortic bifurcation. Coarctation due to Takayasu's disease, other nonspecific types of arteritis, and congenital hypo- or dysplastic disorders is rare (Lipchik and Rogoff 1983a; Kadir 1986). Atherosclerotic lesions are seen predominantly in males over 50 years of age and in postmenopausal women; they appear with a higher incidence and severity in diabetes mellitus and may be accelerated by cigarette smoking, arterial hypertension, and hypercholesterolemia. In the earlier stage of atherosclerosis plaque material develops which can be complicated by ulceration, calcification, or superimposed thrombosis. Abdominal aortic atherosclerosis may involve the orifices of the aortic branches. Acute, complete occlusion of the abdominal aorta is located mostly in below the renal arteries and can be caused by trauma, thromboembolism, aneurysmal thrombosis, acute in situ thrombosis of preexisting atherosclerotic stenosis (Leriche's syndrome), metastatic tumors, coagulation disorders, and iatrogenic lesions due to catheter manipulations or surgical interventions. It clinically manifests with lack of pulse, pallor, pain, paresthesias, and paralysis. Chronic occlusive atherosclerosis also most frequently affects the infrarenal aorta and the aortoiliac bifurcation and often is associated with severe calcifications. Atherosclerotic aortic coarctation is a focal, severe septumlike stenosis in the distal portion of the vessel, typically seen in women 40–50 years of age. Progression of chronic occlusive atherosclerosis is slow and permits the development of extensive collaterals. Symptoms of chronic aortic and aortoiliac occlusive disease depend on its localization and expansion to the branching vessels, including mesenteric ischemia, ischemia of the kidneys with renal failure or arterial hypertension, intermittent thigh and buttock claudication, impotence, paresthesias, ischemic neural pain, and limb weakness. The prognosis of aortic and aortoiliac occlusive disease is poor due to its continuous progression. Surgical management includes thrombendarterectomy and diverse bypass procedures and the implantation of aortoiliac or aortofemoral bifurcation grafts. Of major therapeutic importance today are percutaneous angioplasty and endovascular stenting (Strandness and Van Breda 1994; Nyman et al. 2000).

Diagnostic examination of occlusive or stenotic aortic disease requires characterization of the lesion and exact evaluation of the site and extent, the stenotic grade, the number of collaterals, and the status of adjacent aortic branches proximal and distal to the lesion. The diagnostic tool for detecting and staging occlusive aortic disease includes DSA, US, CT angiography, and MR angiography combined with MR imaging of the aortic wall.

Conventional Angiography. Invasive DSA remains the method of first choice and is considered the gold standard due to its high accuracy in detecting vascular lesions and in evaluating the pathologic vascular anatomy for planning interventional therapy. Although invasive, the risk for the patients is reduced if a transfemoral approach and catheter material of 3 F in diameter are used, which allows an outpatient procedure. The transbrachial approach, required in completely occluded iliac arteries or occlusion of the distal abdominal aorta, involves a greater risk for the patient, particularly when severe atheromatosis of the aortic arch is present. The major advantage of DSA is the possibility of immediate percutaneous management in a large number of patients when occlusive disease is proven and has been found suitable for balloon angioplasty or stent placement.

Ultrasonography. Noninvasive US, particularly color-coded Doppler US, is generally accepted as a fast and simple method of detecting aortic lesions with a high accuracy, including reliable localization of aortic stenosis or occlusion. Occlusive material shows low to medium echogeneity, calcifications are hyperechoic, and color-coded flow information demonstrates accelerated flow rates at the site of stenosis and a loss of flow information in complete occlusion. However, accurate US information of adjacent iliac arteries is obtained in only 50% of cases due to known limitations in this area.

MR Angiography. CT angiography (Prokop et al. 1997; Rubin et al. 1998), which plays only a secondary and complementary diagnostic role in aortic occlusive disease, is useful in analyzing the site and extent of severe thrombus calcifications before percutaneous or surgical intervention. In contrast, breath-hold gadolinium-enhanced 3D MR angiography appears as a true and valid alternative to diagnostic DSA and is well suited for evaluating patients with symptoms suggestive of aortic occlusive disease. In addition to depicting stenoses and inner wall irregularities of the abdominal aorta and the bifurcation, this technique can also display collateral vessels and distal vascular run-off vessels on postprocessed images (Figs. 18.4a–f, 18.5a–d). The problem of distinguishing between complete occlusion and high grade stenosis due to its threshold dependence can be solved by both the analysis of source images and virtual endoscopy (Davis et al. 1997). Using CE breath-hold 3D MR angiography, a correct diagnosis of vascular obstruction has been reported with a sensitivity and specificity of 100% and 100%, respectively, for the infrarenal aorta, and 100% and 97%–98%, respectively, for the common iliac arteries (Snidow et al. 1996; Leung et al. 1998). Complementary to MR angiography, CE or postcontrast T1-weighted MR imaging is able to depict not only location and amount of atheromatous plaque material, which can be distinguished clearly from signal-intense flowing blood, but also inflammatory causes of aortic stenosis, i.e., in Takayasu's arteritis, which shows a pathologic contrast enhancement (Choe et al. 2000). For the characterization of mural thrombi, nonenhanced T1- and T2-weighted MR imaging can differentiate between organized (low signal in T1 and T2), unorganized (high signal in T1 and T2), and mixed (adequate pattern of signal

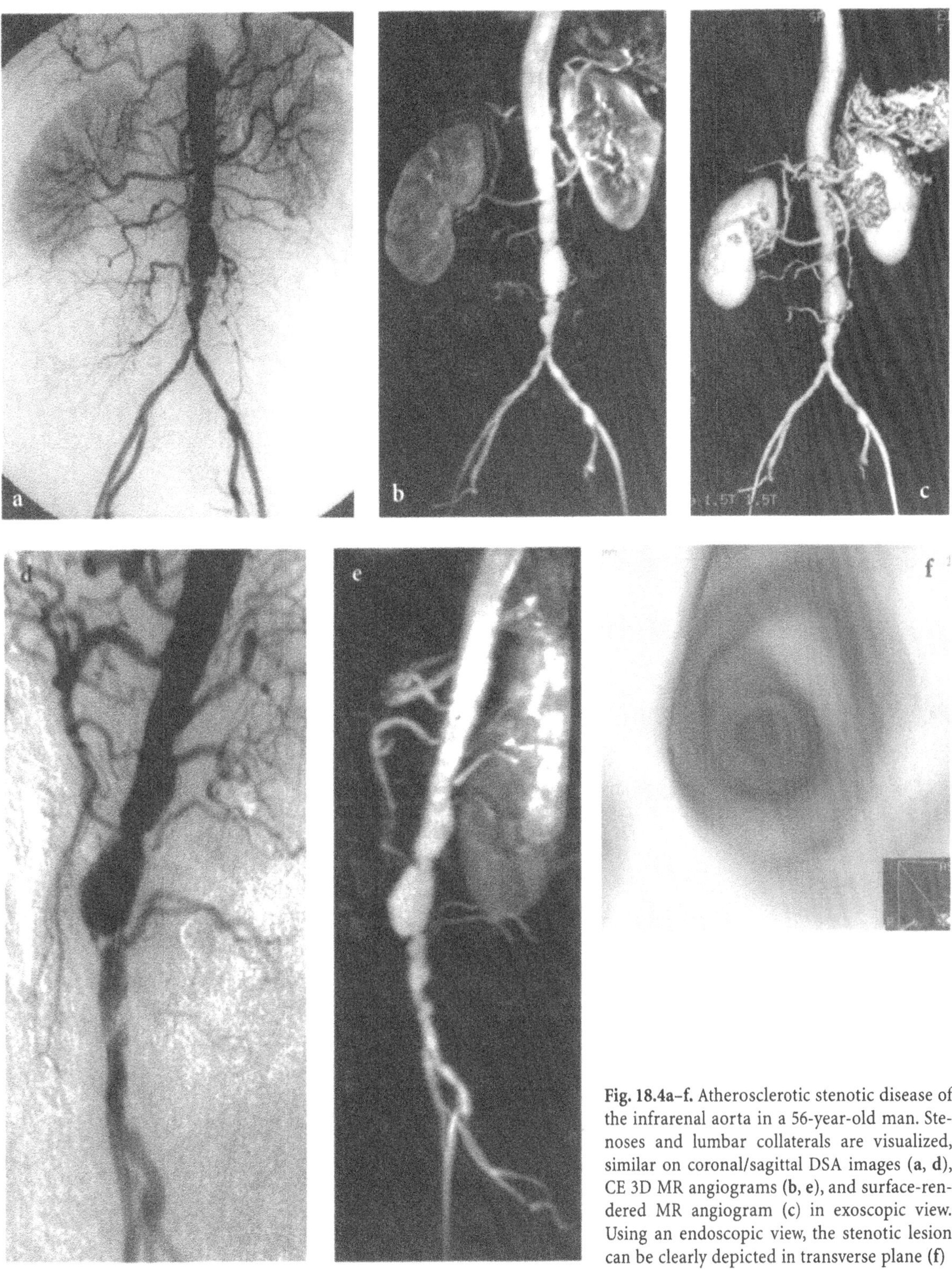

Fig. 18.4a–f. Atherosclerotic stenotic disease of the infrarenal aorta in a 56-year-old man. Stenoses and lumbar collaterals are visualized, similar on coronal/sagittal DSA images (**a**, **d**), CE 3D MR angiograms (**b**, **e**), and surface-rendered MR angiogram (**c**) in exoscopic view. Using an endoscopic view, the stenotic lesion can be clearly depicted in transverse plane (**f**)

intensities) thrombus material (Castrucci et al. 1995). In complete occlusion of the distal aorta, i.e., Leriche's syndrome, CE 3D MR angiography offers a noninvasive alternative to transbrachial arteriography. A correct diagnosis has been reported in 100% of cases (Link et al. 1998), including a better visualization of distal iliac and femoral arteries than in DSA, in which these vascular structures frequently cannot be depicted satisfactorily (Fig. 18.6a–c). Thus, in the preoperative planning prosthetic graft therapy, which requires information about the distal run-off vessels, MR angiography can replace DSA. The useful-

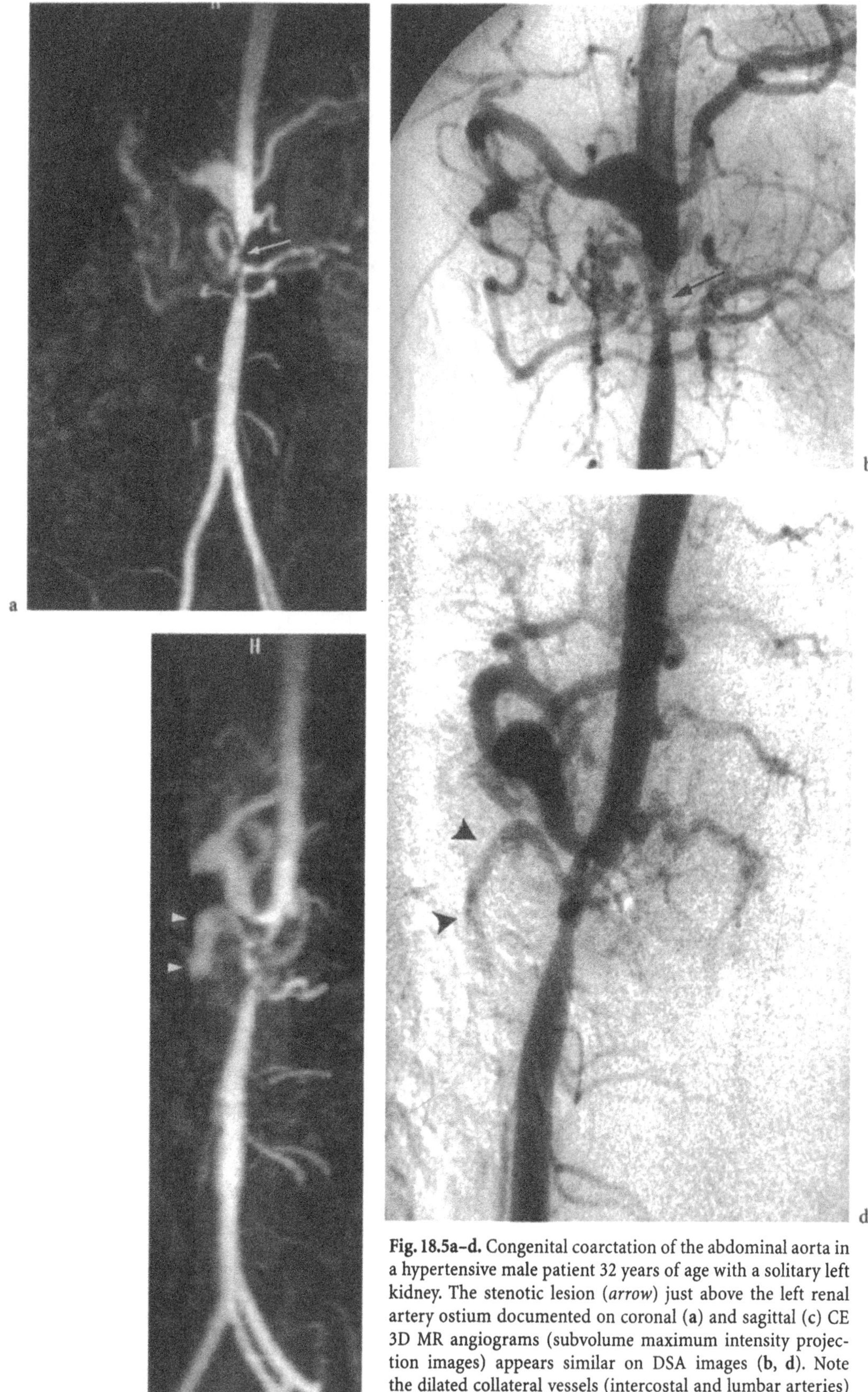

Fig. 18.5a–d. Congenital coarctation of the abdominal aorta in a hypertensive male patient 32 years of age with a solitary left kidney. The stenotic lesion (*arrow*) just above the left renal artery ostium documented on coronal (**a**) and sagittal (**c**) CE 3D MR angiograms (subvolume maximum intensity projection images) appears similar on DSA images (**b, d**). Note the dilated collateral vessels (intercostal and lumbar arteries) and a pseudoaneurysmal dilatation of the celiac trunk. SMA (*arrowheads*) is mainly supplied by collaterals via the gastroduodenal artery

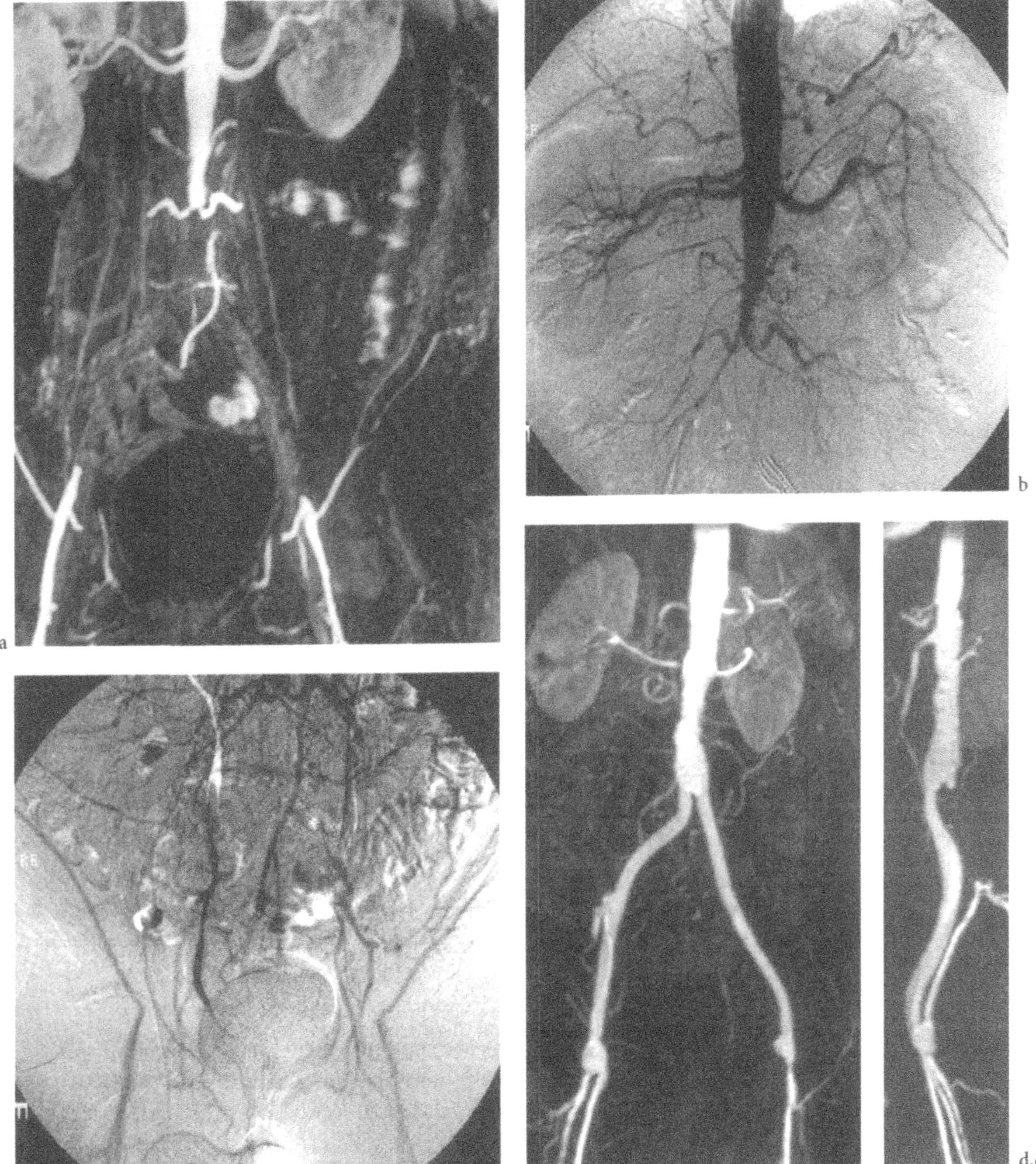

Fig. 18.6a–e. Totally occluded terminal aorta (Leriche's syndrome) in a 62-year-old man with bilateral claudication of the lower extremities and symptoms of impotence. Coronal CE 3D MR angiogram (**a**) clearly shows the aortic occlusion. Collateral vessels and both common femoral arteries can be better visualized than on DSA images (**b, c**) due to higher contrast. Postinterventional CE 3D MR angiography (maximum intensity projection) shows normal patency of the aortofemoral bifurcation prosthesis in the coronal (**d**) and sagittal plane (**e**)

ness of CE 3D MR angiography has been proven in postinterventional follow-up (Carlos et al. 1999), showing an accurate evaluation of critical anastomotic areas, run-off vessels, and the patency of prosthetic grafts, endovascular stent grafts, and the vessel lumen after angioplasty (Figs. 18.6d, e, 18.7a, b). However, diverse metallic graft materials may induce different grades of signal void due to artifacts (Fig. 18.8) that may limit the evaluation of this vascular region on CE 3D MR angiograms (see Chap. 12).

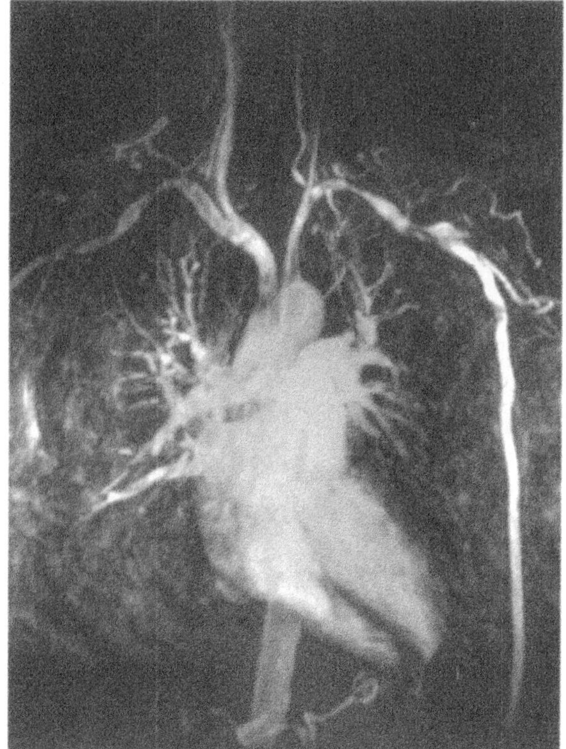

a

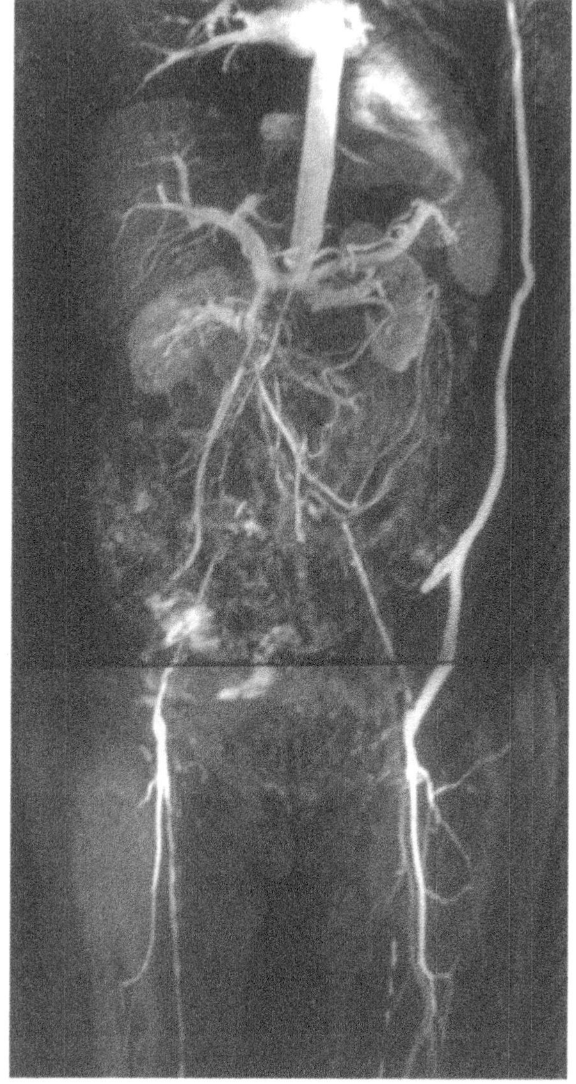

b

Fig. 18.7a, b. A 78-year-old man with Leriche's syndrome surgically treated by extracorporeal left axillo-femoral dacron bypass-graft. The thoracic (**a**) and abdomino-pelvic (**b**) CE 3D MR angiograms performed in two examination steps show a patent graft, including normal anastomoses

18.3.2.1.2
Aneurysmal Disease

A variety of etiological mechanisms have been implicated in the pathogenesis of aneurysms. Atherosclerosis, although most commonly cited, is probably not the only important etiological factor. Other potential contributing factors include arterial hypertension, lateral wall stress, vibratory forces, enzymatic imbalance, trauma, infection – including mycotic lesions and vasculitis in Behcet's disease – and congenital disorders such as Marfan's and Ehlers-Danlos syndrome, which all may reduce the aortic wall stability and resistance to pressure. The prevalence of abdominal aortic aneurysm (AAA) is reported to be increasing. A 2%–6% incidence of AAA has been proven in autopsy studies: approximately 10% of patients in a vascular surgeon's practice suffer from AAA, approximately 28,000 new aneurysms have been reported in the USA every year, and 5000 patients present with rupture. Eighty-five percent of patients are male, the mean age is 67 years, in more than 90% the infrarenal part of the abdominal aorta is involved, and in 30% the aneurysm extends to the iliac arteries (Kadir 1986; Millis et al. 1992). Aneurysmal disease is defined as a localized widening of the vessel lumen up to a diameter more than 50% larger than normal. In the abdominal aorta, aneurysmal disease commonly is considered if the diameter is 4 cm and more. In most cases AAA appears fusiform, whereas saccular aneurysms are rare. In true aneurysms, all layers of the aortic wall are involved, whereas in saccular false aneurysms, the layers are disrupted and surrounded by periarterial tissue. The presence of AAA

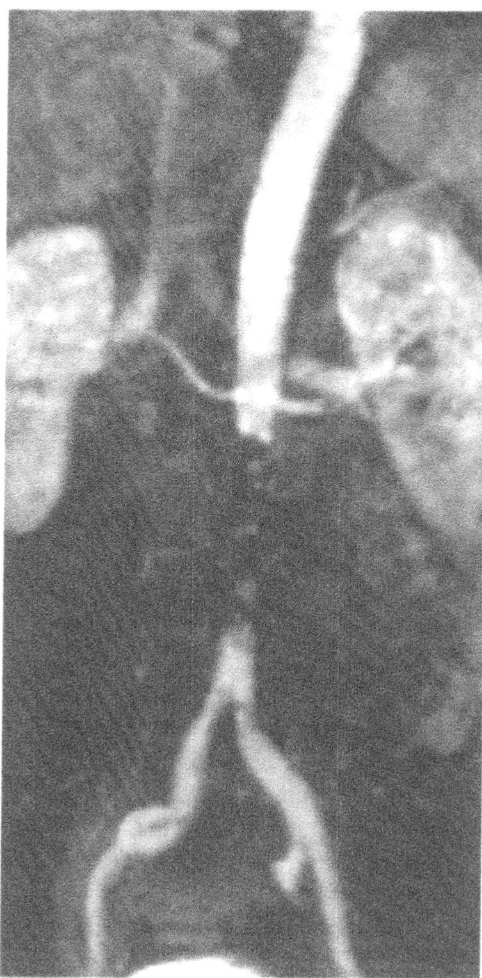

Fig. 18.8. Postinterventional CE 3D MR angiogram of a patient with occlusive disease of the infrarenal aorta treated by endoluminal stent angioplasty (Wallstent). Note the complete signal loss in the stent area due to metallic material artifacts

is associated with an increased probability of aneurysms elsewhere. In the absence of interventional treatment, AAA commonly dilatates until rupture and exsanguination occur. This progression is predicated by Laplace's law, which states that the tension on the wall of a sphere is directly proportional to the radius of its lumen and the pressure exerted from within. Hence, as the radius of an aneurysm increases, so does the wall tension, and rupture will inevitably result. The classic relationship between aneurysm size and 5-year risk of rupture has been described by Szilagyi et al. (1966). Once an aneurysm has attained the size of 6 cm, the risk of precipitous rupture increases significantly. For an aneurysm of 4 cm in size, the risk of rupture is less than 15%, whereas for aneurysms greater than 8 cm the 5-year rupture rate is reported to be 75%. The growth rate of smaller aneurysms is 2–3 mm, of larger aneurysms up to 4 mm per year. In the majority of cases the AAA is asymptomatic; clinical symptoms can be observed in 40% of patients and may indicate rapid growth or imminent rupture. Symptoms are described as abdominal pain located in the epigastrium or flank pain. The atypical location of the aneurysm may cause compression of adjacent structures, inducing different symptoms. Inflammatory AAA accounts for 5%–23% of all aneurysms. The definition of inflammation includes mural thickening, fragmentation, and attenuation of the internal elastic lamina, loss of smooth muscle in the media, dense connective tissue with neovascularity surrounding the aortic wall, and infiltration by lymphocytes, plasma cells, and histiocytes. Adherence of various visceral structures can be observed, e.g., ureter, duodenum, vena cava, and sigmoid colon (Cullenward et al. 1986). Opinions as to the etiology of such inflammatory aneurysms differ. Some have suggested an immunological basis while others have proposed that they form as part of the spectrum of inflammatory aortitis or bear a relationship to retroperitoneal fibrosis. Although the frequency of rupture in inflammatory aneurysms is reported to be not higher than in noninflammatory AAA, indications for surgery or endovascular stent grafts are more restricted because repair is associated with a higher morbidity and mortality. If correctly diagnosed preoperative steroid treatment can be instituted to reduce the inflammatory reaction. In rare cases, mycotic aneurysms of the abdominal aorta can be observed. This is mostly of the saccular type and is associated with septic infectious disease due to endocarditis, spondylitis, or osteomyelitis. Invasive elective treatment of AAA is commonly recommended when the diameter exceeds 5–6 cm, when rapid progression has been found in follow-up studies, or if aneurysms of less than 5 cm in diameter become clinically symptomatic. Because the mortality following elective surgery has progressively decreased to 2%–3% due to improved operative techniques and cardiac preparation, prophylactic graft replacement is advocated in patients in good health. In contrast, aneurysmal rupture is a highly life-threatening event with a mortality of more than 60%. Surgical techniques include endoaneurysmorrhaphy or segmental resection, and the implantation of tubes or bifurcation grafts (Millis et al. 1992). In selected cases with a suitable configuration of the AAA, endovascular stent graft placement can be performed successfully to exclude the aneurysm and prevent rupture (Blum et al. 1996; Dorffner et al. 1997). For planning invasive therapy, preinterventional information is required on the type and localization of the aneurysm, its diameter and craniocaudad extent, the aneurysmal wall structures and the periaortic space, the relationship to renal and iliac arteries, the status of the mesenteric and internal iliac circulation, and the presence of additional iliac occlusive disease. The detection of accessory renal arteries which arise from the aneurysm is of major importance for the prevention of segmental renal infarction following surgery or stent graft placement. Before stent graft therapy, the characteristic parameters have to be measured exactly, such as the lengths of the infrarenal aorta and the proximal aneurysmal neck, and the diameters of the supra- and infrarenal aorta, the aortic bifurcation, and iliac arteries. On the basis of these data, the individual size of a stent graft prosthesis can be planned and manufactured.

Ultrasonography. US has emerged as a highly valuable tool for the detection of suspected AAA, with an accuracy of up to 100%, and has been introduced for screening in the elderly population (Dock et al. 1998). US is useful and accurate for sequential measurement of the diameter of a known asymptomatic AAA; it can detect an intraluminal thrombus and perianeurysmal fibrosis or perivascular masses in ruptured aneurysm. However, due to known limiting factors, the primary role of US is still the identification of an AAA, whereas other diagnostic techniques are more useful to stage AAA for interventional therapy.

CT Angiography. Helical CT angiography, a noninvasive technique combining the advantages of conventional angiography and conventional CT imaging for evaluation and staging of AAA (Zeman et al. 1995), plays the primary diagnostic role today. Using this technique, aneurysmal extent, diameter, mural thrombus, wall calcifications and inflammatory wall thickening, perivascular space, and status of the renal, splanchnic, and iliac arteries can be evaluated. In addition, CT is sensitive in the evaluation of suspected imminent or acute aneurysmal rupture, of postoperative perigraft fluid collections, anastomotic pseudoaneurysms, aortoenteric fistulas, abscess formations, and endoleaks or dislocation of stent material following stent graft treatment (Siegel and Cohan 1994; Dorffner et al. 1997).

Conventional Angiography. For the diagnosis of AAA conventional angiography (Lipchik and Rogoff 1983b) has been replaced by CT angiography, which is less invasive, lower in cost, and can better evaluate the entire aneurysmal extent. Although the aneurysmal diameter and extent into iliac arteries are frequently underestimated, particularly in cases of mural thrombus, angiography is highly accurate in the evaluation of renal, splanchnic, and iliac arteries. Furthermore, conventional calibrated catheter angiography in combination with helical CT examination is of important value for the correct measurement of vascular distances, which is necessary for planning endovascular stent graft therapy (Blum et al. 1996; Qanadli et al. 2000).

MR Angiography. Noninvasive ultrafast CE 3D MR angiography has major advantages over CT angiography and can help overcome its limitations in the group of patients in which AAA is associated with progressive atherosclerotic disease. The use of paramagnetic contrast agents is nearly free from side effects; in particular nephrotoxic effects can be widely excluded (Prince et al. 1996). MR angiography and complementary post-contrast T1-weighted imaging of the AAA combine the advantages of DSA and cross-sectional imaging; it provides information about the condition of the lumen, the aortic wall, and the para-aortic space. The large field of view in 3D MR angiography allows easy visualization of the extent of an aneurysm into the iliac arteries (Davis et al. 1997; Gilfeather et al. 1997). Intraluminal contrast enhancement accurately visualizes the perfused portions of the AAA during the arterial phase (Figs. 18.9a, 18.10a–c). In large aneurysms with slow blood flow the acquisition of two repetitive 3D data sets is useful in order to optimize the visualization of renal arteries during the early and iliac arteries during the late arterial phase. The intraluminal aneurysmal anatomy can be displayed and the exact dimensions of the aneurysm can be determined by using subvolume MIP images and MPR images in any desired plane. The 3D nature of the data set allows ready assessment of the relationship of the aneurysm to the origins of renal and splanchnic arteries. Important information regarding diseases of the renal arteries and their relationship to the proximal aneurysmal neck can be easily obtained from reformatted images. Moreover, the true nature of SR display is sometimes superior to MIP imaging in the preoperative evaluation of abdominal aneurysms, and virtual endoscopy can be helpful in preoperative planning by providing an internal view of the aorta and branch origins (Davis et al. 1997). In comparison with conventional angiography or operative findings of AAA, CE 3D MR

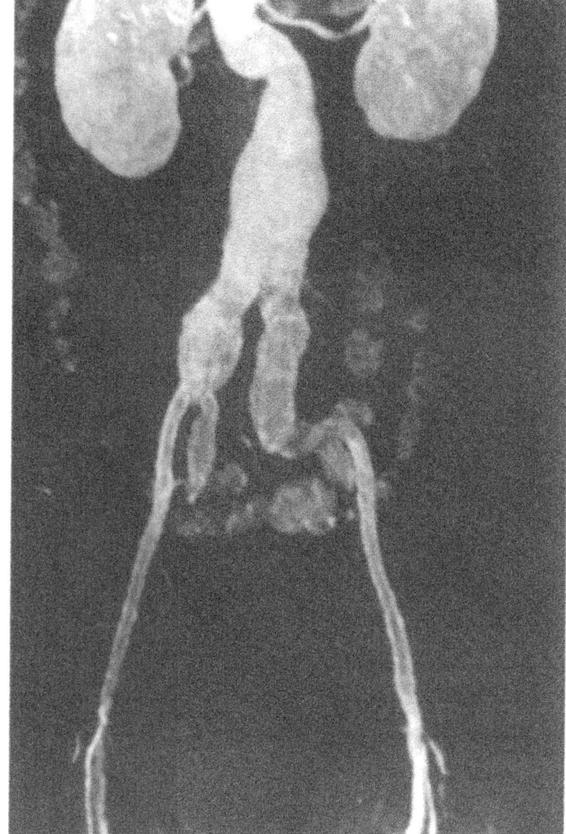

a

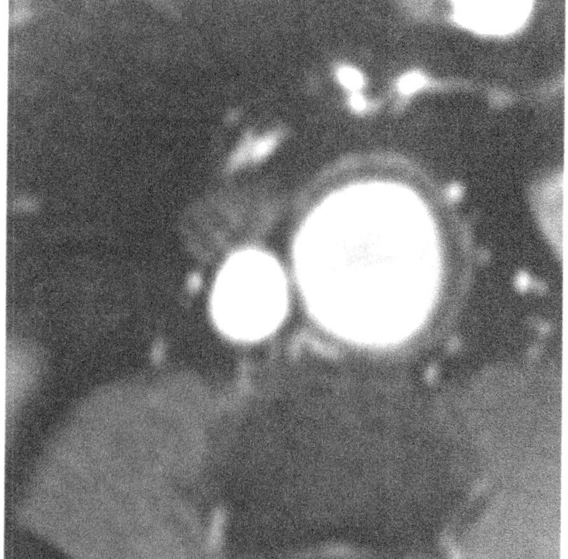

b

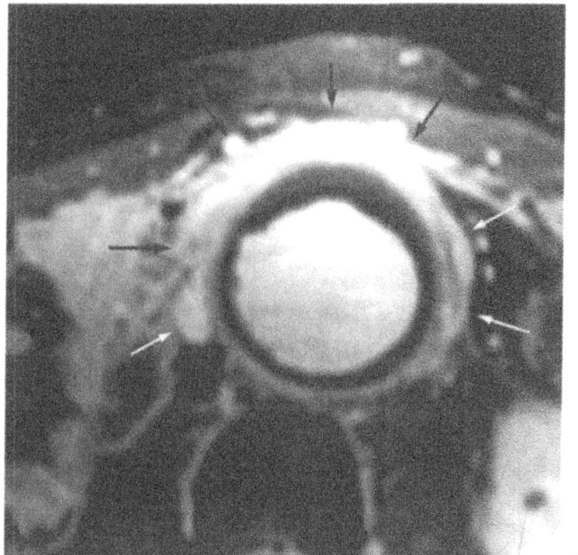

c

Fig. 18.9a–c. CE 3D MR angiogram (maximum intensity projection) of an abdominal aortic aneurysm with aneurysmal extension into both common iliac arteries (**a**). Postcontrast fat-saturated T1-weighted transverse GRE images (150/4.2 ms TR/TE, 75° flip angle, 31.2 kHz bandwidth, 192×256 matrix, 40 cm field-of-view, 6-mm section thickness with a 0.6-mm gap, 1 nex, spectral fat-saturation, 13 sections within a breath-hold) show examples of a thickened inner aortic wall due to thrombotic layers (**b**) and a thickened outer aortic wall tissue with significant contrast enhancement (**c**) (*arrows*) due to inflammatory hypervascularization

angiography has been reported to be highly sensitive and specific in the detection of accessory renal arteries and associated occlusive or stenotic disease of the splanchnic, renal, and iliac arteries (Prince et al. 1995; Thurnher et al. 1997). Compared with CT angiography it is regarded as being superior in assessing visceral and iliac artery disease because of the larger field-of-view, but sometimes inferior in depicting accessory renal arteries and grading renal artery stenosis (RAS).

Fat-saturated, postcontrast T1-weighted fast GRE breath-hold imaging immediately performed after the angiographic study allows the accurate evaluation of aortic wall structures, a clear differentiation of thrombus from intraluminal slow flow, the depiction of intramural hemorrhage and inflammatory changes of the aortic wall, and the evaluation of para-aortic space involvement (Fig. 18.9b, c). CE 3D MR angiography in combination with postcontrast T1-weighted imaging have been shown to be as good as CT angiography and DSA in staging AAA for therapy using suitable software (Arlart et al. 1997; Thurnher et al. 1997). The evaluation of aneurysmal extent, the determination of distances between the aneurysm and renal artery origins or aortic and iliac bifurcations, and the measurement of the aortoiliac

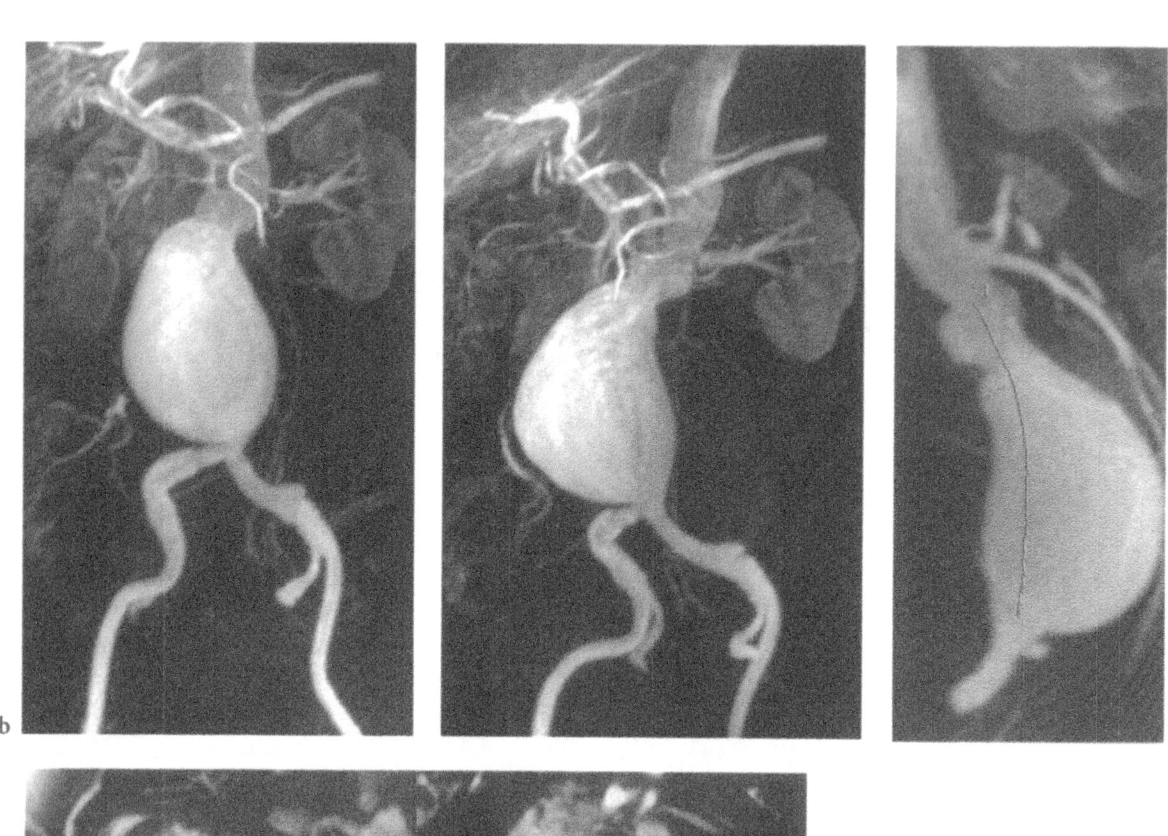

a,b c

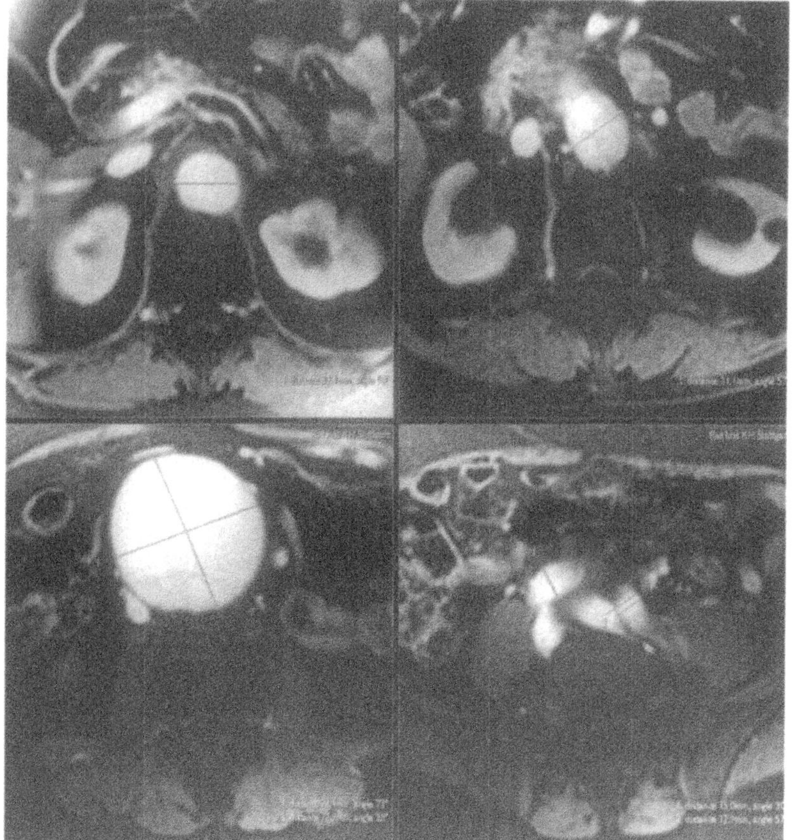

d

Fig. 18.10a–d. Asymptomatic abdominal aortic aneurysm in a 76-year-old man. CE 3D MR angiography (maximum intensity projection images) during the late arterial phase shows the site and extension of the aneurysm and its relationship to renal, mesenteric, and iliac arteries in coronal plane (**a**), 45° LAO projection (**b**), and on sagittal (**c**) reformatted images. On MIP images in the coronal and sagittal plane longitudinal extension of the aneurysm can be determined. Representative vascular diameters can also be measured (levels of suprarenal aorta, proximal aneurysmal neck, aneurysmal sac, aortic bifurcation, and both common iliac arteries) on transverse fat-saturated postcontrast T1-weighted images (**d**)

diameters needed for therapeutic planning can be performed in coronal and transverse sections (Fig. 18.10c, d). In post-treatment follow-up, CE 3D MR angiography is able to provide reliable information about graft patency and vascular complications (Figs. 18.11, 18.12, 18.13). In our experience the sequence protocol combining MR angiography and postcontrast T1-weighted imaging (Fig. 18.14a–d) has shown to be more reliable than CE helical CT studies in depicting endoleaks.

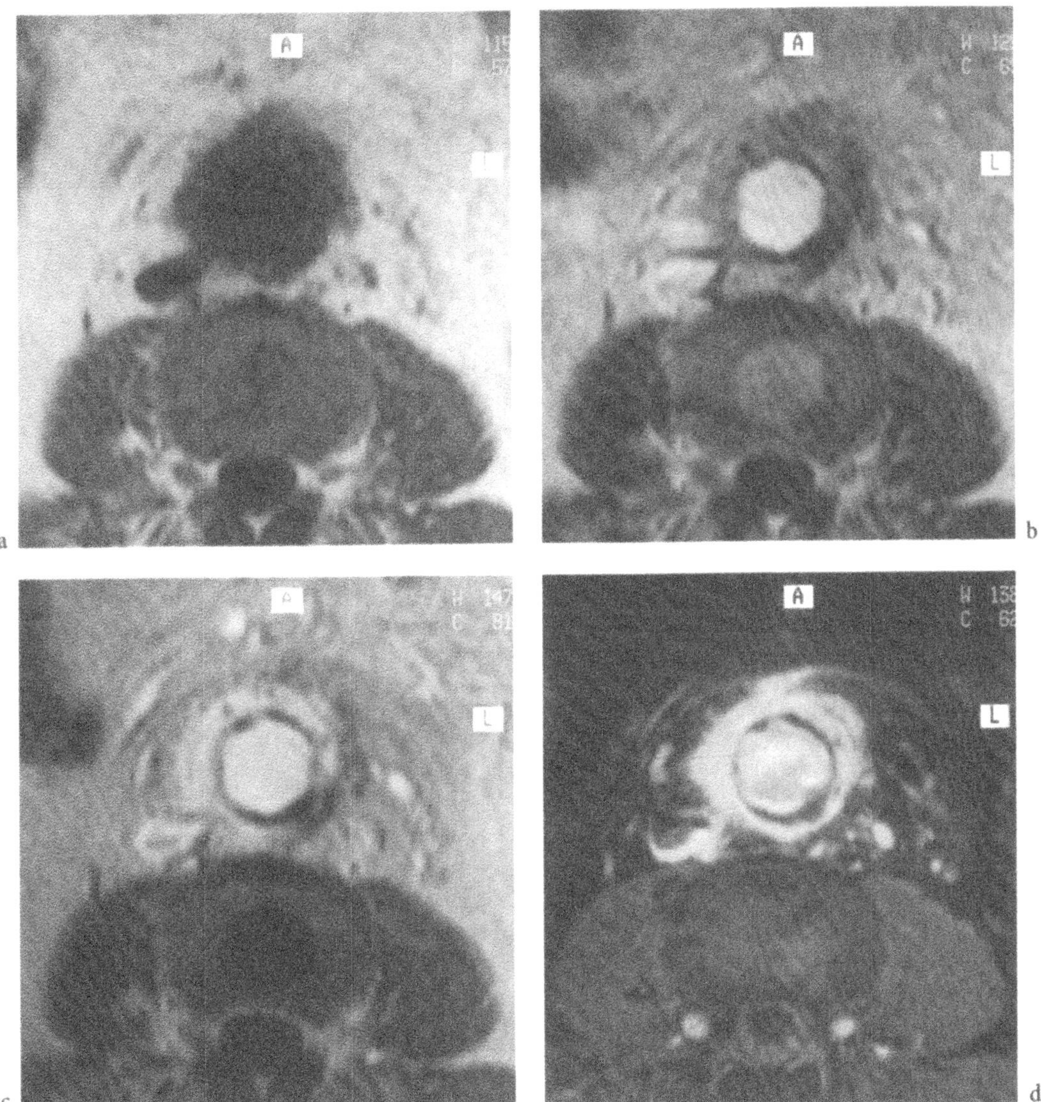

Fig. 18.11a–d. Follow-up study in a 67-year-old man in whom abdominal aortic aneurysm was surgically treated by aortic tube-graft prosthesis. As a complication inflammatory disease is proven by dynamic transverse CE T1-weighted GRE imaging, showing irregular low signal aortic wall thickening on the precontrast image (**a**) with increasing contrast enhancement in the early (**b**) and late (**c**) phase following i.v. administration of gadolinium DTPA (0.2 mmol/kg). The enhanced circular inflammatory aortic wall thickening can be depicted particularly on a postcontrast fat-saturated T1-weighted image (**d**)

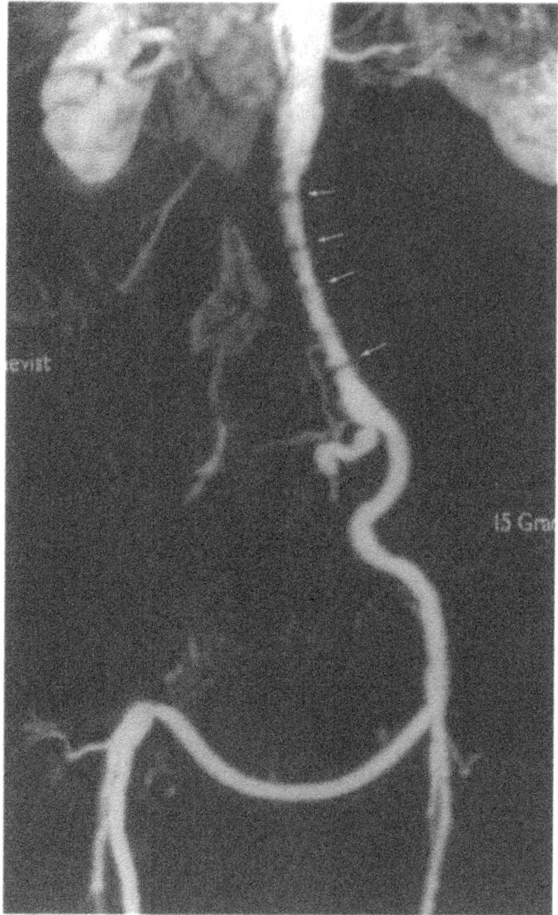

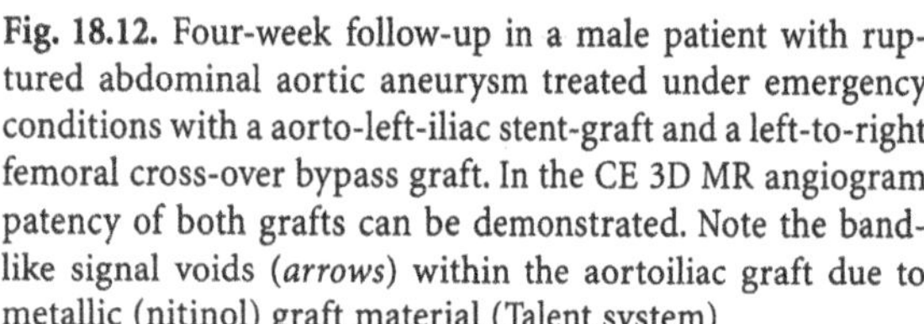

Fig. 18.12. Four-week follow-up in a male patient with ruptured abdominal aortic aneurysm treated under emergency conditions with a aorto-left-iliac stent-graft and a left-to-right femoral cross-over bypass graft. In the CE 3D MR angiogram patency of both grafts can be demonstrated. Note the band-like signal voids (*arrows*) within the aortoiliac graft due to metallic (nitinol) graft material (Talent system)

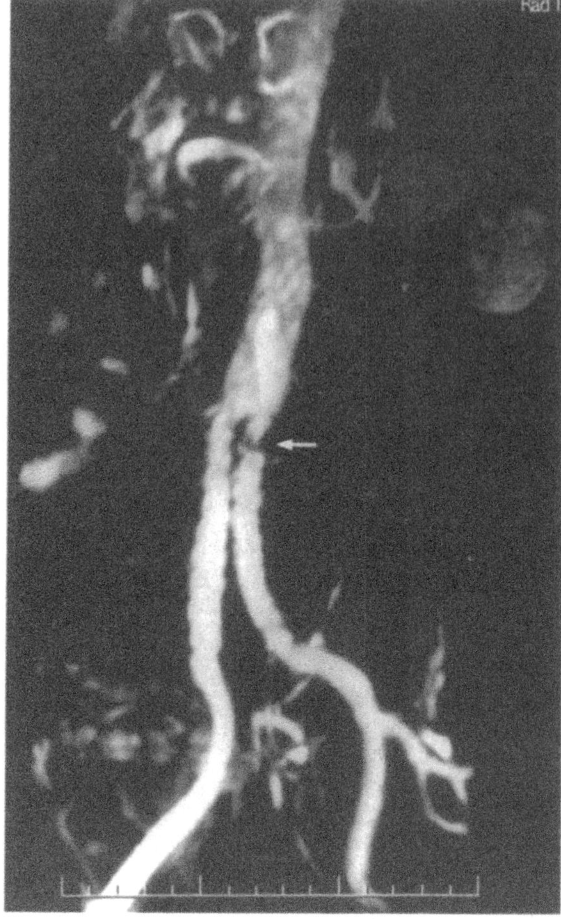

Fig. 18.13. Twelve-month follow-up in a patient with abdominal aortic aneurysm successfully treated by endovascular stent graft placement (Vanguard bifurcation system). The signal void at the left aortoiliac junction (*arrow*) mimicking stenosis is caused by metallic clip material

18.3.2.1.3
Dissection

Aortic dissection is widely recognized as the most common nontraumatic aortic event, with an out-of-hospital mortality of up to 80%, whereas overall in-hospital mortality is still only 15%–25%. Mortality and serious morbidity due to acute aortic dissection result from its attendant complications. In two-thirds of cases type A (Stanford classification) and in one third type B dissection can be observed. The majority of cases of abdominal aortic dissection (AAD) originate in the thoracic aorta, whereas a local aortic or iliac dissection iatrogenically due to arterial catheterization, surgical procedures, or blunt abdominal trauma is rare. Up to 30% of patients with type B dissection sustain a branch vessel occlusion with end-organ ischemia, including the kidneys in 8%, liver or gut in 5%, spine in 3%, and the extremities in 24% of cases (Kadir et al. 1986; Williams et al. 1997). Symptoms of AAD depend on the site of the vascular complication and may include thoracic or lumbar pain, rupture leading to exsanguination, and ischemic complications due to aortic branch occlusion. Ischemia of the viscera and extremities depends on the pathoanatomic conditions following dissection and may be caused either by partial or complete occlusion of the arterial ostia due to compression of the true lumen by an extensively dilated false channel or reduced arterial perfusion of the kidneys or mesenterics when those branches arise from a minimally perfused false channel without the existence of sufficient re-entries. Additionally, intimal flaps can directly occlude these arterial branches. In symp-

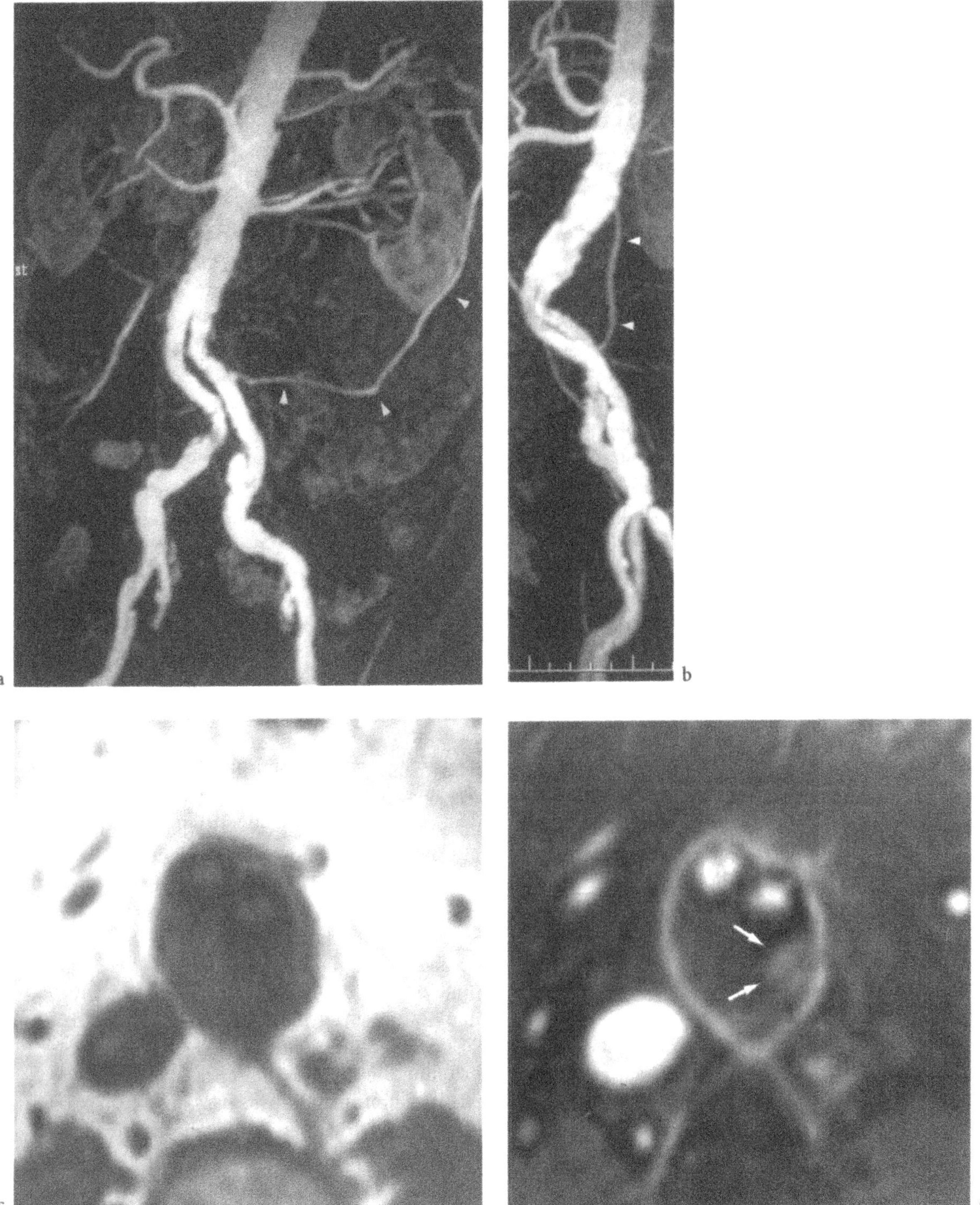

Fig. 18.14a–d. Six-month follow-up in a male patient having obtained endoluminal stent-graft treatment of an abdominal aortic aneurysm (Talent bifurcation system). On coronal (**a**) and sagittal (**b**) CE 3D MR angiograms the patency of the graft can be demonstrated as well as retrograde collateral enhancement of the inferior mesenteric artery (IMA) (*arrowheads*). Transverse pre-contrast T1-weighted GRE image shows homogeneous signal of the excluded aneurysmal sac (**c**), whereas on a fat-saturated post-contrast T1-weighted image a pathologic enhancement of the aneurysmal sac (**d**) can be depicted clearly (*arrows*) due to a leakage via IMA

tomatic cases, immediate interventional therapy is required. Surgery and medical therapy for this condition have shown to be inadequate in many cases, because both are associated with substantial rates of failure and considerable potential morbidity and mortality due to the treatment itself and to subsequent aneurysmal formation. Operative mortality approaches 50% when the acute dissection is complicated by paraplegia or renal and mesenteric ischemia. In addition to expeditious repair of the ascending aorta in the Stanford A type, several treatments for acute branch vessel obstruction have been described, such as resection of the entry tear, placement of an aortic interposition graft, operative fenestration of the dissecting membrane, and bypass grafting (Fann et al. 1995). Recently, percutaneous endoluminal catheter interventions have been introduced which demonstrate significantly lower morbidity and mortality rates. Importantly, balloon fenestration and placement of intraluminal stent grafts in the aorta or ostia of visceral and renal arteries have been recommended in order to avoid ischemic complications (Williams et al. 1997). Chronic AAD is asymptomatic in most cases and may be found in type B dissection of the descending aorta or secondarily following invasive treatment of symptomatic type A dissection of the ascending aorta. Chronic AAD with patency of both channels and no ischemic symptoms is usually managed conservatively and controlled by diagnostic follow-up. However, secondary aneurysmal widening of the false channel can occur with the risk of rupture due to a reduction in aortic wall resistance. In these cases invasive management strategies have to be considered.

In the majority of patients with aortic dissection, two patent channels are found which typically appear as a "double-barrel" aorta when distal re-entries exist at the level of the visceral arteries and the aortic, iliac, or femoral bifurcation. Imaging of the abdominal aorta in cases of dissection has to answer the following questions: is an aortic dissection present with a true and false lumen? If so, the extent of the dissection into pelvic or femoral arteries has to be evaluated, the origins of the visceral arteries from the true or false lumen have to be localized, involvement of the visceral arterial supply has to be excluded, possible re-entries have to be detected, and the flow and pressure condition in the true and false channel may be of interest in order to plan suitable therapy. Because patients with aortic dissection are often in unstable condition and require emergency evaluation, fast diagnostic imaging modalities are favored. Imaging strategies involve cross-sectional modalities such as US, CT angiography, and MR angiography.

Ultrasonography. Transthoracic or transesophageal color-coded duplex Doppler US can usually detect thoracic aortic dissection. Using percutaneous US, characteristic findings of the dissection membrane, which divides the aortic lumen into two channels, can be visualized in AAD and abnormal flow conditions in the aorta and the renal parenchyma can be reliably determined.

CT Angiography. Due to the limitations of US, CE helical CT angiography in combination with a fast thoracoabdominal approach is accepted today as the superior modality in the evaluation of aortic dissection. A high accuracy in the detection of the dissection membrane, the visceral branches originating from the true or false lumen, potential re-entries at the level of visceral arteries and the aortic bifurcation and in the determination of flow conditions in the true and false channel has been reported (Sebastia et al. 1999).

MR Angiography. In patients with ADD, breath-hold CE 3D MR angiography can provide answers to the diagnostic questions, like CT angiography. For complete imaging of the aortic dissection the MR examination requires less than 30 min even when CE MR angiography is combined with a 2D cine PC study to evaluate flow abnormalities (Alley et al. 1998). In suspected type B aortic dissection, both thoracic and abdominal CE 3D MR angiograms can be rendered after a single contrast injection when two separate, contiguous 3D data sets are acquired rapidly under conditions of dynamic table translation (Earls et al. 1998). However, in our experience detailed information of thoracic involvement, including the aortic arch branches, and in abdominal dissection, including the relationship to splanchnic and renal arteries, cannot be provided accurately due to problems of optimizing the contrast bolus. Thus, when a therapeutic decision must be made, both thoracic and abdominal MR angiograms should be performed in two separate studies. Time-resolved, i.e., biphasic high-resolution CE 3D MR angiography of the abdominal aorta allows the evaluation of flow differences between the true and false lumen, the accurate localization of splanchnic, iliac, and renal arterial ostia and their relationship to the dissecting membrane, and the perfusion of parenchymal organs. Vascular diagnostic information is optimized by the multiplanar reformatting capabilities of MR angiography. Oblique coronal and sagittal subvolume MIP images can demonstrate the craniocaudad course of the dissecting membrane, whereas transversely reformatted images and subvolume MIP images at the level of the visceral arteries accurately visualize the complex nature of the intimal flap anatomy and the different vessels arising either from the true or false channel (GILFEATHER et al. 1997; ALLEY et al. 1998) (Fig. 18.15a–l). Compared with conventional angiography and surgical findings, even non-breath-hold 3D MR angiography was able to diagnose correctly the type of aortic dissection, entry and re-entry tears, and the patency of the false lumen in 100% of cases (LEUNG et al. 1996), whereas breath-hold technique has been shown to be superior in evaluating the ostial status of visceral branches.

Direct quantification of blood flow in the true and false lumen is possible using 2D MR PC velocity mapping (INOUE et al. 1996). Different mean flow volumes and average peak velocities can be measured that may occur in the true and false lumen (STROTZER et al. 2000). In two-thirds of their patients the authors found a bidirectional flow in the false lumen with different degrees of reflux volumes which correlated with the MR angiographically proven distal occlusion of the false channel. As an advantage of MR angiography over CT angiography, the examination of the entire aorta without the use of nephrotoxic contrast agent is an important consideration in patients in whom coexisting renal disease is evident. As a drawback of MR imaging, calcifications of the aortic wall or the dissecting membrane, which sometimes may be of interest, cannot be visualized. Because CE MR angiography is able to reliably demonstrate critical vascular conditions in symptomatic patients with AAD, conventional angiography is still indicated in persistent, unclarified angiomorphologic conditions which may occur at the level of splanchnic and renal arteries, particularly in patients in whom catheter-guided intervention is selected for therapy on the basis of cross-sectional imaging techniques.

18.3.2.2
Splanchnic Arteries

In the splanchnic arteries primary and secondary pathologic disorders can be distinguished. Primary disorders of the celiac and mesenteric arteries include aneurysms, peripheral hemangiomas or arteriovenous malformations, and acute or chronic occlusive disease. Splanchnic artery aneurysms are rare (<1%), usually asymptomatic, and found incidentally in the majority of cases. Among the visceral aneurysms, those of the splenic artery are the most common, followed by aneurysms of the hepatic artery (approximately 80% extrahepatic), mesenteric arteries (approximately 8%), and celiac artery (approximately 4%). The cause of visceral aneurysms is primarily atherosclerosis; other etiologies are rare and include arterial dysplasia with medial wall degeneration, inflammatory processes, trauma, and congenital diseases. Symptoms, if present, depend on the site of the aneurysms and may consist of only vague upper abdominal discomfort, abdominal angina, and acute bowel ischemia when thrombosis occurs. However, aneurysmal rupture is a life-threatening event; an incidence of up to 30% has been reported and is significantly more common in aneurysms greater than 2 cm in size (MILLIS et al. 1992). Thus, even asymptomatic aneurysms greater than 2 cm should be repaired on account of the increased risk of rupture. Hemangiomas and arteriovenous malformations located in the peripheral mesenteric arcades as well as tumorous and inflammatory lesions can be a source of life-threatening intestinal bleeding. The clinically most important primary disorder of the mesenteric and celiac artery is acute occlusion due to thombembolic disease, which may lead to ischemia of the small and right large bowel when the superior portion is affected. Ischemia of the left large bowel, including the sigmoid colon, is observed when the inferior portion is affected. Acute mesenteric ischemia is a life-threatening event: the ischemic tolerance of the intestine is estimated to be 2–3 h. The incidence is increasing in accordance with the aging population, mainly in patients with cardiac arrhythmia. Mortality rates in acute mesenteric ischemia are over 60%. However, stenosis or even occlusions in the major branches of the splanchnic arteries may also occur without spectacular abdominal symptoms, such as postprandial pain associated with weight loss or unspecific symptoms mimicking a variety of other gastrointestinal diseases, or completely without any symptoms. In more than 95% of patients, atherosclerotic stenoses which are usually located at the origin of the SMA are responsible for chronic ischemia. The main secondary disorder of the celiac artery and SMA is caused by stenosis or occlusion due to infiltrative invasion of retroperitoneal tumors, particularly in advanced carcinoma of the pancreas. The detection of vascular infiltration is highly important for tumor staging and for planning suitable therapeutic procedures. Hepatic arterial and portal venous supply is of particular inter-

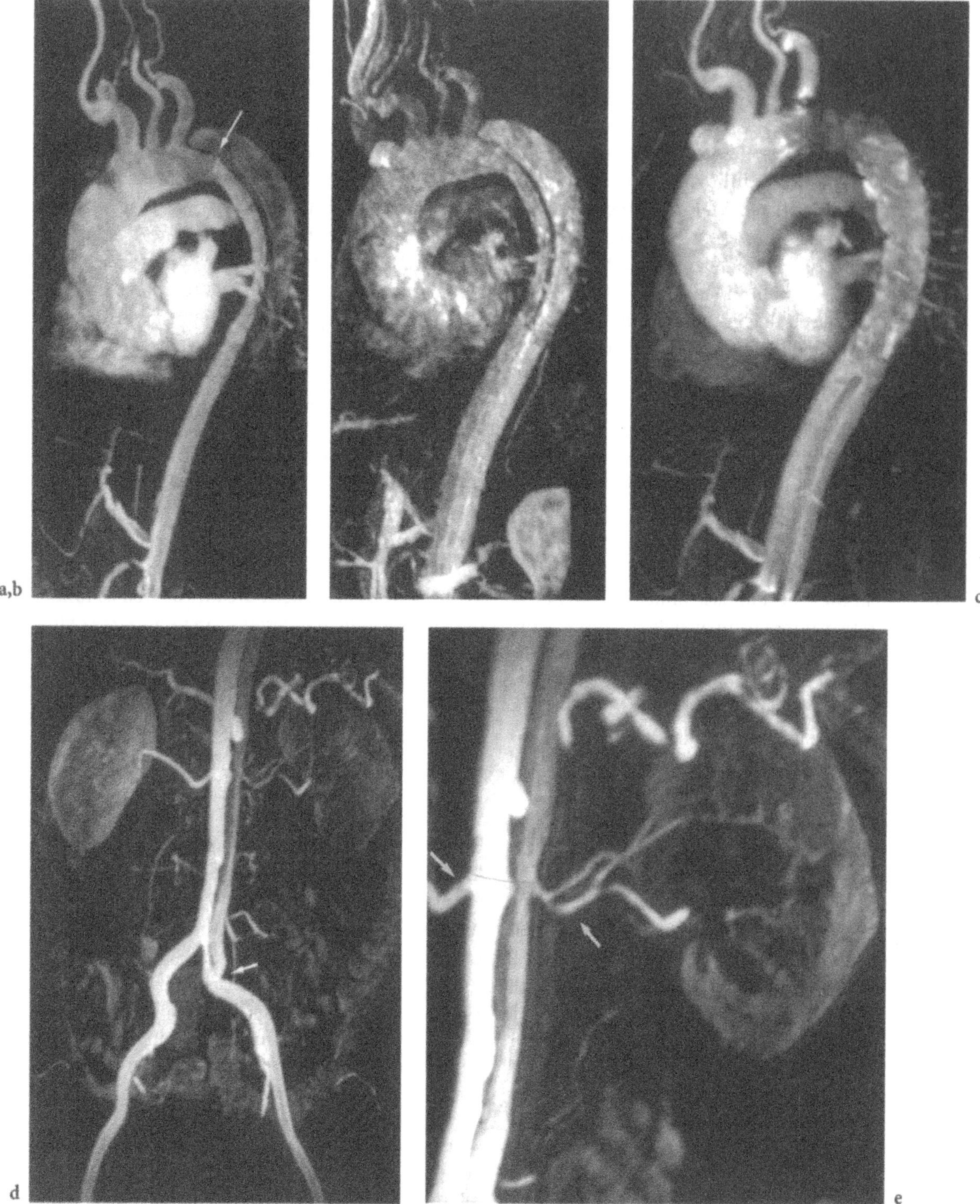

Fig. 18.15a–l. A 64-year-old hypertensive man with subacute symptomatic type B dissection of the thoracic and abdominal aorta. Pathoanatomy shows an entry to the false channel distally of the left subclavian artery, celiac trunk, superior mesenteric artery (SMA), and right renal artery arising from the right true lumen, and left renal artery and inferior mesenteric artery (IMA) arising from the left false lumen. A re-entry was located at the level of the left common iliac artery. Due to progressive aneurysmal dilatation of the descending aorta with imminent rupture, severe reduction of left renal function, and a left lower extremity claudication endoluminal stent-graft placement has been performed in the thoracic aorta, the left renal artery and the left common iliac artery. CE 3D MR angiograms of the thoracic aorta were acquired in the oblique sagittal plane, those of the abdominal aorta in the coronal plane. In a pre-interventional study of the thoracic aorta, the site of the entry to the false lumen can be located distal of the left subclavian artery ostium (*arrow*) during the early (**a**) and late (**b**) arterial phase. In the post-interventional study the entry is covered by the stent-graft (Talent system) and the false lumen has disappeared (**c**). On the pre-interventional ... →→

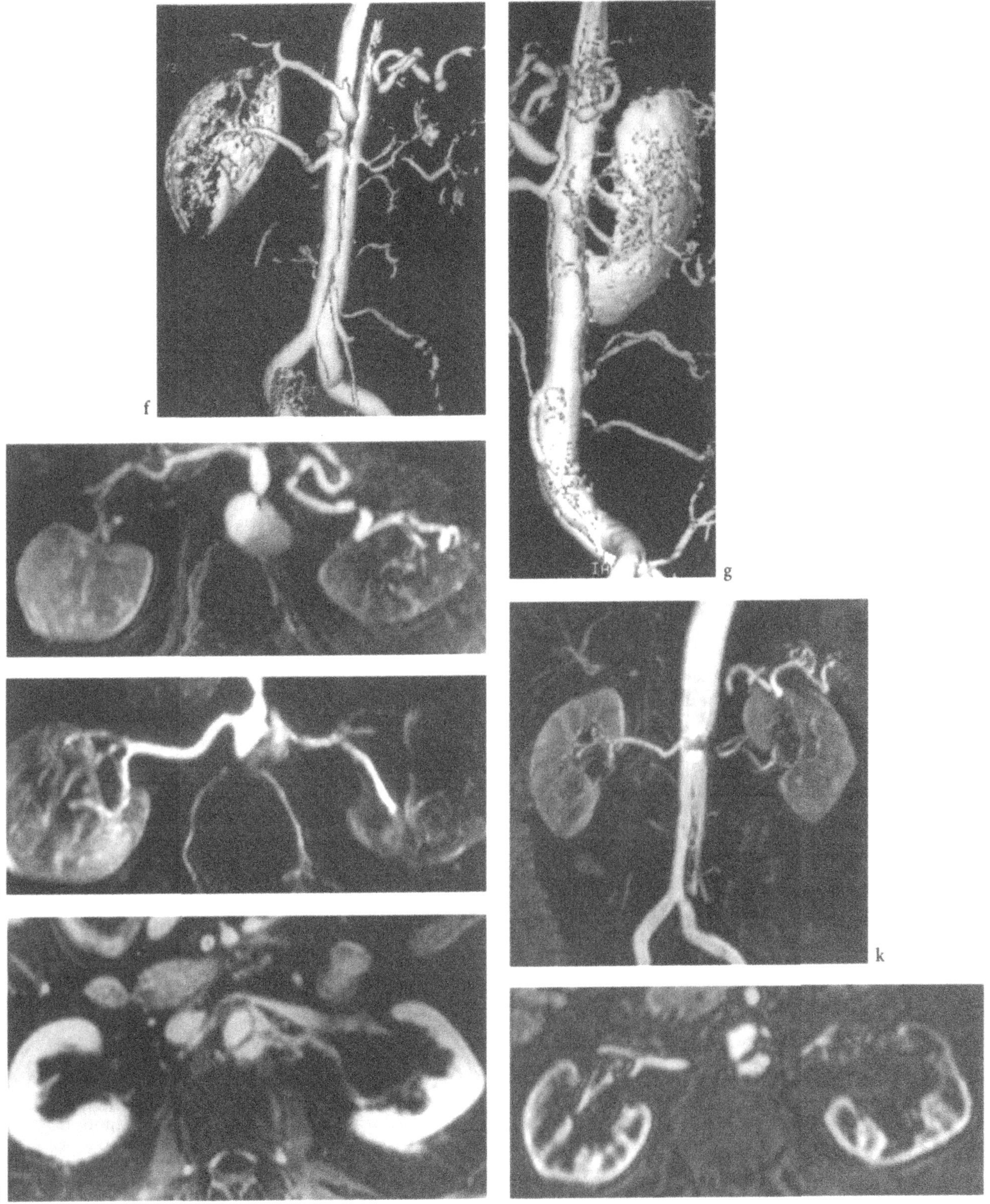

Fig. 18.15a-l (continued) 3D MR (maximum intensity projection, MIP) of the abdominal aorta the dissecting membrane can be clearly depicted separating the right normally perfused lumen from the left false lumen with reduced flow (**d**) which is mainly supplied through a left iliac re-entry (*arrow*). The coronal subvolume MIP image (**e**) allows an evaluation of the extent of the dissecting membrane, the arising right and left renal artery (*arrows*), and the reduced perfusion of the left kidney. The clear relationship between visceral arteries and the dissection membrane can be evaluated on surface-rendered coronal and sagittal MR angiograms (**f, g**) and reformatted transverse images (**h**, celiac trunk; **i**, right and left renal artery with postostial stenosis due to intimal rupture) and postcontrast images (**j**, left renal artery with a separate septum to the ostium). The postinterventional study shows a persistent aortic dissection membrane on the coronal MIP angiogram (**k**), a normalized perfusion of the left kidney after ostial stent-graft placement, and a completely occluded left iliac re-entry after stent-graft implantation. Note the signal void at the level of the left renal artery ostium on coronal (**k**) and reformatted transverse (**l**) images due to metallic stent material

est for planning liver transplantation, characterizing hepatic tumors, localizing tumorous lesions, and establishing the relationship between a hepatic lesion and the adjacent vasculature before planning surgical organ-protective resective therapy. It is accepted that the maximum number of metastatic lesions should not be more than four and at least two to three hepatic segments should be free from tumor.

Conventional Angiography. In disorders such as aneurysms or occlusive disease, the proximal parts of the celiac and mesenteric vascular structures can be visualized accurately (Boijson 1983) by aortography. In most cases aneurysmal lesions are detected accidentally during angiographic work-up, whereas in occlusive disease characteristic symptoms prompt the examination. Conventional angiography provides information for planning surgical or endovascular therapy (Kaleya et al. 1992). Percutaneous interventional procedures such as mesenteric angioplasty, stenting, and thrombolysis may be indicated, particularly in patients who are too frail to undergo surgery. Selective catheter angiography of the hepatic and mesenteric vasculature is also able to detect small and peripheral lesions due to its high spatial resolution (Abrams 1983b; Baum 1983). If they are causing gastrointestinal bleeding, these lesions will be found either directly or can be localized indirectly if the active volume of blood leakage is greater than 2 ml/min.

Ultrasonography. Abdominal US is able to reliably depict larger aneurysms of the central splanchnic arteries when color-coded duplex technique is used. In patients with suspected acute or chronic mesenteric ischemia, immediate diagnosis is required. Duplex Doppler US with color-flow imaging has been suggested as a primary screening procedure in these cases (Roobottom et al. 1993; Moneta et al. 1993; Giovagnorio et al. 1998). Among the Doppler criteria, measurement of the fasting peak systolic velocity is accepted as a reliable parameter (Moneta et al. 1993; Lim et al. 1999). Thus, due to its high accuracy of up to 90%, US may lead to a reduction of unnecessarily invasive angiography (Lim et al. 1999). In addition, collateralized IMA can be depicted and flow can be evaluated by Doppler in cases of superior mesenteric occlusion, demonstrating an increased blood flow volume and a monophasic waveform (Erden et al. 1998).

MR Angiography. With CE 3D MR angiography diverse pathologic entities of the splanchnic vasculature can be depicted, such as visceral aneurysms (Gilfeather et al. 1997; Shirkhoda et al. 1998), and the site of gastrointestinal bleeding detected when larger deposits of contrast material in the intestinal lumen become visible, similar to conventional angiography. However, the chance of demonstrating the cause of gastrointestinal bleeding directly is low due to reduced spatial resolution of MR angiography.

Recent advances in MR imaging techniques permit the evaluation of both vascular anatomic abnormalities and physiologic disorders in small bowel ischemia. Arterial and venous occlusion, both of which are responsible for intestinal hypoperfusion, can be imaged by CE 3D MR angiography with increasing visual fidelity (Prince 1994; Alley et al. 1998) and this technique is regarded as an alternative to conventional angiography, with nearly adequate evaluation of relevant arterial and venous structures in several studies (Holland et al. 1996; Shirkhoda et al. 1997). Stenoses of the SMA and the celiac trunk and its branches, including the gastroduodenal artery, as well as the stump of an occluded artery can be visualized reliably on sagittal, reformatted subvolume images (Davis et al. 1997) (Figs. 18.16a–d, 18.17a, b, 18.18a–c, 18.19a, b). In patients with stenosis of the SMA, the arc of Riolan can be visualized accurately, which reconstitutes the middle portion of the SMA via collaterals from the IMA. In larger series, detection of ostial stenoses of the celiac artery, SMA, and IMA has been reported with an accuracy of up to 100% (Holland et al. 1996; Prince et al. 1995). Furthermore, tumor invasion of the arterial and venous mesenteric structures can be accurately evaluated on CE 3D MR angiograms, comparable to conventional angiography (Shirkhoda et al. 1998) and 3D CT angiography (Kaneko et al. 1997; Novick and Fishman 1998) (Fig. 18.20a–c). Although more experience in the correlation of MR angiography with conventional arteriography is necessary, preliminary results are promising and show that replacement of the invasive method can be expected in a large number of patients, in particular those with symptoms of chronic mesenteric ischemia. However, the exclusive use of MR angiography to evaluate patients with acute symptoms of mesenteric ischemia cannot be advocated at the moment due to insufficient spatial and temporal resolution in depicting nonocclusive low flow states or distal emboli (Gilfeather et al. 1997). Therefore, the combination of CE 3D MR angiography and functional MR imaging is a promising approach in the detection of acute and chronic mesenteric ischemia. Functional MR-based techniques are able to assess chronic mesenteric ischemia. With

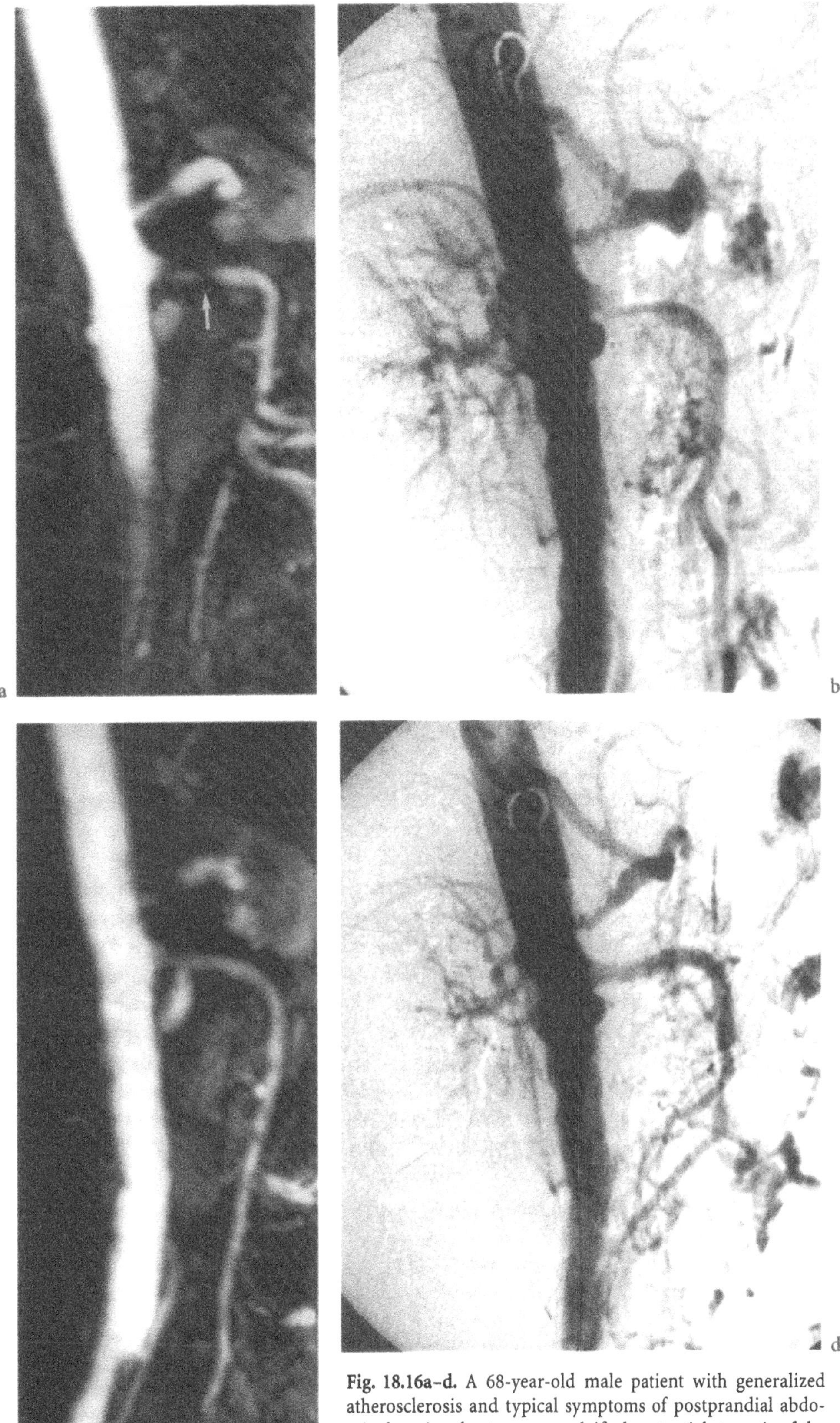

Fig. 18.16a–d. A 68-year-old male patient with generalized atherosclerosis and typical symptoms of postprandial abdominal angina due to severe calcified postostial stenosis of the superior mesenteric artery (*arrow*) and moderate stenosis of the celiac trunk. Sagittal CE 3D MR angiograms (**a, c**) and DSA images (**b, d**) demonstrate stenotic disease before (**a, b**) and after (**c, d**) successful balloon angioplasty

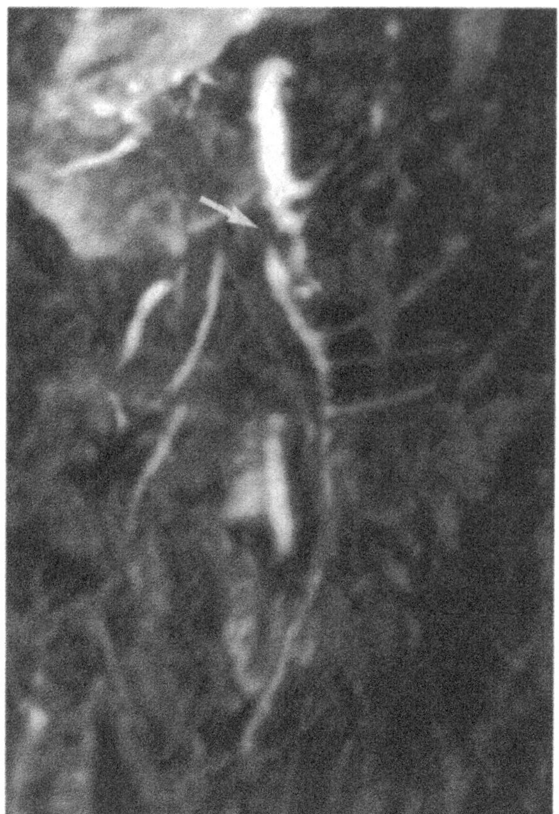

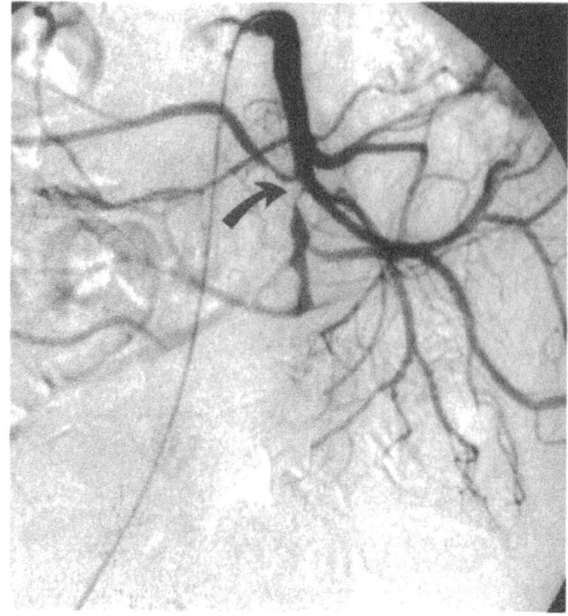

Fig. 18.17a, b. Significant stenosis (*arrows*) of the main trunk of the superior mesenteric artery (SMA) distal to the first-order branching. The lesion is demonstrated on a coronal CE 3D MR angiogram (subvolume maximum intensity projection) (**a**) and on the DSA image (**b**). Note that the poststenotic distal branches of the SMA can be evaluated better on the MR angiogram than on the DSA image

2D PC MR cine flow mapping, flow volumes in the SMA and SMV have been determined successfully (Burkart et al. 1993; Li et al. 1994). A significant arterial and venous blood flow reduction can be found in mesenteric ischemic states, and a consistent relationship exists between MR flow measurements in the SMV and the flow measured in the arteries supplying these veins (Burkart et al. 1993). Thus, flow in the SMV can be regarded as an accurate predictor of flow in the SMA. Moreover, in ischemic states due to high-grade SMA stenosis, a significant reduction in normally occurring postprandial hyperemia has been reported (Li et al. 1994), whereas the discrepancy of increased SMV flow under conditions of >50% SMA stenosis was explained by recruitment of collateral flow. As another convenient marker of mesenteric ischemia, MR oximetry has been suggested (Chan et al. 1999). This method seems to be capable of detecting segmental mesenteric ischemia by a loss of oxygen saturation in the SMV relative to that in the inferior vena cava, caused by increased tissue extraction of blood oxygen. Furthermore, ischemia-induced segmental hypomotility of the small bowel has been visualized with a real-time interactive MR imaging technique based on k-space scanning with interleaved circular echoplanar imaging trajectories (Kerr et al. 1997).

Compared with standard angiographic sequences, CE 3D MR angiography of the hepatic vascular structures can be improved significantly by using an optimized fat-saturated technique (Kopka et al. 1999), with which the arterial hepatic blood supply can be correctly classified in the majority of cases. This technique has demonstrated to be valuable in the detection and functional characterization of hepatic lesions (Hawighorst et al. 1999; Kopka et al. 1999), comparable to CT angiography (Kanematsu et al. 1996). MR angiographic images, including the arterial, hepatovenous, and portal venous phase, have been shown to provide a correct characterization of hepatic lesions which is superior to pre- and postcontrast T1-weighted images, and T2-weighted images. Arterial and portal venous supply of the lesions can be correctly seen on MR angiograms and may provide important information about the localization of focal lesions and their relationship to adjacent vascular structures (Hawighorst et al. 1999; Kopka et al. 1999) (Fig. 18.21a–c).

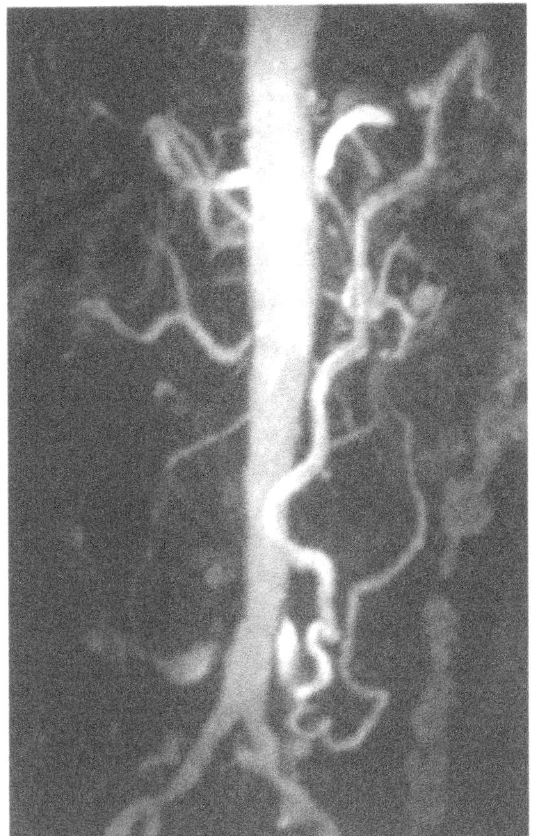

a

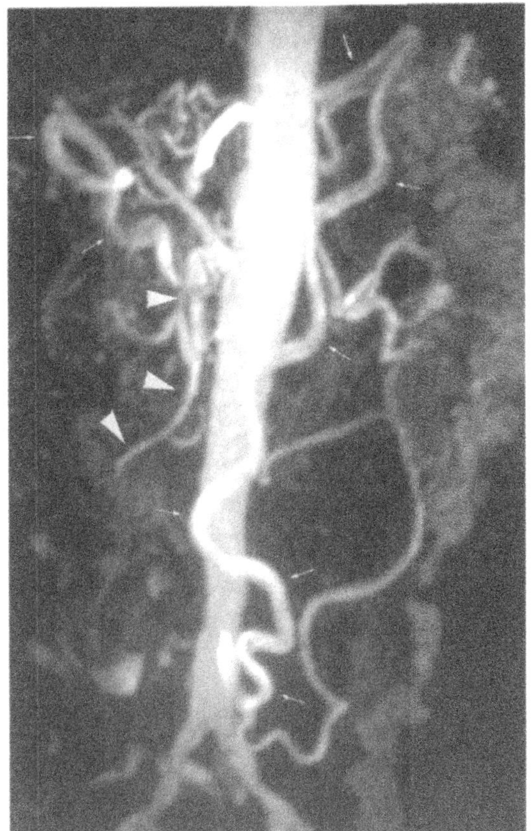

b

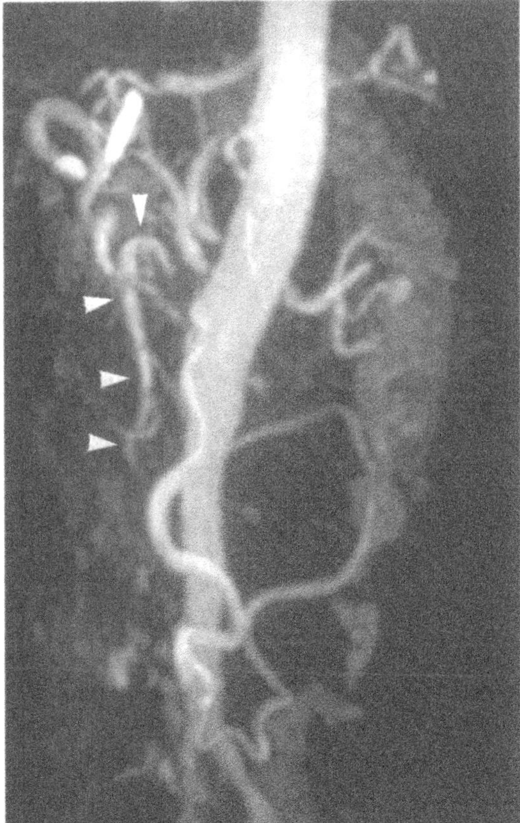

c

Fig. 18.18a–c. Complete chronic occlusion of the proximal superior mesenteric artery (SMA), collateral supply of the postocclusive main trunk of the SMA (*arrowheads*) via the arc of Riolan (*arrows*). This finding is documented on a coronal CE 3D MR angiogram (**a**) in the early phase, and in 30°LA0 (**b**) and 60°LAO (**c**) projection in a delayed arterial phase

Fig. 18.19a,b. In a patient with significant stenosis of the celiac trunk (*arrow*) mesenterico-hepatic arterial collaterals (*arrowheads*) can be depicted on a sagittal (**a**) and coronal (**b**) CE 3D MR angiogram of the splanchnic arteries

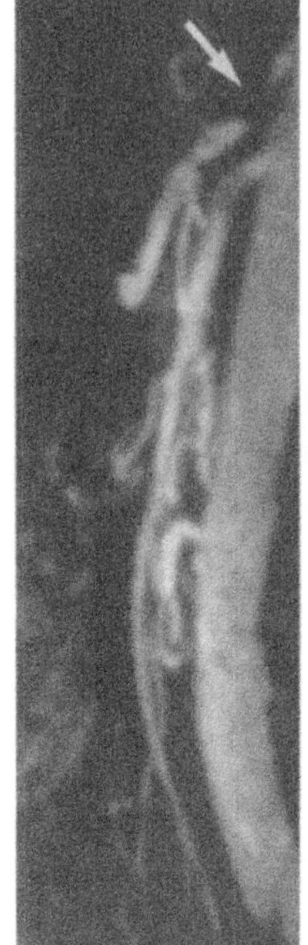

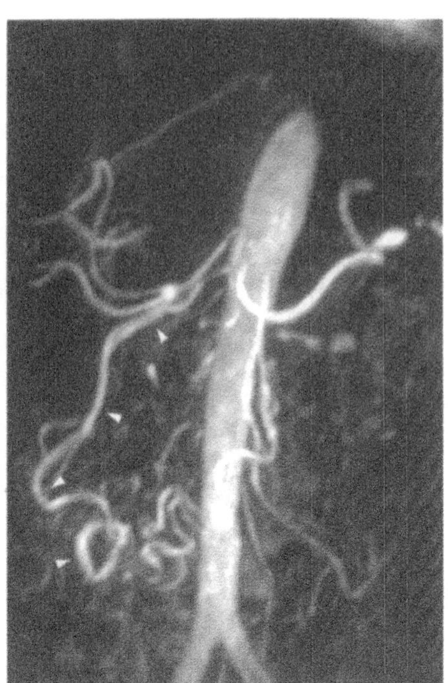

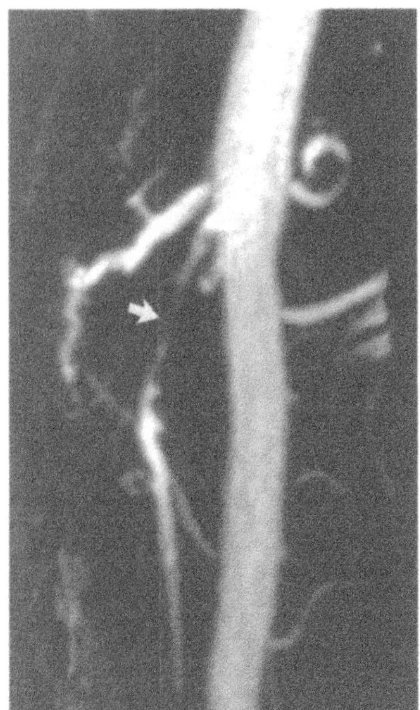

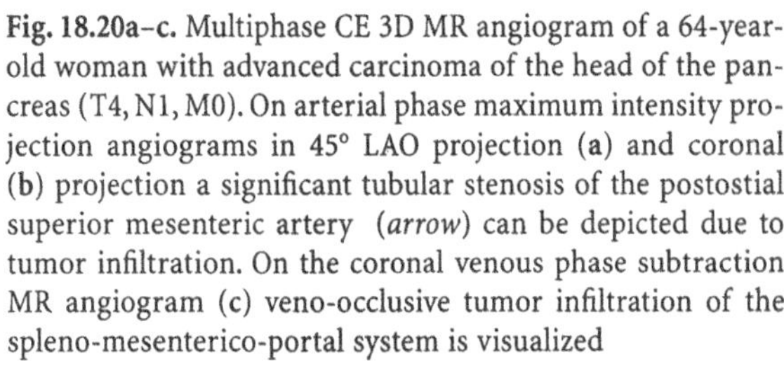

Fig. 18.20a–c. Multiphase CE 3D MR angiogram of a 64-year-old woman with advanced carcinoma of the head of the pancreas (T4, N1, M0). On arterial phase maximum intensity projection angiograms in 45° LAO projection (**a**) and coronal (**b**) projection a significant tubular stenosis of the postostial superior mesenteric artery (*arrow*) can be depicted due to tumor infiltration. On the coronal venous phase subtraction MR angiogram (**c**) veno-occlusive tumor infiltration of the spleno-mesenterico-portal system is visualized

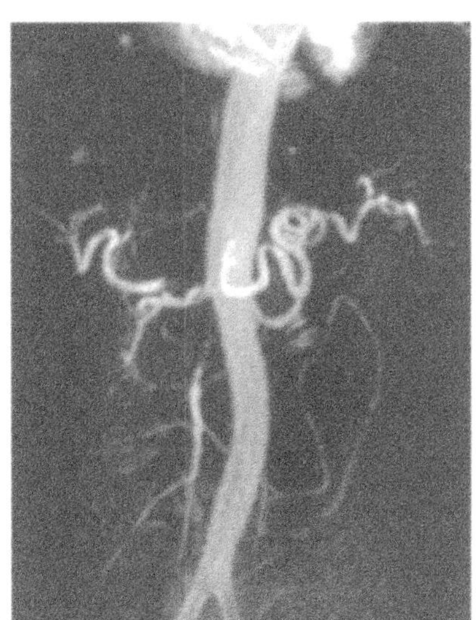

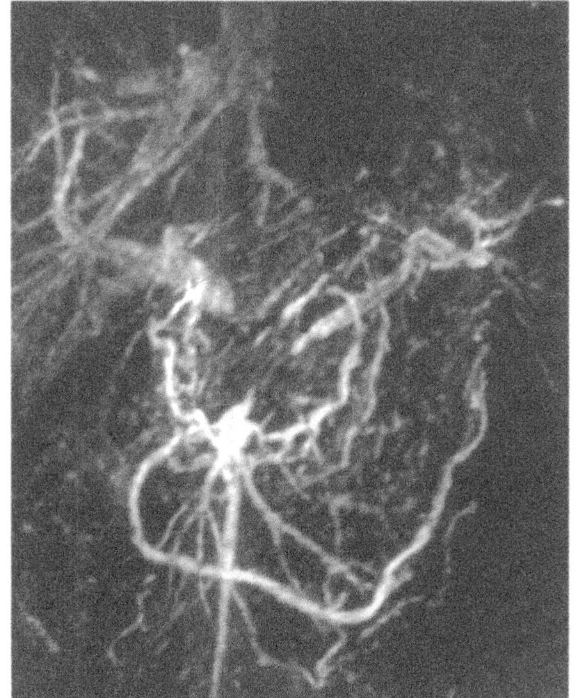

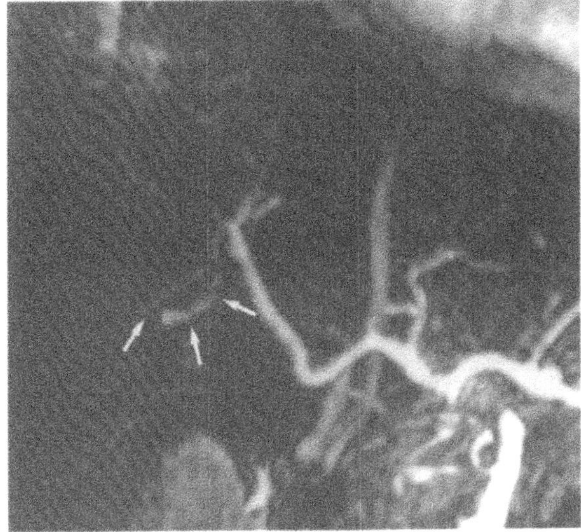
a

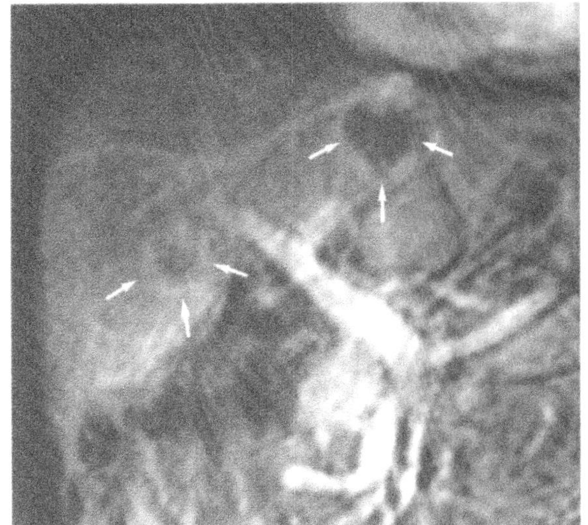
b

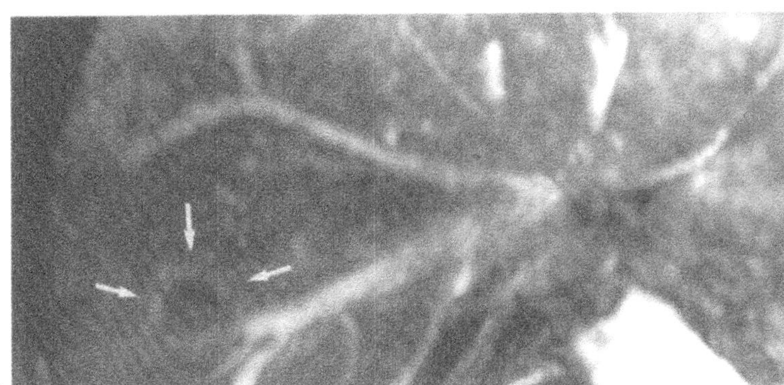
c

Fig. 18.21a–c. A 67-year-old man with hepatic metastases due to colorectal cancer. On the CE 3D MR angiogram in the early arterial phase the hepatic artery, including the left and right branches, is visualized in coronal view (**a**). A first-order branch of the right hepatic artery shows encasement due to metastasis (*arrows*) in segment 5 which can be confirmed on portal venous phase coronal (**b**) and transverse (**c**) reformatted MR angiograms. Another metastasis is located in the left liver lobe (segment 2)

18.3.2.3
Renal Arteries

The renal artery can be involved by a variety of lesions or abnormalities, such as aneurysms, arteriovenous fistulas and malformations, intimal dissection, thromboembolic occlusion, occlusion due to progressive atherosclerosis, stenotic disorders of different etiology, and partial or complete occlusion of the renal arterial ostium due to an intimal flap in aortic dissection (Kadir 1986). The majority of these vascular lesions may cause renal hypoperfusion, initiating arterial hypertension as a results of an activated renin-angiotensin-aldosterone system. The prevalence of renovascular hypertension (RVH) is estimated at 1%–5% of the hypertensive population – approximately10%–15% of the entire population. Despite the low incidence, screening for RVH is useful because enhanced arterial blood pressure can be decreased or normalized in the majority of patients when the renovascular lesion is successfully treated by either surgical or percutaneous endovascular procedures. Other symptoms that may indicate renal arteriography are hematuria, unilateral renal failure, and acute flank pain. Furthermore, renal arteriography is of interest when tumor enucleation in renal cell carcinoma is planned and in follow-up studies after renal artery interventions.

Renal artery aneurysms, which occur in less than 1% of the population, are rarely symptomatic except for the elevated blood pressure values seen in approximately 70% of cases. The majority of aneurysms are diagnosed incidentally in patients undergoing angiography. Etiology includes atherosclerosis, fibromuscular dysplasia, congenital abnormalities, trauma, and polyarteritis nodosa. Rupture may occur in about 5%. Therapeutic intervention is indicated in aneurysms greater than 1.5 cm in diameter and symptomatic aneurysms in association with arterial hypertension of any size in women who are of child-bearing age because pregnancy may increase the incidence of rupture. Arteriovenous fistulas and malformations of the kidney are also rare disorders. Arteriovenous fistulas are mostly caused by percutaneous renal biopsy whereas the arteriovenous malformation is a congenital abnormality which can be classified into a cirsoid type and an aneurysmal type (TAKAHA et al. 1980). When these disorders cause persistent massive hematuria, arterial hypertension, or cardiac failure due to large arteriovenous shunt volumes, therapeutic intervention is required. The management protocols include surgical interventions or percutaneous catheter embolization, depending on the localization and configuration of the lesion. Both larger aneurysms and intrarenal arteriovenous fistulas can be accurately detected using diagnostic modalities such as color-coded duplex Doppler US, CT angiography, and *MR angiography*. In a publication of TAKEBAYASHI et al. (1994) including nine cases of arteriovenous malformations with gross hematuria, 3D PC MR angiography was able to detect all three aneurysmal-type malformations and four of six cirsoid-type malformations. Depending on the size of the abnormalities, sensitivity, specificity, and accuracy have been reported at 78%, 100%, and 91%, respectively. Using CE 3D MR angiography, HOLLAND et al. (1996) in their series depicted one renal artery aneurysm and one renal arteriovenous malformation. Both were obscured on full volume MIP but were correctly diagnosed on subvolume MIP or reformatted images.

The most common cause of RVH is renal artery stenosis (RAS). This lesion can be removed successfully in a large number of cases by percutaneous endovascular interventions, leading to a normalization or improvement in blood pressure – particularly in FMD. However, in atherosclerotic RAS this therapeutic procedure was put to discussion once again due to the disappointing results frequently observed (VAN JAARSVELD et al. 2000). Thus, screening of hypertensive patients for RAS is justified as renal angioplasty is advisable particularly in patients with RAS whose blood pressure cannot be controlled satisfactorily by drug therapy. In addition to the effects of renal balloon angioplasty or stent placement on arterial blood pressure, recanalization of the renal artery can prevent the development of chronic renal failure caused by progressive atherosclerotic occlusive disease (BLUM 1999). In approximately 70%–75% of cases, mainly in the older male population, RVH is caused by atherosclerotic disease. Atherosclerotic RAS can be observed bilaterally in about 30% of cases; in more than 90% the main renal artery is involved near its origin. The morphologic appearance of atherosclerotic RAS is commonly eccentric and irregular, with a poststenotic dilatation. RAS due to FMD of the renal artery is found in approximately15%–25% of patients with RVH, occurs mainly in the younger female population, and is found bilaterally in nearly two thirds of cases. The main renal artery is involved in approximately 80%, segmental arteries additionally in 17%, and peripheral arteries in 3%. The morphology of FMD depends on the type of lesion. In the majority of cases the lesion appears centric with a smooth border and varies from short segmental narrowing to alternating areas of aneurysmal formation and narrowing ("string-of-beads" appearance). Other rare etiologies of RAS include neurofibromatosis, arteritis, intimal dissection, and congenital vascular disorders. In patients in whom RAS is suspected, diagnostic vascular imaging requires reliable visualization of the number of renal arteries, including high-quality imaging of pole arteries, accessory arteries, and segmental branches (Fig. 18.22), as well as reliable detection of the lesion and accurate grading of the stenosis. Because atherosclerotic plaque stenosis of the renal artery is found in a significant number of normotensive individuals, additional noninvasive procedures have been established to clarify the hemodynamic significance of the stenosis in such cases, including renal renin sampling, determination of converting-enzyme inhibitor levels, dynamic radionuclide scanning during converting-enzyme inhibition, and intrarenal Doppler flow measurements.

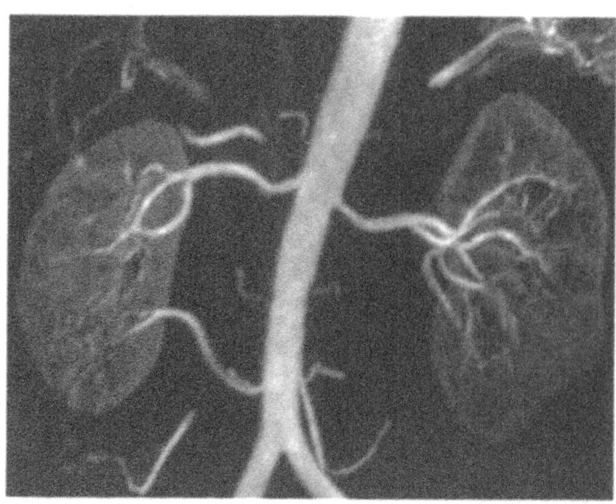

Fig. 18.22. Anatomic variants of the renal arteries. Coronal CE 3D MR angiogram (maximum intensity projection) shows a single left renal artery and two right renal arteries including a lower pole artery

Conventional Angiography. Conventional angiography and DSA as the gold standard for detecting, evaluating, and grading RAS (ABRAMS 1983a) combine the advantages of direct pressure gradient measurement and percutaneous management of a proven RAS within the same procedure. However, due to its invasiveness and costs, other noninvasive and cost-saving modalities have been suggested for screening in the hypertensive population, particularly in view of the low prevalence of the disease. Nevertheless, all these methods have to be oriented to the high diagnostic accuracy of DSA to guarantee that this invasive method is only performed to confirm RAS under aspects of potential percutaneous endovascular therapy.

Current noninvasive screening tests that allow both a direct angiomorphologic depiction of the renal artery and a functional information of the poststenotic kidney include color-coded duplex Doppler US and MR imaging techniques. At the present time, CT angiography is limited to the visualization of renovascular morphology only.

Ultrasonography. Color-coded duplex Doppler US has advanced in recent years to become an important diagnostic tool in the detection of RAS. Several Doppler criteria have been established which can be divided into direct and indirect parameters. Doppler changes that occur directly at the site of the involved renal artery have been reported as being 84%–93% sensitive and 73%–98% specific in optimistic studies (STRANDNESS 1990; AVASTHI et al. 1984; HANSEN et al. 1990; HOFFMAN et al. 1991; RITTGERS et al. 1985), whereas in more critical studies sensitivity and specificity ranged from 0% to 37% and from 37% to 81%, respectively (DESBERG et al. 1990; BERLAND et al. 1990; POSTMA et al. 1992; KLIEWER et al. 1993). As optimum parameters, maximum peak systolic velocity (PSV) (88% sensitive, 93% specific), peak systolic to end-diastolic velocity ratio (94% sensitive, 100% specific), and renal to aortic systolic peak velocity ratio (RAR) (94% sensitive, 93% specific) have been evaluated using endovascular flow wire studies (VAN DER HULST et al. 1996). It was shown that RAR or PSV may provide the best combination of parameters, demonstrating a sensitivity and specificity of 85% and 76%, respectively (HOUSE et al. 1999). Indirect intrarenal Doppler parameters for detecting RAS are determined by the alteration of the intrarenal arterial Doppler-waveform due to the intravascular pressure drop behind the lesion that affects intrarenal circulation. These parameters include acceleration time, acceleration index, pulsatility index (PI), and resistive index (RI). In the literature, data on indirect Doppler accuracy for depicting RAS vary widely. On the one hand, findings with no statistically significant difference between stenotic and normal renal arteries have been reported with respect to diverse parameters (KLIEWER et al. 1993; VAN DER HULST et al. 1996); on the other hand, significantly pathologic delta RI (RI of the normal kidney minus RI of the stenosed kidney) has been measured as being 82% sensitive and 92% specific in RAS >50%, and 100% sensitive and 94% specific in RAS >60%, respectively (SCHWERCK et al. 1994). Both pathologic acceleration time and acceleration index have been observed to be 41% and 56% sensitive and 85% and 62% specific, respectively (HOUSE et al. 1999). Recently, the use of an angiotensin-converting enzyme inhibitor has been advocated to improve the accuracy of Doppler waveform analysis in RAS >50%, resulting in a sensitivity and specificity that increased from 81% to 100% and from 98% to 100%, respectively (OLIVA et al. 1998). The variability of intrarenal Doppler data in the detection of RAS found in the literature has been interpreted and critically discussed by BUDE et al. (1995), who pointed out that poststenotic intrarenal hemodynamics are complex phenomena to measure. Thus, false-negative and false-positive results are not only caused by errors in measuring the Doppler angle between the US beam and the flow velocity due to incompetence of the operator.

CT Angiography. CT angiography of renal arteries on the basis of helical data acquisition has been shown to be very accurate in the angiomorphologic depiction of RAS (Table 18.2). A clear advantage over conventional angiography is provided for the characterization of eccentric stenoses and wall calcifications. However, as a drawback of CT angiography, it necessitates the application of potentially nephrotoxic contrast material.

Table 18.2. Sensitivity and specificity of contrast-enhanced helical CT angiography in renal artery stenosis >50%

Authors	Number of patients	Sensitivity (%)	Specificity (%)
BEREGI et al. 1996	20	88	98
KAATEE et al. 1997	71	96	96
JOHNSON et al. 1999	25		
VR		89	99
MIP		94	87
GALANSKI et al. 1999, different modalities	77	94.8–97.7	78.8–87.9

MR Angiography. MR angiography of renal arteries can be performed using several different 2D and 3D GRE techniques, such as inflow TOF methods, gadolinium-enhanced and non-enhanced PC methods, and breath-hold CE 3D techniques. Although demonstrating different accuracy, all methods are able to visualize renal arteries directly for depicting RAS >50% (see Tables 18.3, 18.4). To optimize the diagnostic accuracy in detecting RAS, a combination of different MR angiographic imaging modalities has been recommended by several authors. Thus, when combining 3D TOF and 3D PC technique, specificity and accuracy in depicting RAS >50% could be increased to 90% and 92%, respectively (Loubeyre et al. 1996a). Cardiac gating in 3D PC MR angiography was able to improve the overall detection of RAS and increased sensitivity from 77% to 93% by systolic gating (De Haan et al. 1996). A 100% sensitivity in detecting RAS >50% has been reported when non-enhanced 3D PC MRA was combined with CE 3D MR angiography (Hahn et al. 1999). Within recent years, breath-hold CE 3D MR angiography was demonstrated in many studies to be superior to all flow-sensitive techniques in detecting RAS >50% (see Tables 18.3 and 18.4; Figs. 18.23a–c, 18.24a–c, 18.25a, b, 18.26a–d, 18.27a–c). Using the time-resolved, multiphase imaging techniques available today (Schoenberg et al. 1999; van Hoe et al. 2000), visualization of distal main renal arteries and segmental arteries could be improved even further and allow the evaluation of intraparenchymal renal hemodynamics on the basis of contrast enhancement. However, although less severe than on nonenhanced flow-related MR angiograms, overestimation of the degree of a stenosis may also occur on CE 3D MR angiograms due to the phenomenon of minimal phase dispersion, reduced spatial resolution and vessel pulsation, and image artifacts (Fig. 18.28a–c). Image

Table 18.3. Sensitivity and specificity of non-enhanced flow-sensitive MR angiography in proximal renal artery stenosis >50%

Authors	Number of patients	Technique	Sensitivity (%)	Specificity (%)
Kim et al. (1990)	25	2D TOF	100	92
Kent et al. (1991)	23	2D TOF	100	94
Arlart et al. (1993)	26	2D TOF	88	85
	26	3D TOF	78	80
Grist et al. (1993)	35	2D TOF/3D PC	89	95
Yucel et al. (1993)	16	2D/3D TOF	100	93
Herzt et al. (1994)	16	2D TOF	91	94
Loubeyre et al. (1994)	53	3D TOF	100	76
Loubeyre et al. (1996a)	46	3D TOF/3D PC	100	90
De Cobelli et al. (1997)	55	3D PC	96	94
Schoenberg et al. (1997)	23	2D PC	100	93
Hahn et al. (1999)	22	3D PC	95	38

Table 18.4. Sensitivity and specificity of gadolinium-enhanced 3D MR angiography in RAS >50%

Authors	Number of patients	Sensitivity (%)	Specificity (%)
Prince et al. (1995)	19	100	93
Grist et al. (1996)	28	88	88
Holland et al. (1996)	63	100	100
De Cobelli et al. (1997)	55	100	97
Rieumont et al. (1997)	30	100	71
Bakker et al. (1998)	50	97	92
Hany et al. (1998b)	39	98	93
Schoenberg et al. (1999)	26	100	95
Hahn et al. (1999)	22	91	79
Thornton et al. (1999)	42	100	98
De Cobelli et al. (2000)	55	100	93

artifacts can occur during the acquisition period as a result of incomplete breath-holding and by image reformatting procedures, particularly when thicker sections have been used, which may demonstrate renal artery lesions mimicking FMD (Fig. 18.29a, b). Thus, in RAS caused by FMD, a high spatial resolution is necessary to depict those lesions accurately, which not uncommonly have a very distinct appearance, showing numerous thin septal stenoses without larger aneurysmal formations. Accurate data on the detection of FMD of the renal artery have only been published with helical CT angiography (BEREGI et al. 1999): different rates of accuracy have been observed, depending on the analysis of transverse images (83%, 53%, 57%), MIP images (75%, 84%, 71%), and SSD images (58%, 74%, 57%) with respect to the aneurysmal appearance, "string-of-bead" appearance or stenotic appearance. Although typical and representative renal FMD appearances have been demonstrated on CE 3D MR angiograms (DE COBELLI et al. 1997; LEUNG and DEBATIN 1998; SCHOENBERG et al. 1999), no systematic evaluation is available similar to that of BEREGI et al. (1999). Thus, the actual number of cases of renal FMD really depicted accurately by CE 3D MR angiography is unknown. On the other hand, CE MR angiography has been shown to be an excellent method for diagnostic postinterventional follow-up (CARLOS et al. 1999) (Fig. 18.30). After stent application, however, metallic material may cause significant signal void at the site of placement (Fig. 18.31), so that recurrent stenosis within the stent can only be confirmed by indirect renal perfusion parameters or direct measurement of renal blood flow.

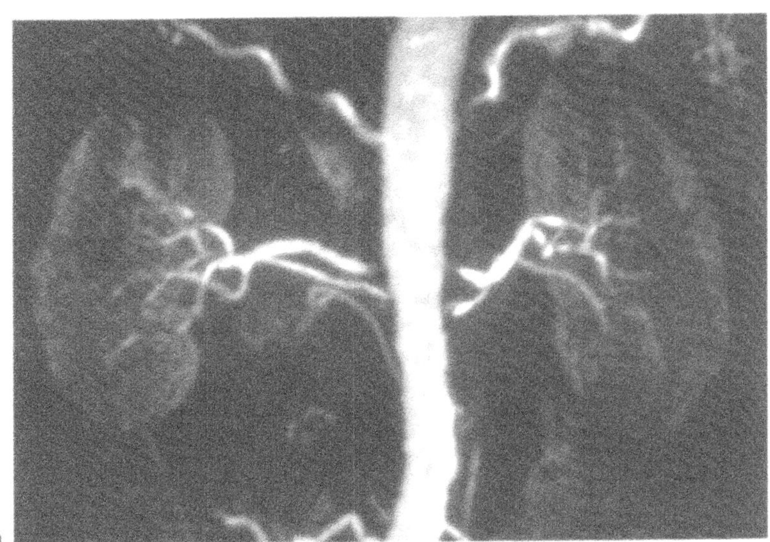
a

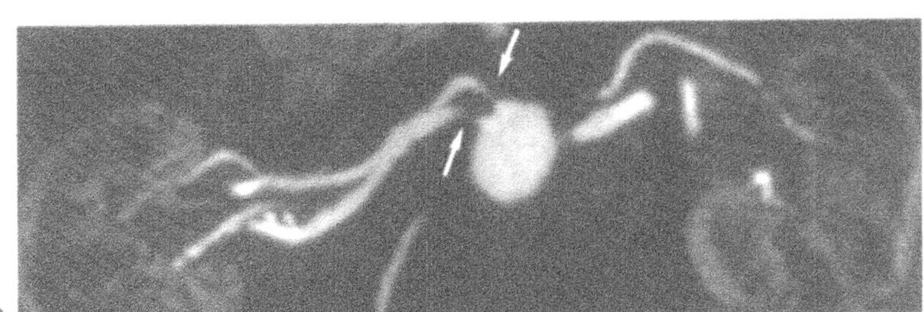
b

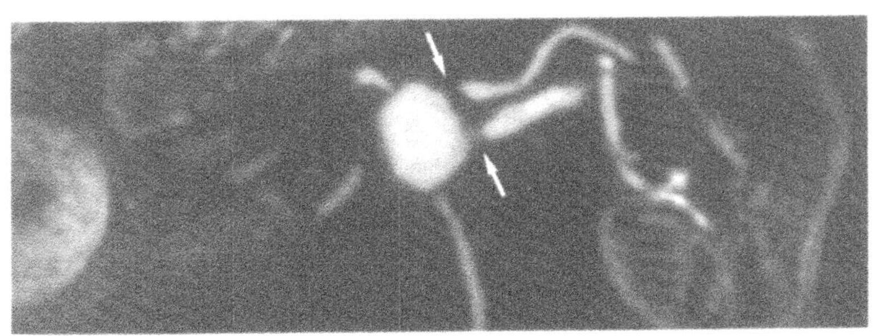
c

Fig. 18.23a–c. Bilateral ostial renal artery stenosis in a hypertensive patient with a two renal artery supply of both kidneys. CE 3D MR angiograms in coronal plane (maximum intensity projection) (**a**) and transverse plane (reformatted images) (**b**, **c**) show a significant signal loss at the ostium of each artery due to stenotic disease (*arrows*). A single data set was acquired during a breath-hold (1.5 T, phased-array coil) using the following sequence parameters: 34×38 cm field-of-view, 41.7 kHz bandwidth, 5.5/1.8 ms TR/TE, 35°flip angle, 36 sections, 1.0–1.1 section thickness after zero filling, 0.5 nex, fat saturation, 23 s acquisition time, 25 ml of gadolinium-DTPA (1.5 ml/s flow rate)

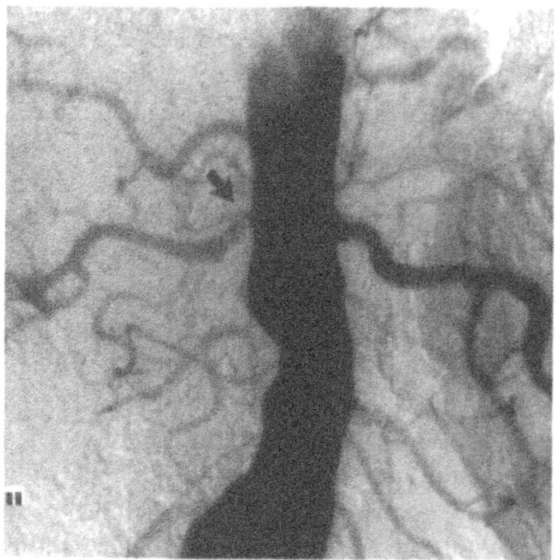

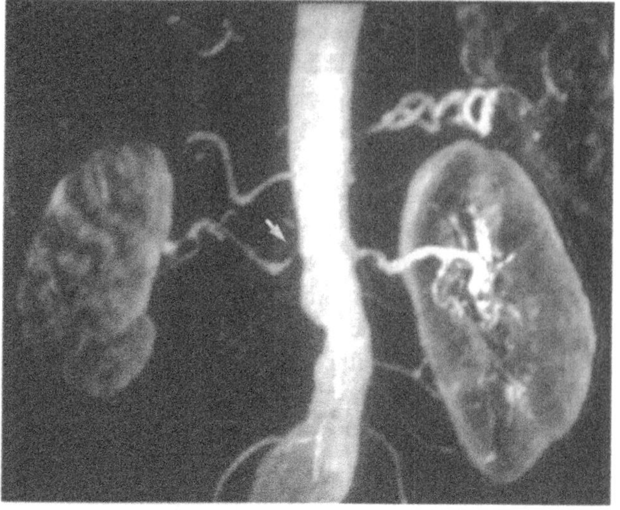

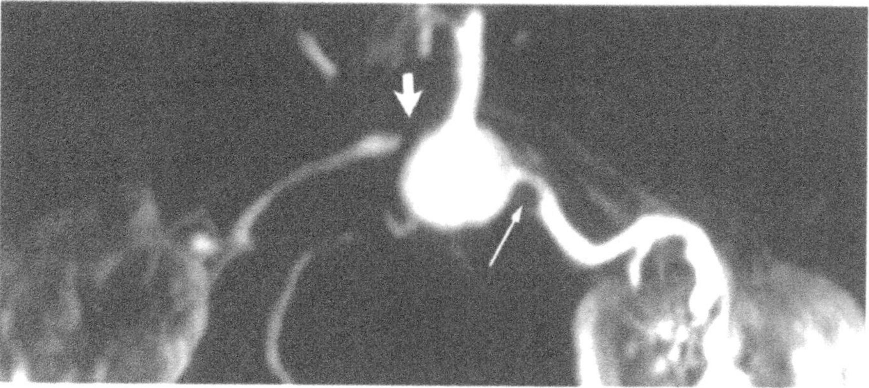

Fig. 18.24a–c. High-grade right atherosclerotic ostial renal artery stenosis in a hypertensive male patient with an abdominal aortic aneurysm. On CE 3D MR angiograms in coronal (**b**) and transverse (**c**) view the stenosis (*arrow*) can be depicted more reliably than on the DSA image (**a**). Compared with the left kidney, the right kidney appears smaller in size and with reduced parenchymal contrast enhancement due to hypoperfusion. Note that the eccentric atherosclerotic plaque in the proximal part of the left renal artery (*thin arrow*) can only be depicted on the MR angiogram in transverse view

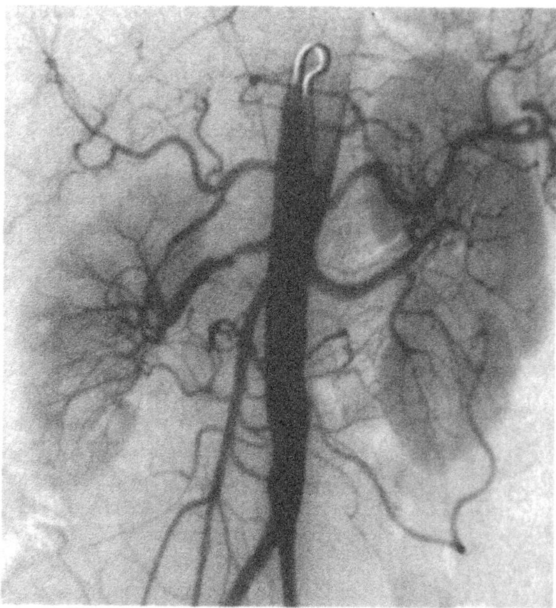

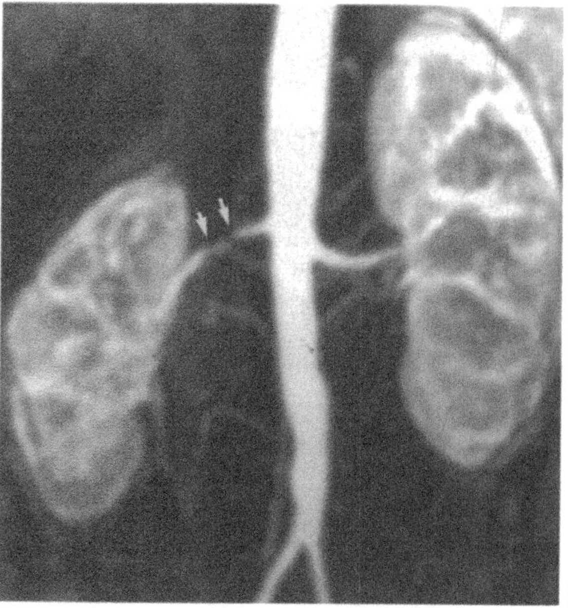

Fig. 18.25a, b. Right renal artery stenosis due to fibromuscular dysplasia in a young female hypertensive patient of 35 years. The characteristic appearance of stenotic and aneurysmal lesions (*arrows*) is demonstrated identically on both the DSA image (**a**) and coronal CE 3D MR angiogram (**b**)

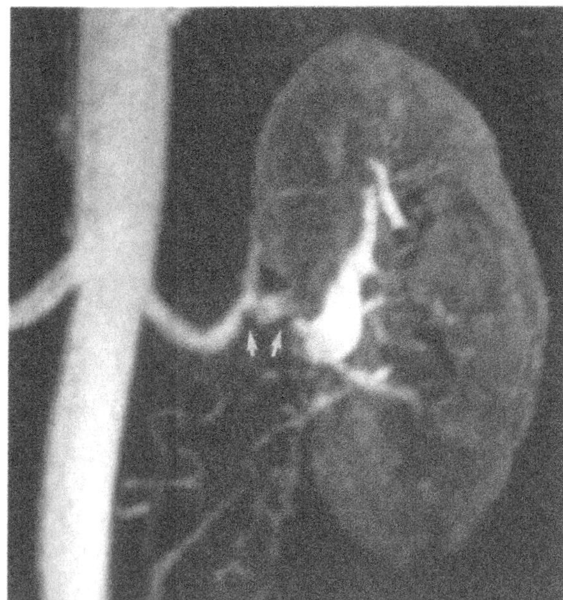

a

b

c

d

Fig. 18.26a–d. A 38-year-old man with arterial hypertension screened for renovascular cause. On CE 3D MR angiograms in the coronal (**a**) and transverse (**b**) plane an aneurysmal dilatation of a left segmental renal artery can be seen that was confirmed by DSA (**c**, **d**). Particularly on the transverse reformatted MR image additional preaneurysmal stenoses can be identified (*arrows*). This vascular lesion histologically proven was caused by Gsell-Erdheims's disease

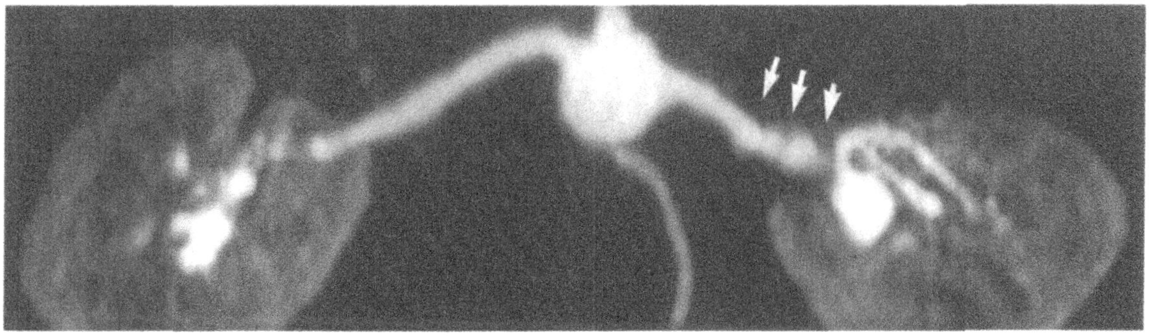

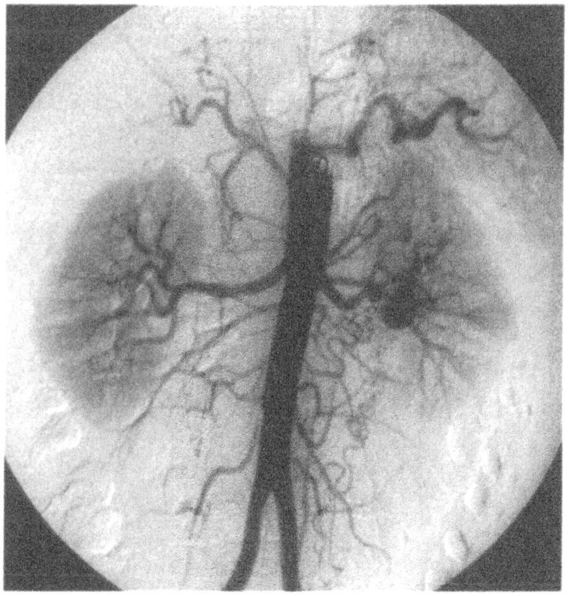

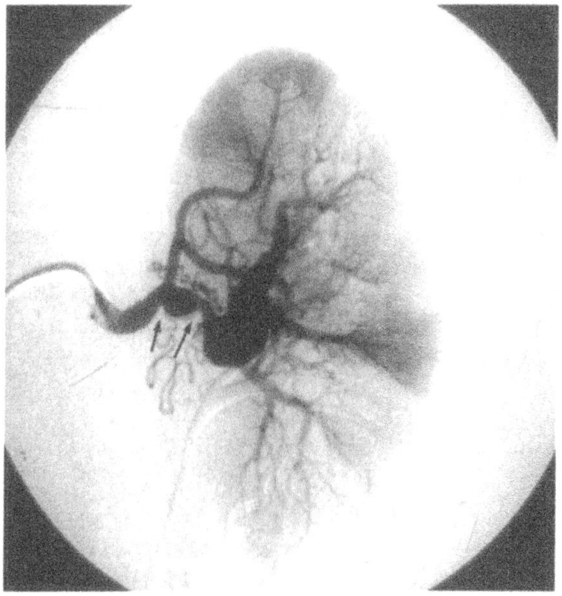

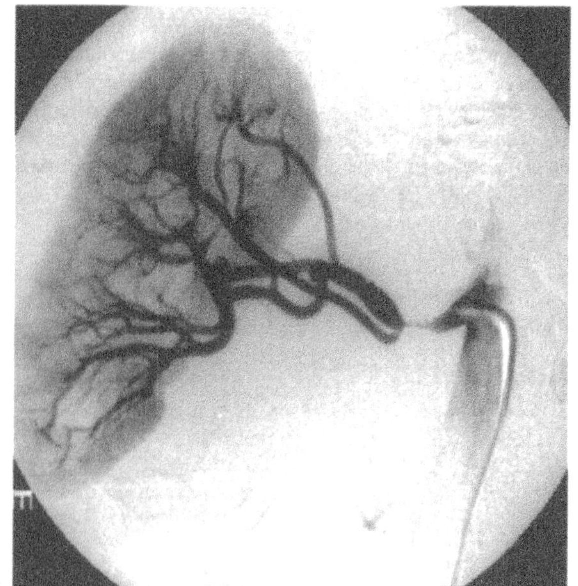

a

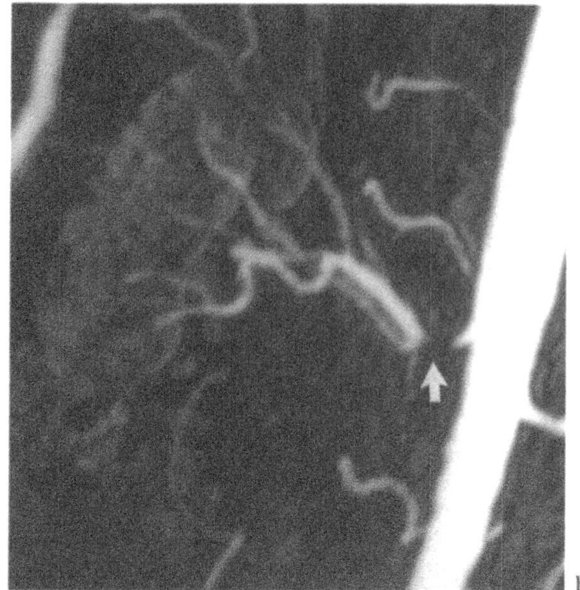

b

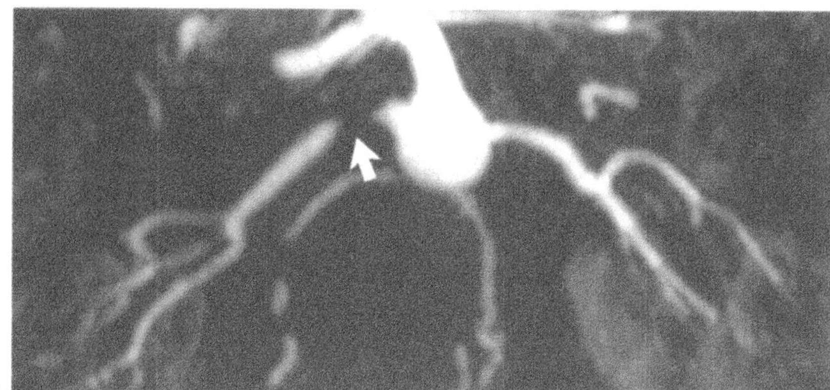

c

Fig. 18.27a–c. Significant stenosis of the right main renal artery just before the segmental bifurcation (*arrow*). Appearance in DSA (**a**) is similar to that on the CE 3D MR angiogram (subvolume maximum intensity projection) in coronal plane (**b**) and on the reformatted transverse image (**c**). Note the slight overestimation of the stenosis with MR angiography

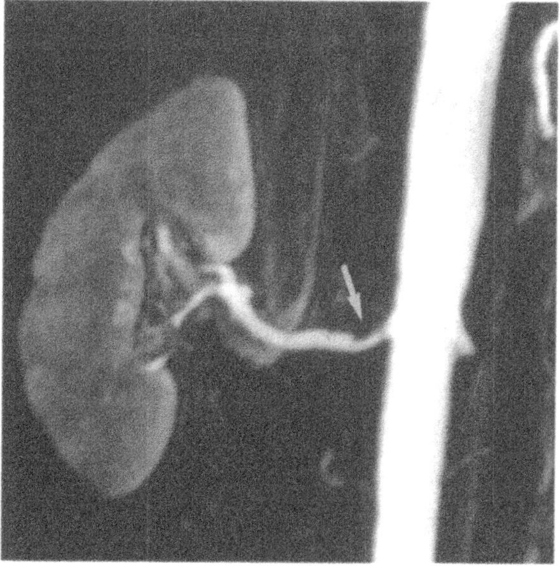

a

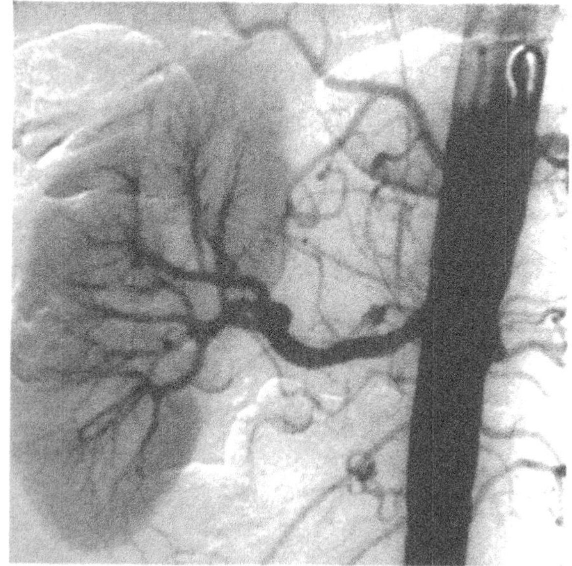

b →→

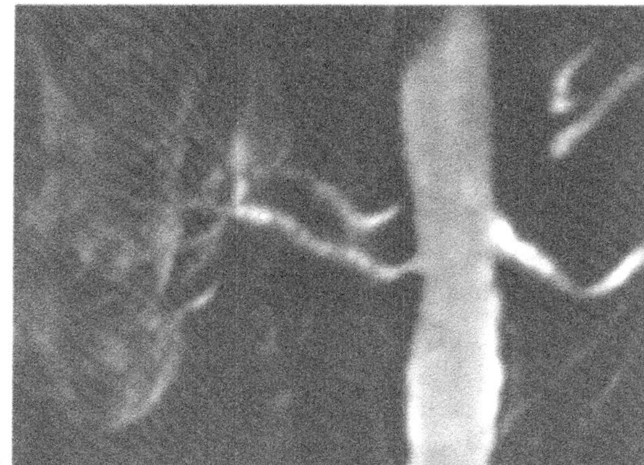

a

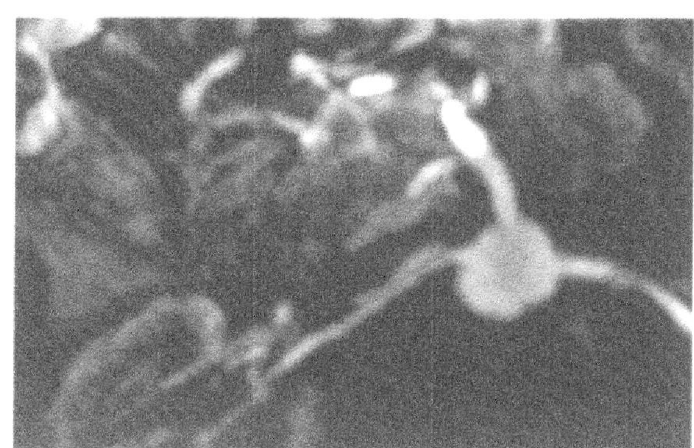

b

← **Fig. 18.29a, b.** A 48-year-old hypertensive woman screened for renal artery stenosis. On the CE 3D MR angiogram in the coronal plane (maximum intensity projection) (**a**) renal arteries show luminal irregularities similar to a string-of-beads appearance mimicking fibromuscular dysplasia. In the transverse plane (reformatted image) (**b**), however, it can be demonstrated that vascular irregularities are caused by thick-section acquisition (4 mm)

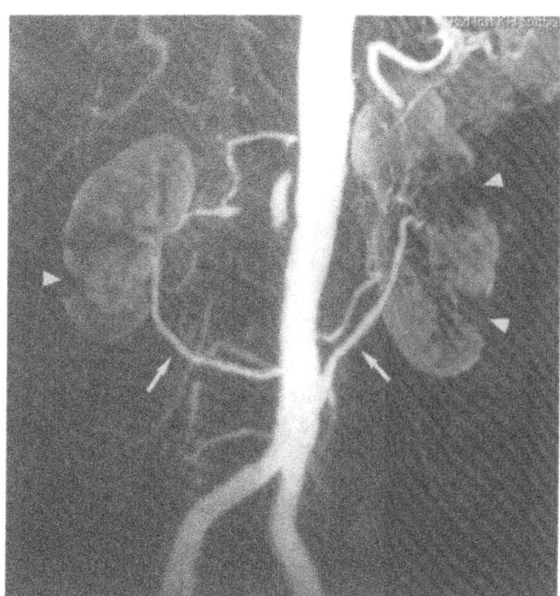

Fig. 18.30. A 54-year-old man with renovascular hypertension due to bilateral renal artery stenosis. CE 3D MR angiography was performed following surgical bilateral aortorenal bypass graft implantation, demonstrating a patent venous graft (*arrows*) to both kidneys and peripheral parenchymal perfusion defects due to renal infarction (*arrowheads*). The left kidney is supplied by an additional accessory artery

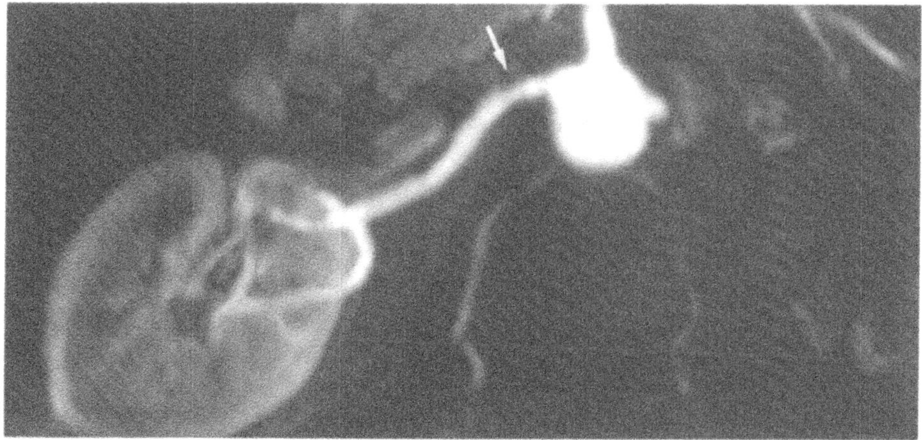

c

Fig. 18.28a–c. Hypertensive male patient with left side nephrectomy due to acute pyonephrosis. On the CE MR angiogram in coronal view (**a**) more pronounced than in transverse view (**b**) an irregular postostial signal void (*arrow*) can be observed suspected of being renal artery stenosis. The simultaneous DSA image (**c**) shows a widely normal lumen of the right renal artery with only distinct atherosclerotic plaque material

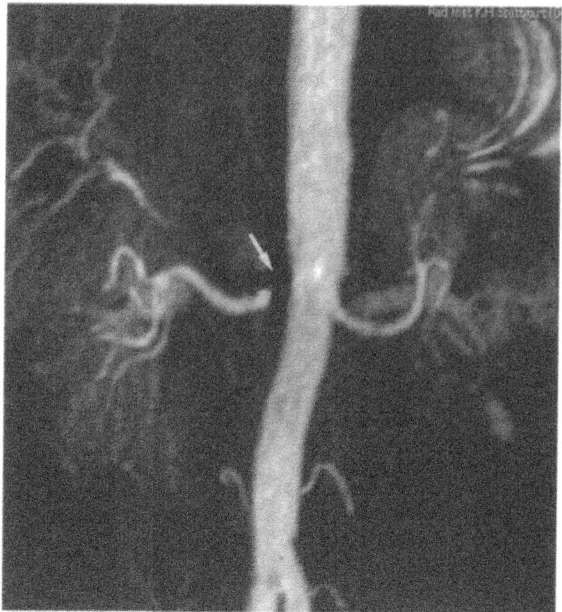

Fig. 18.31. A 53-year-old man with recurrent right renal artery stenosis was successfully treated by metallic stent placement in the right renal artery ostium. Following this procedure renal blood flow and arterial blood pressure normalized. On the CE 3D MR angiogram the peripheral part of the right renal artery shows normal signal, whereas a complete signal void can be seen at the site of the metallic stent (*arrow*)

In the functional evaluation of hemodynamically significant RAS, different MR techniques have been described. Indirect parameters can be found by analyzing the contrast-enhancement of renal parenchyma in time-resolved CE 3D MR angiography, whereas direct functional parameters can be determined by PC methods. Suitable protocols which combine angiomorphologic and functional MR imaging have been recommended by different authors (Prince et al. 1997; Dong et al. 1999; Schoenberg et al. 1997, 1999). Prince et al. (1997) reported diverse collateral signs such as post-stenotic dilatation >20% in 59% of cases, reduction in ischemic kidney length and cortical thickness, and a parenchymal gadolinium enhancement reduced by 15% in the ischemic kidney. Ros et al. (1995) proved the feasibility of combining MR angiography, MR renography, and gadopentate-based measurements of glomerular filtration rate; the results suggest a potential for a comprehensive approach in the detection of significant RAS. Walsh et al. (1996) observed an asymmetric signal in the renal collecting system as a sign of unilateral RAS following administration of gadopentate dimeglumine, confirming the known phenomenon of hyperconcentration of contrast material due to autoregulative mechanisms in hypoperfused kidneys. Grenier et al. (1996) compared captopril-sensitized dynamic CE MR imaging of the kidneys, with captopril scintigraphy revealing similar results in both. However, captopril-induced changes were not present in all patients with proven RAS and scintigraphy could not demonstrate segmental functional involvement. Using 3D PC MR imaging, Prince et al. (1997) described a signal void due to severe dephasing in 87% of patients with significant RAS. For grading RAS on 3D PC images, mild stenosis of 25%–49% showed a normal appearance, moderate stenosis of 50%–75% appeared with or without spin dephasing, and all severe stenoses >75% appeared with severe spin dephasing (Dong et al. 1999). A stenosis score has been established for DSA-proven, significant RAS (intra-arterial pressure measurement) on 3D PC images, which is based on the presence and length of flow void and flow signal intensity in the distal renal artery (Wasser et al. 1997): flow void occurred at rates of 62% sensitivity and 83% specificity, and distal flow signal intensity was impaired at a 92% sensitivity and 75% specificity, respectively. Direct quantification of renal blood flow has been determined using 2D PC MR cine flow mapping (Schoenberg et al. 1997). Hemodynamic parameters in DSA-proven RAS included a decrease in mean flow and a delay and reduction in systolic velocity maximum, revealing a sensitivity of 90% and specificity of 94% in the overall detection of RAS and a sensitivity of 100% and a specificity of 93% in detecting RAS >50%, respectively. Recently, an angiotensin-converting enzyme inhibitor was administered in combination with 2D cine PC MR imaging (Lee et al. 2000) in order to measure renal artery velocity waveforms in suspected RAS. In contrast to a comparable US study of Oliva et al. (1998), which showed significant differences between stenosed and nonstenosed kidneys, this technique was not useful in predicting RAS accurately.

18.3.2.4 Renal Transplants

A renal transplant artery is most commonly anastomosed end-to-end with the proximal internal iliac artery when a living donor kidney is used, whereas arterial anastomosis is located end-to-side at the common or external iliac artery when a cadaver graft is used. Vascular complications in renal transplant allografts have become an important cause of arterial hypertension, graft dysfunction, and graft loss despite improvements in surgical techniques and drug therapy. Its incidence has been observed in up to 12% of patients (Brichaux et al. 1995; Loubeyre et al. 1996b). Complications in the early postoperative period are probably due to technical factors in most cases. Thrombosis of the main renal artery occurs more frequently than venous thrombosis, which is mostly caused by surgical malposition of the graft or extension of an iliac vein thrombosis. The most frequent late vascular complication is RAS, occurring in approximately 10% of cases (GRENIER et al. 1997), whereas complete arterial thrombosis is rare (approximately 1% of grafts) and is usually associated with severe acute rejection. More frequently, segmental artery thrombosis can be observed which may cause segmental renal infarction. Distal arteriovenous fistulas or pseudoaneurysms commonly are caused iatrogenically by graft biopsies. A variety of parenchymal disorders such as acute tubular necrosis and subacute or chronic rejection of the graft may occur, leading to cortical vascular alterations, cortical hypoperfusion, and impaired graft function.

In order to detect vascular and parenchymal disorders as a cause of reduced graft function, noninvasive imaging techniques have been suggested such as color-coded duplex-Doppler US and MR imaging, neither of which depend on the administration of nephrotoxic contrast material (LOUBEYRE et al. 1996b; MARTINOLI et al. 1996; GRENIER et al. 1997; WIESNER et al. 1998).

Ultrasonography. Routinely used Doppler US has been shown to be an accurate and simple method for depicting vascular and parenchymal complications of the renal transplant. With US the entire course of the artery can be visualized and arterial velocities reliably measured. RAS is characterized by elevated peak systolic velocity. Moreover, the intraparenchymal vasculature can be evaluated best by power Doppler technique (MARTINOLI et al. 1996). However, difficulties remain in distinguishing significant from nonsignificant RAS, and in conditions of vessel kinking or coiling. Furthermore, it has been demonstrated that the absence of detectable intraparenchymal flow at the interlobular level does not reliably correspond to cortical perfusion in MR imaging.

MR Angiography. In depicting transplant RAS, 3D PC MR angiography has been shown to be insufficient due to a variety of false-positive findings caused by major intravoxel phase dispersion (LOUBEYRE et al. 1996b). However, correct MR angiographic diagnosis of stenotic and thrombotic lesions of the main renal artery without false negatives or disagreement have been reported by BRICHAUX et al. (1995) when a combination of flow-sensitive 2D and 3D GRE sequences was performed. Since the advantages of CE 3D MR angiography over flow-sensitive methods have been recognized and excellent image quality of arterial and venous structures became available (Fig. 18.32), it could be shown that, in revealing significant arterial stenosis, sensitivity and specificity was 100% and 98% in a prospective study, and 86%–88% and 98%–100%, respectively, in a retrospective study (FERREIROS et al. 1998). The most promising examination protocol should combine CE 3D MR angiography of the renal graft vasculature with postcontrast T1-weighted GRE imaging of the graft parenchyma (GRENIER et al. 1997, WIESNER et al. 1998). This concept allows the reliable detection of transplant RAS (Figs. 18.33, 18.34a–c), arterial occlusion, complications at the anastomosis (Fig. 18.35a–d), renal vein thrombosis, and parenchymal perfusion defects due to renal infarction, cortical necrosis, acute tubular necrosis, and venous ischemia. Fluid collections and dilatation of the collecting system or abnormalities of the surrounding tissues can be documented when an additional fat-saturated T2-weighted sequence is used.

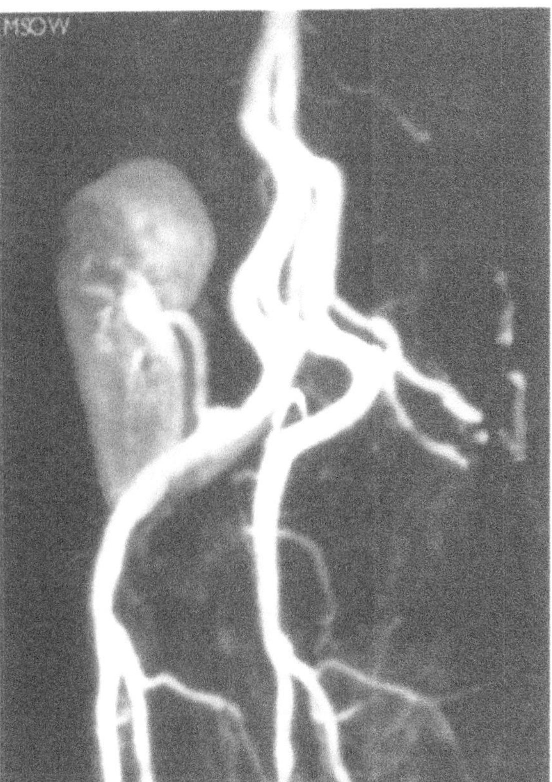

Fig. 18.32. Renal transplant including an artery anastomosed with the right external iliac artery. On the CE 3D MR angiogram (maximum intensity projection) anastomosis and complete course of the normal transplant artery can be evaluated only in a nearly sagittal view. The graft shows normal parenchymal enhancement

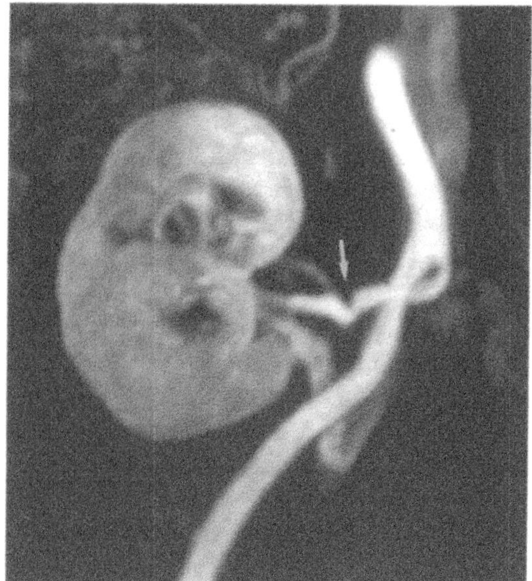

Fig. 18.33. CE 3D MR angiogram (coronal subvolume maximum intensity projection) of an allograft renal transplant showing moderate narrowing of the arterial lumen at the level of anastomosis with the right internal iliac artery (*arrow*). On this image both the arterial and venous structures are visualized

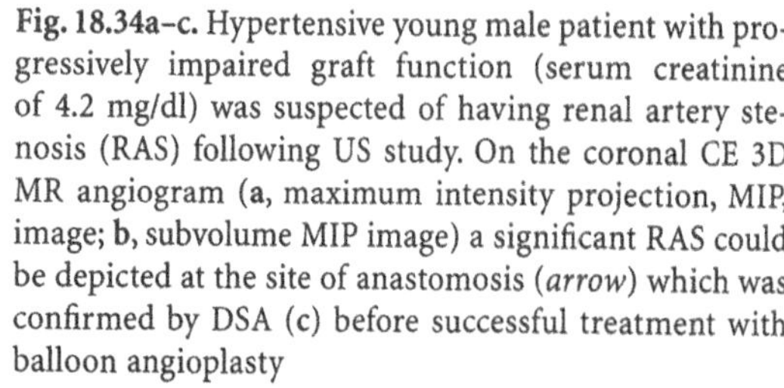

Fig. 18.34a–c. Hypertensive young male patient with progressively impaired graft function (serum creatinine of 4.2 mg/dl) was suspected of having renal artery stenosis (RAS) following US study. On the coronal CE 3D MR angiogram (**a**, maximum intensity projection, MIP, image; **b**, subvolume MIP image) a significant RAS could be depicted at the site of anastomosis (*arrow*) which was confirmed by DSA (**c**) before successful treatment with balloon angioplasty

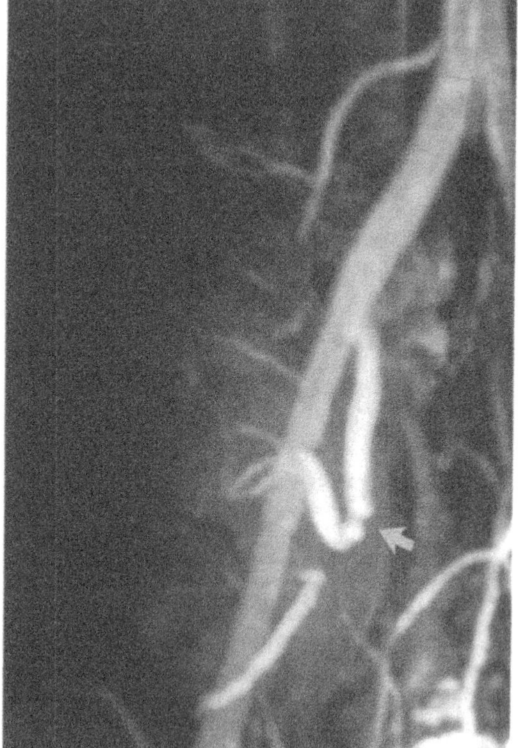

a

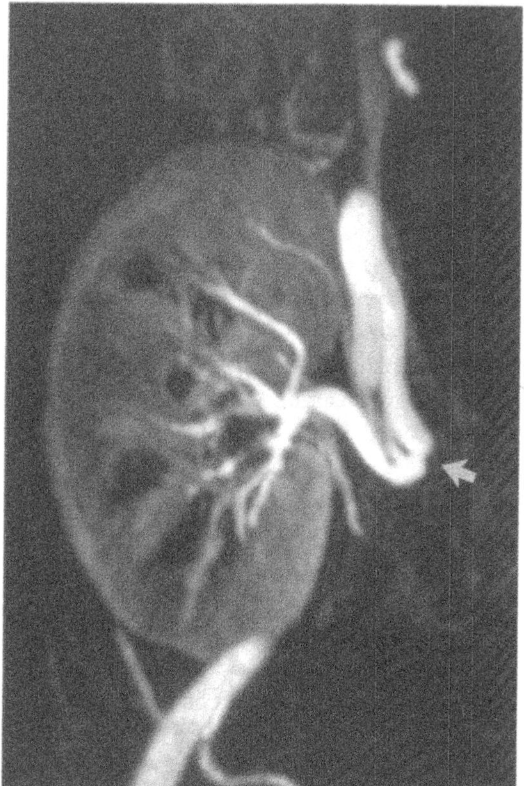

b

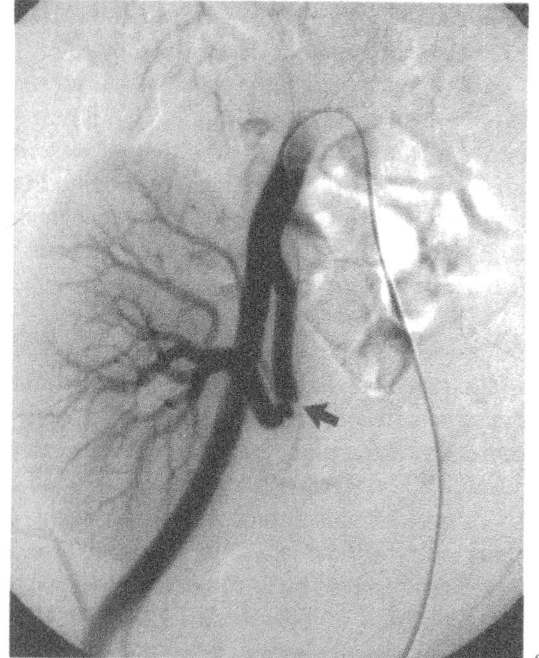

c

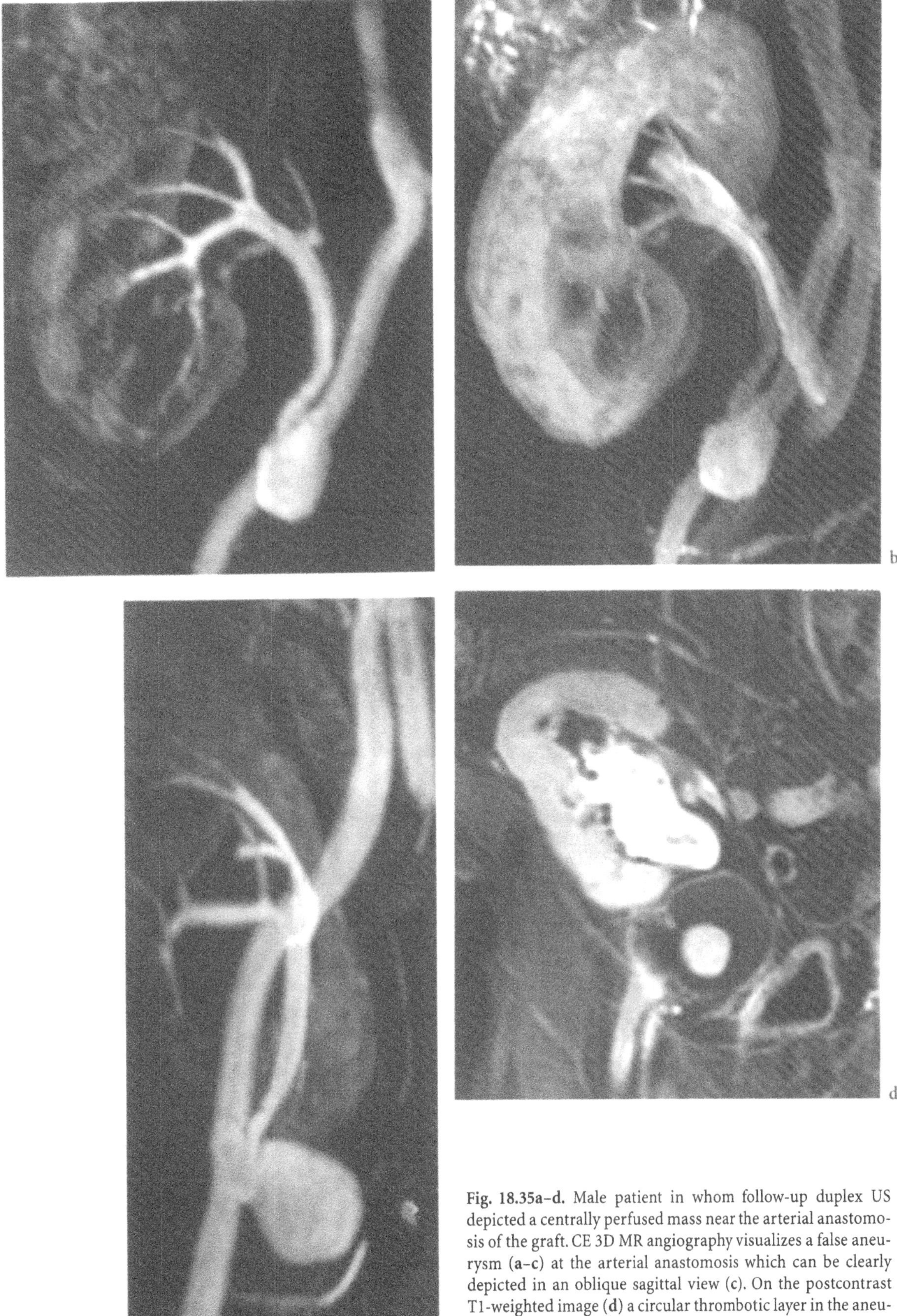

Fig. 18.35a–d. Male patient in whom follow-up duplex US depicted a centrally perfused mass near the arterial anastomosis of the graft. CE 3D MR angiography visualizes a false aneurysm (**a–c**) at the arterial anastomosis which can be clearly depicted in an oblique sagittal view (**c**). On the postcontrast T1-weighted image (**d**) a circular thrombotic layer in the aneurysmal sac is demonstrated; graft parenchyma is normally perfused

18.4 Conclusions

Since the early work of PRINCE and colleagues in 1993 and the method has been optimized, CE 3D MR angiography has been incorporated in clinical practice. Multiple vascular territories can be examined with this technique, which has shown to be particularly useful in abdominal aortic disease such as congenital coarctation, atherosclerotic stenosis, or occlusion, aneurysm, and dissection. Aortic morphology can be completely visualized by using MR angiography in combination with postcontrast T1-weighted MR imaging. Moreover, due to its high accuracy, this technique has been introduced successfully into noninvasive diagnostic imaging of aortic branches, including the splanchnic and renal arteries.

Two standardized CE MR angiographic protocols can be distinguished at the moment that are based either on a single-phase or multiphase, time-resolved technique, by which one or more 3D data sets are acquired within a single breath-hold. Timing of the contrast bolus has been shown to be extremely important when the single-phase technique is used, whereas in the multiphase technique a contrast bolus timing is not really necessary. High-resolution single-phase MR angiograms with excellent arterial image quality can be provided during the first pass of the contrast agent, and late arterial and venous information can be obtained during repetitive breath-holds. Multiphase MR angiographic imaging, although still rather low in spatial resolution, is able to assess the hemodynamic significance of stenotic disease on the basis of arterial as well as parenchymal flow differences due to temporal information. Moreover, with 2D cine PC flow mapping techniques blood flow can be quantified in the main aortic branches, which may be of importance in the functional evaluation of occlusive disorders. In screening for RVH, CE 3D MR angiography has proven to be a reliable method. Its accuracy is similar to that of CT angiography, with the advantage that non-nephrotoxic contrast material is administered.

In splanchnic vascular imaging, CE 3D MR angiography also plays an important noninvasive diagnostic role, particularly in depicting proximal occlusive or aneurysmal disease but also in staging pancreatic and hepatic tumors.

Compared with conventional angiography CE MR angiography is still limited in visualizing distal and peripheral small arteries of the splanchnic system and within the renal or hepatic parenchyma. Thus, the challenge for MR angiography in the future is to further improve temporal and spatial resolution. It can be expected that this technical concept will have become reality within the next few years and lead to an optimized MR angiographic quality which may replace conventional angiography even in the majority of patients with peripheral small vessel disease. Moreover, CE 3D MR angiography of the abdominal aorta, its branches, and abdominal venous structures can already supplement standard MR imaging as well as MRCP when performed in patients with hepatic, pancreatic, or biliary disease with suspected vascular involvement.

Acknowledgements. The authors thank Mrs. Tanja Endres for assistance with data acquisition and preparation of image material.

References

Abrams HL (1983a) Renal arteriography in hypertension. In: Abrams HL (ed) Angiography, vascular and interventional radiology, 3rd edn. Little, Brown, Boston, pp 1247–1298

Abrams HL (1983b) Splenic arteriography. In: Abrams HL (ed) Angiography: vascular and interventional radiology, 3rd edn. Little, Brown, Boston, pp 1531–1572

Alley MT, Shifrin RY, Pelc NJ, Herfkens RJ (1998) Ultrafast contrast-enhanced three-dimensional MR angiography: state of the art. Radiographics 18:273–285

Amanuma M, Mohiaddin RH, Hasegawa M, Heshiki A, Longmore DB (1992) Abdominal aorta: characterization of blood flow and measurement of ist regional distribution by cine magnetic reonance phase-shift velocity mapping. Eur Radiol 2:559–564

Arlart IP, Guhl L, Edelman RR (1992) Magnetic reonance angiography of the abdominal aorta. CIR 15:43–50

Arlart IP, Guhl L, Hausmann R (1993) Evaluation of 2D and 3D time-of-flight MRA in renal artery stenosis. Fortschr Roentgenstr 157:59–64

Arlart IP, Gerlach A, Kolb M, Erpenbach S, Würstlin S (1997) Gadopentate dimeglumine enhanced MR angiography (MRA) for staging AAA: a correlation with DSA and CT. Fortschr Roentgenstr 167:257–263

Avasthi PS, Voyles WF, Greene ER (1984) Noninvasive diagnosis of renal artery stenosis by echo-Doppler velocimetry. Kidney Int 25:824–829

Bakker J, Beutler JJ, et al (1998) Renal artery stenosis and accessory renal arteries: accuracy of detection and visualization with gadolinium-enhanced breath-hold MR angiography. Radiology 207:497–504

Bass JC, Prince MR, Londy FJ, Chenevert TL (1997) Effect of Gadolinium on phase-contrast MR angiography of the renal arteries. AJR Am J Roentgenol 168:261–266

Baum S (1983) Hepatic arteriography. In: Abrams HL (ed) Angiography, vascular and interventional radiology, 3rd edn. Little, Brown, Boston, pp 1479–1504

Beregi J-P, Elkohen M, Deklunder G, Artaud D, Coullet JM, Wattinne L (1996) Helical CT angiography compared with arteriography in the detection of renal artery stenosis. AJR Am J Roentgenol 167:495–501

Beregi J-P, Louvegny S, Gautier C, Mounier-Vehier C, Moretti A, Desmoucelle F, Wattinne L, McFadden E (1999) Fibromuscular dysplasia of the renal arteries: comparison of helical CT angiography and arteriography. AJR Am J Roentgenol 172:27–34

Berland LL, Koslin DB, Routh WD, Keller FS (1990) Renal artery stenosis: prospective evaluation of diagnosis with color duplex US compared with angiography. Radiology 174:421–423

Blum U, Langer M, Spillner G, et al (1996) Abdominal aortic aneurysms: preliminary technical and clinical results with transfemoral placement of endovascular selfexpanding stents-grafts. Radiology 198:25–31

Blum U, Hauer M, Krumme B (1999) Percutaneous revascularization of the kidney: conventional angioplasty versus renal artery stenting. Radiologe 39:135–143

Boijsen E (1983) Superior mesenteric angiography. In: Abrams AL (ed) Angiography: vascular and interventional radiology, 3rd edn. Little, Brown, Boston, pp 1623–1668

Brichaux JC, Grenier N, Douws C, Degreze P, Palussiere J, Trillaud H, Morel D, Potaux L (1995) Time-of-flight angiography of kidney transplants. Eur Radiol 5:406- 413

Bude R, Rubin JM (1995) Detection of renal artery stenosis with Doppler sonography: it is more complicated than originally thought. Radiology 196:612–613

Burkart DJ, Johnson CD, Ehman RL (1993) Correlation of arterial and venous blood flow in the mesenetric system based on MR findings. AJR Am J Roentgenol 161:1279–1282

Buzzas GR, Shield CF, Pay NT, Neuman MJ, Smith JL (1997) Use of gadolinium-enhanced, ultrafast, three-dimensional, spoiled gradient-echo magnetic resonance angiography in the preoperative evaluation of living renal allograft donors. Transplantation 64:1734–1737

Carlos RC, Dong Q, Stanley JC, Prince MR (1999) MR angiography after renal revascularization: spectrum of expected anatomic results and postintervention complications. Radiographics 19:1555–1568

Castrucci M, Mellone R, Vanzulli A, De Gaspari A, Castellano R, Astore D, Chiesa R, Grossi A, Del Maschio A (1995) Mural thrombi in abdominal aortic aneurysms: MR imaging characterization – useful before endovascular treatment? Radiology 197:135–139

Chambers TP, Fishman EK, Bluemke DA, Urban B, Venbrux AC (1995) Identification of the aberrant hepatic artery with axial spiral CT. J Vasc Interv Radiol 6:959–964

Chan FP, Li KCP, Heiss SG, Razavi MK (1999) A comprehensive approach using MR imaging to diagnose acute segmental mesenteric ischemia in a porcine model. AJR Am J Roentgenol 173:523–529

Choe YH, Han B-K, Koh E-M, Kim D-K, Do YS, Lee WR (2000) Takayasu's arteritis: assessment of disease activity with contrast-enhanced MR imaging. AJR Am J Roentgenol 175:505–511

Cullenward MJ, Scanlan KA, Pozniak MA, Acher CA (1986) Inflammatory aortic aneurysm (periaortic fibrosis): radiologic imaging. Radiology 159:75–82

Davis CP, Ladd ME, Göhde SC, Pfammatter T, Fass L, Debatin JF (1996) Virtual intravascular endoscopy in the renal arteries: a new way of reading 3D MR angiography data sets. Fortschr Roentgenstr 165:257–263

Davis CP, Hany TF, Wildermuth S, Schmidt M, Debatin JF (1997) Postprocessing techniques for Gadolinium-enhanced three-dimensional MR angiography. Radiographics 17:1061–1077

Debatin JF, Ting RH, Wegmüller H, Sommer FG, Fredrickson JO, Brosnan TJ, Bowman BS, Myers BD, Herfkens RJ, Pelc NJ (1994) Renal artery blood flow: quantification with phase-contrast MR imaging with and without breath- holding. Radiology 190:371–378

Debatin JF, Wildermuth S, Leung DA, Botnar R, Felbinger J, McKinnon GC (1995) Flow quantification with echo-planar phase-contrast velocity mapping: in vitro and in vivo evaluation. J Magn Reson Imaging 5:656–662

De Cobelli F, Vanzulli A, Sironi S, Mellone R, Angeli E, Venturini M, Garancini MP, Quartagno R, Bianchi G, Del Maschio A (1997) Renal artery stenosis: evaluation with breath-hold, three-dimensional, dynamic, Gadolinium-enhanced versus thre-dimensional phase-contrast MR angiography. Radiology 205:689–695

De Cobelli F, Venturine M, Vanzulli A, Sironi S, Salvioni M, Angeli E, Scifo P, Garancini MP, Quartagno R, Bianchi G, Del Maschio A (2000) Renal arterial stenosis: prospective comparison of color Doppler US and breath-hold, three-dimensional, dynamic, gadolinium-enhanced MR angiography. Radiology 214:373–380

De Haan MW, Kouwenhoven M, Thelissen GRP, Koster D, Kessels AGH, de Leeuw PW, van Engelshoven JMA (1996) Renovascular disease in patients with hypertension: detection with systolic and diastolic gating in three-dimensional phase-contrast MR angiography. Radiology 198:449–456

De Haan MW, Kouwenhoven M, Kessels AGH, van Engelshoven JMA (2000) Renal artery blood flow: quantification with breath-hold or respiratory triggered phase-contrast MR imaging. Eur Radiol 10:1133–1137

Desberg AL, Paushter DM, Lammert GK, et al (1990) Renal artery stenosis: evaluation with color Doppler flow imaging. Radiology 177:749–753

Dock W, Turkof E, Maier A, Metz V, Puig S, Mittelböck M, Eibenberger K, Lechner G, Polterauer P (1998) Prevalence of the abdominal aortic aneurysm: a sonographic sreening study. Fortschr Roentgenstr 168:356–360

Dong Q, Schoenberg SO, Carlos RC, Neimatallah M, Cho KJ, Williams DM, Kazanjian SN, Prince MR (1999) Diagnosis of renal vascular disease with MR angiography. Radiographics 19:1535–1554

Dorffner R, Thurnher S, Polterauer P, Kretschmer G, Lammer J (1997) Treatment of abdominal aortic aneurysms with transfemoral placement of stent-grafts: complications and secondary radiologic intervention. Radiology 204:79–86

Dumoulin CL, Yucel K, Vock P, Souza SP, Terrier F, Steinberg FL, Wegmuller H (1990) Two- and three- dimensional phase contrast MR angiography of the abdomen. J Comput Assist Tomogr 14:779–784

Earls JP, DeSena S, Bluemke DA (1998) Gadolinium-enhanced three-dimensional MR angiography of the entire aorta and iliac arteries with dynamic manual table translation. Radiology 209:844–849

Edelman RR, Wentz KU, Mattle H, Zao B, Lin C, Kim D, Laub G (1989) Projection arteriography and venography: initial clinical results with MR. Radiology 172:351–357

Erden A, Yurdakul M, Cumhur T (1998): Doppler waveforms of the normal and collateralized inferior mesenteric artery. AJR Am J Roentgenol 171:619–627

Ernst O, Asnar V, Sergent G, Lederman E, Nicol L, Paris J- C,

L'Hermine C (2000) Comparing contrast-enhanced breath-hold MR angiography and conventional angiography in the evaluation of mesenteric circulation. AJR Am J Roentgenol 174:433–439

Fann JI, Smith JA, Miller C, Mitchell RS, Moore KA, Grunkemeier G, Stinson EB, Oyer PE, Reitz BA, Shumway NE (1995) Surgical management of aortic dissection during a 30-years period. Circulation 92 [Suppl 2]:113–121

Ferreiros J, Mendez R, Jorquera M, Gallego J, Lezana A, Prats D, Pedrosa CS (1998) Using gadolinium-enhanced three-dimensional MR angiography to assess arterial inflow stenosis after kidney transplantation. Am J Roentgenol 172:751–757

Galanski M, Hoogestraat-Lufft L, Högemann D, Baus S, Schmidt A, Koehler A, Arlart IP, Landwehr P, Huppert P, Hecker H, Chavan A (1999) Detection accuracy of various display modalities in CT angiography of renal artery stenosis. Fortschr Roentgenstr 171:200–206

Gilfeather M, Holland GA, Siegelman ES, Schnall MD, Axel L, Carpenter JP, Golden MA (1997) Gadolinium-enhanced ultrafast three-dimensional spoiled gradient-echo MR imaging of the abdominal aorta and visceral and iliac vessels. Radiographics 17:423-432

Giovagnorio F, Picarelli A, Di Giovambattista F, Mastracchio A (1998) Evaluation with Doppler sonography of mesenteric blood flow in celiac disease. AJR Am J Roentgenol 171:629-632

Grenier N, Trillaud H, Combe C, Degreze P, Jeandot R, Gosse P, Douws C, Palussiere J (1996) Diagnosis of renovascular hypertension: feasibility of Captopril-sensitized dynamic MR imaging and comparison with Captopril scintigraphy. AJR Am J Roentgenol 166:835–843

Grenier N, Claudon M, Trillaud H, Douws C, Levantal O (1997) Noninvasive radiology of vascular complications in renal transplantation. Eur Radiol 7:385–391

Grist TM (1993) A prospective evaluation of renal MRA for detecting renal artery stenosis in 35 consecutive patients [abstract]. In: Proceedings of the 12th Annual Science Meeting of the Society for Magnetic Resonance in Medicine, Berkeley, California, p 187

Grist TM (1996) AR angiography of the renal arteries during a breath-hold using gadolinium-enhanced 3D TOF with k-space zero-filling and contrast timing scan [abstract]. In: Proceedings of the 4th Meeting of the International Society for Magnetic Resonance in Medicine, Berkeley, California, p 163

Hahn U, Miller S, Nägele T, Schick F, Erdtmann B, Duda S, Claussen CD (1999) Renal MR angiography at 1.0 T: three-dimensional (3D) phase-contrast techniques versus Gadolinium-enhanced 3D fast low-angle shot breath-hold imaging. AJR Am J Roentgenol 172:1501–1508

Hansen KJ, Tribble RW, Reavis SW, et al (1990) Renal duplex sonography: evaluation of clinical utility. J Vasc Surg 12:227–236

Hany TF, Schmid M, Schoenenberger AW, Debatin JF (1998a) Contrast-enhanced three-dimensional magnetic resonance angiography of the splanchnic vasculature before and after caloric stimulation. Invest Radiol 33:682–686

Hany TF, Leung DA, Pfammatter T, Debatin JF (1998b) Contrast-enhanced magnetic resonance angiography of the renal arteries. Invest Radiol 33:653–665

Hawighorst H, Schoenberg SO, Knopp MV, Essig M, Miltner P, van Kaick G (1999) Hepatic lesions: morphologic and functional characterization with multiphase breath-hold 3D gadolinium-enhanced MR angiography – initial results. Radiology 210:89–96

Hertz SM, Holland GA, Baum RA, Haskal ZJ, Carpenter JP (1994) Evaluation of renal artery stenosis by magnetic resonance angiography. Am J Surg 168:140–143

Higgins CB (1992) The vascular system. In: Higgins CB, Hricak H, Helm CA (eds) Magnetic resonance imaging of the body, 2nd edn. Raven Press, New York, p 629–678

Hoffman U, Edwards JM, Carter S, et al (1991) Role of duplex scanning for the detection of atherosclerotic renal artery disease. Kidney Int 39:1232–1239

Holland GA, Dougherty LP, Carpenter JP, Golden MA, Gilfeather M, Slossman F, Schnall MD, Axel L (1996) Breath-hold ultrafast three-dimensional Gadolinium-enhanced MR angiography of the aorta and the renal and other visceral abdominal arteries. AJR Am J Roentgenol 166:971–981

Hong KC, Freeny PC (1999) Pancreaticoduodenal arcades and dorsal pancreatic artery: comparison of CT angiography with thre-dimensional volume rendering, maximum intensity projection, and shaded-surface display. AJR Am J Roentgenol 172:925–931

House MK, Dowling RJ, King P, Gibson RN (1999) Using Doppler sonography to reveal renal artery stenosis: an evaluation of optimal imaging parameters. AJR Am J Roentgenol 173:761–765

Inoue T, Watanabe S, Masuda Y, et al (1996) Evaluation of blood flow pattern of true and false lumens in dissecting aneurysms using MR phase-contrast techniques. Clin Imaging 20:262

Johnson PT, Heath DG, Kuszyk BS, Fishman EK (1996) CT angiography with volume rendering: advantages and applications in the splanchnic vascular imaging. Radiology 200:564–568

Johnson PT, Halpern EJ, Kuszyk BS, Heath DG, Wechsler BJ, Nazarian LN, Gardiner GA, Levin DC, Fishman EK (1999) Renal artery stenosis: CT angiography – comparison of real-time volume rendering and maximum intensity projection algorithms. Radiology 211:337–343

Kaatee R, Beek FJA, de Lange EE, van Leeuwen MS, Smits HFM, van der Ven PJG, Beutler JJ, Mali WPTM (1997) Renal artery stenosis: detection and quantification with spiral CT angiography versus optimized digital subtraction angiography. Radiology 205:121–127

Kadir S (1986) Diagnostic angiography. Saunders, Philadelphia

Kadir S (1991) Atlas of normal and variant angiographic anatomy. Saunders, Philadelphia

Kaleya RN, Sammartano RJ, Boley SJ (1992) Aggressive approach of mesenteric ischemia. Surg Clin North Am 72:157–181

Kaneko K, Honda H, Hayashi T, et al (1997) Helical CT- evaluation of arterial invasion in pancreatic tumors: comparison with angiography. Abdom Imaging 22:204–207

Kanematsu M, Imaeda T, Mizuno Y, Sone Y, Iida T, Kato M, Yokoyama R (1996) Value of three-dimensional spiral CT hepatic angiography. AJR Am J Roentgenol 166:585–591

Kent KC, Edelman RR, Kim D, Steinman TI, Porter DH, Skillman JJ (1991) Magnetic resonance imaging: a reliable test for the evaluation of proximal atherosclerotic renal artery stenosis. J Vasc Surg 13:311–318

Kerr AB, Pauly JM, Hu BS, et al (1997) Real-time interactive MRI on a conventional scanner. Magn Reson Med 38:335–367

Kim D, Edelman RR, Kent KC, Porter DH, Skillman JJ (1990) Abdominal aorta and renal artery stenosis: evaluation with MR angiography. Radiology 174:727–731

Kliever MA, Tupler RH, Carroll BA, et al (1993) Renal artery stenosis: analysis of Doppler wave-form parameters and tardus-parvus pattern. Radiology 189:779–787

Kopka L, Rodenwaldt J, Fischer U, Renner B, Lorf T, Graessner J, Ringe B, Grabbe E (1999) Hepatic blood supply: comparison of optimized dual phase contrast- enhanced three-dimensional MR angiography and digital subtraction angiography. Radiology 211:51–58

Kraus BB, Ros PR, Abbitt PI, Kerns SR, Sabatelli FW (1995) Comparison of ultrasound, CT, and MR imaging in the evaluation of candidates for TIPS. J Magn Reson Imaging 5:571–578

Lange H (1989) Die differentialdiagnostische Bedeutung des Laktats bei akuten Baucherkrankungen. Acta Chir 60:356–360

Lee VS, Rofsky NM, Ton AT, Johnson G, Krinsky GA, Weinreb JC (2000) Angiotensin-converting enzyme inhibitor-enhanced phase-contrast MR imaging to measure renal artery velocity waveforms in patients with suspected renovascular hypertension. AJR Am J Roentgenol 174:499–508

Leung DA, Debatin JF (1998) Ultrafast magnetic resonance imaging of the vascular system. In: Debatin JF, McKinnon GC (eds) Ultrafast MRI. Springer, Berlin Heidelberg New York, pp 135–184

Leung DA, McKinnon GC, Divis CP, Pfammatter T, Krestin GP, Debatin JF (1996) Breath-hold contrast-enhanced three-dimensional MR angiography. Radiology 201:569–571

Leung DA, Hany TF, Debatin JF (1998) Three-dimensional contrast-enhanced magnetic resonance angiography of the abdominal arterial system. Cardiovasc Intervent Radiol 21:1–10

Lewin JS, Laub G, Hausmann R (1991) Three-dimensional time-of-flight MR angiography: applications in the abdomen and thorax. Radiology 179:261–264

Li KC, Whitney WS, McDonnel CH, et al (1994) Chronic mesenteric ischemia: evaluation with pahse contrast cine MR imaging. Radiology 190:175–179

Lim HK, Lee WJ, Kim SH, Lee SJ, Choi SH, Park HS, Do YS, Choo SW, Choo IW (1999) Splanchnic arterial stenosis or occlusion: diagnosis at Doppler US. Radiology 211:405–410

Link J, Steffens JC, Brossmann J, Loose R, Heller M (1998) Contrast-enhanced MR angiography in Leriche's syndrome. Fortschr Roentgenstr 169:22–26

Lipchik EO, Rogoff SM (1983a) The abnormal abdominal aorta:atherosclerosis and other diseases. In: Abrams HL (ed) Angiography, vascular and interventional radiology, 3rd edn. Little, Brown, Boston, pp 1057–1078

Lipchik EO, Rogoff SM (1983b) Aneurysms of the abdominal aorta. In: Abrams HL (ed) Angiography, vascular and interventional radiology, 3rd edn. Little, Brown, Boston, pp 1079–1090

Lomas DJ, Britton PD, Alexander GJ, Calne RY (1994) A comparison of MR and duplex Doppler ultrasound for vascular assessment prior to orthotopic liver transplantation. Clin Radiol 5:307–310

Loubeyre P, Revel D, Garcia P, et al (1994) Screening patients for renal artery stenosis: value of three-dimensional time-of-flight MR angiography. AJR Am J Roentgenol 162:847–852

Loubeyre P, Troliet P, Cahen R, Grozel F, Labeeuw M, Tran Minh VA (1996a) MR angiography of renal artery stenosis: value of the combination of three-dimensional time-of-flight and three-dimensional phase-contrast MR angiography sequences. AJR Am J Roentgenol 167:489–494

Loubeyre P, Cahen R, Grozel F, Trolliet P, Pouteil-Noble C, Labeeuw M, Tran Minh VA (1996b) Transplant renal artery stenosis: evaluation of diagnosis with magnetic resonance angiography compared with color duplex sonography and arteriography. Transplantation 62:446–450

Marks B, Mitchell DG, Simelaro JP (1997) Breath-holding in healthy and pulmonary compromised populations: effects of hyperventilation and oxygen inspiration. J Magn Reson Imaging 7:595–597

Martinoli C, Crespi G, Bertolotto M, Rollandi GA, Rosenberg H, Pretolesi F, Derchi LE (1996) Interlobular vasculature in renal transplants: a power Doppler US study with MR correlation. Radiology 200:111–117

Merritt CRB (1992) Doppler Color imaging. Churchill Livingstone, New York

Millis JM, Brown SL, Busuttil RW (1992) Thoracic and abdominal aneurysms. In: Bell PRF, Jamieson CW, Ruckley CV (eds) Surgical management of vascular disease. Saunders, London

Misri H, Pöckler-Schöninger C, Gaa J, Georgi M, Sturm J, Ihle V (1998) Ultrafast contrast-enhanced 3D MRA in preoperative diagnostic imaging of liver tumors. Fortschr Roentgenstr 169:278–283

Moneta GL, Lee RW, Yeager RA, Taylor LM, Porter JM (1993) Mesenteric duplex scanning: a blinded prospective study. J Vasc Surg 17:79–86

Morcos SK, Thomsen HS, Webb JAW, et al (1999) Contrast-media induced nephrotoxicity: a consensus report. Eur Radiol 9:1602–1613

Novick SL, Fishman EK (1998) Three-dimensional CT angiography of pancreatic carcinoma: role of staging extent of disease. AJR Am J Roentgenol 170:139–143

Nyman U, Uher P, Lindh M, Lindblad B, Ivancev K (2000) Primary stenting in infrarenal aortic occlusive disease. Cardiovasc Intervent Radiol 23:97–108

Oliva VL, Soulez G, Lasage D, Nicolet V, Roy MC, Courteau M, Froment D, Rene PC, Therasse E, Carignan L (1998) Detection of renal artery stenosis with Doppler sonography before and after administration of captopril: value of early systolic rise. AJR Am J Roentgenol 170:169–175

Postma CT, van Aalen J, de Boo T, Rosenbusch G, Thien T (1992) Doppler ultrasound scanning in the detection of renal artery stenosis in hypertensive patients. Br J Surg 65:857–860

Prince MR, Yucel K, Kaufman JA, Harrison DC, Geller SC (1993) Dynamic Gadolinium-enhanced three-dimensional abdominal MR angiography. J Magn Reson Imaging 3:877–881

Prince MR (1994) Gadolinium-enhanced MR angiography. Radiology 191:155–164

Prince MR, Narasimham DL, Stanley JC, Chenevert TL, Williams DM, Marx MV, Cho KJ (1995) Breath-hold Gadolinium-enhanced MR angiography of the abdominal aorta and its major branches. Radiology 197:785–792

Prince MR, Arnoldus C, Frazoll JK (1996) Nephrotoxicity of high dose gadolinium compared with iodinated contrast material. J Magn Reson Imaging 6:162–166

Prince MR, Chenevert TL, Foo TKF, Londy FJ, Ward JS, Maki JH (1997a) Contrast-enhanced abdominal MR angiography: optimization of imaging delay time by automating the detection of contrast material arrival in the aorta. Radiology 203:109–114

Prince MR, Schoenberg SO, Ward JS, Londy FJ, Wakefield TW, Stanley JC (1997b) Hemodynamically significant atherosclerotic renal artery stenosis: MR angiography features. Radiology 205:128–136

Prokop M, Shin HO, Schanz A, Schaefer-Prokop CM (1997) Use of maximum intensity projections in CT angiography: a basic review. Radiographics 17:433–451

Qanadli SD, Mesurolle B, Coggia M, Barre O, Fukui S, Goeau-Brissonniere O, Chagnon S, Lacombe P (2000) Abdominal aortic aneurysm: pretherapy assessment with dual-slice helical CT angiography. AJR Am J Roentgenol 174:181–187

Rieumont MJ, Kaufman JA, Geller SC, Yucel EK, Cambria RP, Fang LST, Bazari H, Waltman AC (1997) Evaluation of renal artery stenosis with dynamic Gadolinium-enhanced MR angiography. AJR Am J Roentgenol 169:99–44

Rittgers SE, Norris CS, Barnes RW (1985) Detection of renal artery stenosis: experimental and clinical analysis of velocity waveforms. Ultrasound Med Biol 11:523–531

Roobottom CA, Dubbins PA (1993) Significant disease of the celiac and superior mesenteric arteries in asymptomatic patients: predictive value of Doppler sonography. AJR Am J Roentgenol 161:985–988

Ros PR, Gauger J, Stoupis C, Burton SS, Mao J, Wilcox C, Rosenberg EB, Briggs RW (1995) Diagnosis of renal artery stenosis: feasibility of combining MR angiography, MR renography, and gadopentetate-based measurements of glomerular filtration rate. AJR Am J Roentgenol 165:1447–1451

Rubin GD (1998) 3D spiral CT angiography of the aorta and brances. In: Fishman EK, Jeffrey EK Jr (eds) Spiral CT: principles, techniques, and clinical applications, 2nd edn. Lippincott-Raven, Philadelphia, pp 361–401

Rubin GD, Shiau MC, Leung AN, Kee ST, Logan LJ, Sofilos MC (2000) Aorta and iliac arteries: single versus multiple detector-row helical CT angiography. Radiology 215:670–676

Schoenberg SO, Knopp MV, Bock M, Kallinowski F, Just A, Essig M, Hawighorst H, Zuna I, Schad L, van Kaick G (1997) Renal artery stenosis: grading of hemodynamic changes with cine phase-contrast MR blood flow measurements. Radiology 203:45–53

Schoenberg SO, Bock M, Knopp MV, Essig M, Laub G, Hawighorst H, Zuna I, Kallinowski F, van Kaick G (1999) Renal arteries. Optimization of three-dimensional Gadolinium-enhanced MR angiography with bolus-timing-independent fast multiphase acquisition in a single breathold. Radiology 211:667–679

Schwerk WB, Restrepo IK, Stellwaag M, Klose KJ, Schade -Brittinger C (1994) Renal artery stenosis: grading with image-directed Doppler US evaluation of renal resistive index. Radiology 190:785–790

Sebastia C, Pallisa E, Quiroga S, Alvarez-Castells A, Dominguez R, Evangelista A (1999) Aortic dissection: diagnosis and follow-up with helical CT. Radiographics 19:45–60

Shirkhoda A, Konez O, Shetty AN, Bis KG, Ellwood RA, Kirsch MJ (1997) Mesenteric circulation: three-dimensional MR angiography with gadolinium-enhanced multiecho gradient- echo technique. Radiology 202:257–261

Shirkhoda A, Konez O, Shetty AN, Bis KG, Ellwood RA, Kirsch MJ (1998) Contrast-enhanced MR angiography of the mesenteric circulation: a pictorial essay. Radiographics 18:851–861

Siegel CL, Cohan RH (1994) CT of abdominal aortic aneurysm. AJR Am J Roentgenol 163:17–29

Snidow JJ, Johnson MS, Harris VJ, Margosian PM, Aisen AM, Lalka SG, Cikrit DF, Trerotola SO (1996) Three-dimensional gadolinium-enhanced MR angiography for aortoiliac inflow assessment plus renal artery screening in a single breath-hold. Radiology 198:725–732

Strandness DE (1990) Duplex scanning in diagnosis of renovascular hypertension. Surg Clin North Am 70:109–117

Strandness DE Jr, Van Breda A (eds) (1994) Vascular diseases: surgical and interventional therapy. Churchill Livingstone, New York

Strotzer M, Aebert H, Lenhart M, Nitz W, Wild T, Manke C, Völk M, Feuerbach S (2000) Morphology and hemodynamics in dissection of the descending aorta: assessment with MR imaging. Acta Radiol 41:594–600

Szilagyi DE, Smith RF, DeRusso FJ, et al (1966) Contribution of abdominal aortic aneurysmectomy to prolongation of life. Ann Surg 164:678

Takaha M, Matsumoto A, Ochi K, Tekeuchi M, Takemoto M, Sonoda T (1980) Intrarenal arteriovenous malformations. J Urol 315–318

Takebayashi S, Ohno T, Tanaka K, Kubota Y, Matsubara S (1994) MR angiography of renal vascular malformations. J Comput Assist Tomogr 18:596–600

Thornton MJ, Thronton F, O´Callaghan J, Varghese JG, O'Brien E, Walshe J, Lee MJ (1999) Evaluation of dynamic gadolinium-enhanced breath-hold MR angiography in the diagnosis of renal artery stenosis. AJR Am J Roentgenol 173:1279–1283

Thurnher SA, Dorffner R, Thurnher MM, Winkelbauer FW, Kretschmer G, Polterauer P, Lammer J (1997) Evaluation of abdominal aortic aneurysm for stent-graft placement: comparison of gadolinium-enhanced MR angiography versus helical CT angiography and digital subtraction angiography. Radiology 205:341–352

Van der Hulst VPM, van Baalen J, Schultze Kool L, van Bockel JH, van Erkel AR, Ilgun J, Pattynama PMT (1996) Renal artery stenosis: endovascular flow wire study for validation of Doppler US. Radiology 200:165–168

Van Hoe L, De Jaegere T, Bosmans H, Stockx L, Vanbeckevoort D, Oyen R, Fagard R, Marchal G (2000) Breath-hold contrast-enhanced three-dimensional MR angiography of the abdomen: time-resolved imaging versus single-phase imaging. Radiology 214:149–156

Van Jaarsveld BC, Krijnen P, Pieterman H, Derkx FHM, Deinum J, Postma CT, Dees A, Woittiez AJJ, Bartelink AKM, Man in't Veld AJ, Schalekamp MADH (2000) The effect of balloon angioplasty on hypertension in atherosclerotic renal-artery disease. N Engl J Med 342:1007–1014

Walsh P, Rofsky NM, Krinsky GA, Weinreb JC (1996) Asymmetric signal intensity of the renal collecting system as a sign of unilateral renal artery stenosis following administration of gadopentate dimeglumine. J Comput Assist Tomogr 20:812–814

Wasser MN, Geelkerken RH, Kouwenhoven M, et al. (1996) Systolically gated 3D phase contrast MRA of meseneteric arteries in suspected mesenteric ischemia. J Comput Assist Tomogr 20:262–268

Wasser MN, Westenberg J, van de Hulst VPM, van Baalen J, van Bockel JH, van Erkel AR, Pattynama PMT (1997) Hemodynamic significance of renal artery stenosis: digital subtraction angiography versus systolically gated three-dimensional phase-contrast MR angiography. Radiology 202:333–338

Weishaupt D, Ruehm SG, Binkert CA, Schmidt M, Patak MA, Steybe F, McGill S, Debatin JF (2000) Equilibrium-phase MR angiography of the aortoiliac and renal arteries using a blood pool contrast agent. AJR Am J Roentgenol 175:189–195

Wiesner W, Pfammatter T, Krestin GP, Debatin JF (1998) MRI and MRA of kidney transplants – evaluation of vessels and perfusion. Fortschr Roentgenstr 169:290–296

Williams DM, Lee DY, Hamilton BH, et al (1997) The dissected aorta: percutaneous treatment of ischemic complications – principles and results. J Vasc Interv Radiol 8:605–625

Wilman AH, Riederer SJ, King BF, Debbins JP, Rossman PJ, Ehman RL (1997) Fluoroscopically triggered contrast-enhanced three-dimensional MR angiography with elliptical centric view order: application to the renal arteries. Radiology 205:137–146

Winter TC III, Freeny PC, Nghiem HV, et al (1995) Hepatic arterial anatomy in transplantation candidates: evaluation with three-dimensional CT arteriography. Radiology 195:363–370

Wright GA, Nishimura DG, Macovski A (1991) Flow- independent magnetic resonance projection angiography. Magn Reson Med 17:126–140

Yucel EK, Kaufman JA, Prince M, Bazari H, Fang LST, Waltman AC (1993) Time-of-flight MR angiography: utility in patients with renal insufficiency. Magn Reson Imaging 11:925–930

Zeman RK, Silverman PM, Berman PM, Weltman D, Davros WJ, Gomes MN (1995) Abdominal aortic aneurysms: findings on three-dimensional display of helical CT data. AJR Am J Roentgenol 164:917–922

19 Arteries of the Extremities

Matthias Boos

CONTENTS

19.1 Introduction

Although the prevalence peripheral arterial occlusive disease (PAOD) of the lower extremities is a widespread, the clinical importance of this disease is still underestimated compared with other atherosclerotic manifestations such as coronary heart disease or cerebrovascular disease. In the United States, the treatment of PAOD accounts for more than 100,000 surgical procedures annually (Rutkow and Ernst 1986; Rofsky and Adelman 2000). PAOD may cause a wide range of symptoms with substantial morbidity, including claudication, rest pain, tissue loss, and gangrene. Up until 1992, prevalence and incidence studies mostly considered only the symptomatic forms of PAOD (Dagenais et al. 1991; Fowkes 1991). Two research groups, led by Vierodt in Tübingen and Jaquet in Paris (Vierordt 1855), found an angiographically proven high percentage of oligosymptomatic patients without claudication and with well-compensated stenoses or occlusions due to an immobile lifestyle.

Thus, even before the manifestation of symptoms, PAOD can be detected by using simple clinical tests such as palpation of the pulse wave, auscultation of the arteries, and Doppler pressure measurements (Basel study III) (Da Silva and Widmer 1959–1978). The prevalence data of the Basel study I group and the incidence data have both shown that the asymptomatic form of this disease is three times more common than the symptomatic form with claudication. If both forms are taken into consideration, the incidence of PAOD is the same as coronary heart disease: 7.1% for PAOD and 6.2% for coronary heart disease in a 5-year period (Nissen et al. 1981). The easy accessibility of arteries of the extremities or the carotid bifurcation (Henerici et al. 1985) for color-coded duplexultrasonography (CCDS) makes it possible to depict systemic atherosclerosis in the asymptomatic stage. It can be assumed that patients with early-detected PAOD will be at risk of developing coronary heart disease and stroke that will presumably reduce their life expectancy by 5 years compared with individuals with healthy arteries (Barras et al. 1989). Thus, early detection of PAOD is extremely important in this target group in order to prevent severe complications of atherosclerotic disease. The occurrence of PAOD is three times higher in men than in women. In symptomatic patients claudication has been proven to be three times more common in smokers and six times more common in heavy smokers. PAOD is found in 25% of patients suffering from arterial hypertension compared with 8% of the control group. A further correlation can be seen between hyperlipidemia (high-density lipoproteins) and PAOD. PAOD is often associated with diabetic disease, causing the most nontraumatic lower extremity amputations in the industrialized world. In total, 40% of diabetics suffer from advanced ischemic states compared with only 18% of subjects without diabetes. The risk of lower extremity amputation is 15–46 times higher in diabetic patients than in nondiabetics (Armstrong and Lavery 1998).

M. Boos, M.D.
IRN - Institute of Radiology and Nuclear Medicine Ltd., Krankenhausstrasse 70, 85276 Pfaffenhofen, Germany

In symptomatic PAOD, information about the number, length, and severity of vascular lesions is essential when a revascularization procedure is planned. Invasive conventional angiography with the use of iodinated contrast material is accepted as the gold standard in this regard. However, the diagnostic problem in PAOD is not only the precise grading of stenotic disease, but also the overall evaluation of various additional parameters, such as the residual vessel diameter at different vessel localizations, the run-off conditions, and the clinical symptoms, including the results of basic examinations such as ankle-brachial pressure index, walking distance, and oscillography. When the conclusive diagnosis has been made, suitable therapeutic procedures can be planned.

As a true noninvasive alternative to conventional angiography and a method which shows a variety of advantages over CCDS (Widmer et al. 1994), peripheral magnetic resonance angiography (pMRA) now is playing an increasing role in the detection and evaluation of PAOD. Since the introduction of MRA in 1986 by Wedeen et al., angiographic MR imaging of the peripheral vessels has been focussed on the diagnostic evaluation of specific regions of the extremities (Wedeen et al. 1986). Although time-of-flight (TOF) and phase contrast (PC) MRA techniques provided relatively high sensitivities and specificities in the detection and grading of stenoses responsible for PAOD (Edelman 1992), the clinical use of these flow-sensitive MR angiographic methods in the visualization of the entire vascular system of the lower extremities was restricted due to long investigation times, a small field of view (FOV), and several artifacts caused by motion, dephasing phenomena, and in-plane saturation. Since the successful introduction of contrast-enhanced MR angiography (CE MRA) in 1994 by Prince, the problems associated with flow-sensitive methods on the basis of TOF and PC techniques have been overcome. In addition, many studies have shown that the arterial system from the aorta down to the lower legs can be visualized by CE MRA with a satisfactory diagnostic quality (Prince 1994). If contrast-enhanced peripheral MRA (CE pMRA) is to become a true alternative to conventional angiography (including the purpose of replacing this invasive technique), the display of various vessel diameters ranging from 10 mm to less than 1 mm on a diagnostic confidential angiogram must also be possible on pMRA images to allow a decision on the most effective therapy for PAOD patients to be made. In the case of long occlusions or high-grade stenosis, the entire collateral system has to be visualized by CE pMRA (Fig. 19.1). During the past 3 years, CE pMRA has received increasing attention due to the development of improved examination protocols using faster sequence techniques and dedicated peripheral coils (Rofsky and Adelman 2000). Thus, CE pMRA has become a fast technique that is safe and easy to use, and whose image impression is comparable to that of intra-arterial digital subtraction angiography (i.a. DSA).

19.2 Peripheral MR Angiography: Technical Considerations

19.2.1 3D/2D TOF MRA

TOF methods are principally able to display peripheral arteries on the basis of the inflow effect. However, over longer distances the flow-sensitive signal will be saturated within the acquired volume or section. When a 3D TOF technique is used, only small volumes can be acquired in the craniocaudal direction to avoid saturation effects of the spins. This results in extensive scan times for peripheral arteries, making this technique unfeasible for the visualization of the entire peripheral vasculature. In comparison with the 3D technique, the sequential 2D technique with transverse slice acquisition is more useful in visualizing slow flow and acquiring data over a long vessel segment without saturation effects (Vosshenrich et al. 1998; Reimer et al. 1998). Although several study groups used the 2D TOF technique to establish MR angiograms of the peripheral vascular system, disadvantages became obvious such as signal voids due to diastolic back flow, and low background suppression and saturation effects due to in-plane flow in the case of curved vessels that may mimic stenotic disease. The larger voxel size (2D slices are relatively thick compared with the effective slice thickness of 3D volumes) combined with a longer echo time (TE) results in an increased intravoxel phase dispersion. One of the main drawbacks of the 2D TOF technique is the long scan time of about 40–60 min needed for an axial acquisition of the complete arterial system of the pelvic and lower extremity region. Saturation effects due to retrograde flow may be overcome with ECG gating, but the examination time is extended (Vosshenrich et al. 1998; Reimer et al. 1998).

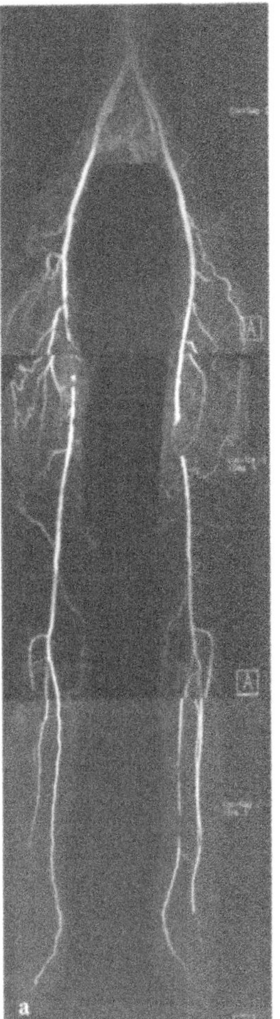

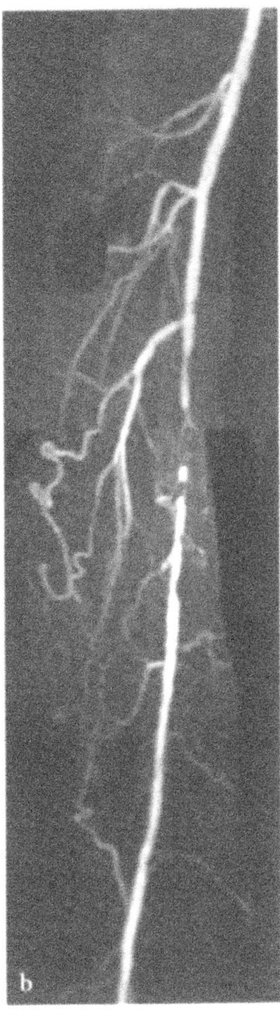

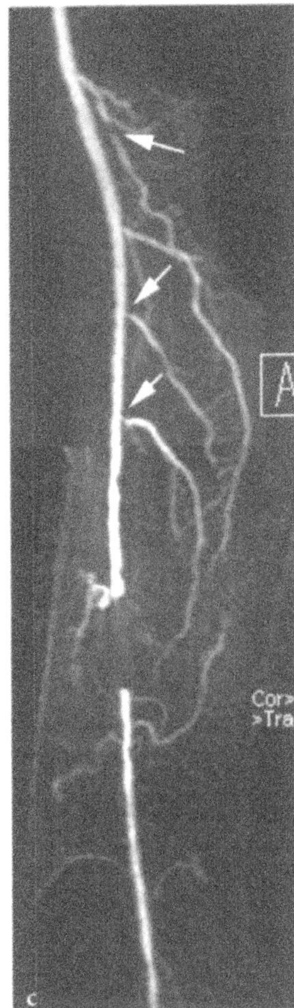

Fig. 19.1. 3D CE MRA (panoramic table hybrid technique; **a**) of a patient suffering from claudication and rest pain (Fontaine stadium II; **b**). It is very important to also visualize the details of the collateral system in the case of these 4-cm-long occlusions at both sides of the femoral artery. The collateral system at left side (**c**) is not sufficient for blood supply to the tibial region due to multiple stenoses (*arrows*) of the deep femoral branches (normal variant without common deep femoral branches) as compared to the left side with more sufficient collateralization (**b**)

19.2.2
3D/2D PC MRA

The movement of transverse magnetization in the direction of a magnetic field gradient results in phase shifts which can be encoded as a signal intensity difference when compared to those in stationary tissue. This phase shift is directly proportional to the flow velocity and can be displayed in an angiographic image. A thick slab is typically acquired with 2D PC MRA and displayed as a projection image, while 3D PC MRA offers the option of displaying the data set from different viewing angles. Due to scan times of more than 15 min when 3D PC MRA is used for visualization of a FOV of up to 450 mm, this technique is not feasible for clinical use in PAOD (Prince 1998). To achieve fast overviews of the peripheral vasculature, 2D PC MRA can be used as an alternative (Fig. 19.2). The 2D acquisition slabs are thus comparable to projections achieved with i.a. DSA. Compared with sequential inflow MRA, this technique is more time efficient (Boos et al. 1997; Reimer et al. 1997), and saturation effects do not affect the vessel contrast of PC MRA images. With phase contrast techniques a coronal position of the slab is possible, resulting in a larger FOV than in TOF MRA (Jones et al. 1998; Steinberg et al. 1990). However, there are major disadvantages: a velocity-encoding (VENC) parameter has to be prospectively selected for the acquisition; artifacts occur from pulsatile flow, breathing, and peristalsis; and the highly anisotropic image voxel of this projection technique results in destructive phase interference in the case of overlapping vessels, sometimes mimicking stenosis or occlusion (Fig. 19.2).

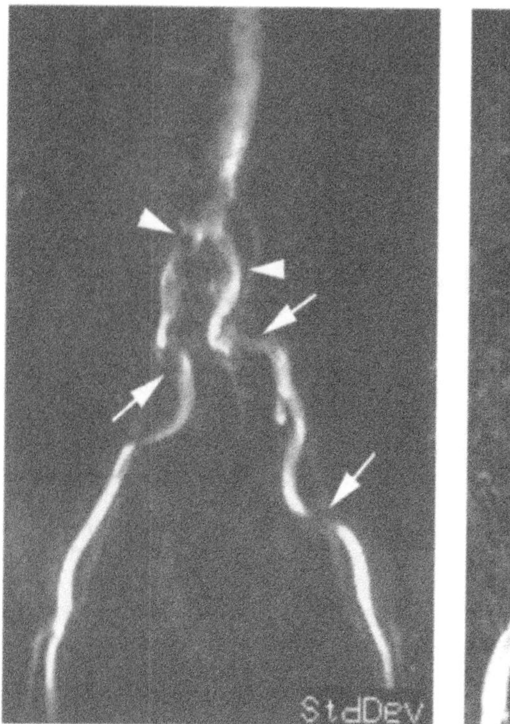

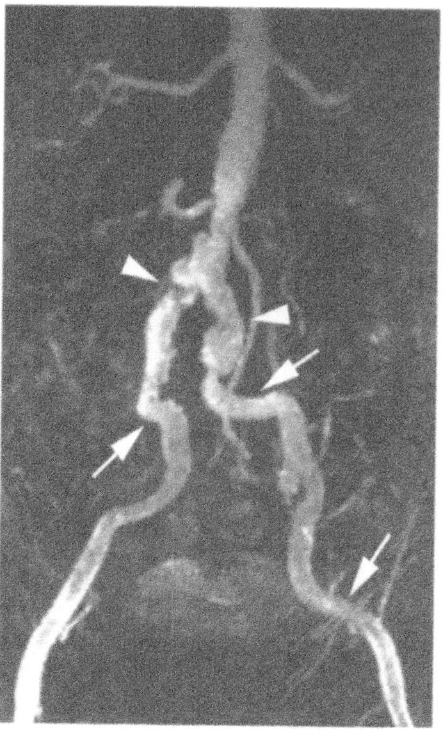

Fig. 19.2. 2D PC (**a**) and 3D CE (**b**) MRA of a patient with ulcerated stenoses of the distal abdominal aorta and the left common iliac artery. The stenoses were overestimated on the PC MRA image (*arrowheads*). In addition, the PC MRA image shows flow voids due to overlaying signals from the iliac artery and vein (*large arrows*) simulating stenoses. However, the CE MRA image shows luminal contrast-enhanced signals demonstrating no stenoses in these locations

19.2.3 Contrast-Enhanced Peripheral MR Angiography

19.2.3.1 General Considerations

With the hardware improvements and sequence optimizations that have been made during the last 2–3 years in the field of CE pMRA, this technique now plays the dominant role in MR imaging of the arteries of the extremities. The CE MRA technique is based on shortening the T1-relaxation time of blood by injecting a paramagnetic contrast medium (CM). This results in large signal intensity differences between the background and vessels on images acquired with heavily T1-weighted sequences. The acquired 3D data set contains high signal intensity voxels ideally corresponding to arteries and can be postprocessed using the maximum intensity projection (MIP) algorithm to achieve different projections of the vascular tree. In addition, multiplanar reformation (MPR) programs allow the evaluation of the cross-sectional vessel areas. As with PC MRA, CE MRA is not affected by saturation effects due to inflowing spins. Therefore, the acquisition of a 3D slab in the coronal plane is one of the main advantages of this method (Vogl et al. 1994; Maki et al. 1998). For the diagnosis of PAOD an optimal image quality is required: the technology should offer a maximum of image resolution, and vessels up to 120 cm in length should be displayed clearly and rapidly to cover the peripheral arterial system. CE pMRA seems to be able to fulfill these demands during an acceptable examination time, and therefore offers an alternative which is superior to previously implemented flow-sensitive MR angiographic techniques (Fig. 19.3).

Different attempts have been discussed concerning the selection of the coil for visualizing of the entire pelvic and lower leg vascular region (Rodenwaldt et al. 2000; Hadley et al. 2000; Vosshenrich et al. 1997). In principal, CE pMRA can be performed with the standard body coil (SBC) with which a FOV of approximately 450 mm can be applied in head-feet extension (Fig. 19.4). The investigation profits from the use of a 512 matrix size (Fig. 19.5) and from surface coils, such as the body phased-array coil, due to

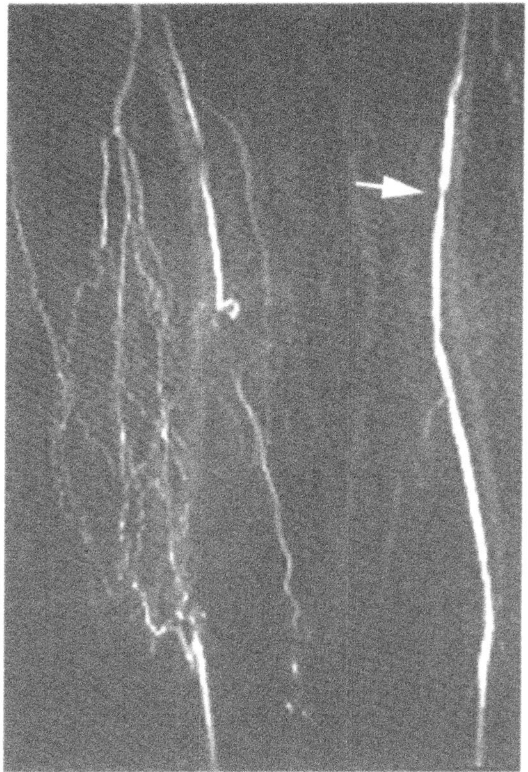

a

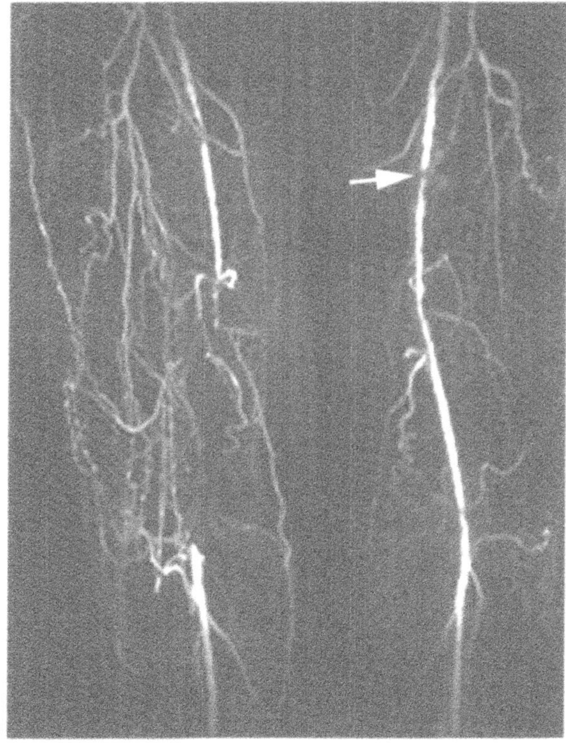

b

Fig. 19.3. The 10-cm-long occlusion of the well-collateralized right SFA is similarly demonstrated by both the 2D PC MRA (**a**) and the 3D CE MRA (**b**) method. However, the collateral branching from the deep femoral artery is visualized much better by CE MRA than PC MRA. Sometimes the grade of stenosis can be overestimated by using CE MRA technique. Note that the PC MRA image shows only a 50% stenosis, whereas a high-grade stenosis (>90%) was detected on the CE MRA

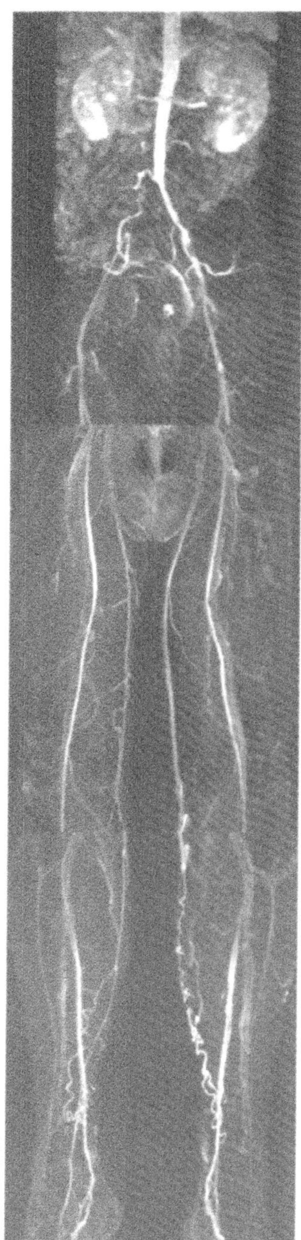

Fig. 19.4. A patient with a complete occlusion of the common iliac artery at the right side (well collateralized) and a 70% stenosis of the proximal external iliac artery at the left side. No stenosis at the femoropopliteal arteries. The calf arteries are not sufficiently assessable due to overlay of venous structures [constant CM infusion technique (0.5 ml/s) and panoramic table technique (3-step; standard body coil) was used]

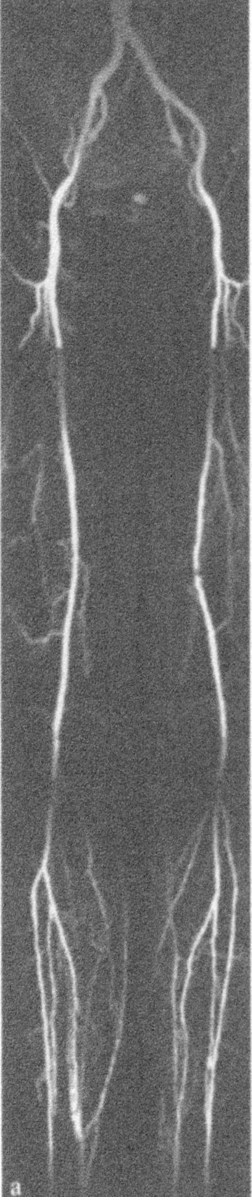

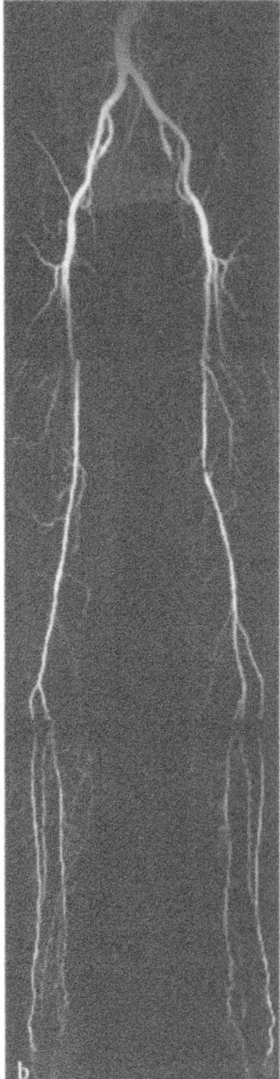

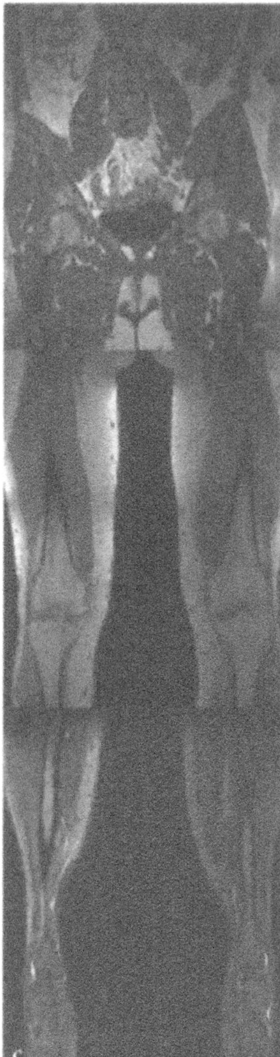

Fig. 19.5. Comparison of the multi/separate bolus injection technique using body phased-array coils (256×196 matrix, FOV=370 mm) for all three stations (**a**) and body phased-array coil combined with the dedicated pMRA coil (512×392 matrix, FOV=400 mm; **b**). The proximal stenosis of the left dorsal pedal artery was only detected by using pMRA coil images due to larger FOV. However, it is also important to give the clinician anatomical landmarks by presenting a selection from the 3D data set (**c**)

an improved signal-to-noise ration (SNR; Fig. 19.6), but simultaneously the FOV decreases to approximately 350–400 mm. The lower SNR of the SBC can theoretically be improved by using a higher CM concentration. In addition, the use of specially designed peripheral vascular phased-array coils can improve the SNR such that a lower concentration of gadolinium (Gd) within the arteries achieves identical vessel contrast (Fig. 19.6).

19.2.3.2 Examination Protocols

In contrast to MR angiography of the abdominal arteries, longer acquisition times are possible in CE pMRA due to fewer or no breathing movement artifacts. Measurement time limits are only expected only in the most peripherally localized vessels due to a faster arteriovenous transit time, which may result in the overlay of the vascular signal from enhanced veins producing poorer arterial image quality. A breath-hold CE MRA measurement of the iliac arteries is not absolutely necessary. Usually, in diagnosis of PAOD, CE pMRA protocols should include the aortic bifurcation, iliac arteries, and the arteries of the extremities. On the other hand, the visualization of renal arteries in peripheral angiography is still standard clinical practice when conventional techniques are used to exclude renal artery stenosis in hypertensive patients with PAOD or to depict progressive atherosclerotic renal occlusive disease with the potential risk of kidney loss which can be prevented by endovascular or surgical therapy. Thus, in hypertensive patients the routine evaluation of the entire abdominal aorta should be included in the CE pMRA protocol using either the multi-station evaluation with bolus chase technique or the dynamic table movement technique. However, if renal arteries are

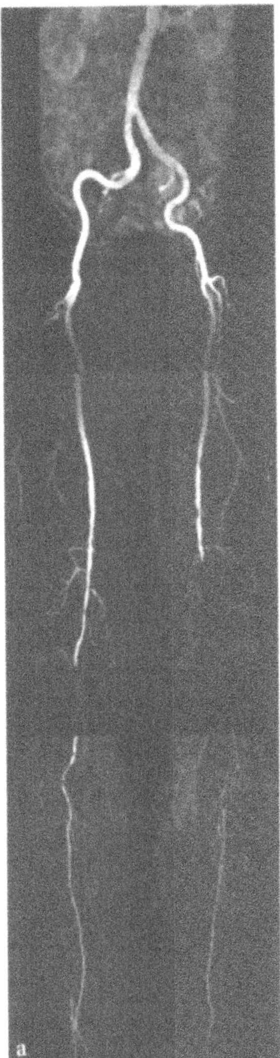

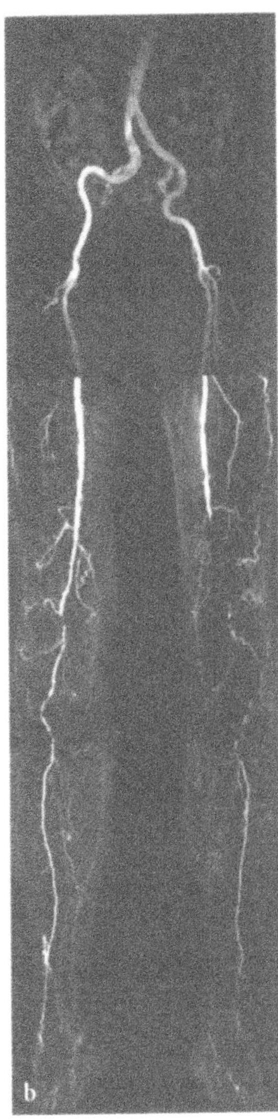

Fig. 19.6. Comparison of a 3D CE pMRA using body phased-array coils for all three stations (**a**) and a body phased-array coil combined with the dedicated pMRA coil (**b**). The pMRA coil provides larger FOVs and a more homogenous SNR, especially at the edges of the FOV. In addition, due to the special design of the pMRA coil, the proximal feet vessels can also be visualized. Findings: High-grade stenosis of the right popliteal artery, long and complete occlusion of the left popliteal artery (moderate collateralized via deep branches) and poor one vessel run-off on both sides

included in the aortoiliac evaluation of patients with PAOD, three consecutive 3D data sets have to be acquired using a FOV larger than 40 cm, a standard body coil, and a breath-hold imaging technique with short acquisition times. A drawback of this procedure is that it may reduce spatial resolution in the abdominal region. If a high-resolution CE MRA image of the renal arteries is desired, a separate CM bolus should be used with a smaller FOV or a phased-array coil to achieve better resolution than a comprehensive study (Rofsky and Adelman 2000).

19.2.3.2.1
Sequence Parameters

The vessel scout protocol for preparation of the 3D data set is based on a 2D TOF sequence. Vessels can be identified as points of high signal intensity due to inflow enhancement. Alternatively, a 2D PC MRA protocol can be used. The sequence parameters have to be determined in order to cover the entire vessel region of interest with respect to the clinical requirement. To increase spatial resolution, more phase-encoding steps are needed, hence a longer acquisition time and a weaker SNR. The best resolution is imperative for stenosis grading.

Although in principle acquisition times as short as possible should be used with current equipment, this may lower the spatial resolution in the slice select direction because there are fewer partitions. Slice interpolated sequences do not really overcome this problem, because the calculated resolution cannot be considered as real spatial resolution. However, considering the sequence parameters, it does not make sense to define high resolution if the bolus is not large enough to cover the high frequency k-lines at the outer k-space which define the resolution of the image (see Chap. 6). Therefore, the bolus geometry has to correspond to predefined parameters in order to optimize the vessel contrast (Maki et al. 1998; Boos et al. 1998; Prince et al. 1997). Thick 3D volumes (approximately 100–120 mm) in coronal orientation are mandatory to cover the complete internal iliac region as well as the common femoral region (Fig. 19.7). The partition thickness must be reduced to at least 1.5 mm. In our experience, an isotropic resolution of 1.5 mm is sufficient to estimate reliably the therapeutically relevant grade of iliac artery stenosis.

19.2.3.2.2
Imaging Philosophies

At present there is no standardized examination strategy for imaging the arterial system of the lower extremities on the basis of CE pMRA. In principle, one can differentiate between a multi-station technique and a dynamic technique which is based on a stepwise movement of the table on which the patient is placed. For CE pMRA, a large FOV of up to 120 cm or more is necessary to perform a run-off study. This requires three steps, as the FOV is restricted to approximately 45 cm by the homogeneity of the magnet. Thus, three separate acquisitions of 3D data sets have to be repeated in different patient positions.

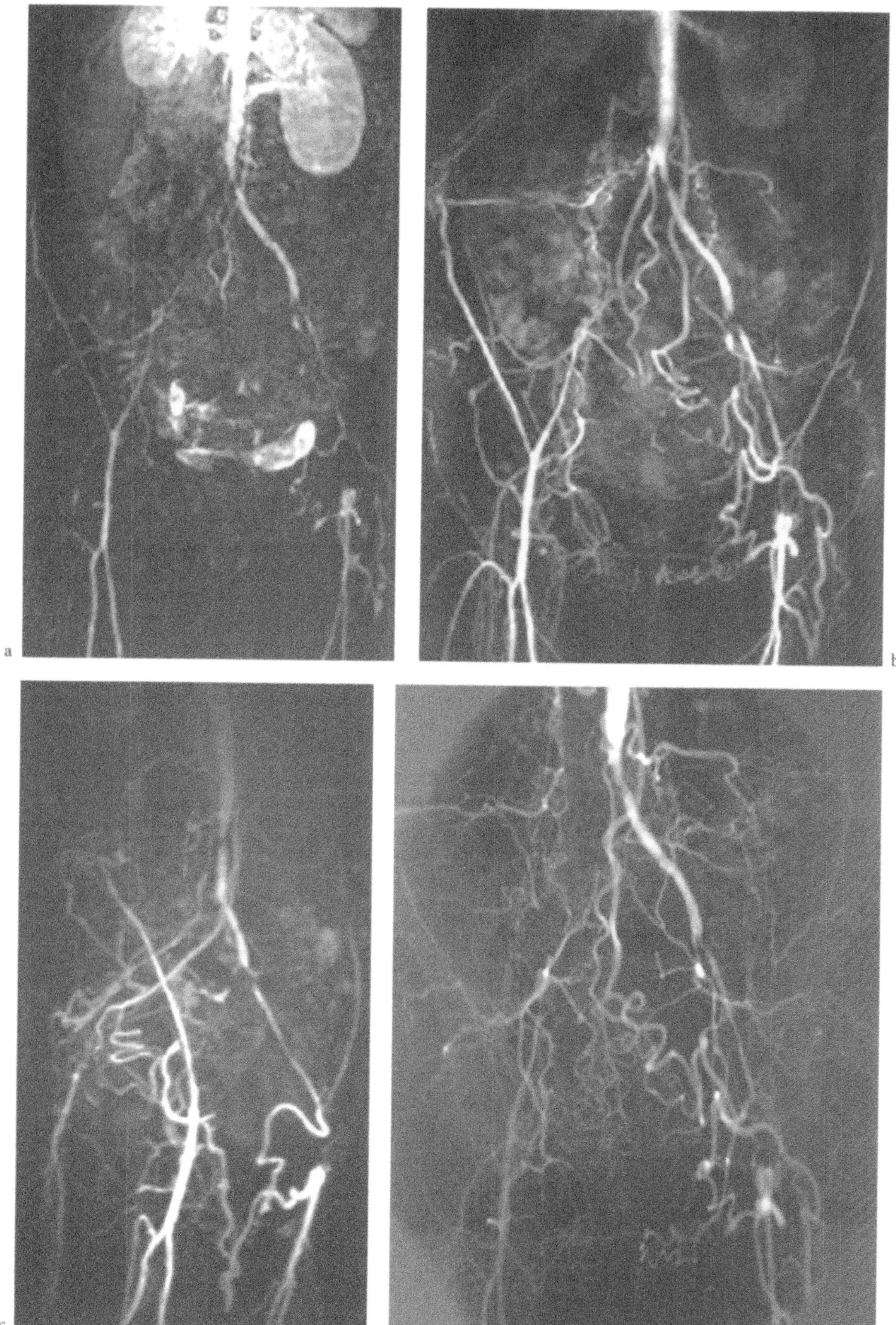
a
b
c
d

Multi-station Technique. In the multi-station technique approach the coil position has to be changed twice (iliofemoral, popliteocrural) or three times (aortoiliac, femoropopliteal, cruropedal) in order to acquire the entire peripheral arterial system (Fig. 19.8). Commonly, the iliac region is examined first; otherwise, disturbance of the overlay by the filled bladder and other contrast material (CM)-enhancing structures may be expected. However, it is also possible to cut the enhanced structure of the bladder after scanning by using predetermined postprocessing methods. Alternatively, the lower legs can be examined first, avoiding enhancement from the veins. A significant improvement of the vessel contrast can be achieved by the application of a fat-saturation and subtraction technique (Leung et al. 1998). In addition, a nonenhanced 3D data set has to be acquired before the Gd-enhanced study which is subtracted from the CE 3D data set (Fig. 19.9).

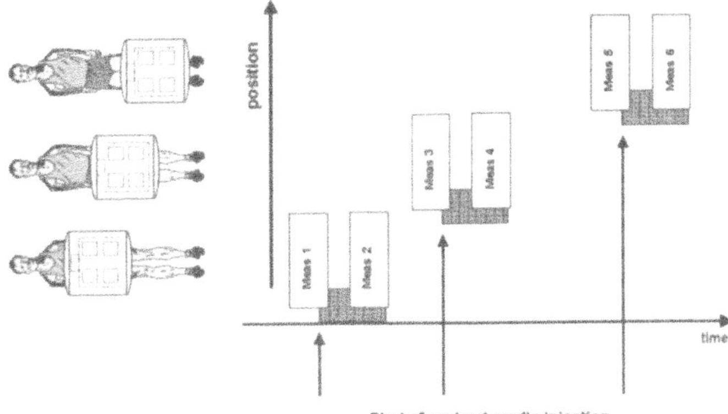

Fig. 19.8. Multi-station pMRA technique (without table movement). All three stations were measured separately applying single-dose Gd three times. The native scan is performed immediately before the enhanced scan. The bolus time can be evaluated only once (e.g., at the common femoral artery). For the femoral and calf region, 5 s and 10 s, respectively, have to be added to the BAT of the pelvic region

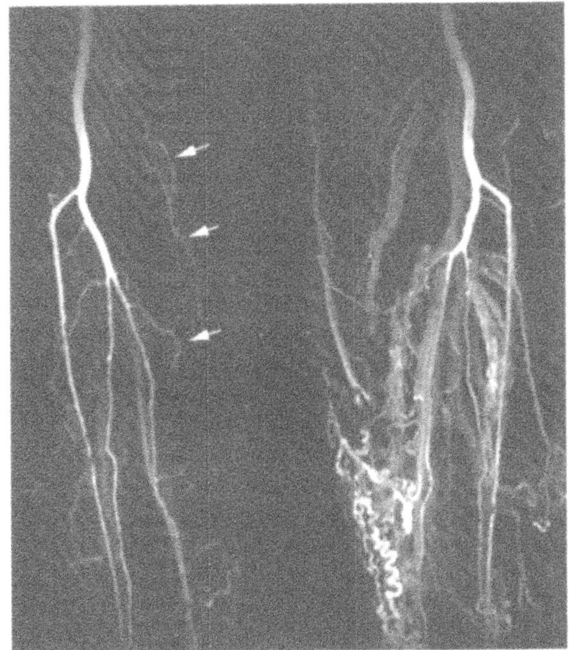
a

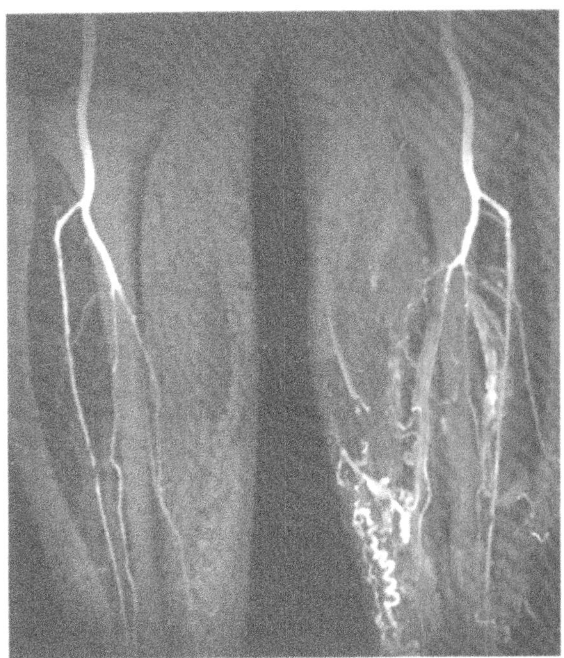
b

Fig. 19.9. This example of a patient with arteriovenous malformation at the left calf shows that the background suppression is improved for digital subtraction (DS) MIP (**a**) as compared to the MIP reconstructed on the basis of the nonsubtracted CE MRA data set (**b**). Therefore, more details are visualized by DS CE MRA (*arrows*) which cannot be detected on the nonsubtracted

Fig. 19.7. A 78-year-old woman with iliac occlusions at both sites demonstrated also by the "conventional" 3D CE MRA (single dose of CM, 80 mm coronal slab; **a**). However, the thick slab and high-resolution CE MRA (**b**, coronal MIP; **c**, –60° MIP) visualize all details of the extensive collateral system (branches of internal iliac and also of inferior mesenteric arteries). Identical findings were demonstrated by i.a. DSA (**d**), but only providing 2D information

The acquisition time in the multi-station technique can be readily prolonged allowing the application of a smaller voxel size with an improved spatial resolution. The diameter of the three main arteries of the lower leg range between 1 and 3 mm. Therefore, the voxel dimensions in all three directions should be adjusted to 1.0–1.5 mm (Fig. 19.10). To achieve a sufficient SNR, the use of a body phased-array or a dedicated peripheral vascular coil is required (Fig. 19.6). High-resolution images with a high SNR of the crural and pedal arteries can be acquired by an additional second separate investigation, applying a second Gd injection of at least 0.2 mmol/kg body weight. Obviously, more details such as collateral circulation and digital vessels can be visualized by using a 512 matrix size and a double dose of CM. The disadvantages of this technique are the increase of acquired data, resulting in longer image calculation times, and the higher CM doses required. Therefore, the decision between low- and high-resolution CE pMRA must be made with respect to the clinical question.

Dynamic Table Movement Technique. The purpose of the dynamic table movement technique (i.e., panoramic table technique, step-by-step technique, stepping-table technique, moving-bed technique) is to allow several measurements at different patient table positions with automatic table movement using a single contrast injection or infusion. The basic idea of the table movement technique is shown in Fig. 19.11. Two or three 3D data set acquisitions are performed without image reconstruction in between the measurements. After measurement of the first vascular region, the patient table moves a certain distance in order to allow the acquisition of the next vascular region exactly at the same location relative to the magnet's isocenter. After the second measurement the patient table moves again, and the third vascular region of the patient is scanned. When the last measurement has been finished, the patient table moves back to its original position.

Because CE pMRA studies are performed typically by subtraction technique, all the required measurements are performed twice, with and without CM injection. Due to the minimal delay between the acquisition of pre-contrast and contrast-enhanced images, gross patient motion artifacts are minimized. When the equipment does not offer automatic table movement, a surface coil combination can be used. Under these limited conditions it is possible to move the table manually. Another limitation may be the lower random access memory of the image reconstruction computer.

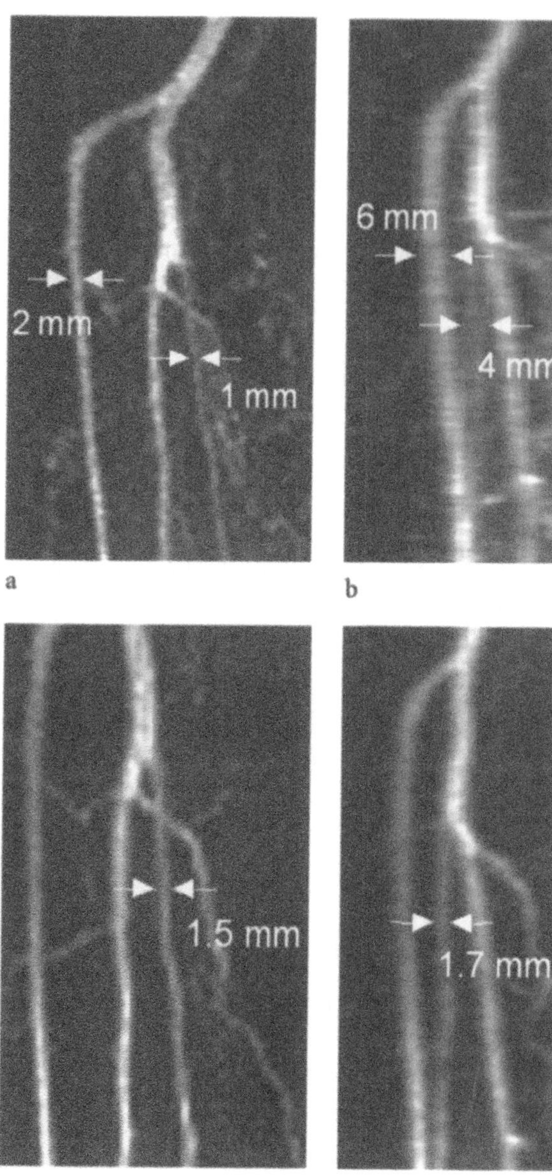

Fig. 19.10. This patient was investigated twice, first using the dynamic table movement technique (**a** and **b**) 512×396 matrix size and 3 mm interpolated partition, and, secondly, using the multi-station technique with separate CM injection, (**c** and **d**) 256×196 matrix size but 1.5-mm partition thickness) were performed. All figures are zoomed clippings of the 3D CE MRA MIP in coronal view and 60° projection to sagittal view. Note that the in-plane spatial resolution is quite similar (compare **a** with **c**; insignificant advantages of panoramic table technique), but on the 60° projection images the vessels appear less sharply delineated and are three times larger than the multi-station technique using thinner partitions (compare **b** with **d**)

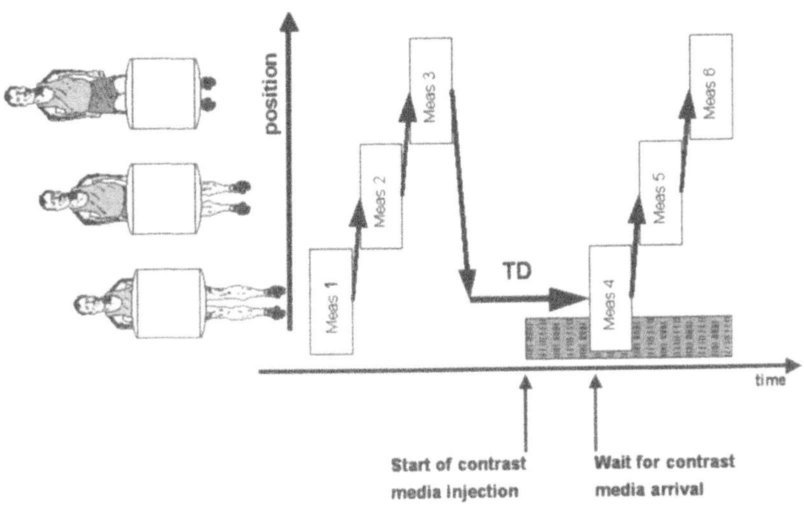

Fig. 19.11. Table moving procedure for dynamic table movement technique (panoramic table technique) using standard body coil and a continuous CM injection protocol. All native 3D CE MRA scans are performed first. After (bolus timing and) CM injection the enhanced scans are acquired. The table can be moved through the body coil without changing the patient's position

Table 19.1. Sequence parameter (example) of the multi-station and the dynamic table movement technique

Number of step		TR	TE	FA	k-space ro	FOV	FOVph	No part/th	Matrix size	Voxel dim.
	Multi-station technique									
2	Iliac arteries	3.85	1.5	25	asym (33%)	450	75%	56/1.5	256/512×192	1.6×1.0×1.5
3	Femoral arteries	3.85	1.5	25	asym (33%)	450	75%	56/1.5	256/512×192	1.6×1.0×1.5
1	Tibial arteries	4.57	1.95	25	asym (33%)	450	75%	72/1.0	512×268	1.3×0.9×1.0
	Dynamic table movement start by using care bolus									
1	Iliac arteries	4.45	1.74	25	asym (33%)	450	75%	64/1.5	512×192	1.8×0.9×1.5
2	Femoropopliteal arteries	4.47	1.74	25	centric	450	75%	56/1.4	512×211	1.6×0.9×1.4
3	Calf arteries	4.63	1.77	25	centric	450	68.8%	56/1.2	512×246	1.3×0.9×1.2
	Panoramic table hybrid start by using BAT evaluation									
1	Calf arteries (selective measure) go on using care bolus	4.63	1.77	25	centric	450	75%	72/1.0	512×268	1.3×0.9×1.0
2	Iliac arteries	4.45	1.74	25	asym (33%)	450	75%	64/1.5	512×192	1.8×0.9×1.5
3	Iliac arteries	4.47	1.74	25	centric	450	75%	56/1.4	512×211	1.6×0.9×1.4

k-space ro, k-space reordering; FOV, field of view; FOVph, FOV in phase encoding direction; No part/th, number of partition/slice thickness; Voxel dim., voxel dimension.

In Table 19.1, representative sequence parameters are recommended that have been shown to be useful for the acquisition of both multi-station and dynamic table movement pMRA.

19.2.3.3
Administration of Contrast Material in CE pMRA

It should be kept in mind that paramagnetic Gd chelates used as the CM in MR angiographic studies can be administered intravenously without the nephrotoxic effects and other adverse reactions that are known from X-ray CM (Prince et al. 1996; Haustein et al. 1992; Nelson et al. 1995). Thus, these substances have a variety of advantages compared with iodinated agents used in conventional angiography and computed tomographic angiography.

In order to optimize MR angiographic results in patients with PAOD (Prince et al. 1997; Westenberg et al. 1999), imaging protocols are of importance, including sequence designs and techniques of CM administration as well as clinical information on the patient's condition. Concerning the CM administration, several infusion schemes have been developed and used in clinical studies. As T1-shortening of the arterial blood during the first pass of the CM depends on its concentration, the aim of the CM administration is to obtain the highest concentration in the arteries during the acquisition of the central part of k-space (see Chap. 6). The CM bolus geometry depends on several parameters such as flow rate, CM dose, saline flush volume, and additionally on cardiac output, blood flow characteristics, and blood volume. The following criteria should be considered in order to optimize vessel contrast:

- ↓ Flow rate (<1 to 0.5 ml/s) → bolus length ↑ (vessel contrast ↓) (Fig. 19.13)
- ↑ Saline flush volume → bolus length ↑ (no change of vessel contrast)
- ↑ CM dosage → bolus length ↑ (vessel contrast ↑)

Our own study results demonstrated that the vascular contrast benefits from increasing flow up to 2–3 ml/s. Faster injections mainly shorten the bolus without having an effect on the resulting contrast. Enlarging the saline flush volume evidently caused a lengthening of the bolus through wash-out effects of the brachial and subclavian vein after cubital injection. Physiologically the CM bolus is diluted by the passage through the heart and lungs, the distribution of blood into proximal vessel branches, and the diffusion into interstitial tissue. Central CM bolus dilution effects are identical for all peripheral vessels (Maki et al. 1998; Boos et al. 1998; Prince 1998). The concentration and length of the CM bolus is influenced by the number of branching vessels, blood flow velocity, and the caliber of proximal vessels at the targeted peripheral vessel region. Additionally, lesions in proximal vessels may have a negative effect on the CM bolus.

The assessment of the bolus arrival time (BAT) has been shown to be an important parameter for receiving high-quality angiograms of the peripheral vasculature (Maki et al. 1996, 1998; Boos et al. 1998; Prince et al. 1999).

19.2.3.3.1
Timing of the Contrast Bolus

The determination of CM BAT within the region of interest can be achieved either automatically by using a continuous fast 2D sequence or by the test-bolus technique.

In order to visualize all the peripheral vessels, including the iliac, femoropopliteal, crural, and pedal arteries, the determination of the BAT is recommended in the region of the common femoral artery (CFA). The determination of the BAT in the distal vessel regions has the advantage that even in the case of iliac occlusions or an extremely slow run-off a satisfactory distribution of the CM may occur in small arterial branches and collateral vessels within the entire FOV before the contrast-relevant low-frequency k-lines are acquired (Fig. 19.7). For bolus timing in the femoropopliteal and lower leg region, 5 and 10 s, respectively, should be added to the BAT value determined in the region of the CFA in order to avoid having to perform a second test bolus for this region. Following a CM dose of 2 ml (0.5 mmol Gd/ml) for the test bolus, a saline flush of 30 ml applied at the identical injection rate (IR) should be performed for the CE angiographic 3D data acquisition (Boos et al. 1998). By means of a test bolus and a timing scan, the scan time and the first pass of the CM through the region of interest (ROI) being investigated can be coordinated.

As an alternative to the test-bolus technique, the CM BAT in the distal abdominal aorta can be automatically determined using the care bolus or smart prep technique simultaneously at the start of the 3D MR angiography by continuous 2D scan in a particular vessel region (Foo et al. 1997; Ho and Foo 1998). In particular, this may be necessary in cases of occluded femoropopliteal arteries (Fig. 19.12). The application of a time-resolved MR angiographic sequence as another alternative seems to be useful in determining CM dynamics in vascular areas which are limited (i.e., run-off vessels in the lower leg region), as with this technique a significantly lower resolution is observed.

19.2.3.3.2
Separate CM Injection in the Multi-station Technique

When using the multi-station technique, repeated separate CM injections are sufficient. The CM has to be administered at a relatively higher injection rate of 1–2 ml/s in order to achieve an optimal first pass enhancement for all three stations (Boos et al. 1998; Westenberg et al. 1999). Alternatively, it is possible to use a continuous CM injection for each of the three stations if all three stations were imaged in a continuous way (Boos et al. 1998; Janka et al. 1999 Vosshenrich et al. 1998; Ho 1999; Lenhart et al. 1999). Thus, for distal run-off vessels the acquisition of a separate 3D data set has been shown to be useful, administering at least 0.1–0.2 mmol/kg of Gd when a spatial resolution of 1.0+1.0+1.0 mm^3 voxel size is required.

The more peripherally arteries are localized, the more the CM bolus will be diluted (spread of the bolus). Therefore, preliminary results suggest varying the injection rate (IR) in relation to a bolus dilution factor of the CM (Fig. 19.13). This dilution factor depends on the passage of flowing blood into the

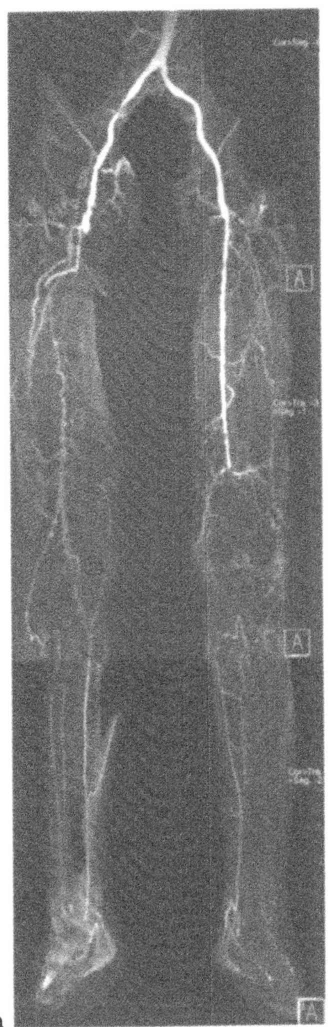

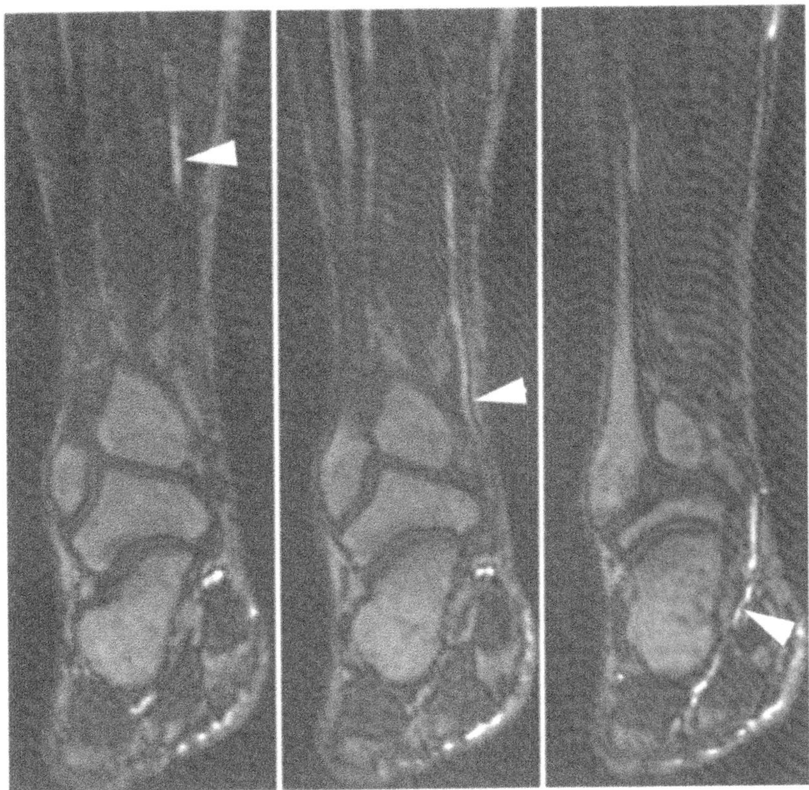

a b

Fig. 19.12. This patient has a severe PAOD with long femoropopliteal occlusion on the right and a complete popliteal occlusion on the left side (**a**). Due to the lack of popliteal arteries, a sufficient timing at this location was impossible, therefore the dynamic table movement technique using pMRA coils was performed, although the stage of Fontaine IV indicated the use of the panoramic table hybrid technique with separate CM injection at the lower leg region. When venous overlay occurrs, sometimes the source images help to identify distal parts of the posterior tibial artery at the right side, which can be used for a bypass approach (**b**, *arrowheads*)

more peripheral vessel region.

19.2.3.3.3
CM Injection in the Dynamic Table Movement Technique

When the dynamic table movement technique is used, the contrast agent can be injected by a constant infusion procedure to maintain high signal intensity in all vessels throughout the entire study (Figs. 19.1, 19.4 and 19.13). After injection in the cubital vein, the CM circulates several times through the body. Only 20% of the CM dose will arrive in the peripheral arteries during the first pass. The remaining CM volume flows through the head (20%), the heart (20%), the intestine (20%), and the kidneys (20%). A certain part of this CM will re-appear in the arteries after a secondary vein/lung passage. In the case of a constant infusion technique, this secondarily appearing CM will add to the primary concentration of CM and increase the signal intensity of the arteries. As a result, the later steps of dynamic table movement MR angiography may show a higher arterial signal than the first step during constant infusion.

In cases with significantly delayed blood flow due to proximal occlusive disease, the BAT should be either recalculated by using a second test bolus in the region of the popliteal artery or prolonged by more than the 5 s usually selected in the pelvic region. If there is a significant unilateral blood flow delay in the lower leg arteries, it may be useful to acquire the calf region twice in succession as part of the three-step table movement CE pMRA. This effect can be reduced when a biphasic injection scheme is used with different injection rates during the examination. Initially, a higher injection rate produces a high contrast during the first acquisition, whereas in the delayed second phase the injection rate of the CM

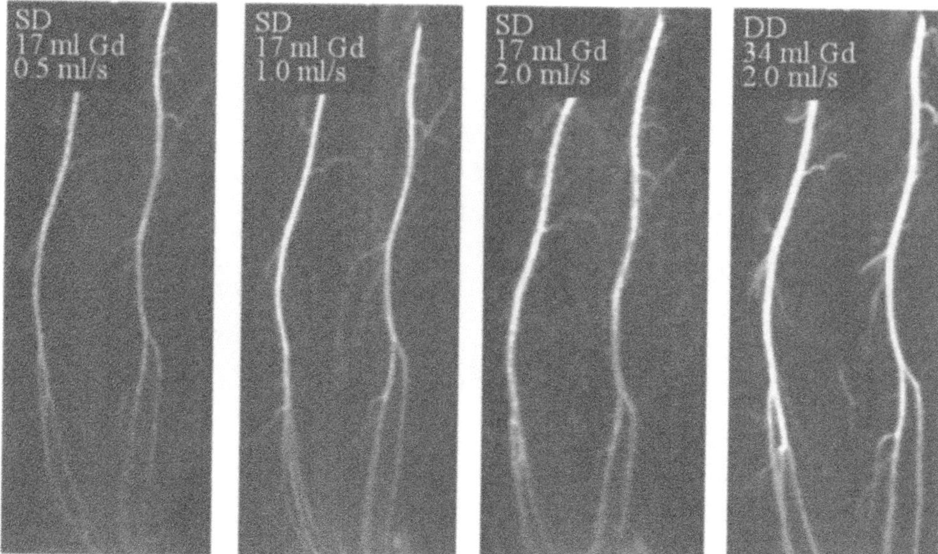

Fig. 19.13. High resolution (1 mm³ voxel size) CE MRA of the calf arteries of a normal volunteer using different injection rates (IR=0.5, 1.0 and 2.0 ml/s) and applying a single-dose (SD) CM volume (*first three images from the left*). The vessel edges are depicted much sharper using lower flow rates but with lower SNR. This can be compensated using a higher Gd volume (double dose, IR=2.0 ml/s) which results in better delineation of the vessels and benefits also from a higher SNR (*right image*)

administration can be reduced to a value which keeps the CM concentration at the initial level (Janka et al. 1999; Ho 1999; Lenhart et al. 1999; Amanuma et al. 1999; Hayashi 1999; Wang et al. 1998) utilizing the second contrast peak that results from the venous return of the renal and splanchnic vessel region (Fig. 19.1).

CM injection schemes in dynamic table movement techniques (bolus chase technique) are demonstrated in Table 19.2.

Via a tube filled with 10 ml of saline, 10 ml of Gd are primarily administered intravenously with an IR of 1.0 ml/s, followed by an infusion of 10 ml of Gd with an IR of 0.5 ml/s over 20 s. Providing a higher CM concentration at the level of the calf arteries, the remaining 10 ml of Gd are injected with a faster IR of 1.0 ml/s and flushed by an additional 20 ml of saline (1.0 ml/s). This injection scheme can be used for MR scanners providing automatic table movement and an acquisition time of about 20–25 s for a 3D data acquisition.

Another technique, which we called the *panoramic table hybrid technique*, involved performing a 3D CE pMRA by using a test bolus (1 ml Gd); secondly, 8–10 ml Gd (1.0 ml/s) and 25 ml NaCl were administered, measuring the 3D data set at the calf position. Thirdly, the pelvic and the femoropopliteal region were scanned by using the motion table technique and the three-phasic CM administration protocol. (Table 19.2, Fig. 19.1a).

Table 19.2. CM injection protocols (example) for the dynamic table movement technique

No	injection		IR (ml/s)	Vol (ml)
		Triphasic protocol		
1	1	Gd	1	20
	2	Gd	0.5	10
	3	NaCI	1	30
		Panoramic table hybrid		
1		Test bolus (PA)		
	1	Gd	1	1
	2	NaCI	1	25–30
2		Selective injection (calf)		
	1	Gd	1	8–10
	2	NaCI	1	25–30
3		Care bolus (IA, SFA, PA)		
	1	Gd	1	10
	2	Gd	0.5	2–6
	3	NaCI	0.5	6–2
	4	NaCI	1.5	25–30

IR, injection rate; Vol, Gd volume; PA, popliteal artery; IA, iliac artery; SFA, superficial artery.

19.2.3.4
Tips and Tricks for CE pMRA

An automatic power injector is highly recommended for CE pMRA, as it provides a higher reproducibility of the image quality compared with a manual injection of the CM.

- When the visualization of renal arteries is required, breath-hold 3D CE MRA should be performed in order to minimize motion artifacts.
- A noncontrast 3D data set should be acquired before the administration of CM to allow for a subtraction technique which improves both image quality and vascular signal.
- If high-resolution imaging is required to visualize run-off vessels of the lower leg area, a higher dosage of CM should be used. In a number of cases, a separate contrast study of the lower leg arteries using a phased-array surface coil is recommended.
- CM should be injected into the antecubital vein. A wrist vein will not transport the CM in a way as expected by the selected injection rate. The arm should be positioned erect over the head to allow a free contrast flow and to avoid phase-encoding wrap.

19.3 Applications of MR Angiography

19.3.1 Normal Anatomy

19.3.1.1 Iliac Arteries

The paired common iliac arteries are the terminal branches of the aorta, which descend to supply the organs of the pelvis, the pelvic wall, and the lower extremities. At the level of L5-S1 both common iliac arteries divide into the external iliac artery, which supplies the lower extremities, and the internal iliac artery. The branching of the internal iliac artery is variable and includes four main branches: superior and inferior gluteal artery to the pelvic wall, obturator, and internal pudendal arteries to the viscera (genitourinary tract). Branches of the external iliac artery are the deep iliac circumflex artery and the inferior epigastric arteries which arise behind the inguinal ligament. These vessels supply muscles and skin in the lower abdominal wall. Below the inguinal ligament the external iliac artery continues as the common femoral artery (Fig. 19.14a).

19.3.1.2 Femoral and Popliteal Arteries

From the common femoral artery arise the superficial iliac circumflex artery, the superficial epigastric artery, and the external pudendal artery. The common femoral artery bifurcates into the superficial femoral (SFA) and the deep femoral artery (DFA). Sometimes a high bifurcation can occur in a very short or absent common femoral artery. In approximately 40% of cases the DFA lies behind the SFA. From the DFA originate several branches: the medial and lateral femoral circumflex artery, including ascending, descending, and transverse muscular branches, and a branch to the femoral head; and separate branches to the muscles of the thigh. These branches have small communications to distal muscular branches of the SFA and to branches of the popliteal artery which can serve as potential collaterals in occlusive disease of the SFA joint. When the femoral artery reaches the space behind the knee, known as the popliteal fossa, it continues as the popliteal artery. Typical branches of the popliteal artery are the superior and inferior lateral, and the superior and inferior medial genicular arteries. These branches supply the knee joint and muscles of the thigh and calf. Many of its branches also join the connecting nerve network of the knee and can provide alternative routes in the case of popliteal artery obstruction (Fig. 19.14b).

19.3.1.3 Arteries of the Lower Leg and Foot

The popliteal artery divides at the lower margin of the popliteus muscle in 95% of individuals into two main branches: the anterior and the posterior tibial artery. In the remainder, one branch originates above this margin. The anterior tibial artery passes down between the tibia and the fibula and continues directly to the dorsalis pedis artery. The posterior tibial artery descends beneath the calf muscles. Both the anterior tibial and the posterior tibial artery divide into branches to supply the skin, muscles, and other tissues of the lower leg. Some of these join the neural networks behind the knee and around the ankle. The largest branch of the posterior tibial artery is the fibular artery, which distally divides into perforating branches that may serve as important collaterals to the dorsalis and plantaris pedis artery in the case of anterior or posterior tibial artery occlusion (Fig. 19.14c).

The anterior tibial artery continues as the dorsal and plantar pedis artery and forms the arcuate artery of the foot, branching into four dorsal metatarsal arteries. The plantar arch is formed by the lateral plantar artery originating, from the posterior tibial artery and the deep plantar branch of the dorsal

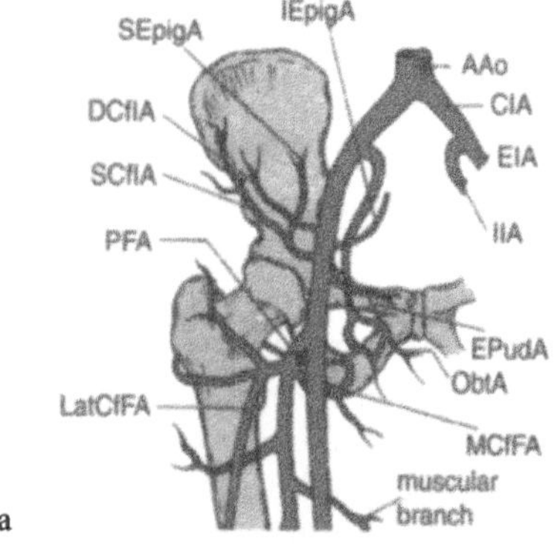

a

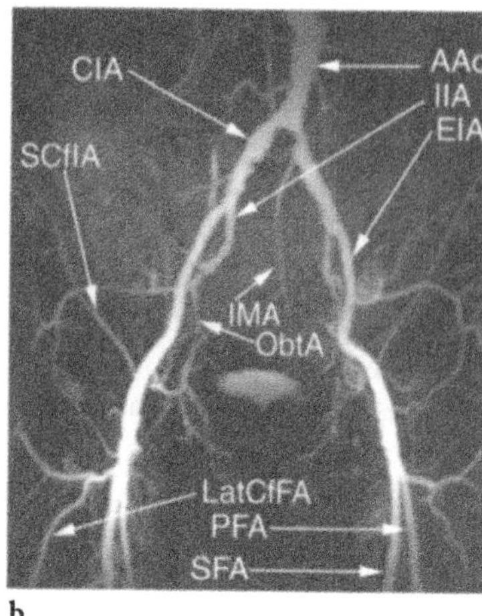

b

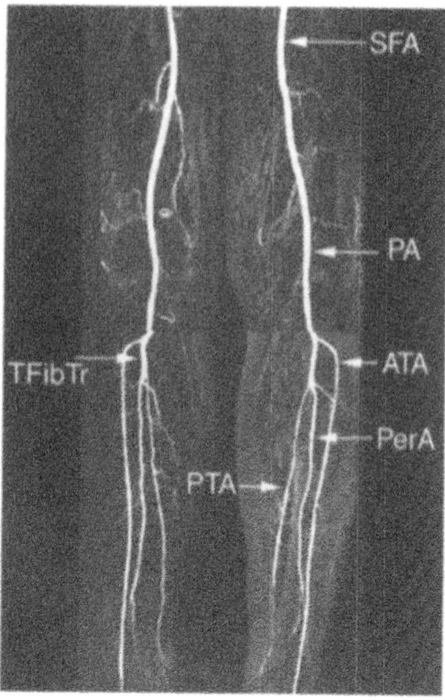

c

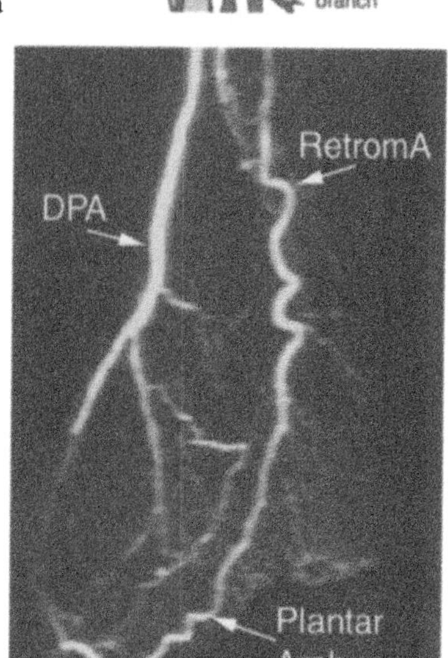

d

Fig. 19.14. Anatomy of the peripheral vasculature. (*AAo* abdominal aorta, *CIA* common iliac artery, *EIA* external iliac artery, *IIA* internal iliac artery, *EPudA* external pudenda artery, *ObtA* obturator artery, *MCfFA* medial circumflex femoral artery, *LatCfFA* lateral circumflex femoral artery, *SFA* superficial femoral artery, *PFA* profunda femoral artery, *SCflA* superficial circumflex iliac artery, *DCflA* deep circumflex iliac artery, *SEpigA* superficial epigastric artery, *IEpigA* internal epigastric artery, *IMA* inferior mesenteric artery, *PA* popliteal artery, *TFibTr* tibiofibular trunc, *ATA* anterior tibial artery, *PerA* peroneal artery, *PTA* posterior tibial artery, *RetromA* retromaleolar artery, *DPA* dorsal pedal artery)

pedal artery which provides the predominant blood supply to the plantar arch. The dorsal digital arteries receive blood from the dorsal metatarsal arteries and communicate with the plantar digital arteries in the clefts between the toes. The superficial veins form a "plantar cutaneous venous arch" that extends across the root of the toes and continues at both sides of the foot into medial and lateral veins (Fig. 19.14d).

19.3.2 Peripheral Arterial Occlusive Disease

19.3.2.1 Characteristic Appearance and Vascular Morphology

The etiology of peripheral arterial occlusive disease (PAOD) is complex, but in the majority of cases atheromatosis is the leading factor. Concerning the site of PAOD, typical patterns can be distinguished such as terminal aortic obstruction, common and external iliac, superficial and popliteal, crural and pedal obstructions. The location of the lesion and the inflow and outflow conditions may influence clinical symptoms, which include intermittent claudication, rest pain, ischemic gangrene of the foot, and acute limb-threatening ischemia. Limb-threatening ischemia in the majority of cases occurs in acute embolic or thrombotic occlusive disease which may affect all parts of the involved extremity. In these cases the prognosis is worse, leading to a high rate of amputations, particularly when the lower leg arteries are involved (Humphrey et al., 1994; Criqui et al. 1985; Imarato et al. 1975). Lower extremity ischemia can be divided into two groups: intermittent claudication and limb-threatening ischemia. Prognosis is good for patients with intermittent claudication, with the disease running a benign course with a low rate of amputation and a limited need for surgical interventions.

19.3.2.2
Basic Diagnostic Concepts

The diagnosis of PAOD is primarily based on the patient's history (risk factors, clinical development of symptoms) and clinical examination, including a precise evaluation of clinical symptoms (classification following stress test), pulse status, and vessel auscultation. In cases with pathologic clinical findings that may suggest PAOD, the noninvasive diagnostic procedure primarily used is Doppler technique by which the perfusion pressure can be determined and the so-called Doppler indices can be established. In clinical practice the following diagnostic tools are typically applied and standardized in most institutions; the PAOD, the localization of the vascular lesions, and the determination and grading of stenoses or occlusions as well as their functional effects can be evaluated in symptomatic patients:

a) High-resolution color-coded duplex ultrasonography (CCDS) allows reliable judgment of the localization and grade of stenoses. Drawbacks of CCDS in the pelvic region are problems in adipose patients due to bowel gas. In addition, considerable calcifications of the vessel wall can reduce the accuracy in evaluating the perfused vessel lumen. In the diagnosis of PAOD of the tibial fibular or the pedal arteries, this method is usually not sufficient.
b) Conventional angiography and i.a. DSA are still regarded as the standard procedures in PAOD. The advantages, particularly of i.a. DSA, are a high temporal and spatial resolved imaging of peripheral arteries, including the small branches of the lower leg region, and the subtraction technique, which eliminates interfering bone structures. A drawback of X-ray angiography is that the procedure is invasive, involving a well-known rate of complications, particularly when a transbrachial access is used in occlusive disease of the terminal aorta or both iliac arteries. However, when a transfemoral fine-needle technique is used, which allows excellent imaging of the iliac artery as well as the leg arteries, the procedure is relatively acceptable for the patient and can be performed in an outpatient setting.

It should be noted that iodinated contrast material used in DSA is potentially nephrotoxic, particularly in patients with reduced renal function and diabetes mellitus. Moreover, there is a risk of image manipulation due to electronic image processing that may cause an underestimation of atherosclerotic disease compared with intraoperative findings.

19.3.2.3
Therapeutic Concepts

The decision on a suitable therapeutic procedure depends on the findings made from the diagnostic procedures mentioned above and may involve a vascular surgeon, an interventional radiologist, or an angiologist giving conservative treatment.

19.3.2.3.1
Surgical Procedures

Surgical procedures in PAOD include Fogarty -catheter maneuvers in embolic occlusive disease. In chronic occlusive disease, aortoiliacal and iliaco-femoro-popliteo-crural-pedal bypass grafting in long distance occlusions is performed, whereas thromboendarterectomy in combination with patch plastic or stripping maneuvers is preferred in short occlusions and severe calcified stenoses. Synthetic allograft prosthesis is mainly used in the aortoiliac region, whereas for bypassing the femoral or popliteal artery, autologous venous material (e.g., reversed bypass using saphenous vein material) has advantages over synthetic materials due to higher patency rates (Fig. 19.15). Patch plastic is indicated in ostial stenoses of the superficial and deep femoral as well as in stenoses of the common femoral artery. Only in cases with multiple crural vessel occlusion and lack of distal vessels for cruro-pedal bypass reconstruction is a primary conservative procedure indicated.

19.3.2.3.2
Percutaneous Endovascular Interventions

Percutaneous endovascular interventions most commonly performed by the interventional radiologist include a variety of techniques using different devices. In the majority of patients with chronic obstructions, balloon angioplasty is performed in the iliac, femoropopliteal, and even in the crural region, whereas stent placement has been shown to be most successful in iliac artery occlusions or excentric calcified stenoses. Occlusive disease of the aortic bifurcation can be treated successfully using the "kissing balloon" technique or stent placement. However, stent placement in the femoropopliteal region yields no acceptable results using the material available today. The length, type, and site of stenosis may influence the results of PTA (Percutaneous transluminal angiography): the more proximal and shorter the stenosis, the more successful the result (Pentecost et al. 1994). In acute and subacute PAOD due to embolic or thrombotic disease, procedures such as low-dose fibrinolysis and clot or thrombus aspiration via spe-

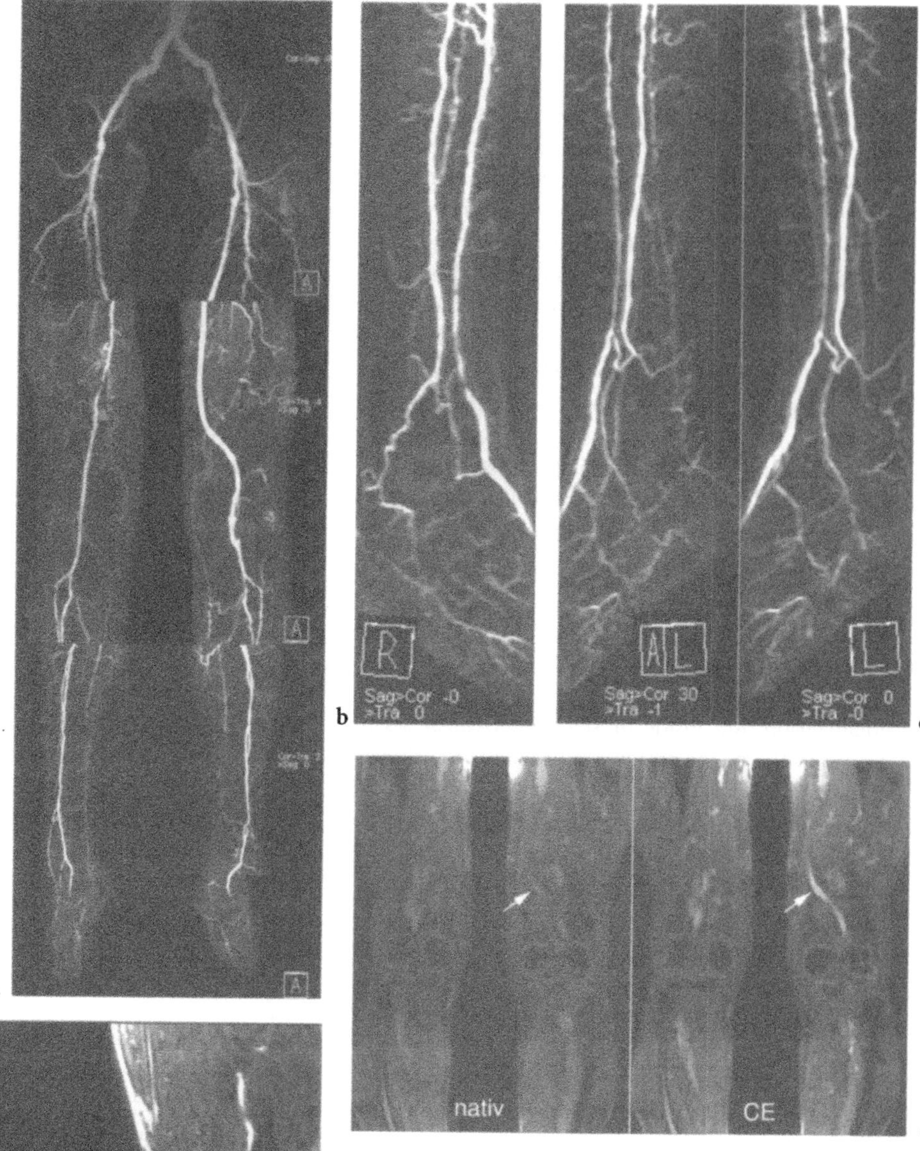

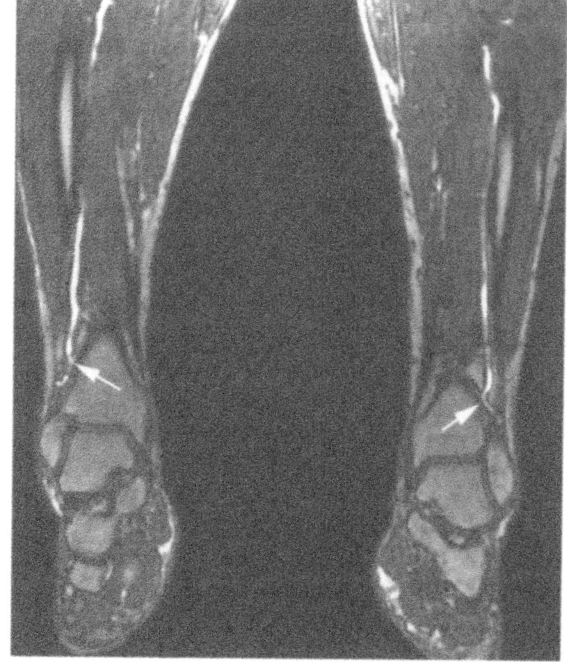

Fig. 19.15a–e. CE MRA follow-up of a patient with a patent femoropopliteal bypass at the left site (sufficient anastomoses), but claudication symptoms at the right leg due to a high-grade stenosis of the SFA which is not well compensated by collaterals from the deep artery (**a**). Note that the coronal MIP image alone does not allow one to interpret the run-off. Therefore, calculations were made on a 60° (**b**) and a sagittal view of the right (**b**) and a sagittal view of the left calf (**c**), showing the important right peroneal artery with collaterals running to the dorsal pedal artery (see also **d**; the source images may help to identify the perforating branches). The proximal left dorsal pedal artery stenosis can also be identified on the sagittal MIP image, the retro-malleolar artery gets its blood supply via collaterals from the peroneal artery (**b**). **e** The native and contrast-enhanced source images of the 3D data set (femoral region) are demonstrated. Some enhancement from the CM administered during the first calf measurement using separate CM injection can be seen within the arterial bypass (*arrow*). But there is enough signal increase after the second injection for a sufficient MIP after subtraction

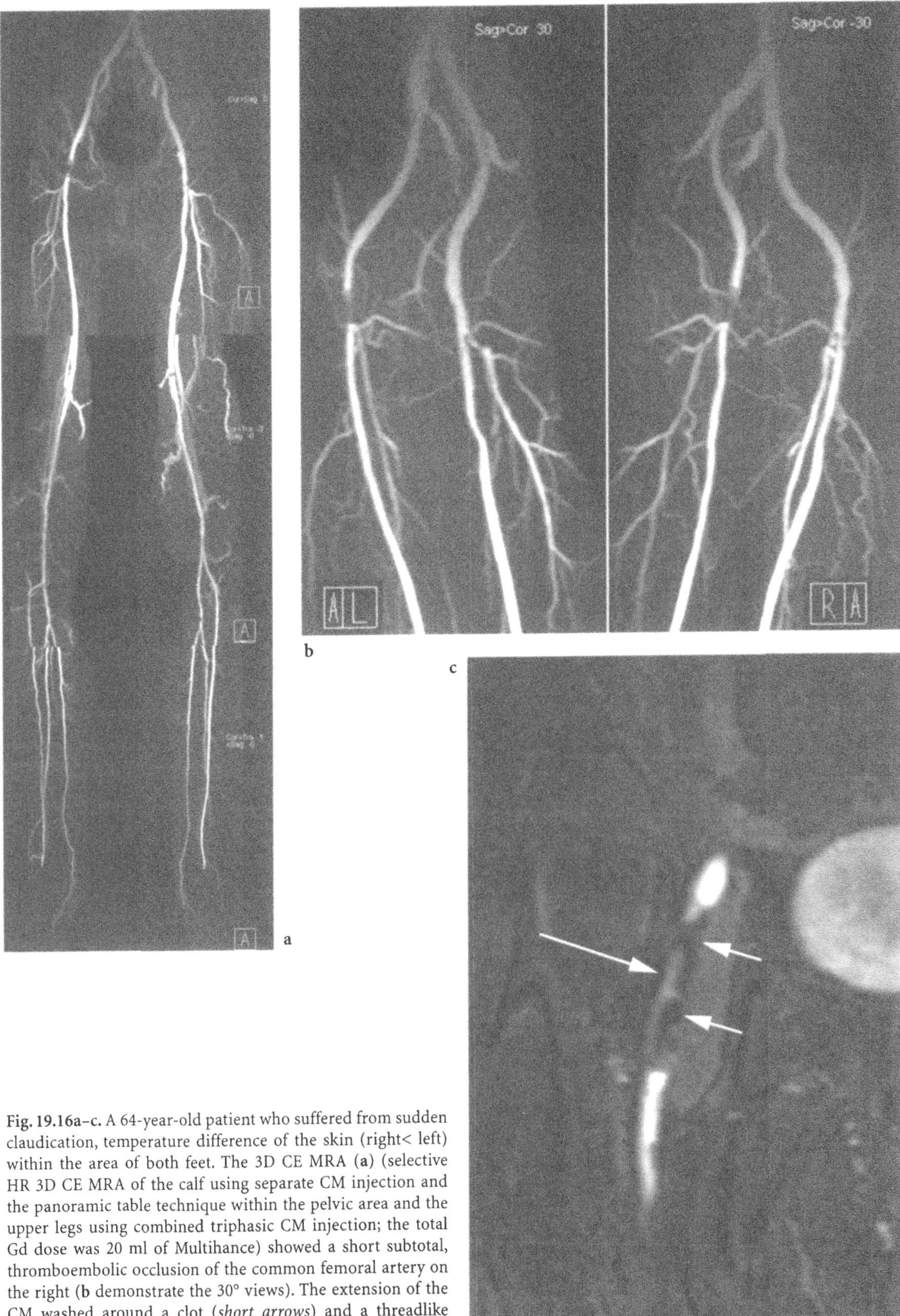

Fig. 19.16a–c. A 64-year-old patient who suffered from sudden claudication, temperature difference of the skin (right< left) within the area of both feet. The 3D CE MRA (**a**) (selective HR 3D CE MRA of the calf using separate CM injection and the panoramic table technique within the pelvic area and the upper legs using combined triphasic CM injection; the total Gd dose was 20 ml of Multihance) showed a short subtotal, thromboembolic occlusion of the common femoral artery on the right (**b** demonstrate the 30° views). The extension of the CM washed around a clot (*short arrows*) and a threadlike lumen (*large arrow*, **c**) is demonstrated on the source image

cially developed devices can be used successfully (McPhail et al. 1983) (Fig. 19.16).

Bypass or prosthetic surgery is usually confined to extreme cases with limb-threatening ischemia in which short-term interventional therapy is immediately required. All the procedures that may preserve the extremity are more cost-effective than amputation.

19.3.2.3.3
Conservative Therapeutic Management

The conservative therapeutic regimen of PAOD in the majority of cases is reserved for patients with compensated claudication or when invasive procedures cannot be performed due to technical limitations or have not been clinically successful. In these cases training programs can be recommended in combination with systemic or locally applied drug therapy (e.g., prostavasine) and other adjuvant methods.

19.3.3
Evaluation of pMRA

In patients with PAOD the planning of revascularization processes requires a precise anatomic mapping of the site and severity of the lesion. Because conventional angiography, to date the standard of reference for investigation of PAOD, is an invasive technique with some risk for the patient, noninvasive examinations such as CCDS or MR angiography are increasingly beeing used in the diagnostic work-up of patients with PAOD. Although vascular MR imaging is still a complex and relatively expensive method because of its exclusive technology, its clinical role is continuously expanding due to systematic development and improvement. The aim of pMRA is to substitute invasive conventional angiography.

Multiple reports have been published within the last 10 years in which pMRA, as compared to conventional angiography, has become the accepted reference standard (Table 19.3). A generally valid evaluation of the diagnostic accuracy of pMRA is difficult to perform due to the inhomogeneous spectrum of studies which included different techniques and equipment, resulting in a wide range of varying sensitivities and specificities (Nelemans et al. 2000) (Table 19.1). Clinical experience in pMRA has been gained with the 2D TOF technique, 2D PC technique, and CE 3D MR angiography.

19.3.3.1
Flow-Sensitive Versus CE pMRA Versus Conventional Angiography

The different techniques described above represent the current status of pMRA in clinical use. The main problems and drawbacks of inflow techniques are potential imaging artifacts and the inability to visualize the entire peripheral arterial vasculature within an acceptable examination time because contiguous transverse thin sections have to be acquired with the 2D technique. Vascular stenosis can be falsely suggested by in-plane saturation effects. Although 2D

Table 19.3. Study reports of PMRA, as compared to conventional angiography as the accepted reference standard

MR angiographic study results							
Author	Year of publication	MRA modality	Coil setup	CM administration	Anatomical sites studied	Sensitivity	Specificity
Snidow et al.	1995	Single-step	SBC	NA, BAT	IA-peroneal artery	92	74
Glickerman et al.	1996	TOF	SBC	NA	IA-peroneal artery	87	96
Ho et al.	1997	Single-step	SBC	NA, BAT	IA-SF	71	87
Davis et al.	1997	TOF	NA	NA	PA-peroneal artery	94	94
Poon et al.	1997	Single-step	NA	NA	IA-SF	100	90
Rofsky et al.	1997	2-Step	SBC	NA	IA-ankle	97	96
Ekiof et al.	1998	TOF	NA	NA	PA-peroneal artery	81	94
Hany et al.	1998	Single-step	BPA	NA	IA-CF	96	91
Ho et al.	1998	3-Step TM	SBC	0.5ml/s cont.	IA-peroneal artery	93	98
Yamashita et al.	1998	NA	NA	NA	IA-peroneal artery	96	83
Kai Yiu et al.	1998	3-Step TM	SBC	NA cont.	IA-peroneal artery	93	98
Meany et al.	1999	3-Step TM	SBC	0.5ml/s cont.	IA-peroneal artery	81	91
Sueyoshi et al.	1999	3-Step	BPA	hm, cont.	IA-peroneal artery	97	99
Ruehm et al.	2000	3-Step	pMRA	0.5–0.7 ml/s cont.	IA-peroneal artery	92	96

SBC, standard body coil; BPA, body phased-array coil; pMRA, pMRA coil; NA, not available; cont., continuous CM infusion; BAT, bolus arrival time; IA, iliac artery; SF, superficial artery; PA, popliteal artery; CF, common femoral artery.

PC pMRA permits coronal slice orientation using a larger FOV along the flow direction and a shortened acquisition time, this technique also shows a variety of limitations mainly due to phase dispersion and difficulties in determining of velocity-encoding (VENC) values (Boos et al. 1995). A false-positive diagnosis of stenotic disease can be made due to the aliasing phenomenon.

Compared with flow-sensitive techniques, CE pMRA has a significantly higher and more stable intravascular signal in all parts of the peripheral arteries, including, in particular, an increased visualization of distal vessels. However, in practice, CE pMRA of the entire lower leg circulation suffers because a total vessel distance of more than 100 cm has to be covered. Thus, to date study results have only shown that there is a high sensitivity and specificity in the iliac and femoropopliteal arteries, whereas the optimized technique in lower leg artery visualization is still in development. Using the dynamic table movement technique, the prolonged CM infusion may sometimes degrade image quality of the lower leg arteries, because veins and soft tissue may still be enhanced from the first pass CM bolus during acquisition of the pelvic and upper leg. This phenomenon can be avoided when a noncontrast 3D data set is acquired before a second CM injection under consideration of a separate bolus timing for the tibial arteries that can be subtracted from the contrast-enhanced data set. This procedure may be useful in side-different run-off conditions. Moreover, by using dedicated peripheral vascular phased-array coil systems, the spatial resolution of crural and pedal arteries can be significantly improved. High-resolution CE pMRA, which requires a large number of phase-encoding and partition-encoding steps, may influence both the acquisition time and the dynamic memory store. This technique has been shown to be useful only in lower leg artery acquisition in order to limit strong venous enhancement, particularly in the calf region. This approach can be recommended in the case of surgical planning and run-off studies. In CE pMRA follow-up studies, the presence of indwelling stents can cause severe artifacts that make it impossible to decide whether the vessel segment is patent or not.

Both the test bolus and automatic bolus finding techniques in CE pMRA have advantages and drawbacks. Care bolus or smart prep techniques do not require a test bolus, are time-saving and mostly easy to use. Otherwise, the test bolus can be examined over a longer period, allowing one to distinguish accurately between inflow artifacts and actual CM arrival. In addition, the decision when to start the acquisition of 3D CE pMRA can be made within 1 or 2 s, whereas the test bolus series can only be evaluated by a mean curve.

A meta-analysis published by Nelemans et al. (2000) had the purpose of summarizing the overall diagnostic performance of MR angiography in the detection or exclusion of arterial stenoses of 50%–99% or occlusions in the peripheral vascular tree, and identifying the most important sources of variations in diagnostic accuracy between different studies. In this meta-analysis, flow-sensitive 2D TOF MRA was compared with 3D CE pMRA concerning the accuracy in depicting lesions in different vascular segments such as aortoiliac, femoropopliteal, and below-knee lesions. Conventional angiography was used as the standard of reference. The sensitivities and specificities found in this analysis have been described as follows:

a) 2D TOF MRA: aortoiliac ranging from 83% to 100% and 23% to 98%, femoropopliteal ranging from 88% to 92% and 82% to 98%, and crural ranging from 86% to 98% and 91% to 95%
b) 3D CE pMRA: aortoiliac ranging from 92% to 100% and 91% to 98%, femoropopliteal ranging from 94% to 100% and 97% to 99%, and crural ranging from 91% to 94% and 100%

From this meta-analysis it can be concluded that 3D CE pMRA is superior to 2D TOF MRA in the detection and grading of PAOD. Moreover, the additional evaluation of transverse source images or multiplanar reformations provides diagnostic gain as compared with interpretations based only on MIP images (Hany et al. 1998). It has been hypothesized that the accuracy of MR angiography may vary according to the anatomic level, with a higher accuracy of 2D TOF MRA at lower anatomic levels (Huber et al. 1997). Using CE pMRA, distal arteries are considered to be more difficult to study than proximal vessels due to a reduction of the CM concentration, a delayed arrival of the CM bolus, particularly if proximal vessels are diseased (Rofsky et al. 1997), and a venous filling of the CM which causes an overprojection, making images more difficult to interpret. 2D TOF MRA and 3D CE pMRA in this meta-analysis showed no clear trend in diagnostic accuracy with varying anatomic levels, considering that it was not possible to study the effect of verification bias on diagnostic accuracy.

Usually, MR angiography is performed because of its ability to depict hemodynamically significant stenoses. However, for the selection of the optimal surgical treatment and distal run-off vessels, the ability to detect patent vessels is also important. Several reports documented better visualization of patent vessel segments in 2D TOF MR angiograms than in conventional angiograms, varying between 13% and 23% (McDermott et al. 1995; Carpenter et al. 1992; Owen et al. 1992, 1993). On the other hand, recently available CE pMRA imaging modalities may contribute to these findings because a more reliable bolus timing is possible and spatial resolution can be significantly improved in the area of crural and pedal vessels. More recently, experience with the dynamic table movement technique has been gained in combination with dedicated peripheral coils found to be useful for the positioning of patients and accurate in the visualization of the entire peripheral arterial system.

For postprocessing of the CE 3D data set mainly MIP imaging is used. Arterial bifurcations of the iliac and femoral region can be evaluated in the majority of cases by using the MIP technique. Multiplanar reformatted imaging and the analysis of source images are able to improve significantly the accurate analysis of vessels (Nelemans et al. 2000). MR angiographic determination of the degree of a stenosis usually involves the subjective interpretation of image findings on the basis of a visual impression. Thus, numerical statements of stenotic grading should be viewed critically.

19.3.3.2
pMRA Versus CCDS

For patients with PAOD, planning of revascularization procedures requires precise anatomic mapping of the site and the severity of the lesion. CCDS has been successfully introduced in clinical routines to select patients with clinical symptoms of PAOD for invasive conventional angiography combined potentially with percutaneous angioplasty or vascular surgery. CCDS has been shown to be a reliable modality with a fairly good sensitivity and specificity in PAOD, and the investment cost for the equipment is acceptable. However, the method is operator-dependent, in difficult cases the examination may be time consuming, lower leg arteries are sometimes limited to investigation, and the modality does not provide a road map equivalent to that of angiography.

As an alternative noninvasive diagnostic procedure, CE pMRA provides high-quality 3D images of the vascular system within a short time and with a high diagnostic accuracy. As a drawback of CE pMRA, the investment cost of the MR equipment is much higher than that of CCDS, the examination comfort for the patient is reduced, and a number of contraindications have to be considered.

The role of pMRA or CCDS in the diagnostic work-up of patients with PAOD is to distinguish between diseased and nondiseased vascular segments, to grade a vascular lesion, and to provide information useful for making the correct therapeutic decision. Besides diagnostic accuracy, the evaluation of both methods has to include clinical reliability and cost-effectiveness. In a meta-analysis published by Vissier and Hunink (2000), the authors compared the diagnostic accuracy of CE pMRA and CCDS in PAOD (Visser and Hunink 2000). In comparison with conventional angiography, both imaging modalities showed good diagnostic performance. With a random effects model used in this study, pooled sensitivity was higher for pMRA (97.5%) than for CCDS (87.5%), whereas the pooled specificities were similar for both techniques (96.2% for pMRA and 94.7% for CCDS). However, using the analysis of the summary of receiver operating characteristics, the pooled value of the natural logarithm of the diagnostic odds ratio was 6.43 for pMRA and 4.99 for CCDS, indicating that pMRA has a better discriminatory power than CCDS.

Considering cost-effectiveness at the present state of technical development, CCDS may be more cost-effective than flow-sensitive pMRA techniques. However, when ultrafast 3D CE pMRA with dynamic table movement technique is used, this modality is more effective than CCDS in overall diagnostic accuracy, including the site and the degree of a lesion (Fig. 19.17). Due to its superior informative character and the ability to cover the entire peripheral vascular system and to depict accurately the lower leg run-off vessels, CE pMRA is more reliable in planning suitable interventional therapeutic procedures. On the other hand, particularly in patients with symptoms of advanced PAOD that have already been diagnosed by a previous angiogram, CCDS appears useful in depicting new lesions. In a simple and fast procedure, CCDS can help to evaluate iliofemoral lesions and to determine the puncture site for a planned percutaneous intervention. Furthermore, CCDS is a very fast and accurate modality for follow-up studies after endovascular intervention or bypass surgery.

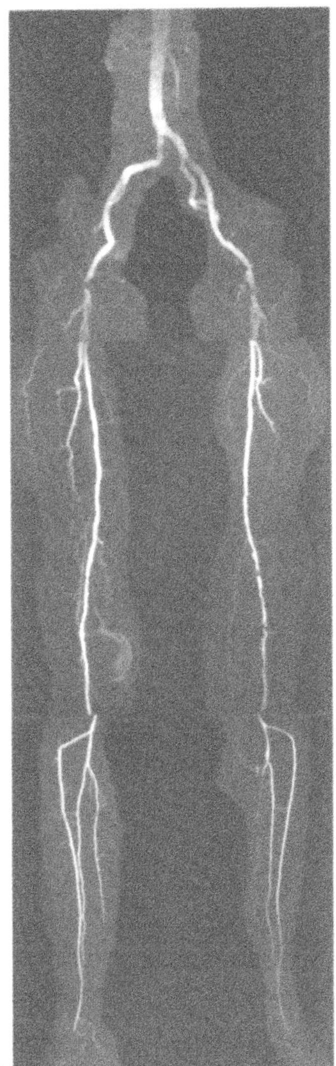

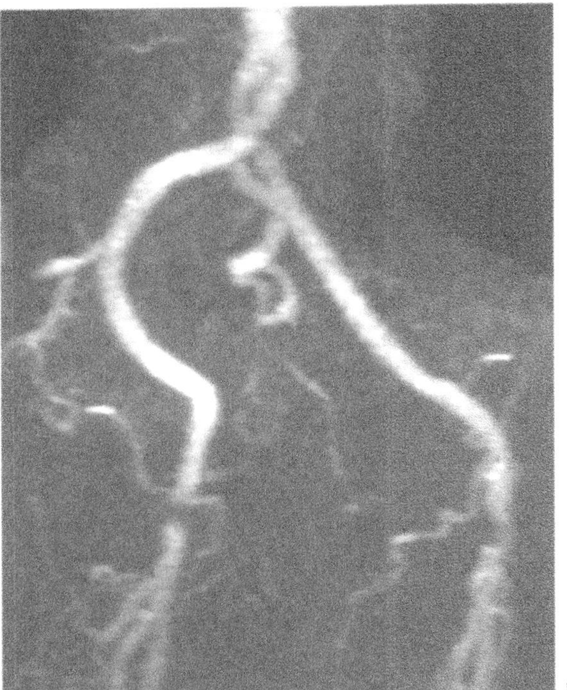

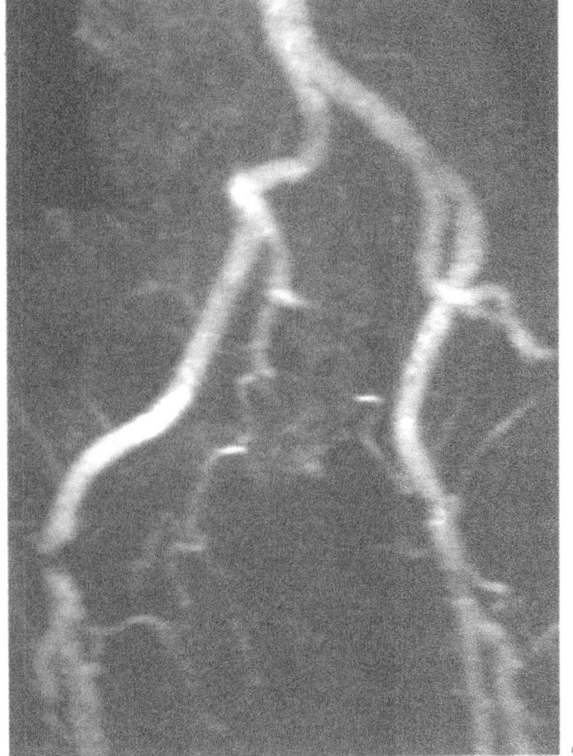

Fig. 19.17. Peripheral MRA (**a**: coronal MIP) of a patient with PAOD (Fontaine III) and restricted run-off below the ankle (no CM filling of the dorsal of plantar arch) because of diabetes mellitus: Due to calcified plaques the high-grade stenosis of the common femoral arteries on both sites was not correctly identified by CCDS. Note that the details of the femoral bifurcations can only be seen at the 45° and -45° rotated MIPs (**b** and **c**): no stenosis at the left and mild stenosis at the right site of the deep femoral artery. In addition, multiple high-grade and eccentric stenoses of the SFA were detected on the left which have to be treated for improvement of the run-off. PMRA technique: three-step MRA with separate CM injections (3× single-dose Gd) and pMRA coil; the calf was imaged first, subsequently the iliac arteries and the femoral region were scanned

19.3.4 pMRA: Relationship to Symptomatology and Therapy

It is essential that diagnostic radiologists are familiar with the clinical symptoms of PAOD and the range of therapeutic procedures, including vascular surgery, endovascular interventions, and conservative treatment options, in order to decide which the MR angiographic technique is suitable (ROFSKY and ADELMAN 2000). For therapy, the following diagnostic targets in PAOD have to be considered: the inflow to the lesion, the outflow from the lesion, and the nature of the lesion itself. The inflow is characterized as the nonrestricted blood flow proximal to the lesion of interest directly entering the lesion itself or bypassing the lesion via a collateral system. If the inflow is restricted by another more proximally located obstruction, a distal arterial recanalization or reconstruction procedure may be limited. The outflow or run-off of a lesion is defined as the arterial blood flow and vascular tree, respectively, distal to the lesion of interest. By the term "run-off" most authors understand the arterial flow below the knee. In case of a limited outflow caused by high resistance and distal occlusive disease, the success of arterial reconstruction of the proximal lesion may be compromised. It is important to characterize the nature of the lesion (Fig. 19.18). Acute occlusions usually show fresh and soft thrombotic material, a reduced amount of collateral vessels, mostly a sudden and significant clinical onset, and severe symptoms of ischemia. A chronic lesion is characterized by fibrotic tissue difficult to traverse mechanically, calcification, and a large degree of collaterals.

19.3.4.1 Intermittent Claudication

The inability to sufficiently increase blood flow as a response to exercise is defined as intermittent claudication. The pain must be located in a functional

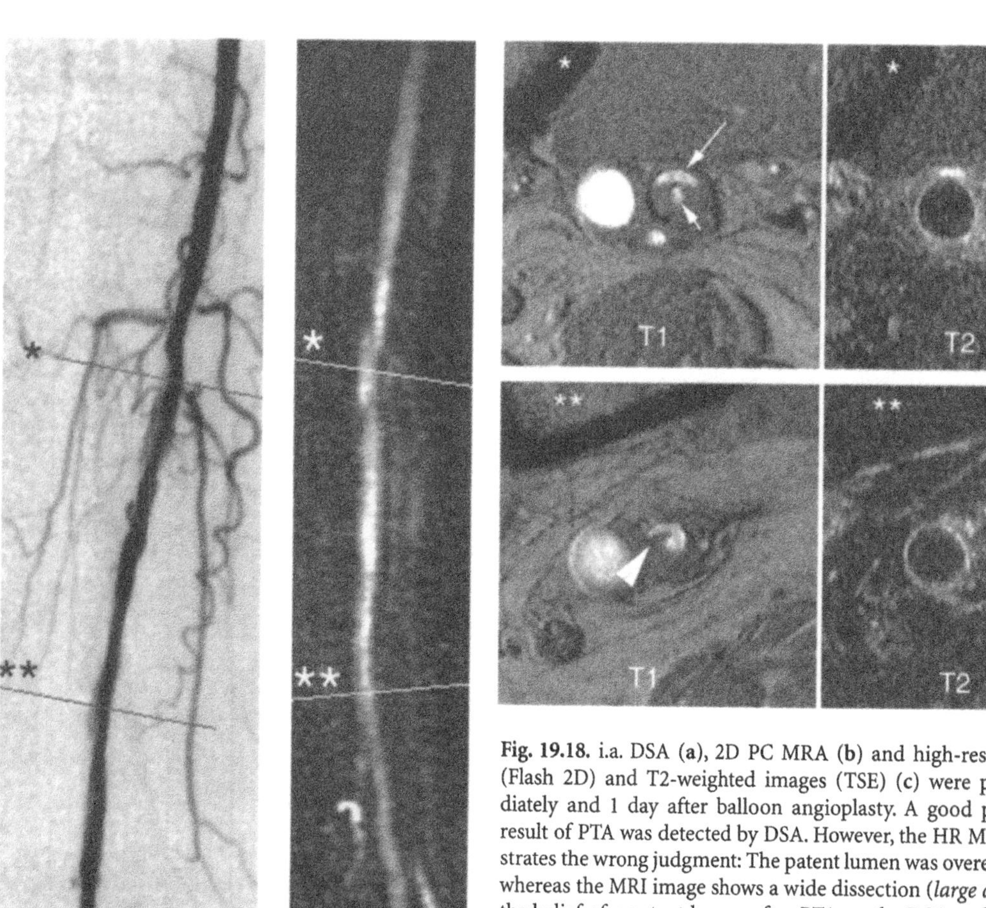

Fig. 19.18. i.a. DSA (**a**), 2D PC MRA (**b**) and high-resolution (HR) T1-(Flash 2D) and T2-weighted images (TSE) (**c**) were performed immediately and 1 day after balloon angioplasty. A good primary technical result of PTA was detected by DSA. However, the HR MRI image demonstrates the wrong judgment: The patent lumen was overestimated by DSA, whereas the MRI image shows a wide dissection (*large arrow*; supporting the belief of a patent lumen after PTA on the DSA and PC MRA image) and demonstrates the actually stenosed lumen (*short arrow*). Distal to this lesion a heavy intimal flap was detected (*arrowhead*). As expected from these HR MR images, there was reocclusion 14 days after PTA

muscle group, reproducible with consistent muscle work load, and be promptly relieved by stopping exercise. The level of PAOD will dictate the symptomatic segment of the extremities. Symptoms typically occur below a stenotic vascular lesion.

Segmental iliac artery stenosis commonly presents with buttock and thigh pain from claudication (DeBakey et al. 1985). One third of all arterial stenoses or occlusions of the lower extremities can be depicted in the aorto-iliac region. More than 90% of stenoses are caused by atherosclerosis. Eighty percent to 90% of patients with PAOD consult their physician because of intermittent claudication, whereas rest pain or ischemic gangrene are rare and occur mostly in the presence of additional femoropopliteal or crural occlusions. Patients with superficial femoral artery (SFA) disease most commonly have a calf claudication. Deep femoral artery (DFA) disease often results in an isolated thigh claudication. The SFA and DFA are the most frequently affected vessels at an incidence of approximately 50% of all patients with PAOD.

An obstruction of the SFA can be compensated over years when the iliac segment is patent and an extensive collateral circulation to the postobstructive segment has developed via branches of the DFA. On the other hand, even when claudication occurs unilaterally, in more than 50% of patients the contralateral SFA is similarly involved.

The first treatment aspect of patients with claudication is to prevent progression of the disease, which may result in a limb-threatening situation. Although the amputation rate for this patient group is low (1%–2% per year), up to 80% will be improved during a 2.5–6-year period (Imarato et al. 1975; Jonason and Ringqvist 1985). The second aspect is to find a suitable treatment strategy considering the degree of discomfort. Because of the relatively benign course, most commonly these patients have a Doppler examination and are then treated conservatively. Otherwise, in intermittent claudication, balloon angioplasty of an isolated stenosis of the SFA or popliteal artery is a simple procedure and therefore a useful alternative option for improving the patient's comfort. At the moment, stent placement is recommended in iliac artery lesions, whereas in the femoral segment there is no proven benefit for the patient as compared with simple PTA (Martin et al. 1995; Murphy et al. 1998; Long et al. 1995; Vorwerk et al. 1996; Henry et al. 1995). Thus, considering these aspects, aortoiliofemoral vascular imaging in intermittent claudication seems to be useful and is recommended. This can be confirmed by the fact that, statistically, patients with clinically relevant short segment lesions (>50%) are referred for PTA. In symptomatic longer occlusions up to 10 cm, PTA is still a matter of discussion because long-term patency rates are limited, particularly in cases with restricted run-off below the lesion. In these cases, femoropopliteal bypass surgery is a suitable alternative presenting far better patency rates.

19.3.4.1.1 MR Angiographic Considerations

The purpose of pMRA in intermittent claudication is to determine the location, degree, and length of an obstruction, differentiating a stenosis from an occlusion. The iliac and femoral bifurcation can be reliably visualized by using oblique MIP views or multiplanar reformatted imaging (Fig. 19.19). The evaluation of the DFA origin is of particular interest in evaluating wheather is the collateral system sufficient in SFA obstruction (Peabody et al. 1974). Stenoses and occlusions of the SFA, the DFA, and their branching vessels can be precisely depicted using CE pMRA. Even collaterals originating from the DFA can generally be reliably depicted. Another goal of pMRA is to separate patients who should receive PTA from those who should be treated conservatively or by bypass surgery.

When using pMRA for the diagnosis in intermittent claudication, the aortoiliac segment is best evaluated with the 3D contrast-enhanced technique. In comparison to CE pMRA, the 2D TOF method cannot claim any relevant advantages in the diagnosis of PAOD (Rofsky et al. 1997; Snidow et al. 1995; Poon et al. 1997; Quinn et al. 1997). Although simple iliac or femoral stenoses can be depicted, the collateral circulation cannot be satisfactorily visualized. Depending on the flow patterns (turbulence or accelerations), the level of stenosis can be over- or underestimated. Under particular circumstances, the 2D PC MRA can be a viable alternative in cases in which CM has to be saved or in postinterventional follow-up studies.

When CE pMRA is used, a time-efficient examination is possible by the application of a bolus chase technique (Adelmann and Jacobowitz 1998). However, for this technique an automatic table movement feature of the MR system must be available. Alternatively, CE pMRA with separate injections (10–5 ml of Gd-DTPA; 0.5 mmol/ml) administered for the aortoiliac, femoropopliteal, and tibial segments can be performed in two or three steps. Iliac and femoropopliteal stenoses and occlusions can be accurately detected using this technique.

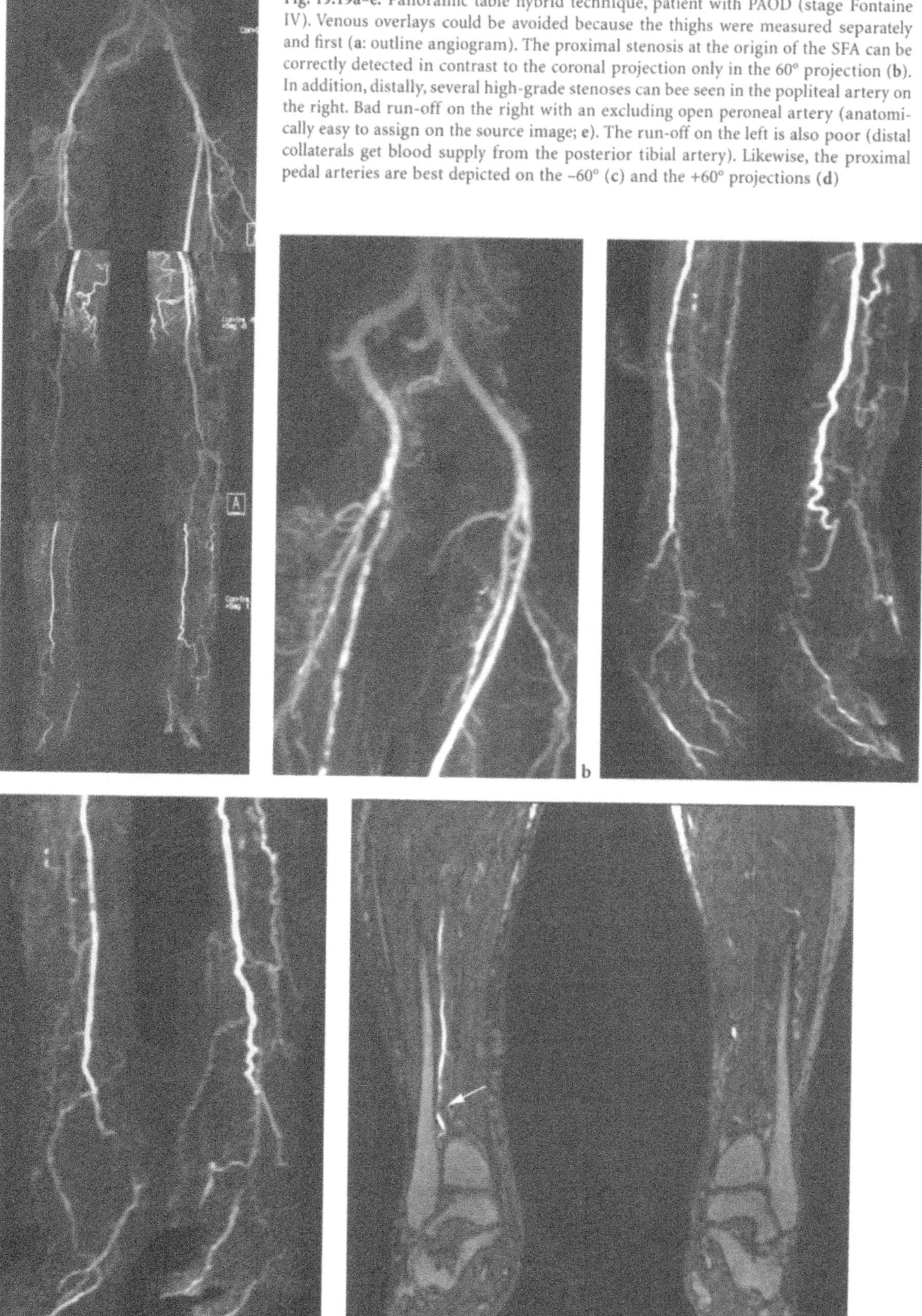

Fig. 19.19a–e. Panoramic table hybrid technique, patient with PAOD (stage Fontaine IV). Venous overlays could be avoided because the thighs were measured separately and first (**a**: outline angiogram). The proximal stenosis at the origin of the SFA can be correctly detected in contrast to the coronal projection only in the 60° projection (**b**). In addition, distally, several high-grade stenoses can bee seen in the popliteal artery on the right. Bad run-off on the right with an excluding open peroneal artery (anatomically easy to assign on the source image; **e**). The run-off on the left is also poor (distal collaterals get blood supply from the posterior tibial artery). Likewise, the proximal pedal arteries are best depicted on the -60° (**c**) and the +60° projections (**d**)

The correct setting of the 3D volume in the anterior–posterior direction is of importance; both the common femoral and the internal iliac artery must be covered by selecting a suitable volume of up to 120 mm in thickness. However, the extension of the imaging volume will cause either longer acquisition times or decreased spatial resolution.

In particular, thicker 3D volumes should be chosen when collateral vessels originating from the internal iliac artery branches are to be depicted in external iliac occlusion. The 3D character of CE pMRA provides information regarding the luminal configuration of a stenosis, which requires isotropic resolutions lower than 1.5 mm in all three directions. As a postprocessing method, MPR provides the endovascular therapist with important information for intra-arterial guidance of the catheter (Fig. 19.20).

As a drawback of the dynamic table movement technique, similar to that observed in conventional angiography when the table step-by-step technique is used, delayed or retrograde flow cannot be reliably visualized, leading to limitations in the depiction of the true length of an occlusion. This problem can be solved by the multi-station CE pMRA technique (Poon et al. 1997; Ho et al. 1997; Hertz et al. 1993; Swan et al. 1993).

19.3.4.2
Limb-Threatening Ischemia

Limb-threatening ischemia is defined as the inability of blood flow to fulfill baseline metabolic demands under rest conditions. This restriction of blood flow results in rest pain, usually affecting the forefoot, and tissue necrosis may begin to develop. Patients typically have multisegmented PAOD usually including both proximal and crural lesions. Thus, a complete evaluation of the arterial system from the infrarenal abdominal aorta to the foot is necessary. These lesions may be observed in advanced states of atherosclerosis, Buerger's disease, and particularly in diabetic angiopathy (60%–70%).

Since limb-salvage surgery has become available, primary amputations can be successfully avoided (Samson et al. 1999). This therapeutic procedure includes different bypass variants (aorto-ilio-femoral, femoro-popliteo-cruro-pedal), which are able to increase the arterial perfusion of the threatened segment. Bypass patency rates are maximized if the supra- or infragenicualate segments are used for bypass insertion. Autologous venous material is preferred when performing a femoropopliteal bypass with the distal anastomosis below the knee, whereas the proximal popliteal segment has been shown to be superior when prosthetic graft material is used. Gangrenous peripheral arterial disease requires a restoration of pulsatile flow to the lower leg or foot arteries via femorocrural or femoropedal bypass (LoGerfo et al. 1992; Andros 1995; Pomposelli et al. 1995). In long femoral occlusions without sufficient collateralization via DFA and a non-occluded popliteal artery but segmentally stenosed tibial vessels (Adelmann and Jacobowitz 1998; Kaufman et al. 1982), the bypass graft ideally should be inserted beyond the stenosed tibial segments. There are different surgical approaches to the anterior, posterior tibial, and peroneal artery. If the tibial artery is selected as a recipient vessel for bypass insertion, it must be in continuity with the pedal arch. Direct inflow into the pedal arch facilitates pulsatile flow to reach the level of tissue loss, increasing nutritive perfusion. Unrestricted flow within this peripheral arterial bed reduces the risk of bypass occlusion, whereas poor outflow speaks for a lower patency rate (Pomposelli et al. 1995; Andros 1995; Dardik et al. 1981). Nevertheless, in patients who are considered as candidates for amputation, distal bypass surgery should be performed even when the patency of the pedal arch is limited. Although distal arterial bypass insertion usually succeeds without any problem, arterial wall calcifications may complicate the bypass approach. On the other hand, the presence of vascular calcifications is not considered as a definitive contraindication to bypass (Ascer et al. 1986).

19.3.4.2.1
MR Angiographic Considerations

Because the main principle of bypass surgery is the reconstruction of a vessel segment with unrestricted inflow to a vessel segment with a free outflow, the determination of a suitable blind popliteal segment for bypass insertion requires comprehensive imaging of the associated collateral bed of the popliteal artery and accurate measurement of its length. The blind popliteal segment should measure 7–10 cm in length and be associated with a sufficient geniculate collateral system (Samson et al. 1999). Thus, the popliteal artery and crural arteries are the key vessels which have to be evaluated using pMRA in cases of limb-threatening PAOD because they are frequently targeted for bypass insertion. For imaging of the popliteal artery in SFA occlusion, 2D TOF MRA is not suitable because it may underestimate the patent length of popliteal artery in case of retrograde filling (Poon et al. 1997). The MR angiographic technique of choice, however, is CE pMRA because it

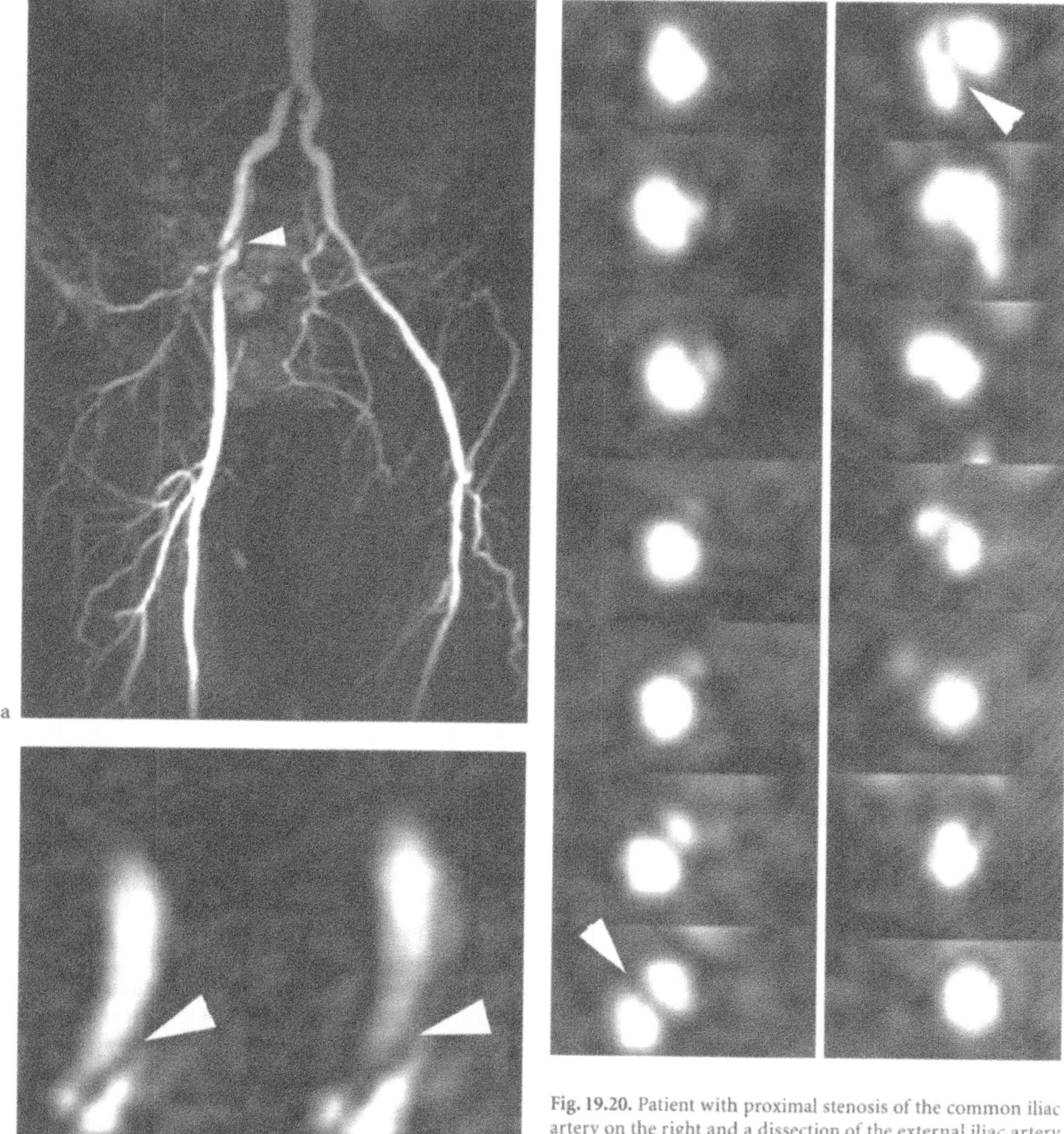

Fig. 19.20. Patient with proximal stenosis of the common iliac artery on the right and a dissection of the external iliac artery after PTA (**a**: 3D CE MRA MIP, high-resolution technique). The dissection can be detected on the MIP images; the exact extent is defined, however, only on the source image (**b**, *arrowhead*) and on the reformatted MPR images (**c**, *arrrowhead*). The turn of the dissection membrane and the distinction of the false and true lumen are only possible on the MPR image

better defines all of the patent segments if properly performed. Although CE pMRA has been shown to be useful in the diagnostic work-up of PAOD, indications for conventional angiography persist in acute limb-threatening severe arterial ischemia, which requires rapid intervention, in particular when catheter-guided low-dose fibrinolysis or endovascular thrombectomy is planned.

Osseous landmarks on MR images are important. These should include the hip (puncture site for PTA) and femoral condyles, tibial head, and the ankle in order to facilitate the surgical approach for an appropriate distal bypass insertion (Rofsky et al. 1999). Imaging of the run-off vessels is necessary if a bypass graft is planned so as to optimize long-term patency. As a prerequisite, tibial vessels should be patent in continuity with the popliteal artery, and there should be a free outflow to the pedal arch (Fig. 19.21). MR angiographic imaging of tibial and pedal circulation requires special anatomic knowledge of this vascular area because a misdiagnosis of poor pedal run-off may result in unnecessary interventions or suboptimal therapeutic results. For this reason, pMRA image resolution quality has to be optimized in the visualization of crural and pedal arteries. As the diameters of the lower leg and foot arteries range from less than 1 to 3 mm, a resolution of less than 1.5 mm in all three directions is required if the grade of stenosis is to be assessed accurately. In the literature, the MR angiographic approach to tibial vessels is described as being dominated by the use of 2D TOF techniques (Rofsky and Adelman 2000), particularly when the acquisition has been performed with head coils (Hoch et al. 1999; Cambria et al. 1993) or dedicated peripheral vascular phased-array coils (Kojima et al. 1995; Hoch et al. 1996), providing high-resolution imaging but with a smaller field-of-view. 2D TOF pMRA has been described as a reliable method in the detection of distal occlusions in calf arteries, sometimes being superior to i.a. DSA (Baum et al. 1995; Cortell et al. 1996; Glickerman et al. 1996). This advantage of 2D TOF MRA, however, may be coun-

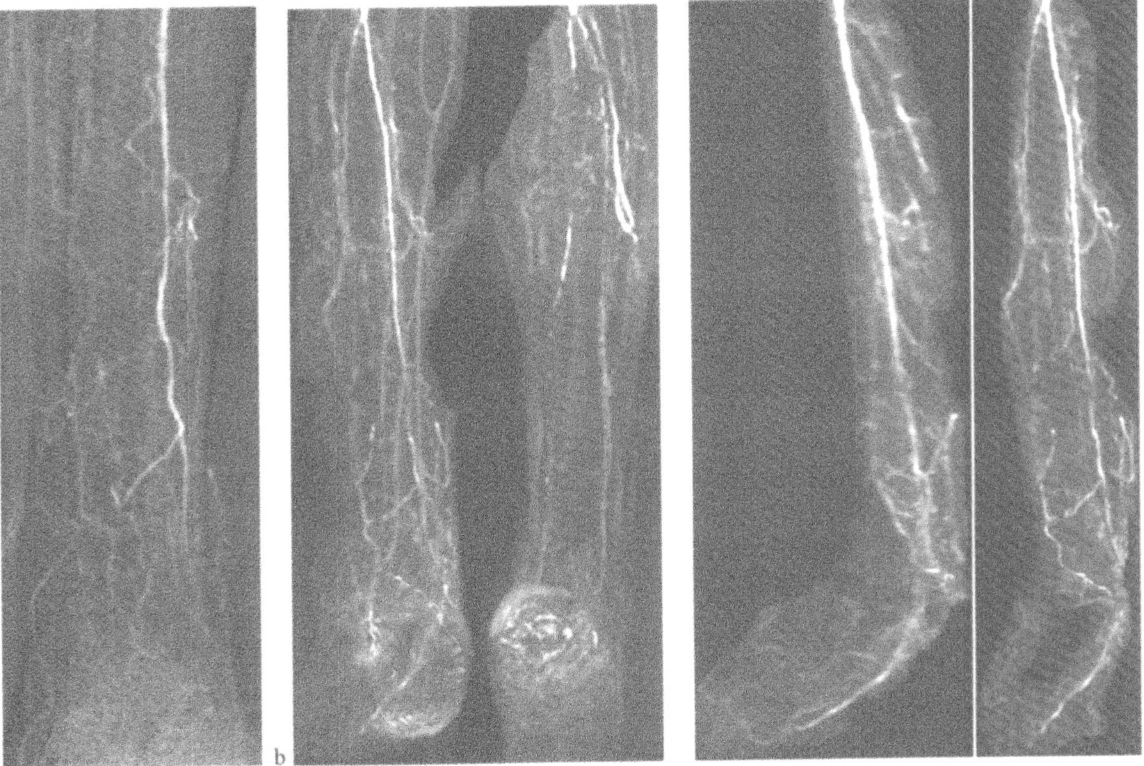

Fig. 19.21. i.a. DSA (**a**) of a patient suffering from diabetes mellitus for many years shows the difficult situation of searching for a bypass-linkable artery at the foot area. The evaluation of the 3D CE MRA (**b**, coronal outline MIP) is disturbed due to overlay of venous enhancement (a-v shunts due to ulcus cruris). Therefore, very selective MIP and complex segmenting of the 3D CE MRA data set were made, allowing a better evaluation. The sagittal and 30° MIP image permit a more exact and very good representation of the foot arteries, too (**c**). In this way a bypass-linkable artery could be found within the area of the plantar arch. The findings were confirmed intra-operative and the extremity was saved

teracted by its known drawbacks and by the fact that the standard quality of i.a. DSA has to be considered under optimized selective antegrade conditions which permit accurate depiction of occult distal vessels (Jacob et al. 1996).

Although the reliability of CE pMRA in depicting lower leg vascular lesions has not yet been proven in similar studies, preliminary results and personal experience show that, similar to i.a. DSA, this method is able to visualize all the run-off vessels, including the collateral net, the plantar arch, and the proximal digital arteries (Rofsky et al. 1997; Winterer et al. 1999). With CE pMRA acquisitions are faster and examination times decreased and the option of high resolution in all three directions offers further benefits. As the resolution in this vessel area should be 1 mm or less for the depiction of run-off prior to surgery, the use of body coils is not sufficient in this vessel area (Glickerman et al. 1996; Carriero et al. 1998). However, this can be realistically achieved by using a dedicated phased-array surface coil, a separate CM injection, and an acquired volume with very thin partitions. As a consequence, examination time will be prolonged and the single CM bolus must cover this longer acquisition time. Due to the lower signal-to-noise ratio, it may be necessary to administer a double or triple CM dose. On the other hand, under conditions of rapid venous return or the presence of arteriovenous shunts, arterial image quality can be optimized by a second CM injection and a separate acquisition of a 3D data set of the lower leg arteries using additional image subtraction (Fig. 19.22). In some cases, the additional application of 2D TOF pMRA has been shown to be useful in imaging the proximal foot region when CE pMRA of tibial and pedal vessels does not provide sufficient information.

MR imaging does not prevent problems that may occur when bypasses should be inserted at recipient vessel segments because of its inability to demonstrate vascular wall calcifications. In this regard, diabetic patients and patients undergoing dialysis more often present a problem.

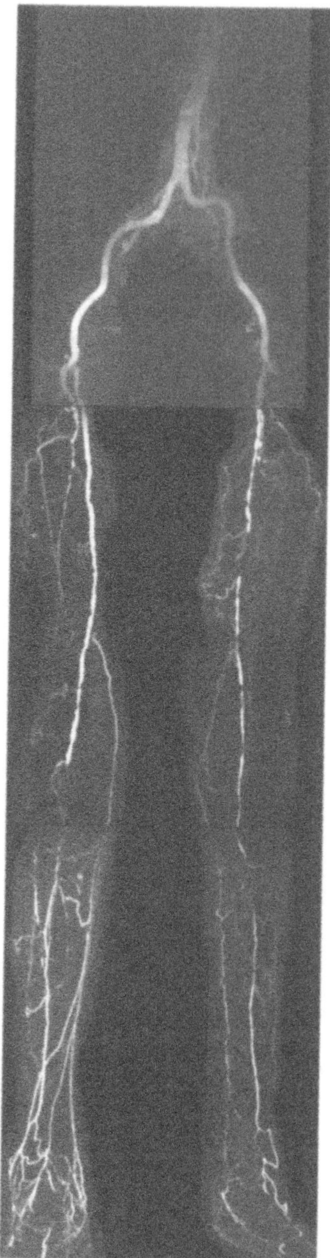

Fig. 19.22. A 78-year-old woman with PAOD (Fontaine IV) and diabetes mellitus. The pMRA (panoramic table technique with three-phase CM injection protocol) shows a complete occlusion on both sides at the level of the popliteal artery/tibial trunk. No sufficient collateralization was found by MRA. Due to chronic venous insufficiency and ulcers at the right side, a rapid venous return occurred after CM administration. The overlay of venous structures inhibits the judgment of the run-off at the right side

19.3.4.3 Diabetic Angiopathy

The incidence of lower extremity amputation is significantly higher in diabetic patients than in nondiabetics. Risk factors for foot amputation in diabetics include peripheral neuropathy, structural foot deformities, infection, ischemic tissue loss due to microangiopathy, and PAOD. Advanced surgical revascularization techniques in patients with limb-threatening ischemia require precise preoperative imaging of the peripheral vasculature.

19.3.4.3.1 MR Angiographic Considerations

As discussed in the previous sections, some studies have shown that, compared with 2D TOF MRA, i.a. DSA may fail to reveal occult vessels of the lower leg that are suitable for distal bypass surgery in patients with severe PAOD (Carpenter et al. 1992; Owen et al. 1992; Baum et al. 1995; Kreitner et al. 2000). More recently, CE pMRA has been recommended for evaluating arteries of the distal calf and foot in diabetic patients who were scheduled to undergo distal bypass surgery. In one of the current studies, CE pMRA was found to be significantly better than i.a. DSA in revealing peripheral run-off vessels and demonstrating occult pedal vessels suitable for distal bypass grafting in 38% of cases that were not depicted by DSA (Kreitner et al. 2000). However, as a bias of the study, in only 10 of 24 patients was a selective DSA performed, whereas in the other 14 subjects nonselective or fine-needle DSA was used. Apart from the problem of spatial resolution in CE pMRA, arterial overlap due to enhanced veins may be another problem leading to a reduced diagnostic image quality. Tissue necrosis, gangrene, and chronic venous insufficiency may induce the development of arteriovenous shunts that cause early venous CM return. Distal venous enhancement can be prevented by using short 3D data acquisition at the expense of a decreased number of partitions, resulting in a lower through-plane resolution. In addition, the k-space should be scanned in a centric order, enabling longer acquisition times without venous enhancement of veins as opposed to measuring the higher frequencies of the k-space at first. Using these options, acquisition times up to 40 s are possible, giving thin partitions of 1 mm, following the evaluation of bolus arrival time by a test bolus. When a time-resolved MR angiographic technique with a scan time of 18–25 s is used without any test bolus, a slight venous enhancement of 15%–20% can be observed (Kreitner et al. 2000). Other authors who also used a 2D time-resolved MR technique found that CE pMRA with image subtraction was superior to 2D TOF pMRA in the depiction of distal calf and pedal circulation without the appearance of overlaying veins (Lee et al. 1998; Lee and Wang 1998). Problems only occurred in the evaluation of the pedal arch, which however is considered as a prerequisite for planning distal bypass surgery in diabetic patients.

In diabetic PAOD patients, we prefer a combined MRA technique for the evaluation of the entire peripheral vasculature: Following a test bolus at the level of the knee and adding 5 s to define the bolus arrival time, a nonenhanced and a Gd-enhanced 3D data set of the distal calf and proximal foot region are acquired in the coronal plane. A total of 10–15 ml of CM is injected mechanically with an injection rate of 1.0 ml/s, centering the low frequencies of the k-space to the CM bolus arrival. After subtraction and image reconstruction the table is moved to the aortoiliac position. Using the bolus chase technique, two other 3D data sets of the aortoiliac and the femoropopliteal vascular region are acquired (Ho et al. 1998; Meaney et al. 1999). Although this procedure is a little more time consuming than the bolus chase technique alone, superimposition of venous vessels can be prevented in most cases.

19.3.4.4 Aneurysm and Other Pathologies

When claudication occurs in younger patients, it may be caused by anatomical anomalies which are occasionally a congenital. Entrapment syndrome (1%–3%), cystic degeneration of the adventia (1%–2%; Fig. 19.23), and aneurysmal disease (3%–7%; Fig. 19.24) of the popliteal artery can be observed in addition to atherosclerosis, which has already been discussed (Yucel et al. 1992; Kolb et al. 1997). Other causes of nonatherosclerotic lesions of the popliteal artery are very rare. Although in such cases CCDS is the primary diagnostic method in clinical routine, angiographic visualization of the involved vessels is needed in the majority of cases. As all the lesions mentioned above show typical perivascular findings, the use of slice scanning methods is preferred for accurate detection and evaluation. 3D CE pMRA can be recommended as the method of choice for evaluating the vessel wall, the extent of an aneurysm including thrombotic parts, and the existence of abnormal insertions of the gastrocnemius muscle heads as well as their relation to the popliteal artery (Sameshima et al. 1999). Thus, the MR technique as a single method is able to provide information about the vascular lesion, the perivascular space, and the adjacent soft tissue conditions that can be used to make correct therapeutic decisions.

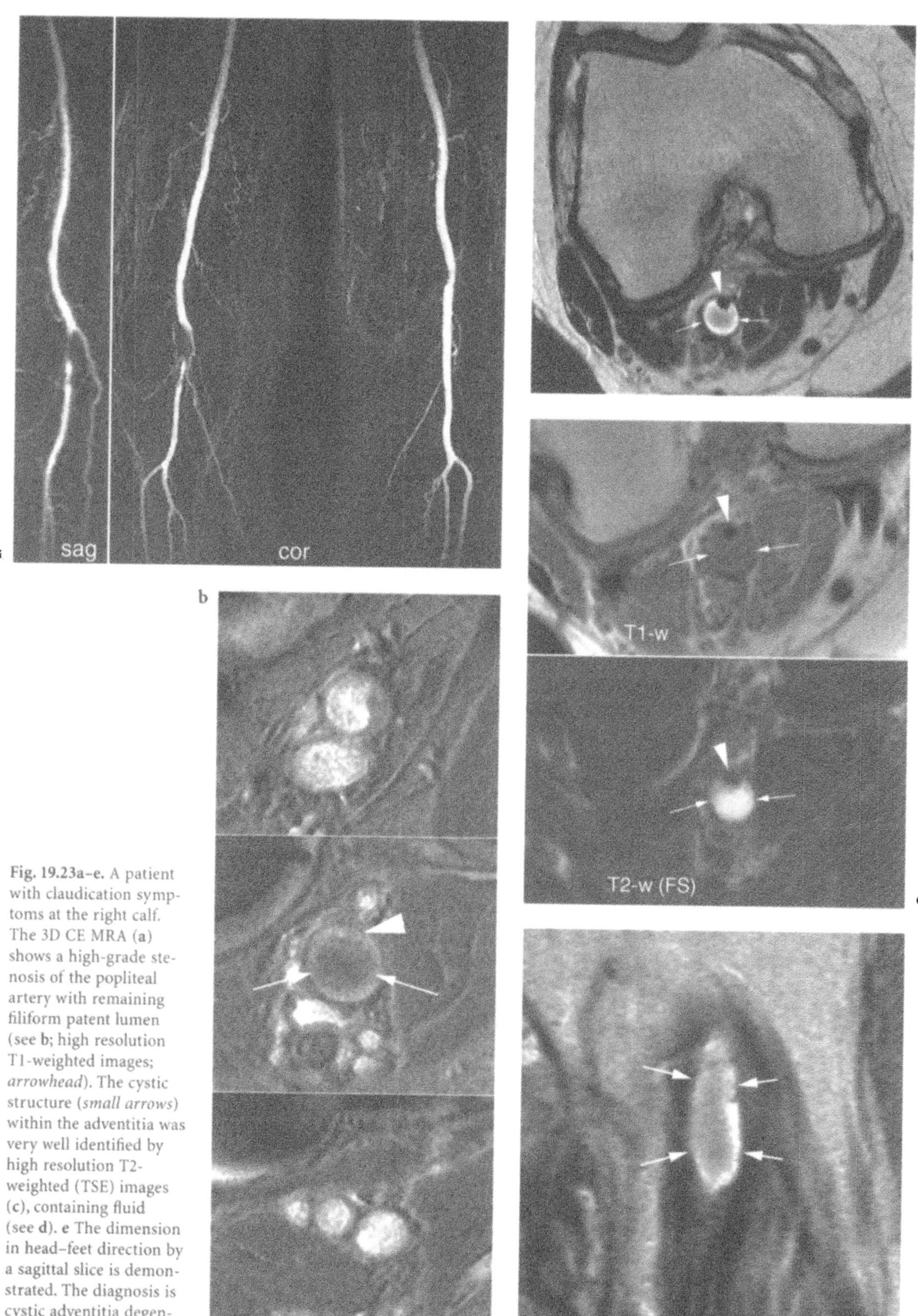

Fig. 19.23a–e. A patient with claudication symptoms at the right calf. The 3D CE MRA (a) shows a high-grade stenosis of the popliteal artery with remaining filiform patent lumen (see b; high resolution T1-weighted images; *arrowhead*). The cystic structure (*small arrows*) within the adventitia was very well identified by high resolution T2-weighted (TSE) images (c), containing fluid (see d). e The dimension in head–feet direction by a sagittal slice is demonstrated. The diagnosis is cystic adventitia degeneration

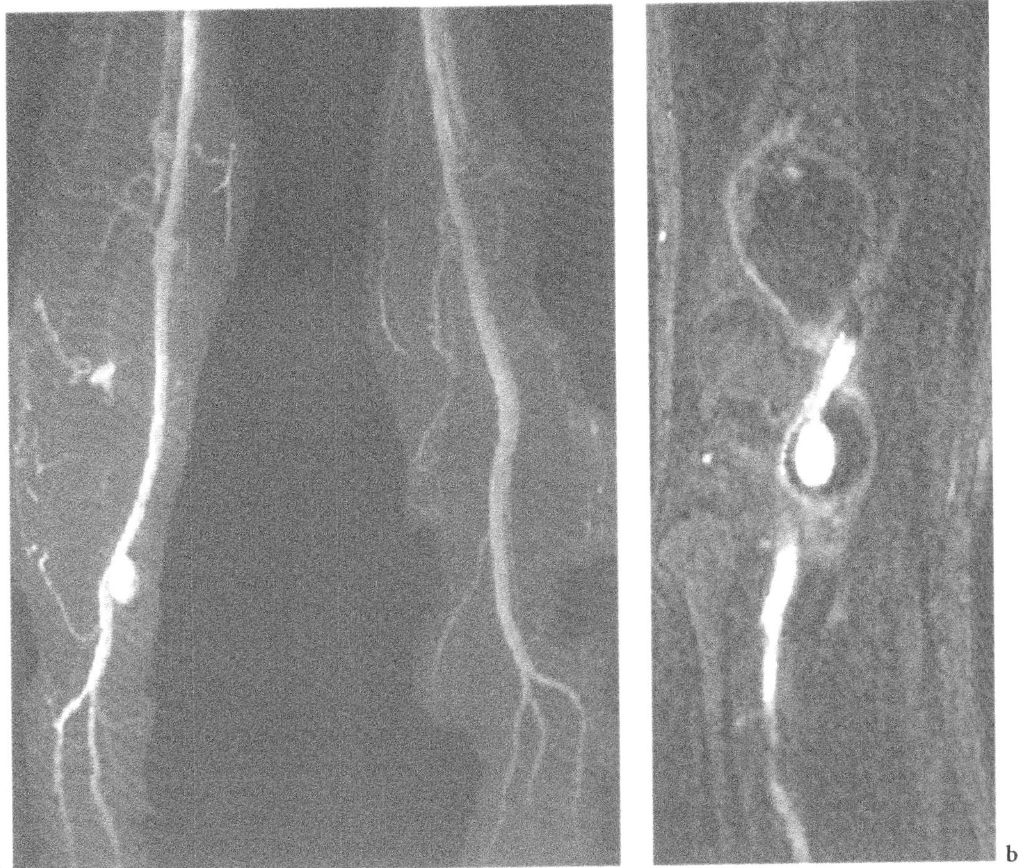

Fig. 19.24. The 3D CE MRA (**a**) of this patient shows a 2-cm perfused aneurysm. The real size of the aneurysm is 3.5 cm. The thrombotic part of the aneurysm (*dark*) can only be demonstrated by the source images (**b**)

19.4 Conclusion

3D CE pMRA is preferred over 2D TOF or PC MRA in the imaging of the lower extremity arterial system because this method is widely independent of flow signal and the problem of providing artifacts is fairly well solved. Using the CE 3D technique, the entire peripheral vascular tree can be visualized within a short acquisition time of only some minutes. Technical innovations improving both image quality and the ability to evaluate different segments of the peripheral arterial system have been established during the last 2 years. Sequence designs with short repetition times and echo times allow a further reduction of the acquisition time of the 3D data sets, the application of time-resolved MR angiography, and the acquisition of high-resolution angiograms. Increased temporal resolution may effectively eliminate venous enhancement, especially in the lower leg region. Dedicated lower extremity phased-array coils are able to improve significantly the signal-to-noise ratio and the contrast-to-noise ratio. Two types of MR angiographic applications are available today: the multistation technique and the dynamic table movement technique. Both methods have advantages and drawbacks, and more clinical experience is needed before making a conclusive evaluation of which technique is superior. Of particular interest is the highly resolved visualization of crural and pedal arteries on the basis of ce pMRA, which has to be standardized by reference to i.a. DSA. There have been rapid developments in ce pMRA over the last few years and the results to date are promising, suggesting that this MR technique will substitute conventional diagnostic angiography and i.a. DSA in the near future.

References

Adelmann MA, Jacobowitz GR (1998) Body MR angiography: a surgeon's perspective. Magn Reson Imaging Clin North Am 6:397–416

Amanuma M, Hirata H, Tanaka J, et al (1999) [Table-moving contrast-enhanced MR angiography of abdominal aortic aneurysm]. Nippon Igaku Hoshasen Gakkai Zasshi 59:760–764

Andros G (1995) Bypass grafts to the ankle and foot: a personal perspective. Surg Clin North Am 75:715–729

Andros G (1995) Bypass grafts to the ankle and foot: expanded role of arterial reconstruction. Surg Clin North Am 75:715–729

Armstrong DG, Lavery LA (1998) Diabetic foot ulcers: prevention, diagnosis and classification. Am Fam Physician 15:1325–1332

Ascer E, Veith FJ, Flores SA (1986) Infrapopliteal bypasses to heavily calcified rock-like arteries: management and results. Am J Surg 152:220–223

Barras JP, da Silva A, Widmer MT, Zemp E, Jäger K, Widmer LK (1989) Evolution de l'artériopathie précocement décelée – mortalité et causes de décès. Vasa Suppl 27:265

Baum RA, Rutter CM, Sunshine JH, et al (1995) Multicenter trial to evaluate vascular magnetic resonance angiography of the lower extremity. American College of Radiology Rapid Technology Assessment Group. JAMA 274:875–880

Boos M, Böttcher U, Brechtelsbauer D, Goyen M, Heuser L (1995) Clinical Potentials of phase contrast MRA, magnitude contrast MRA and high resolution MRI before and after PTA. Proc Soc Magn Reson Eur Soc Magn Reson Med Biol 1:541

Boos M, Scheffler K, Jacob A, Böttcher U, Bongartz G (1997) Development of a suitable clinical MRA protocol for planning and follow-up of PTA using 2D phase contrast, ECG gated 2D TOF and contrast enhanced techniques. In: Oudkerk M, Edelman R (eds) High-power gradient MR-Imaging, Advances in MRI II. Blackwell Science, Vienna, pp 365–371

Boos M, Lentschig M, Scheffler K, Bongartz GM, Steinbrich W (1998) Contrast-enhanced magnetic resonance angiography of peripheral vessels. Different contrast agent applications and sequence strategies: a review. Invest Radiol 33:538–546

Cambria RP, Yucel EK, Brewster DC, et al (1993) The potential for lower extremity revascularization without contrast arteriography: experience with magnetic resonance angiography. J Vasc Surg 17:1050–1056; discussion 1056–1057

Carpenter JP, Owen RS, Baum RA, et al (1992) Magnetic resonance angiography of peripheral runoff vessels. J Vasc Surg 16:807–813; discussion 813–815

Carriero A, Gatta S, Baratto M, Marano R, Aulisa R, Bonomo L (1998) [Angiography compared to high resolution magnetic resonance and digital angiography in atherosclerosis of the iliac-femoral arteries]. Radiol Med (Torino) 95:165–169

Cortell ED, Kaufman JA, Geller SC, Cambria RP, Rivitz SM, Waltman AC (1996) MR angiography of tibial runoff vessels: imaging with the head coil compared with conventional arteriography. AJR Am J Roentgenol 167:147–151

Criqui MH, Fronek A, Klauber MR, Barrettt-Connor E, Gabriel S (1985) The senisitivity, specificity, and predictive value of traditional clinical evaluation of peripheral arterial disease: results from noninvasive testing in a defined population. Circulation 71:516–522

Dagenais GR, Maurice S, Robitaille NM, Gingras S, Lupien PJ (1991) Intermittent claudication in Quebec men from 1974–1986: the Quebec cardiovascular study. Clin Invest Med 14:93–100

Dardik H, Ibrahim IM, Sussman B, et al (1981) Morphologic structure of the pedal arch and its relationship to patency of crural vascular reconstruction. Surg Gynecol Obstet 152:645–648

Da Silva A, Widmer A (1959–1978) Periphere arterielle Verschlusskrankheit: Frühdiagnose, Häufigkeit, Bedeutung, Verlauf. Beobachtungen bei 2630 Männern. In: Widmer LK, Stähelin HG, Nissen C, da Silva A (eds) Venen-Arterienkrankheiten, koronare Herzkrankheit bei Berufstätigen, Basler Studie I-III. Huber, Berne

DeBakey ME, Lawrie GM, Glaeser DH (1985) Patterns of atherosclerosis and their surgical significance. Ann Surg 201:115–131

Edelman RR (1992) Basic principles of magnetic resonance angiography. Cardiovasc Intervent Radiol 15:3–13

Foo TK, Saranathan M, Prince MR, Chenevert TL (1997) Automated detection of bolus arrival and initiation of data acquisition in fast, three-dimensional, gadolinium-enhanced MR angiography. Radiology 203:275–280

Fowkes FGR (1991) Epidemiology of peripheral vascular disease. Springer, Berlin Heidelberg New York

Glickerman DJ, Obregon RG, Schmiedl UP, et al (1996) Cardiac-gated MR angiography of the entire lower extremity: a prospective comparison with conventional angiography. AJR Am J Roentgenol 167:445–451

Hadley JR, Chapman BE, Roberts JA, et al (2000) A three-coil comparison for MR angiography. Magn Reson Imaging J 11:458–468

Hany TF, Leung DA, Pfammatter T, Debatin JF (1998) Contrast-enhanced magnetic resonance angiography of the renal arteries. Original investigation. Invest Radiol 33:653–659

Haustein J, Niendorf HP, Krestin G, et al (1992) Renal tolerance of gadolinium-DTPA/dimeglumine in patients with chronic renal failure. Invest Radiol 27:153–156

Hayashi H (1999) Composition of vascular tree using moving-table MR angiography: development and preliminary clinical experience with a semi-automated program combining stacks of MR angiographic images [in process citation]. Nippon Igaku Hoshasen Gakkai Zasshi 59:409–411

Henerici M, Rautenberg W, Trockel U, Kladetzky RG (1985) Spontaneous progression and regression of small carotid vessels. Lancet 1:1415–1419

Henry M, Amor M, Ethevenot G, et al (1995) Palmaz stent placement in iliac and femoropopliteal arteries: primary and secondary patency in 310 patients with 2–4-year follow-up. Radiology 197:167–174

Hertz SM, Baum RA, Owen RS, Holland GA, Logan DR, Carpenter JP (1993) Comparison of magnetic resonance angiography and contrast arteriography in peripheral arterial stenosis. Am J Surg 166:112–116; discussion 116

Ho VB (1999) Automated bolus chase peripheral MR angiography: initial practical experiences and future directions of this work-in-progress [in process citation]. J Magn Reson Imaging 10:376–388

Ho VB, Foo TK (1998) Optimization of gadolinium-enhanced magnetic resonance angiography using an automated bolus-detection algorithm (MR SmartPrep). Original investigation. Invest Radiol 33:515–523

Ho KY, de Haan MW, Oei TK, et al (1997) MR angiography of the iliac and upper femoral arteries using four different inflow techniques. AJR Am J Roentgenol 169:45–53

Ho KY, Leiner T, de Haan MW, Kessels AG, Kitslaar PJ, van Engelshoven JM (1998) Peripheral vascular tree stenoses: evaluation with moving-bed infusion-tracking MR angiography. Radiology 206:683–692

Hoch JR, Tullis MJ, Kennell TW, McDermott J, Acher CW, Turnipseed WD (1996) Use of magnetic resonance angiography for the preoperative evaluation of patients with infrainguinal arterial occlusive disease. J Vasc Surg 23:729–800; discussion 801

Hoch JR, Kennell TW, Hollister MS, et al (1999) Comparison of treatment plans for lower extremity arterial occlusive disease made with electrocardiography-triggered two-dimensional time-of-flight magnetic resonance angiography and digital subtraction angiography. Am J Surg 178:166–172

Huber TS, Back MR, Ballinger RJ, et al (1997) Utility of magnetic resonance arteriography for distal lower extremity revascularization. J Vasc Surg 26:415–423; discussion 423–424

Humphrey LL, Palumbo PJ, Butters MA, et al (1994) The contribution on non-insulin-dependent diabetes to lower-extremity amputation in the community. Arch Intern Med 154:885–892

Imarato AM, Kim GE, Davidson T, Crowley JG (1975) Intermittent claudication: its natural course. Surgery 154:795–799

Jacob AL, Stock KW, Proske M, Steinbrich W (1996) Lower extremity angiography: improved image quality and outflow vessel detection with bilaterally antegrade selective digital subtraction angiography. A blinded prospective intraindividual comparison with aortic flush digital subtraction angiography. Invest Radiol 31:184–193

Janka R, Fellner F, Requardt M, et al (1999) Contrast enhanced MRA of peripheral arteries with the automatic "floating table". Rontgenpraxis 52:15–18

Jonason T, Ringqvist I (1985) Factors of prognostic importance for subsequent rest pain in patients with intermittent claudication. Acta Med Scand 218:27–33

Jones L, Pressdee DJ, Lamont PM, Baird RN, Murphy KP (1998) A phase contrast (PC) rephase/dephase sequence of magnetic resonance angiography (MRA): a new technique for imaging distal run-off in the pre-operative evaluation of peripheral vascular disease. Clin Radiol 53:333–337

Kaufman JL, Whittemore AD, Couch NP, Mannick JA (1982) The fate of bypass grafts to an isolated popliteal artery segment. Surgery 92:1027–1031

Kojima KY, Szumowski J, Sheley RC, Quinn SF (1995) Lower extremities: MR angiography with a unilateral telescopic phased- array coil. Radiology 196:871–875

Kolb M, Guhl L, Arlart IP (1997) [Magnetic resonance tomography and magnetic resonance angiography in diagnosis of complicated popliteal artery aneurysm]. Radiologe 37:145–151

Kreitner KF, Kalden P, Neufang A, et al (2000) Diabetes and peripheral arterial occlusive disease: prospective comparison of contrast-enhanced three-dimensional MR Angiography with conventional digital subtraction angiography. AJR Am J Roentgenol 174:171–179

Lee HM, Wang Y (1998) Dynamic k-space filling for bolus chase 3D MR digital subtraction angiography. Magn Reson Med 40:99–104

Lee HM, Wang Y, Sostman HD, et al (1998) Distal lower extremity arteries: evaluation with two-dimensional MR digital subtraction angiography. Radiology 207:505–512

Lenhart M, Djavidani B, Volk M, et al (1999) [Contrast medium-enhanced MR angiography of the pelvic and leg vessels with an automated table-feed technique]. Rofo Fortschr Geb Röntgenstr Neuen Bildgeb Verfahr 171:442–449

Leung DA, Pelkonen P, Hany TF, Zimmermann G, Pfammatter T, Debatin JF (1998) Value of image subtraction in 3D gadolinium-enhanced MR angiography of the renal arteries. J Magn Reson Imaging 8:598–602

LoGerfo FW, Gibbons GW, Pomposelli FB, et al (1992) Trends in care of diabetic foot: expanded role of arterial reconstruction. Arch Surg 127:617–620

Long AL, Sapoval MR, Beyssen BM, et al (1995) Strecker stent implantation in iliac arteries: patency and predictive factors for long-term success. Radiology 194:739–744

Maki JH, Prince MR, Londy FJ, Chenevert TL (1996) The effects of time varying intravascular signal intensity and k-space acquisition order on three-dimensional MR angiography image quality. J Magn Reson Imaging 6:642–651

Maki JH, Prince MR, Chenevert TC (1998a) Optimizing three-dimensional gadolinium-enhanced magnetic resonance angiography. Invest Radiol 33:528–537

Maki JH, Chenevert TL, Prince MR (1998b) Contrast-enhanced MR angiography. Abdom Imaging 23:469–484

Martin EC, Katzen BT, F. BJ, et al (1995) Multicenter trial of the wallstent in the iliac and femoral arteries. J Vasc Interv Radiol 6:843–849

McDermott VG, Meakem TJ, Carpenter JP, et al (1995) Magnetic resonance angiography of the distal lower extremity. Clin Radiol 50:741–6

McPhail NV, Fratesi SJ, Barber GG, Scobie TK (1983) Management of acute thromboembolic limb ischemia. Surgery 93:381–385

Meaney JF, Ridgway JP, Chakraverty S, et al (1999) Stepping-table gadolinium-enhanced digital subtraction MR angiography of the aorta and lower extremity arteries: preliminary experience. Radiology 211:59–67

Murphy TP, Khwaja AA, Webb MS (1998) Aortoiliac stent placement in patients treated for intermittent claudication. J Vasc Interv Radiol 9:421–428

Nelemans PJ, Leiner T, Henrica de Vet CW, Joseph van MA (2000) Peripheral arterial disease: meta-analysis of the diagnostic performance of MR angiography. Radiology 217:105–114

Nelson KL, Gifford LM, Lauber-Huber C, Gross CA, Lasser TA (1995) Clinical safety of gadopentetate dimeglumine. Radiology 196:439–443

Nissen C, Schweizer W, Burkart F, Renngli I (1981) Koronare Herzkrankheit. In: Widmer LK, Stähelin HG, Nissen C, da Silva A (eds) Basler Studie. Huber, Berne

Owen RS, Carpenter JP, Baum RA, Perloff LJ, Cope C (1992) Magnetic resonance imaging of angiographically occult runoff vessels in peripheral arterial occlusive disease. N Engl J Med 326:1577–1581

Owen RS, Baum RA, Carpenter JP, Holland GA, Cope C (1993) Symptomatic peripheral vascular disease: selection of imaging parameters and clinical evaluation with MR angiography [see comments]. Radiology 187:627–635

Peabody CN, Kannel WB, McNamara PM (1974) Intermittent claudication: surgical significance. Arch Surg 109:693–697

Pentecost MJ, Criqui MH, Dorros G, et al (1994) Guidelines for peripheral percutaneous transluminal angioplasty of the abdominal aorta and lower extremity vessels: a statement for health professional from a special writing group of the Councils on Cardiovascular Radiology, Arteriosclerosis, Cardio-Thoracic and Vascular Surgery, Clinical Cardiology, and Epidemiology and Prevention, the American Heart Association. Circulation 89:511–531

Pomposelli FB, Marcaccio EJ, Gibbons GW, et al (1995) Dorsalis pedis arterial bypass: durable limb salvage for foot ischemia in patients with diabetes mellitus. J Vasc Surg 21:375–384

Poon E, Yucel EK, Pagan-Marin H, Kayne H (1997) Iliac artery stenosis measurements: comparison of two-dimensional time-of-flight and three-dimensional dynamic gadolinium-enhanced MR angiography. AJR Am J Roentgenol 169:1139–1144

Prince MR (1994) Gadolinium-enhanced MR aortography. Radiology 191:155–164

Prince MR (1998a) Renal MR angiography: a comprehensive approach. J Magn Reson Imaging 8:511–516

Prince MR (1998b) Contrast-enhanced MR angiography: theory and optimization. Magn Reson Imaging Clin North Am 6:257–267

Prince MR, Arnoldus C, Frisoli JK (1996) Nephrotoxicity of high-dose gadolinium compared with iodinated contrast. J Magn Reson Imaging 6:162–166

Prince MR, Chenevert TL, Foo TK, Londy FJ, Ward JS, Maki JH (1997) Contrast-enhanced abdominal MR angiography: optimization of imaging delay time by automating the detection of contrast material arrival in the aorta. Radiology 203:109–114

Prince MR, Anzai Y, Neimatallah M, Dong Q, Rubin JM (1999) MRA contrast bolus timing with ultrasound bubbles. J Magn Reson Imaging 10:389–394

Quinn SF, Sheley RC, Szumowski J, Shimakawa A (1997) Evaluation of the iliac arteries: comparison of two-dimensional time of flight magnetic resonance angiography with cardiac compensated fast gradient recalled echo and contrast-enhanced three-dimensional time of flight magnetic resonance angiography. J Magn Reson Imaging 7:197–203

Reimer P, Wilhelm M, Lentschig M, et al (1997) [Phase-contrast MR angiography of the lower extremity. Comparison of methods and clinical application]. Radiologe 37:572–578

Reimer P, Wilhelm M, Lentschig M, et al (1998) [Combined use of ECK-triggered 2D-phase contrast MR angiography and 2D-time-of-flight MR angiography for planning and follow up before and after vascular intervention of pelvic and leg arteries]. Rofo Fortschr Geb Röntgenstr Neuen Bildgeb Verfahr 168:243–249

Rodenwaldt J, Kopka L, Vosshenrich R, Fischer U, Grabbe E (2000) 3D MR angiography of the entire aorta: modified application of the body-phased array coil for a single-shot technique. Eur J Radiol 33:41–49

Rofsky NM, Adelman MA (2000) MR angiography in the evaluation of atherosclerotic peripheral vascular disease. Radiology 214:325–338

Rofsky NM, Johnson G, Adelman MA, Rosen RJ, Krinsky GA, Weinreb JC (1997) Peripheral vascular disease evaluated with reduced-dose gadolinium-enhanced MR angiography. Radiology 205:163–169

Rofsky NM, Morana G, Adelman MA, Lee VS, Krinsky GA (1999) Improved gadolinium-enhanced subtraction MR angiography of the femoropopliteal arteries: reintroduction of osseous anatomic landmarks. AJR Am J Roentgenol 173:1009–1011

Rutkow IM, Ernst CB (1986) An analysis of vascular surgical manpower requirements and vascular surgical rates in the United States. J Vasc Surg 3:74–83

Sameshima T, Futami S, Morita Y, et al (1999) Clinical usefulness of and problems with three-dimensional CT angiography for the evaluation of arteriosclerotic stenosis of the carotid artery: comparison with conventional angiography, MRA, and ultrasound sonography. Surg Neurol 51:301–308; discussion 308–309

Samson RH, Showalter DP, Yunis JP (1999) Isolated femoropopliteal bypass graft for limb salvage after failed tibial reconstruction: a viable alternative to amputation. J Vasc Surg 29:409–412

Snidow JJ, Aisen AM, Harris VJ, et al (1995) Iliac artery MR angiography: comparison of three-dimensional gadolinium-enhanced and two-dimensional time-of-flight techniques. Radiology 196:371–378

Steinberg FL, Yucel EK, Dumoulin CL, Souza SP (1990) Peripheral vascular and abdominal applications of MR flow imaging techniques. Magn Reson Med 14:315–320

Swan JS, Kennel TW, Wojtowycz MM, Grist TM (1993) Increased presaturation pulse gaps in two-dimensional time-of-flight MR angiography: a pitfall in diseased lower extremities. J Vasc Interv Radiol 4:569–571

Vierordt K (1855) Die Lehre vom Arterienpuls in gesunden und kranken Zuständen, gegründet auf eine neue Methode der bildlichen Darstellung des menschlichen Pulses. Vieweg, Braunschweig

Visser K, Hunink MGM (2000) Peripheral arterial disease: gadolinium-enhanced MR angiography versus color-guided duplex US – a meta-analysis. Radiology 216:67–77

Vogl TJ, Hoffmann Y, Muhler A, Felix R (1994) [Contrast medium enhanced MR angiography]. Radiologe 34:423–429

Vorwerk D, Gunther RW, Schurmann K, Wendt G (1996) Aortic and iliac stenoses: follow-up results of stent placement after insufficient balloon angioplasty in 118 cases. Radiology 198:45–48

Vosshenrich R, Kopka L, Grabbe E (1997) [Contrast medium enhanced MR angiography of peripheral blood vessels]. Radiologe 37:579–586

Vosshenrich R, Kopka L, Castillo E, Bottcher U, Graessner J, Grabbe E (1998a) Electrocardiograph-triggered two-dimensional time-of-flight versus optimized contrast-enhanced three-dimensional MR angiography of the peripheral arteries. Magn Reson Imaging 16:887–892

Vosshenrich R, Castillo E, Kopka L, Rodenwaldt J, Grabbe E (1998b) [Contrast media-enhanced 3D MR angiography of the peripheral vessels using a "tracking technique": preliminary results]. Rofo Fortschr Geb Röntgenstr Neuen Bildgeb Verfahr 168:90–94

Wang Y, Lee HM, Avakian R, Winchester PA, Khilnani NM, Trost D (1998a) Timing algorithm for bolus chase MR digital subtraction angiography. Magn Reson Med 39:691–696

Wang Y, Lee HM, Khilnani NM, et al (1998b) Bolus-chase MR digital subtraction angiography in the lower extremity. Radiology 207:263–269

Wedeen VJ, Rosen BR, Buxton R, Brady TJ (1986) Projective MRI angiography and quantitative flow-volume densitometry. Magn Reson Med 3:226–241

Westenberg JJ, Wasser MN, van der Geest RJ, et al (1999a)

Gadolinium contrast-enhanced three-dimensional MRA of peripheral arteries with multiple bolus injection: scan optimization in vitro and in vivo. Int J Card Imaging 15:161-73

Westenberg JJ, Wasser MN, van der Geest RJ, et al (1999b) Scan optimization of gadolinium contrast-enhanced three-dimensional MRA of peripheral arteries with multiple bolus injections and in vitro validation of stenosis quantification. Magn Reson Imaging 17:47-57

Widmer LK, da Silva A, Widmer M-T (1994) Epidemiologie und sozialmedizinische Bedeutung der peripheren arteriellen Verschlusskrankheit. In: Alexander K (ed) Gefäßkrankheiten. Urban and Schwarzenberg, Munich

Winterer JT, Laubenberger J, Scheffler K, et al (1999) Contrast-enhanced subtraction MR angiography in occlusive disease of the pelvic and lower limb arteries: results of a prospective intraindividual comparative study with digital subtraction angiography in 76 patients. J Comput Assist Tomogr 23:583-589

Yucel EK, Dumoulin CL, Waltman AC (1992) MR angiography of lower-extremity arterial disease: preliminary experience. J Magn Reson Imaging 2:303-309

20 Large Veins of the Body and Extremities

Anna Gerlach, Ingolf P. Arlart, Gabriel P. Krestin

CONTENTS

20.1 Introduction

The large veins of the extremities, the abdominal parenchymal organs, the retroperitoneum, and the mediastinum are responsible for the transport of deoxygenated blood back to the right atrium and the pulmonary arteries for it to become oxygenated again during the lung passage. Compared with the arteries of the body, the venous system shows a larger number of anatomic variants in vascular course and caliber. Venous blood flow and pressure conditions are completely different from those of arteries, leading to different specific pathologies. One of the main venous disorders is acute thrombosis most frequently located in the deep lower extremity and pelvic veins, which may be a serious and life-threatening complication when pulmonary embolism occurs. Thrombotic disease of the upper extremity and central mediastinal veins in the majority of cases is caused by temporary vein catheters or access devices. Occlusion of the vena cava is mostly due to extravascular tumor compression. Other lesions such as congenital malformations, varicose disease, and acquired abnormalities may also compromise blood flow in venous vessels. To cover all the clinically relevant venous disorders, a diagnostic tool with alternative imaging techniques has to be provided that is able to evaluate both the intravascular lumen of the veins and the perivenous space.

A. Gerlach, M.D.
Radiologisches Institut Stuttgart, Katharinenhospital, Kriegsbergstrasse 60, 70174 Stuttgart, Germany
I. P. Arlart, M.D.
Professor, Radiologisches Institut Stuttgart, Katharinenhospital, Kriegsbergstrasse 60, 70174 Stuttgart, Germany
G. P. Krestin, M.D.
Department of Radiology, University Hospital Rotterdam, P.O. Box 2040, 3000 CA Rotterdam, The Netherlands

20.1.1 Conventional Contrast Venography

Before noninvasive cross-sectional imaging modalities were introduced, conventional contrast venography was the main tool for diagnosing venous pathologies and it is still considered as the gold standard (Abrams 1983; Bettmann and Steinberg 1983; Rabinov and Paulin 1983; Ferris 1983, 1990; Naidich et al. 1988; Redman 1988). Although rarely, complications may occur in conventional venography, such as allergic and nephrotoxic reactions and intraluminal lesions due to catheter manipulations. Moreover, tissue necrosis after extravasation of the contrast material, postvenographic thrombosis, and pulmonary embolism have been described in association with peripheral venography.

In order to avoid potential risks for the patient, noninvasive methods such as *impedance plethysmography* and *radionuclide studies* have been introduced yielding variable results. Both techniques have not been proven sufficiently accurate to warrant the abandonment of venography (Hayt and Binkert 1990; Cronan et al. 1991).

Since ultrasonography has been introduced in the diagnostic work-up of veins permitting visualization of both intraluminal and perivascular disorders that may cause veno-occlusive disease, indications for conventional venography have changed. They have been restricted to those disorders in which ultrasonography is limited due to bowel gas, bone structures, and obesity. Thus, conventional venography is still indicated for visualizing detailed intraluminal changes, evaluating collaterals or venous malformations, clarifying equivocal findings made by noninvasive techniques, and when percutaneous interventional procedures are planned such as local fibrinolysis in acute occlusive disease, placement of vena cava filters in recurrent pulmonary embolism, balloon angioplasty, and implantation of endoluminal stents in chronic occlusive disease as well as catheter-guided in venous malformations.

20.1.2 Ultrasonography

Ultrasonography (US) as a real-time gray-scale technique, with or without a color-coding or continuous-wave Doppler technique, has a high accuracy in detecting venous thrombosis in the pelvis, thigh, and knee region, whereas sensitivity in detecting calf vein thrombosis is lower. On the other hand, some areas hidden to conventional venography can be evaluated, such as the deep femoral vein, internal iliac vein, and jugular vein. The function of venous valves can be well demonstrated by US. US has the capability of visualizing not only the vascular lumen but also adjacent soft tissue that potentially may compress the vein, such as hematoma, lymphocele, Baker's cyst, inflammation, or malignant tumors. US is often the first modality in evaluating renal transplant vascular drainage (Merritt 1992) and arteriovenous shunts (dialysis fistula or traumatic shunts) in the extremities. However, despite its advantages and the ability to provide both morphological and functional information, US does not have the potential of replacing conventional venography completely.

For instance, in the diagnostic approach of intrathoracic veins, US plays only a limited role due to anatomical and technical limitations.

20.1.3 Computed Tomography

Contrast-enhanced (CE) helical computed tomography (CT) is able to visualize venous structures with high accuracy. When a biphasic acquisition technique is used, second-phase imaging allows the evaluation of venous structures after contrast material is intravenously administered in both the abdominopelvic and the femoropopliteal region. Moreover, large veins of the proximal upper extremities and the central chest veins can be visualized directly with excellent image quality when the contrast agent is injected directly into both antecubital veins and immediate acquisition during a breath-hold is performed (Tello et al. 1993; Qanadli et al. 1999). Using this technique, CT angiographic images can be established on the basis of two- (2D) and three-dimensional (3D) reformatting algorithms. Thus, CE CT is accepted today as a modality for diagnostic imaging of intrathoracic, mediastinal, retroperitoneal, and pelvic venous structures, particularly when extravascular tissues have to be evaluated involving the venous system (Fishman et al. 1998).

20.1.4 Development of MR Venography

In the early 1990s, MR venography based on a 2D sequential time-of-flight (TOF) technique was already shown to be a reliable method that enables to visualize the venous structures of the body (Edelman et al. 1989; Arlart et al. 1991; Finn et al. 1993). By using presaturation of the arterial flow, selective pure MR venograms can be obtained. Moreover, perivascular space and adjacent soft tissue structures can be evaluated by cross-sectional MR imaging. This technique has been valuable over the years in the detection of abnormalities of the large veins of the trunk (Arlart 1997; Hartnell et al. 1995).

Although 2D and 3D phase-contrast (PC) MR imaging techniques are feasible in visualizing venous structures (Tavares et al. 1989; Dumoulin et al. 1990), these techniques have never been successfully introduced into clinical practice due to several limitations such as signal voids by artifacts and phase-dispersion and long examination times.

Using flow-sensitive MR techniques, successful functional qualitative and quantitative determination of blood flow velocities has been made possible (Mohiaddin et al. 1990; Debatin et al. 1995). 2D PC imaging is able to determine the direction of blood flow distinguishing craniocaudad from caudocranial venous flow (White et al. 1997).

When the contrast-enhanced (CE) 3D MR angiographic technique based on spoiled 3D GRE sequences was introduced, it was initially applied to image the arterial system (Prince et al. 1993). However, with growing experience CE 3D MR angiography was secondarily also used for imaging of veins. Recently published data on ultrafast 3D MR venography utilizing indirect (Lebowitz et al. 1997; Shinde et al. 1999) or direct (Li et al. 1998; Thornton et al. 1999; Ruehm et al. 2000, 2001) contrast enhancement of the venous system demonstrate a new diagnostic approach. With this technique, MR venograms of excellent quality, similar to conventional angiograms, can be established by using 3D reformation techniques and maximum intensity projection (MIP) algorithms. The development of blood pool contrast agents may have the potential of improving CE MR venography in the near future.

Currently, MR venography is capable of providing answers to a variety of clinical questions in venous diseases. However, it is not widely used and the feasibility of MR venography in the lower extremities has not yet been sufficiently proven compared with alternative methods that are well established for this region.

20.2 Technical Considerations of MR Venography

MR imaging has been proven to be able to provide an excellent visualization of venous structures, the delineation of abnormal vessels, and the relationship of veins to adjacent tissue. Thus, MR imaging using conventional sequences complementary to MR venography is recommended when extrinsic causes of venous occlusive disease are suspected. In these cases, T1- and T2-weighted images in transverse and coronal planes may be extremely valuable (Arrive et al. 1991; Sonin et al. 1992; White et al. 1997; Lutterbey et al. 1998) particularly when fat saturation is used that may optimize diagnostic accuracy. Non-enhanced conventional spin-echo (SE) or gradient-echo (GRE) techniques are sufficient, in many cases, to demonstrate the normal or aberrant venous and perivenous anatomy. However, on gadolinium-enhanced T1-weighted images acquired on the basis of a fat-saturated GRE sequence, intraluminal thrombi or tumor extension can be depicted with far better reliability.

20.2.1 2D TOF MR Venography

20.2.1.1 Chest and Abdominal Veins

Central chest veins and retroperitoneal venous structures can be visualized by using a flow-sensitive 2D spoiled GRE acquisition resulting in a stack of sequential images. MR venograms of the chest and upper abdominal region without blurring can only be acquired during suspended respiration, whereas veins of the lower abdomen and pelvis can be examined without breath-holding. Because venous flow is sufficiently steady during breath-holding, cardiac gating is not necessary and the presence of ghosting artifacts is not a problem. Flow compensation is routinely applied along the slice-select and readout directions. In the coronal acquisition plane, arterial flow signal and arterial phase-encoding ghost artifacts can be eliminated by application of an additional transverse presaturation pulse (5–8 mm presaturation band) through the supravalvular ascending aorta to create pure venograms in the mediastinum and the abdomen (Edelman et al. 1989). The major advantage of coronal slice acquisition is the visualization of the vascular anatomy over a large field of view up to 45 cm. In-plane saturation can be limited in most cases by a slightly oblique course of the vessels through the sections, and in the case of focal signal voids, inflow signal can be optimized by selecting additional acquisition planes perpendicular to the venous flow direction (Fig. 20.1a–c).

Using transverse multislice acquisition, the arterial flow signal can be eliminated by implementing a migrating parallel saturation pulse. This technique allows the acquisition of up to seven sections during a single breath-hold of approximately 30 s. Nevertheless, the acquisition time is prolonged due to the number of transverse slices when the entire vena cava and iliac veins are examined.

Analysis of both the source images and the MIP angiogram is mandatory for the accurate identification of a vascular lesion and its etiology. In addition, subvolume MIPs can reduce disturbing vascular overlap. Peristaltic motion can be reduced by the administration of glucagon or scopolamine-*n*-butylbromide. Optimization of signal-to-noise is possible using a multichannel phased-array coil. This equipment allows the display of even smaller veins especially when slice orientation is perpendicular to the course of the vessel. As a drawback of 2D TOF MR venography, perivascular fat may degrade flow con-

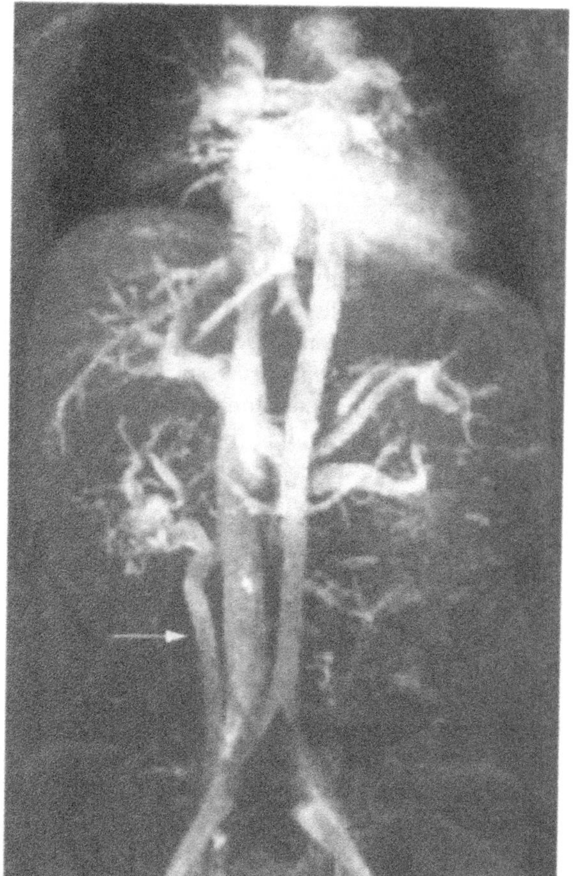
a

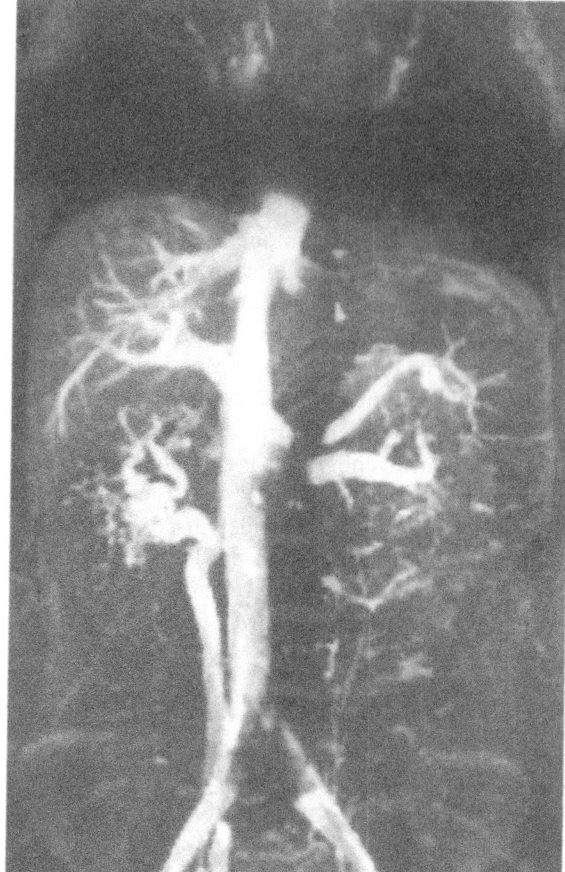
b

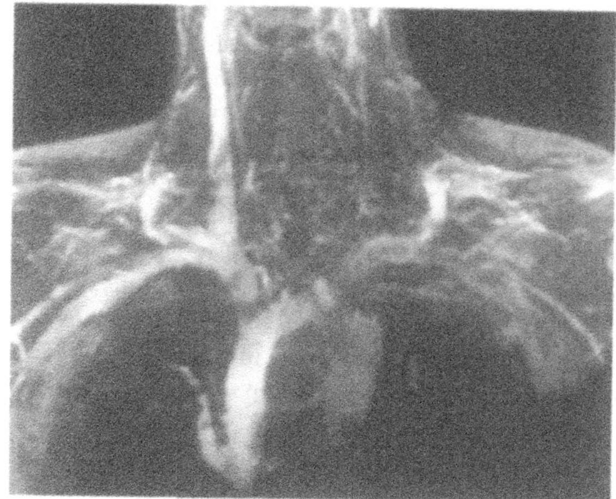
c

Fig. 20.1a–c. Normal individual MR projection angiogram on the basis of a coronal 2D TOF GRE FLASH sequence of the chest and abdomen without (**a**) and with (**b**) presaturation in order to obtain pure MR venograms. By localization of a presaturation band through the aortic root, arterial low signal can be eliminated in the abdomen (**b**) and chest (**c**). Note the atypical course of the right renal vein (*arrow*)

trast as well as ascites or perivascular hematoma containing methemoglobin.

20.2.1.2
Veins of the Pelvis and Lower Extremity

2D TOF MR venography of the pelvis and lower extremities does not require breath-holding. First-order motion flow compensation in slice-select and read-out direction, and a superior traveling saturation pulse should be applied to eliminate arterial flow signal. Using four series of multisectional sequential acquisitions in the transverse plane, the venous system from the inferior vena cava (IVC) through the popliteal veins can be covered. Sequence parameters suitable for 1.0-T MR equipment are presented in Table 20.1.

Table 20.1. Sequence parameters of 2D TOF MR venography of the pelvis and lower extremities (LAISSY et al. 1996)

Plane	Transverse
Field of view (cm)	35
Number of frequency-encoded steps	256
Number of phase-encoded steps	150
Repetition time (ms)	32
Echo time (ms)	8
Flip angle (degree)	40
Number of sections	40–50
Section thickness (mm) 1.5–2	Femoral 2–4, iliac
Number of excitations	2
Acquisition time (min)	7

Compared with lower extremity examination, a smaller section thickness should be selected for the assessment of pelvic veins, otherwise edge artifacts may be disturbing due to their oblique direction. The combination of 2D TOF sequence parameters with an off-resonance magnetization transfer contrast technique has been shown to be able to improve significantly the signal-to-noise ratio (YOSHIZAKO et al. 1996).

In order to improve visualization of calf veins, a variety of flow-enhancement techniques have been reported. Flow velocities can be increased by saline drip infusion before data acquisition (KÖNIG et al. 1997) leading to a more than 50% increase of the signal. A compression of superficial veins and diameter reduction of the deep veins using foam pads have been described by EVANS et al. (1993) utilizing the resultant accelerated flow for data acquisition. Venous flow volume can be increased by flow augmentation following venous occlusion of the thigh for 3 min (HOLTZ et al. 1996). The resulting augmentation of mean flow velocity improves the intravascular signal of deep venous structures. Immediately after termination of the flow-augmentation maneuver, MR venograms of the calf have to be acquired.

20.2.2 Other MR Venographic Techniques with Bright Signal

The True-FISP sequence, which can be favorably applied in the abdomen, is a T2-weighted 2D GRE sequence simultaneously utilizing a FISP and PSIF echo with three balancing echoes. During a single breath-hold of 15 s, six coronal sections in the abdomen can be acquired (TR/TE/flip angle/slice thickness=6.32/3.0 ms/70°/6 mm). Because of its rapidity and the ability of inherent flow compensation, vessels appear in the True-FISP sequence with bright signal. This phenomenon can be used for MR angiographic studies. MIP angiograms can be reconstructed from source images, non-vascular structures with bright signal can be eliminated using fat saturation. As a drawback, the true-FISP technique is sensitive to inhomogeneities of the magnet.

Another MR imaging technique, which is able to visualize particularly smaller extremity veins with slow flow, is based on a flow-independent heavily T2-weighted fast SE sequence, optimized for MR venography (BLUEMKE et al. 1997). Using a body coil, after transverse localizing images, the examination includes flow compensation of first-order gradient-moment nulling along a single axis and fat saturation. Acquisition of 20–30 coronal sections within 3-10 min at 1.5 T requires the following sequence parameters: TR/TE/slice thickness=6000–8000/50–300 ms/3 mm, echo train length of 16, 30–34 cm field of view, 256×256 matrix. The final high-quality MR venogram can be obtained in multiple projections by means of MIP techniques and multiplanar reconstructions. As a drawback, a prolonged acquisition time is necessary.

20.2.3 Contrast-Enhanced 3D MR Venography

To overcome the limitations of flow-sensitive MR venography, CE 3D MR angiography, which is widely accepted in arterial imaging, was also introduced for the imaging of veins (KRESTIN 1992; PRINCE et al. 1999). The administration of paramagnetic contrast material significantly improves the MR angiographic contrast-to-noise ratio particularly in vessels with slow flow, since shortening of T1 relaxation achieved by the contrast agent abolishes the signal loss due to saturation effects. Although flow-related dephasing artifacts are not completely eliminated in CE MR angiography (MARCHAL et al. 1990), the intravenous presence of gadolinium chelates allows excellent delineation of venous structures. CE MR venography can be performed in two different ways which are described in Sects. 20.2.3.1 and 20.2.3.2.

20.2.3.1 Indirect (high dose) 3D CE MR Venography

The use of indirect MR venography has been described by KAUFMAN et al. (1995) and LEBOWITZ et al. (1997) for the abdominal examination, and by SHINDE et al. (1999) for the examination of the upper extremities and central chest veins. Dynamic CE MR venography is performed using a spoiled 3D GRE sequence. The data sets have to be acquired during repetitive breath-holds when the chest and abdomen is examined, whereas no suspending of respiration is necessary for imaging of the extremity veins. The venographic phase following a CE arterial study can be selected indirectly by repetitive acquisition of 3D data sets (LEBOWITZ et al. 1997; SHINDE et al. 1999). Venous MR angiographic quality can be optimized by image subtraction technique. Twelve to 15 s after the primarily performed arterial imaging using a test bolus or preferably a sequence that automatically synchronizes 3D data acquisition with the arterial phase of the contrast bolus, the GRE sequence is repeated three to four times imaging both the arteries and veins. In the upper chest, the jugular veins are typically imaged in an earlier data set than the subclavian veins, brachiocephalic veins and the superior vena cava. In the abdomen, contrast material appears earlier in the renal and hepatic veins than in the IVC. The CE 3D data set with the best venous signal is chosen for subtraction from the arterial 3D data set to generate pure venograms that can be established by MIP algorithm. Because motion can degrade the subtracted data set especially in the abdomen and chest, identical breath-hold procedures are mandatory. For abdominal studies glucagon or scopolamine-*n*-butylbromide is advisable to minimize motion of the GI tract. Source images of the arterial, arteriovenous and subtracted data sets should be revised for image analysis. A 30-ml flush of saline is recommended following the power injection of contrast material by a machine which allows the precise application with a flow rate of 1.0 ml/s via the antecubital vein. The contrast dose chosen should be higher (0.3 mmol/kg) than in arterial MR angiography because of its dilution when passing the arteries and the capillary bed before the appearance within the venous system. Concerning the selection of contrast agent, in our experience gadolinium-BOPTA is more suitable for indirect angiographic imaging of veins than gadolinium-DTPA because its remains longer in the vascular system (Fig. 20.2a–c).

A representative examination protocol for application in the chest, abdomen, and pelvis is presented in Table 20.2 including sequence parameters useful for a 1.5-T MR unit.

20.2.3.2
Direct (low dose) 3D CE MR Venography

Direct CE MR venography displays all vessels containing T1-shortenting contrast material, regardless of the underlying flow characteristics. Thus, imaging along the vessel axis is possible, and the acquired 3D data set provides high spatial resolution which permits the delineation of small vessels. This technique can be employed to evaluate the deep and superficial venous system of the upper and lower extremities as well as the pelvic and the central chest veins (LI et al. 1998, THORNTON et al. 1999, RUEHM et al. 2000/2001).

Table 20.2. Sequence parameters of indirect CE MR venography

Plane	Coronal
Field of view (cm)	25–44
Number of frequency-encoded steps	256
Number of phase-encoded steps	192
Repetition time (ms)	5
Echo time (ms)	1.7
Inversion time (ms)	18
Flip angle (degree)	25–35
Number of sections	32–36
Section thickness (mm)	2–3
Bandwidth (kHz)	41–62
Number of excitations	0.5
Acquisition time (s)	16–20

20.2.3.2.1
Lower Extremity Veins, Iliac Veins, and IVC

For the lower extremity veins, iliac veins, and IVC, a surface coil is favorable, i.e., a multichannel quadrature phased-array peripheral vascular coil, which covers a territory of 3×44 cm with slight overlap. When the venous system of both extremities is examined, both dorsal veins of the foot are punctured, a tourniquet is wrapped around each ankle, and diluted contrast medium is continuously injected by hand or power injector with a flow rate of 1 ml/s (RUEHM et al. 2000, 2001). Dilution of the contrast material with saline in a ratio of 1:10–1:20 prevents T2* effects occurring in the veins and is cost saving. The contrast volume recommended is up to 240 ml to assure complete vein filling from the ankle up to the IVC. Data acquisition should be started approximately 60 s after beginning of the contrast infusion. Table movement is accomplished by automatic table translation. Image acquisition is performed with a 3D spoiled GRE sequence. Each 3D data set should be acquired twice, initially before contrast injection and in a repetitive study during contrast injection in order to obtain high-quality subtraction phlebographic images of the deep venous system. In order to image the superficial veins, the tourniquet has to be removed and the sequence has to be started once more. Parameters suitable for a 1.5-T MR unit are recommended in Table 20.2. For the calf veins, we prefer a higher spa-

a
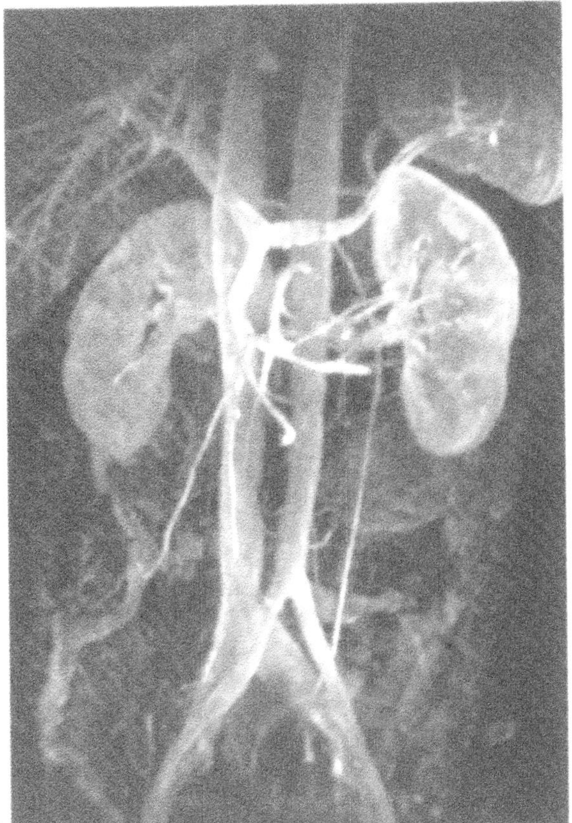

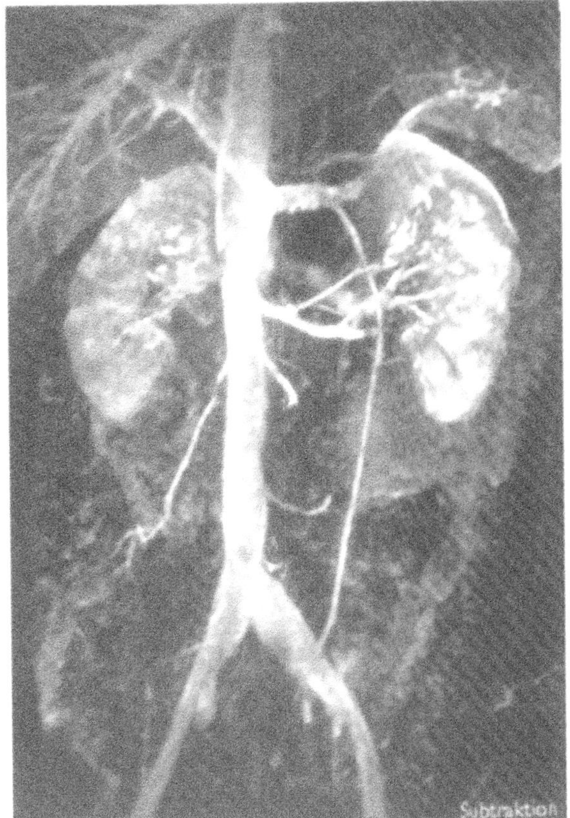

b

c
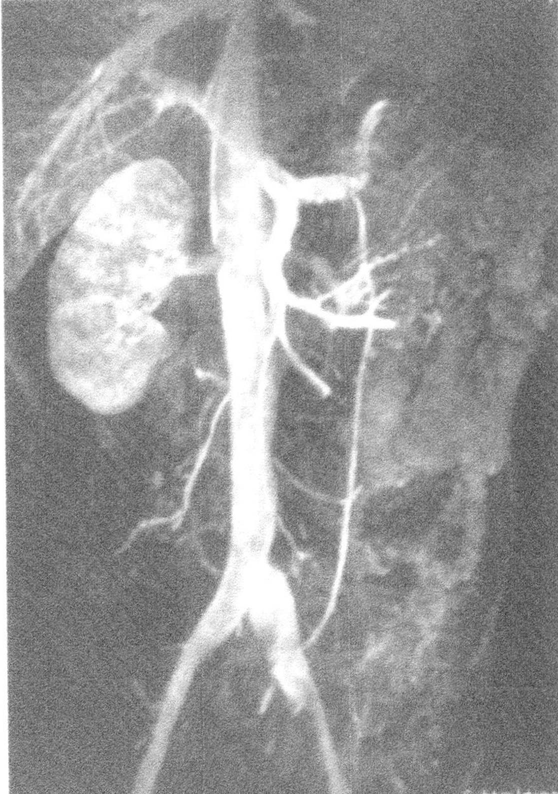

Fig. 20.2a–c. Normal individual indirect 3D CE MR venography of the abdomen. **a** Mixed arterial-venous phase. **b, c** Subtraction technique. The arterial phase data set is subtracted from the arterial-venous data set with the best venous signal. MIP reconstruction is performed and displayed in coronal and oblique views

tial resolution which can be achieved by increasing the number of phase-encoding steps to 512 and the number of excitations to 1, leading to prolongation of the acquisition time of up to 1 min. Source images have to be reconstructed using MIP and reformatting techniques in order to obtain MR venograms. Besides the MIP images, source images have to be evaluated, especially in thrombotic venous disease.

20.2.3.2.2
Upper Extremity and Central Chest Veins

In the MR angiographic imaging of upper extremity veins and central thoracic veins, two concepts have been reported in the literature. RUEHM and co-workers (2001) describe an examination technique similar to that reported for the lower extremity veins. The patient is placed in a prone position, his arms are elevated along the head, and the peripheral vascular coil is wrapped around the arms and head. In an alternative examination protocol (THORNTON et al. 1999), the patient is investigated in a supine position, 30–40 ml of gadopentetate-dimeglumine is injected unilaterally (affected side) by hand within approximately 15 s. Our own examination protocol includes parameters such as the supine position of the patient, the MR angiographic study of the affected side, the use of a surface phased-array coil with a field of view of 40 cm, and the application of 40 ml of diluted (1:10) contrast material by power injector with a flow rate of 1 ml/s. Contrast injection is followed by a 20-ml flush of saline. The delay from starting the injection to starting the sequence is about 20 s. If contrast in the SVC is not sufficient or both sides should be examined, both forearm veins are punctured and contrast material is administered simultaneously. When occlusive disease is suspected including slow flow collateral pathways, a repetitive study is recommended. An improvement of image quality can be obtained by the initial acquisition of a non-CE 3D data set that is subtracted from the CE 3D data set (SHINDE et al. 1999).

On the basis of a breath-hold 3D spoiled GRE sequence, the acquisition parameters useful for a 1.5-T MR unit are presented in Table 20.3.

Table 20.3. Scan protocol of direct CE 3D MR venography of the upper extremities and the central chest veins

Plane	Coronal
Field of view (cm)	40×40
Number of frequency-encoded steps	256–512[a]
Number of phase-encoded steps	192–256[a]
Repetition time (ms)	5.1
Echo time (ms)	2
Inversion time (ms)	20
Flip angle (degree)	35
Number of sections	32
Section thickness (mm)	3.2–2.0[a] (1.6–1.0 with interpolation)
Bandwidth (kHz)	31
Number of excitations	0.5–1[a]

[a]Forearm protocol.

20.3 Applications of MR Venography

20.3.1 Normal Anatomy and Variants

20.3.1.1
Upper Extremity and Central Chest Veins

As the main mediastinal vein, the superior vena cava (SVC) is formed by venous drainage of the head and neck and the upper extremities. The SVC and brachiocephalic veins have no valves. The second important venous system of the mediastinum includes the azygos and hemiazygos vein. At the level of T4 the azygos vein joins the SVC, and at the level of T8 the hemiazygos vein normally joins the azygos vein (KADIR 1986).

Congenital anomalies of the thoracic veins are infrequent often incidental findings. A duplicated and left SVC, respectively, is found in approximately 0.3% of healthy individuals and 4.4% of patients with congenital heart disease, representing persistence of the embryonic left anterior cardinal vein. The left SVC normally drains to the coronary sinus, which is typically enlarged in these patients. In a minority of patients this anomalous vessel drains to the left atrium, creating a right-to-left shunt. A left SVC is associated with absence of the left brachiocephalic vein in 65%, and absence of the right SVC in 10%–18% of cases, and may be associated with azygos continuation of the IVC. Isolated congenital anomalies of the right SVC are rare and include drainage to the left atrium, a low insertion of the vessel, and aneurysmal dilatation. Uncommon venous variants include absence of the left brachiocephalic vein with venous return of the left upper extremity through the left superior intercostal vein to the hemiazygos and azygos veins, and abnormal hepatic venous connection to the right or left atrium (WHITE et al. 1997).

MR imaging reliably provides the delineation of the central thoracic veins, its variants, and congenital abnormalities. Conventional T1-weighted SE sequence shows blood flow as a signal void and is sufficient for demonstrating the aberrant venous anatomy and vessel wall in most cases. Fast GRE techniques, which show flowing blood with high signal intensity, are useful to evaluate intraluminal blood flow (White et al. 1997). In normal volunteers, GRE MR venography based on a 2D TOF technique provides diagnostic quality images of the internal and external jugular veins, brachiocephalic, subclavian and axillary veins, and the SVC without variation of interobserver interpretations (Rose et al. 1996). In addition, PC MR images have been shown to be valuable for ascertaining the direction of blood flow and thus providing a physiological method of distinguishing normal from abnormal venous structures of similar location (White et al. 1997). Indirect or direct CE 3D MR venographic images of excellent quality can be obtained following systemic i.v. administration or injection of diluted contrast material into the antecubital veins revealing images similar to conventional venography (Shinde et al. 1999; Thornton et al. 1999).

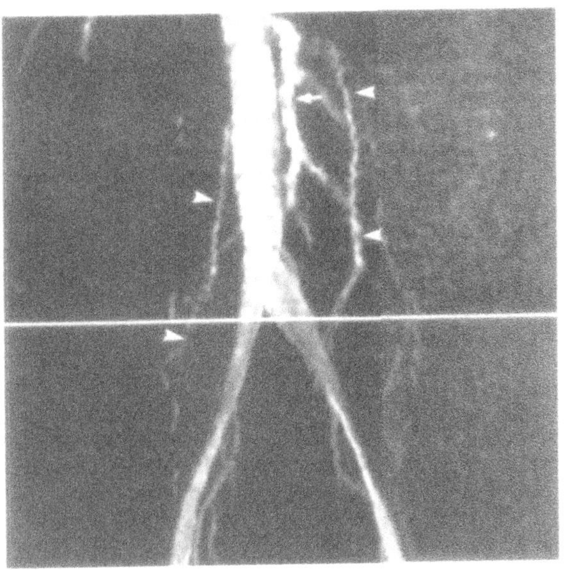

Fig. 20.3. Normal 2D TOF MRA of pelvic and lower abdominal veins (combination of two acquisition volumes) in a woman in the postpartum period showing the iliac veins (external, internal, and common), the inferior vena cava, the distal superior mesenteric vein (*arrow*), and the patent ovarian veins (*arrowheads*) draining into the inferior vena cava on the right and into the renal vein on the left. The renal veins are not visualized due to in-plane saturation effects

20.3.1.2
IVC and Its Tributaries. Pelvic Veins

The main tributaries of the IVC are the left and right common iliac vein, the renal and lumbar veins, the right gonadal, right adrenal, inferior phrenic vein, and the hepatic veins. In the pelvis, the internal iliac veins receive the venous drainage of the gluteal, the internal pudendal, and the obturator veins and merge with the external iliac veins to form the common iliac veins. Testicular and ovarian veins drain at a higher level. During pregnancy and in the postpartum period, ovarian veins may be markedly enlarged. The left spermatic vein may be enlarged in varicocele disease.

Variations in venous topography are common in the IVC, but relatively rare in the pelvis. Congenital anomalies of the IVC reported in the literature can be classified into five groups:

1. Transposition of the IVC (0.2%–0.5%) due to persistence of the left supracardinal vein
2. Duplication of the IVC (1%–3%) due to persistence of both supracardinal veins (Fig. 20.3)
3. Circumaortic venous ring (8.7%)
4. Retroaortic left renal vein (1.8%–2.4%)
5. Absence of the hepatic segment with azygos continuation (0.6%)

Occasionally, a left single renal hilar vein bifurcates before entering the IVC. Multiple renal veins are seen in approximately 28% of individuals (Kadir 1986; Sonin et al. 1992). Knowledge on duplications and transpositions of the IVC as well as on the circumaortic and retroaortic left renal vein is important before performing retroperitoneal surgery. In particular, duplications of the deep venous trunks have to be considered in order to assess accurately thrombotic occlusion of only one branch.

US (Derchi et al. 1991), helical CT (Trigaux et al. 1998), and conventional SE MR imaging (Friedland et al. 1992) are able to visualize normal findings and congenital anomalies of the IVC and its tributaries including the pelvic veins. Compared with SE MR imaging, GRE MR venography has been shown to be superior in the evaluation of retroperitoneal venous structures (Edelman et al. 1989; Arlart et al. 1992). All anatomical variants and abnormalities can be clearly detected on MR venograms and normally do not require further examinations (Finn et al. 1993; Friedland et al. 1992). In the pelvis, common, external, and internal iliac veins can be adequately visualized in all patients by inflow MR venography (Gehl et al. 1990; Richter et al. 1993; Siewert et al. 1992). Even the branches of the internal iliac vein are detectable in 60% (pudendal veins) to 90% (gluteal veins) of cases. The normal testicular and ovarian veins are usually depicted only in their proximal third. Visualization is better on the right side, where drainage occurs directly into the IVC, than on the left side, where these veins empty into the left renal vein. These normal vascular structures can be visualized regardless of the position of the patient (RICHTER et al. 1993). However, artifacts that may occur in inflow MR venography have to be considered, such as short areas of signal loss of the left common iliac vein due to compression by the overlying artery (LANZER et al. 1991), low or inhomogeneous signal due to a common slow flow condition, inhomogeneities of the signal at the junction of large veins due to flow turbulences (GEHL et al. 1990), and signal voids in the large iliac veins and the IVC due to flow reversal during respiration and flow stasis during Valsalva maneuver.

In particular, indirect CE 3D MR angiographic techniques are able to provide accurate depiction of the renal veins and IVC without loss of signal from saturation of in-plane flow (PRINCE et al. 1993; KAUFMAN et al. 1995) promising a further improvement in the MR angiographic evaluation of these vascular structures.

20.3.1.3
Lower Extremity Veins

The veins of the lower extremities can be classified into three categories: deep veins including the main trunks and muscle veins, superficial veins, and perforating veins.

The deep veins are enclosed by the deep fascia. The three main pairs of deep veins (anterior tibial, posterior tibial, and peroneal) of the calf form the popliteal vein, which may be paired in up to 20% of individuals. Multiple muscle veins (soleus, gastrocnemius) empty into the posterior tibial, peroneal, or popliteal veins. The superficial femoral vein and the profunda femoris vein drain into the common femoral vein at the level of the groin. The lesser saphenous vein drains into the popliteal vein, the greater saphenous vein into the femoral vein at the level of the groin. Above this level, superficial veins play a clinical role only as collaterals following obstruction of the deep trunks. The perforating veins of the lower extremities penetrate through the deep fascial planes and connect the deep veins with the superficial veins allowing the blood flow normally only from the superficial to the deep veins.

When using inflow MR angiography for imaging the veins of the lower extremity, specific characteristics of the anatomy and blood flow have to be considered. It has been demonstrated to be reliable in the visualization of venous structures in the pelvis and in the limbs above the knee including the greater saphenous vein. However, this technique shows problems in accurately depicting deep veins below the knee, although improvements of the examination technique have been recommended (HOLTZ et al. 1996) using flow augmentation. MR imaging on the basis of an optimized heavily T2-weighted fast SE sequence has been described to allow a routinely good depiction of venous anatomy of the calf with relatively high resolution (BLUEMKE et al. 1997). Using indirect gadolinium-enhanced subtraction MR venography of the pelvis and lower extremity initialized by LEBOWITZ et al. (1997) routinely, high-quality and high-resolution images of the venous system with excellent suppression of the background signal have been reported. Since the introduction of direct CE 3D MR venography by bilateral pedal administration of the contrast material, the problems of inflow MR venography seem to have been widely solved, and excellent visualization of both the deep and superficial venous system of the limbs has been reported (LI et al. 1998; RUEHM et al. 2000) comparable to that of conventional venograms. Even small vessels have been delineated in the calf as well as perforating and superficial veins containing slow or even retrograde flowing blood, resulting in the assessment of the status of the greater and lesser saphenous vein being 98% sensitive and 92% specific (RUEHM et al. 2000).

20.3.2
Pathologies

20.3.2.1
Upper Extremity and Central Chest Veins

Although occlusive disease of the subclavian veins, the brachiocephalic veins, and the SVC accounts for only 1%–2% of overall deep venous thromboses, this disorder plays an important clinical role, whereas thrombotic disease of peripheral veins normally has no clinical relevance. In approximately 40% of cases the most common cause of central vein thrombosis is due to temporary vein catheters or access devices for hemodialysis, drug or chemotherapy infusion, and hyperalimentation (Fig. 20.4). Other less common causes include idiopathic thrombosis, hyperviscosity syndromes, local trauma and compression of the vascular lumen. Central mediastinal veins are slightly compressible due to the thin-walled anatomy and low intraluminal pressure. Thus, these veins can be occluded by several extrinsic factors such as tumor compression or

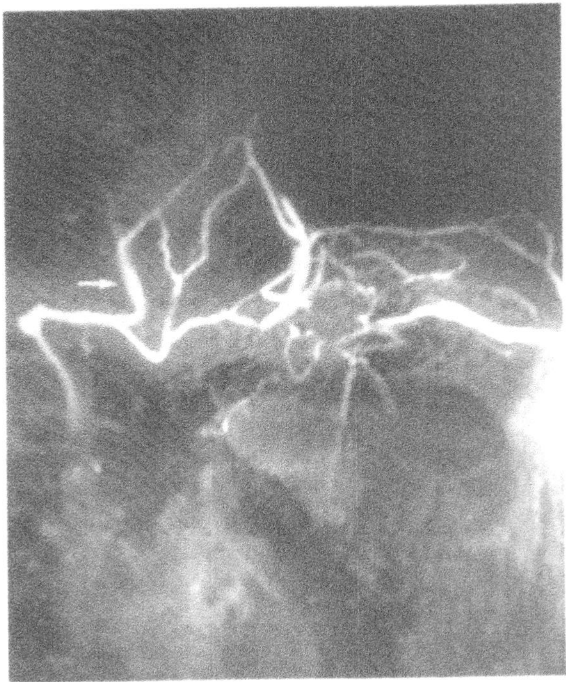

Fig. 20.4. Direct low-dose 3D CE MR venography. A 29-year-old male patient with implanted port system for chemotherapy that led to occlusion of the subclavian, brachiocephalic and left jugular vein with collaterals to the right external jugular vein (*arrow*)

tumor infiltration of the venous wall in rare cases, and most commonly by compression due to preexisting pathoanatomical narrowing of the thoracic inlet.

20.3.2.1.1 Thoracic Inlet Syndrome

In *thoracic inlet syndrome (TIS)* the subclavian vein is typically compressed at the costoclavicular triangle, in rare cases at the interscalene triangle and the subcoracoid space. Because the complete upper extremity neurovascular bundle traverses these narrow spaces, a combined appearance of TIS and thoracic outlet syndrome has been observed. The compression of the subclavian vein may be provoked by hyperabduction of the arm, resulting in acute thrombosis due to mechanical involvement of the vessel wall on the basis of chronic microtrauma of the vascular intima (Fig. 20.5a, b). In patients with thrombotic occlusion of the subclavian or brachiocephalic vein, clinical symptoms may include paresthesias, painless or painful swelling of the arm, and superficial venous collaterals at the upper arm and shoulder as well as at the lateral thorax. The symptoms are limited to the involved extremity and are far less severe than those of superior vena cava syndrome.

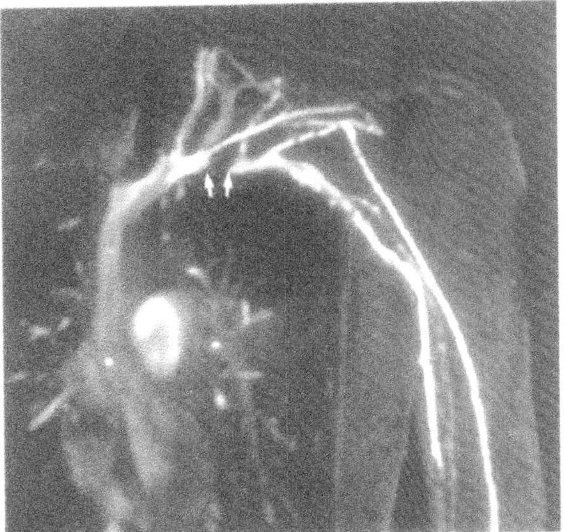

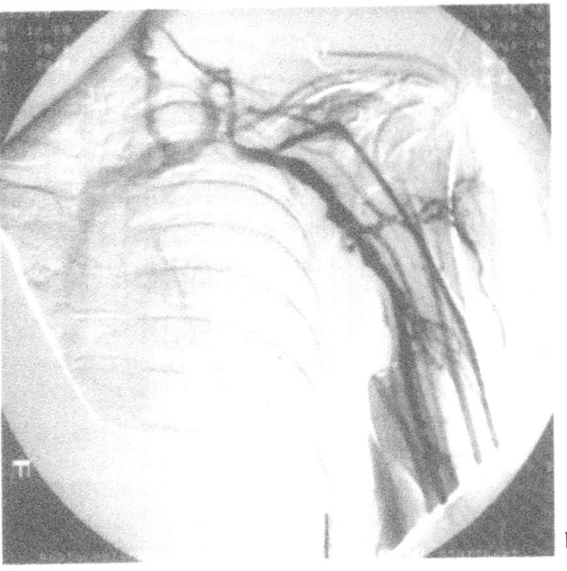

Fig. 20.5a, b. A 20-year-old female with swelling of the left arm. **a** Low-dose direct 3D CE MR venography of the left axilla and the thoracic inlet. Occlusion of the subclavian vein at the costoclavicular triangle (*arrows*), collaterals to the neck veins. **b** Digital subtraction venography of the same patient with good correlation to the MRV

In patients undergoing hemodialysis, venous obstruction can occur anywhere along the venous outflow tract, which extends from the venous anastomosis of the hemodialysis graft to the SVC, and appears as stenotic disease in the majority of cases. Apart from puncture trauma of the shunt veins, it is suspected that elevated intraluminal pressure in the arterialized vein may support the development of central stenotic disease. This venous obstruction is a common cause of access dysfunction and thrombosis. The therapeutic regimen of TIS associated with thrombotic occlusion of the subclavian vein includes conservative treatment with heparin, and systemic or local fibrinolysis in acute states (Sheeran et al. 1997; Kee et al. 1998). In subacute states endovascular recanalization procedures are useful (Kee et al. 1998) and should be combined with an operative resection of the first rib in order to remove the causal factor of compression. Thereby, self-expanding endoluminal metallic stent placement has been shown to be superior to simple percutaneous balloon angioplasty (Vesely et al. 1997). Direct surgical treatment of the diseased deep thoracic veins is of limited value due to high morbidity.

20.3.2.1.2 Superior Vena Cava Syndrome

Compared with TIS, clinical symptoms of the *superior vena cava syndrome (SVCS)* are more dramatic and demonstrate a characteristic appearance. The classical constellation of clinical findings associated with SVCS includes facial, periorbital, neck, and bilateral arm swelling, cyanosis and dilated superficial veins over the chest wall. Although SVCS is rarely life-threatening, it is often associated with distressing complications such as dysphagia, dyspnea, and cognitive dysfunction due to cerebral venous hypertension. The severity of clinical symptoms of central venous obstruction depends on its site and degree, and the development of collateral pathways in chronic states including suprascapular, lateral thoracic, internal thoracic, and intercostal veins to the azygos/hemiazygos system. More than 85% of SVCS cases are due to an underlying malignancy, either primary thoracic malignancy, lymphoma, or metastatic tumor, with an obstruction caused by tumor invasion or extrinsic compression of the SVC. Up to 15% of patients with mostly small-cell bronchogenic carcinoma and 20% with malignant lymphomas may develop SVCS. Metastatic disease to the thorax is seen in a variety of solid tumors, with breast and testicular cancer having the highest frequency. In approximately 15% of cases, SVCS has a benign cause, with the frequency increasing recently due to the more frequent use of the central veins for vascular access. Benign causes include compression from granulomatous or fibrosing mediastinitis, thoracic aortic aneurysm, pericardial disorders, dermoid or bronchogenic cysts, substernal goiter, hematoma, and thrombosis secondary to invasive cardiac pacemaker electrodes, pulmonary artery and central venous monitoring catheters, or vascular access devices for hyperalimentation, chemotherapy, and infusion of fluids and antibiotics (Hirsh et al. 1986; White et al. 1997).

Surgical management of SVCS necessitates open sternotomy, is invasive and usually limited to patients with benign disease, while malignant disease involving the SVC is associated with a poor prognosis. However, palliative treatment with radiation therapy alone or in combination with chemotherapy may provide symptomatic relief. Common side effects include dysphagia, nausea, and vomiting. General medical treatment such as systemic anticoagulation, steroids, and diuretic therapy has limited clinical benefit and is restricted to alleviating symptoms after other treatments have been unsuccessful. Catheter-directed thrombolysis with endovascular stent placement has been shown to be a safe and effective treatment for SVCS in both benign and malignant disease (Gross et al. 1997; Nicholson et al. 1997; Kee et al. 1998).

When clinically symptomatic acute central venous obstruction occurs, it demands a rapid diagnostic evaluation in order to institute suitable management strategies. Furthermore, since more and more hospitalized patients depend on chronic indwelling central venous access lines for total parenteral nutrition and drug delivery, in cases with multiple sites of central venous occlusion and their resultant complex drainage patterns, it is of importance to find out which central venous access sites have remained patent with adequate size, and to require precise determination of the underlying pathology. Radiological diagnostic work-up includes a variety of methods such as conventional venography, duplex Doppler US, contrast-enhanced CT, and MR imaging in order to clarify the site and severity of venous obstruction and to detect vessels accessible to cannulation.

Conventional Venography

Conventional venography of the central chest veins, considered as the gold standard, allows an evaluation of the site and extent of venous occlusion (Benenati et al. 1986) to be made by uni- or bilateral contrast injection via the antecubital veins. The method is time- and highly spatial-resolved, which allows a reliable visualization of collateral circulation and even the depiction of discrete abnormalities of the vessel wall present in postthrombotic disease. Drawbacks of contrast venography include the inability to visualize extraluminal processes that may cause the occlusion, radiation exposure to the patient, and potential side effects of the contrast material.

Ultrasonography

The advances of noninvasive US in gray-scale resolution and color Doppler technology permit direct visualization of thrombus, stenoses, occlusions, and collateral vessels as well as sensitive spectral waveform analysis. Sonographic results are excellent for peripheral veins. Abnormal findings in the thoracic inlet include locally elevated velocities at stenoses with low velocities peripherally (NAZARIAN and FOSHAGER 1995). The sensitivity and specificity of color-coded duplex Doppler US in detecting axillary and subclavian vein thrombosis is reported to range from 92% to 100% (BAXTER et al. 1991; LONGLEY et al. 1992). Although duplex US is technically limited in the direct evaluation of central thoracic veins (HAIRE et al. 1991) due to constraints created by the clavicle, rib cage, and sternum, abnormal cardiac pulsatility and respiratory phasicity can be used as an indirect predictor of complete central venous occlusion, particularly when the lesion cannot be visualized directly (PATEL et al. 1999). Potential pitfalls of US are abnormal waveforms seen with deep inspiration or snoring, slow flow mimicking a thrombus, confusion of a collateral vein with the subclavian vein, and turbulent flow from indwelling catheters or ipsilateral hemodialysis fistulas (NAZARIAN and FOSHAGER 1995).

CT Venography

CE helical CT gives excellent mediastinal soft-tissue details, and the limitations of conventional axial imaging have been overcome with helical CT venographic imaging of the central thoracic veins on the basis of reconstruction modalities. Thus, CT venography has become an important approach in the evaluation of upper chest veins when occlusive disease is suspected (TELLO et al. 1993). In addition, CT-guided fine-needle aspiration biopsy offers the advantage of a percutaneous technique with low morbidity and high accuracy. CT venography is simple to perform by simultaneous bilateral injection of iodinated contrast material via antecubital veins, and can directly provide all the information necessary to diagnose and treat obstruction of the SVC and its tributaries (QANADLI et al. 1999). As a drawback, CT suffers from artifacts caused by flow turbulences within the central veins, and has unwanted side effects due to a relatively high radiation dose of the spine and the contrast material.

MR Venography

MR imaging of the upper mediastinum using a conventional SE sequence is able to depict extravascular disorders which may obstruct the SVC as accurately as single-slice CT (WEINREB et al. 1986). Compared with SE imaging, flow-compensated 2D inflow GRE MR venography has been shown to be more sensitive and specific in detecting venous thrombosis and in visualizing collateral circulation (HANSEN et al. 1990). 2D MR venography with sequential slice acquisition within a breath-hold can demonstrate the vascular lesion with an efficacy similar to CE helical CT venography (TELLO et al. 1993), and findings are comparable to those of conventional venography for the diagnosis of venous occlusion and non-occlusive thrombosis (FINN et al. 1993; HANSEN et al. 1990; ROSE et al. 1996). Acute venous thrombosis can be diagnosed as a filling defect outlined by flow-intense signal. Stenoses are identified as areas of narrowing with or without proximal dilatation or collateral veins. In chronic occlusive disease of the central veins, 2D TOF MR venography was reported to be as diagnostically adequate as US and conventional contrast venography in 95% of cases (ROSE et al. 1996), having a sensitivity and specificity of 97% and 94%, respectively. Furthermore, MR venography predicted 100% of successful line placements and 80% of failures. As a major advantage of inflow MR venography, the evaluation of the SVC is not limited by vascular overlap due to presaturation of the arterial signal. Moreover, MR venography is able to show altered blood flow readily with selective presaturation or bolus tracking, and provides more comprehensive information than conventional venography on central venous anatomy, blood flow, collateral pathways, and extravascular structures (FINN et al. 1993). Despite these positive reports, this imaging modality has several drawbacks. Interpretation of pathologic findings appears to be difficult, as indicated by the high degree of interobserver disagreement of 44% in the study of ROSE et al. (1996). Signal voids can occur simulating stenotic or occlusive disease due to saturation effects within the imaging plane. As a consequence, imaging may be required in different additional planes, resulting in a prolonged examination time of up to 30 min.

Recently introduced direct and indirect CE 3D MR venography of the upper extremity and central chest veins, acquiring 3D data sets during intravenous injection of paramagnetic contrast medium, has been evaluated by THORNTON et al. (1999), SHINDE et al. (1999), and RUEHM et al. (2000, 2001). These techniques could facilitate comprehensive evaluation of abnormalities of the central veins in the thorax demonstrating the image information similar to conventional venography. As a result, arteriovenous graft placement or catheterization of central veins could be guided successfully (SHINDE et al. 1999), and axillary and subclavian vein thrombosis was correctly diagnosed as well as mediastinal vein compression in all reported cases with a 100% sensitivity, specificity, and accuracy (THORNTON et al. 1999). Compared with TOF MR venograms, direct CE MR technique is more reliable, easy to perform, well tolerated, and more accurate in depicting central venous abnormalities due to a constant signal that is not influenced by flow effects. Thus, direct and indirect CE 3D MR venography have become accurate techniques for the evaluation of the majority of abnormalities of the upper arm veins and the central thoracic veins including their tributaries that may replace inflow MR techniques.

However, compared with conventional venography, all MR venographic techniques available today suffer from limitations due to reduced spatial resolution including the depiction of collaterals in the shoulder and neck area as well as the detection of distinct intraluminal postthrombotic alterations such as intimal irregularities and intraluminal septa.

20.3.2.2
IVC and Its Tributaries

20.3.2.2.1
Occlusive Disease of the IVC

Radiologic evaluation of the IVC is important in many clinical scenarios. Recognition of congenital IVC anomalies is important in the differentiation of a pathologic condition from acquired caval disease. In cases of suspected or known thrombosis of the iliac veins, the IVC has to be assessed for proper therapeutic planning, particularly if a caval filter is an option. Staging of tumors that can extend into the IVC lumen or compress it extrinsically can be accomplished. The presence, size, and type of collateral venous pathways in caval occlusion can be determined (Fig. 20.6a, b). A thrombus is the major cause of IVC obstruction and represents a potential source of life-threatening pulmonary embolus (Fig. 20.7a, b). Thrombus can be primarily due to idiopathic thrombosis of the femoroiliac vein, and secondarily to more generalized conditions such as dehydration, sepsis, localized inflammation, hypercoagulopathy, congestive heart failure, immobility, trauma, or severe exertion. Iatrogenic thrombosis may be due to surgery or to direct caval manipulation. Tumor invasion of the IVC is most frequently associated with renal tumors. It is seen in approximately 10% of renal cell carcinoma and origi-

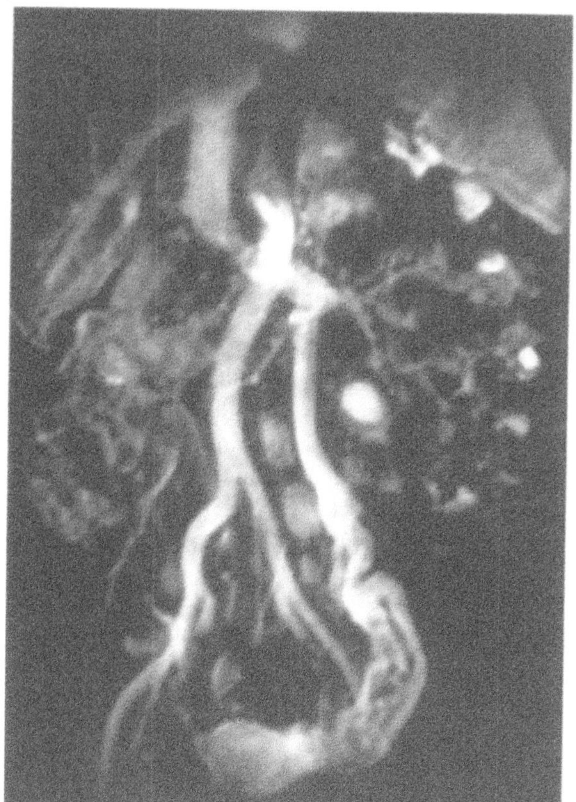
a

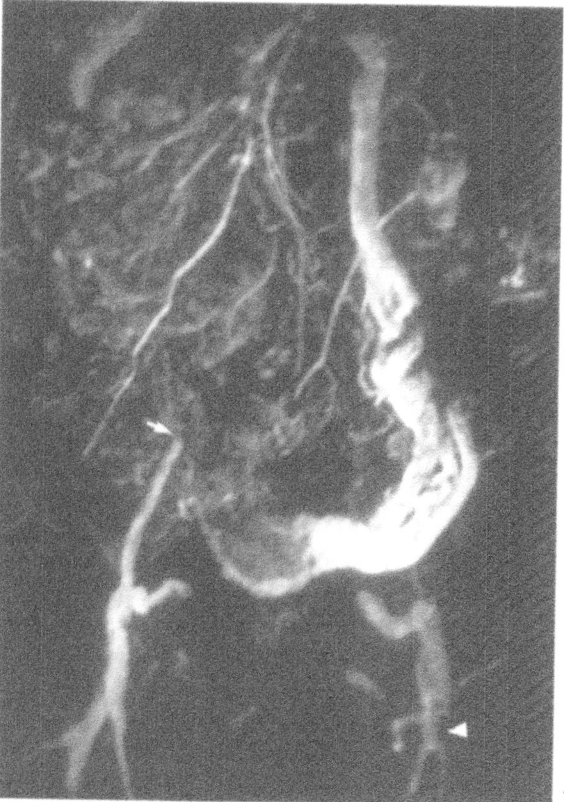
b

Fig. 20.6a, b. A 55-year-old female patient with surgically closed infrarenal VCI. Indirect CE MR venography. **a** The arterial venous phase shows a normal anatomy of the arteries. Drainage of the lower extremities is performed via the ovarian plexus and the ovarian vein up to the left renal vein which drains into the proximal VCI. **b** Late phase subtracted image showing occlusion of the right iliac vein (*arrow*) and postthrombotic disease of the left femoral vein

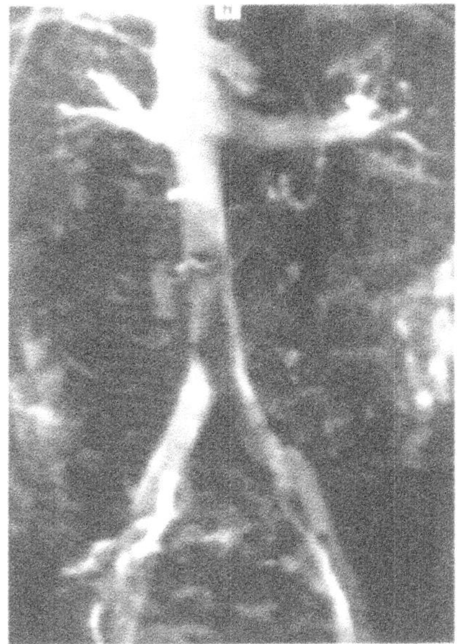

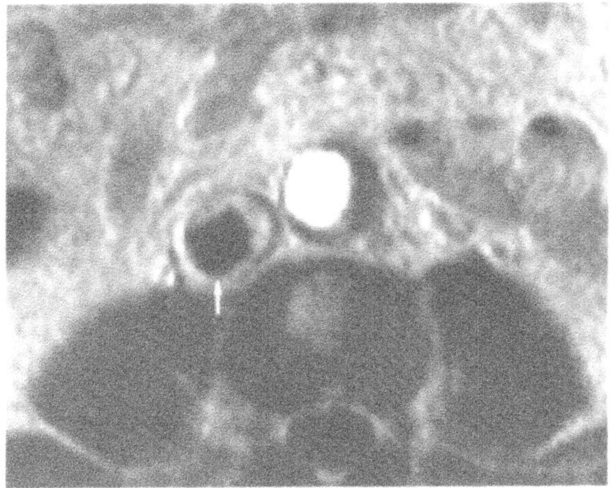

Fig. 20.7a, b. A 60-year-old male patient with pulmonary embolism from thrombotic disease of the left common iliac vein and the IVC. **a** 2D TOF MIP image shows thrombus in the IVC. **b** 2D TRA GRE sequence of the aorta and IVC demonstrates signal void in the IVC (*arrow*)

nates more frequently from the right kidney. Other tumors can extend into the IVC, such as adrenal carcinoma, pheochromocytoma, and Wilms' tumors. Intrinsic obstruction or thrombosis of the IVC are more frequently caused by malignancies than by non-neoplastic disorders, and include rare primary tumors such as leiomyoma, leiomyosarcoma, or endothelioma (Harris 1976; Sonin et al. 1992) (Fig. 20.8a–c). Extrinsic compression of the IVC may occur at any level and is usually due to retroperitoneal lymphadenopathy. Most frequently the mid-IVC is involved at the L2–3 level. Other sources of external compression or displacement include hepatic, renal, adrenal, and pancreatic tumor masses, aortic aneurysms, retroperitoneal masses and fibrosis.

Conventional Angiography

Conventional angiography of the IVC in occlusive disease has been regarded as the method of choice for many years. Although the sensitivity and specificity of detecting tumor thrombus in the IVC with venacavography has been reported to be 100% (Hietala et al. 1988; Kallman et al. 1992), the extent of thrombus may be estimated incorrectly due to early filling of collaterals and the lack of opacification of the vessel behind the occlusion.

Ultrasonography

Under suitable conditions, occlusive disease of the IVC can be reliably detected by US on the basis of echogenic thrombotic material and a vessel narrowing or complete loss of flow signal. In tumor occlusion of the IVC, the upper border of echogenic tumor can be delineated in most cases, resulting in a reported sensitivity and specificity ranging from 33% to 100% and 92% to 100%, respectively.

CT Angiography

CE CT can delineate a tumor thrombus in the IVC more reliably, with a sensitivity and specificity ranging from 66% to 100% and 76% to 100%, respectively (Schwerk et al. 1985; Giuliani et al. 1987; Hietala et al. 1988; London et al. 1989; Kallman et al. 1992). However, CT pitfalls occur and include difficulties in delineating the superior extent of the tumor thrombus when it is near the right atrium or the hepatic venous confluence, and the risk of mistaking unopacified blood or streaming of contrast material in laminar blood flow for clot-like filling defects.

MR Venography

The IVC can be visualized by MR imaging in the majority of cases using a conventional T1-weighted SE sequence. In occlusive disease, a sensitivity and specificity of 82%–100% and 97%, respectively, have been reported in the evaluation of tumor extension within the IVC (Horan et al. 1989; Goldfarb et al. 1990). Inflow 2D GRE MR venograms have been shown to be more accurate in detecting IVC obstruction, where complete signal void can be observed. Since the extension is frequently overestimated on MIP images, a reliable evaluation of the true extension of the lesion is possible using additional analysis of the source images (Arlart et al. 1991). Collateral pathways which become visible even shortly after occlu-

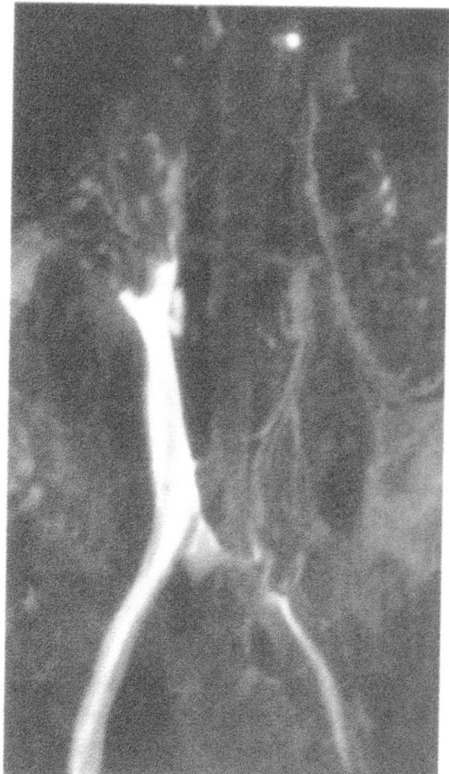

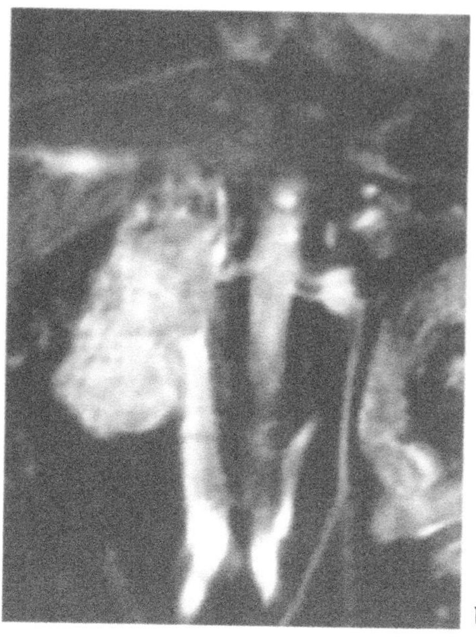

Fig. 20.8a, b. A 66-year-old female patient with a sonographically detected tumor of the IVC, histology: malignant fibrous histiocytoma. **a** Direct low-dose CE MR venography with diluted (1:15) contrast media injected in a punctured right foot vein. Subtotal occlusion of the suprarenal IVC. **b** Breath-hold FSPGR with fat saturation image showing the contrast enhancing tumor

sion of the IVC can be well documented with MR venography.

The protective insertion of a vena cava filter in patients with recurrent pulmonary embolism due to acute or subacute deep venous thrombosis (DVT) of the lower extremities does not preclude the use of MR imaging. Dislodging of the filter during MR examination is unlikely when it has been in place for more than 6 weeks. However, severe susceptibility artifacts may occur due to the filter material obscuring clot material adjacent to or within the filter.

Indirect MR venography based on the delayed venous phase of CE 3D MR angiography of the abdomen has been shown to be also useful in visualizing different variations, anomalies, and pathologies of the renal veins and IVC (Kaufman et al. 1995), particularly when technically optimized by subtracting the arterial from the arteriovenous phase in order to obtain pure venograms. However, there are only preliminary results, allowing no validation of this method compared with inflow MR venography.

20.3.2.2.2
Occlusive Disease of the Pelvic Veins

Besides intrinsic causes of iliac vein thrombosis, both intraluminal venous spurs and extravascular processes may cause acute thrombotic disease or clinically relevant venous narrowing. In about 20% of patients, sail-shaped folds or spurs may be found in the left common iliac vein at the junction with the IVC. The formation of spurs may originate in a reaction of the venous wall to the local compression of the overlying right common iliac artery.

At least partially, spurs may be the cause of the threefold higher incidence of thrombus in the left lower extremity veins. These spurs protrude from either the medial or the lateral venous wall into the vascular lumen, leading to stenoses. Other spurs may present as cords aligned sagittally, and dividing the venous lumen. The spurs develop with age and have to be distinguished from congenital abnormalities of the iliocaval junction.

Compression of the iliac axis due to enlarged uterus in pregnancy and tumorous masses of different etiology can impair venous drainage associated with edema and venous stasis. In accelerated cases, venous compression may induce acute thrombotic disease. Pelvic masses with consequent venous obstruction are visualized only by means of cross-sectional imaging methods such as US, CT, or MR imaging. The therapeutic regimen in thrombotic iliac vein occlusion includes medical anticoagulation and fibrinolytic treatment or surgical thrombectomy with or without femoral arteriovenous fistula in acute states, whereas percutaneous revascularization procedures such as thrombectomy and endovascular self-expanding stent placement is indicated in subacute and chronic stenotic or occlusive disease (Vorwerk et al. 1996).

Conventional Venography

Acute thrombotic occlusion as well as chronic occlusive disease of pelvic veins show a characteristic appearance in conventional venography, such as lack of contrast within the iliac vein, occasional thrombus material which is seen as an intraluminal filling defect depending on the age and site of the occlusion, and typical collateral pathways. In occlusion of the external iliac vein, collateral flow runs from branches of the deep femoral vein via the obturator vein to the internal iliac vein, whereas in occlusion of the common iliac vein collateral vessels can be visualized in the suprapubic and presacral region running to the contralateral iliac veins, and in the epigastrium. However, frequently these vascular conditions cannot be sufficiently visualized in conventional venograms due to slow flow and dilated veins distally of the occlusion despite the application of large volumes of contrast material.

Ultrasonography

Iliac venous occlusions can be reliably detected by using US in most cases utilizing functional Valsalva maneuver studies. However, in this region, even color-coded duplex US may be limited in depicting accurate localization of an occlusion and in evaluating collateral pathways due to obesity and bowel gas.

MR Venography

At the level of venous spurs blood flow is altered, which may cause signal loss in flow-sensitive MR venography, and the differentiation from simple venous compression by the overlying artery may be difficult (Lanzer et al. 1991; Richter et al. 1993). In CE 3D MR venography, venous spurs can be delineated more accurately than with inflow MR techniques, appearing as a wall-standing sail-like filling defect. The hemodynamic relevance of the spur can be quantified by flow measurements and comparison with the contralateral vein.

In pelvic venous occlusive disease, 2D TOF MR venography has been shown to be even more accurate than conventional venography and duplex US (Evans et al. 1993). The presence of intraluminal clot material is characterized by low signal compared with bright signal of adjacent flowing blood. Accurate diagnosis of the site and extension of the iliac thrombus can be made particularly in transverse slices resulting in a sensitivity and specificity of 100% and 94%, respectively (Catalano et al. 1997). One of the most important alterations that may be detected by flow-sensitive MR venography is a thrombus in the internal iliac vein and its branches as well as in the ovarian vein. Some authors described such clinically unsuspected findings in 20%–25% of examined cases (Gehl et al. 1990; Richter et al. 1993) which cannot be detected by conventional venography or direct CE 3D MR venography following pedal injection of the contrast agent. However, despite the usefulness of pelvic 2D TOF MR venography, it should be kept in mind that signal voids may occur due to in-plane saturation, and fresh thrombus material may appear with bright signal due to the content of methemoglobin which may lead to confusion in the diagnosis of DVT in some cases. Thus, in unclear cases with suspected disorders in the external and common iliac vein, direct CE 3D MR venography, which has been shown to be able to depict also smaller lesions due to higher signal and spatial resolution, can be recommended (Li et al. 1998; Ruehm et al. 2000).

20.3.2.2.3 Occlusive Disease of Hepatic Veins

Obstruction of the hepatic veins that can arise due to a space-occupying intrahepatic mass, and at the level of the IVC due to thrombus or tumor invasion, may cause the Budd-Chiari syndrome (BCS). BCS comprises several features including ascites, hepatomegaly, and jaundice.

Ultrasonography

US has been reported as the method of choice for initial diagnosis of BCS (Menu et al. 1985). In addition, the results of pulsed Doppler US have been found to correlate well with angiographic findings in cases of hepatic venous outflow obstruction, demonstrating characteristic blood flow signal from the IVC and/or hepatic veins that changes from phasic to absent, reversed, turbulent, or continuous flow (Hosoki et al. 1989).

MR Venography

A characteristic appearance of BCS has been reported by Stark et al. (1986), when employing MR imaging with SE sequences. However, typical patterns of hepatic vein occlusion and IVC involvement can be identified more reliably by use of indirect CE 3D GRE MR venography. Although characteristic MR venographic signs can be found, such as luminal narrowing and partial or complete signal void in the hepatic veins, very similar findings may also occur in different forms of cirrhotic liver disease. MR angiography has been shown to be extremely useful in the mapping of the intrahepatic venous anatomy in tumorous disease before surgical intervention, or when transjugular intrahepatic portosystemic shunt (TIPS) procedures are planned. In these cases both coronal and transverse acquisition planes should be selected for MR venography in order to optimize flow signal and to obtain multidimensional information on the intrahepatic vasculature (Fig. 20.9a, b).

20.3.2.2.4
Occlusive Disease of Renal Veins

Thrombosis of the renal veins may occur spontaneously in renal disease, hypercoagulopathy, dehydration, paraneoplastic states, and following trauma or surgical intervention. However, more often secondary involvement of the renal veins can be observed as a result of tumor- and lymphoma-induced vascular compression or intravascular extension of a tumor thrombus in patients with renal cell carcinoma (Fig. 20.10a–c). Clinical manifestations of renal vein thrombosis (RVT) may develop gradually and depend on the degree of occlusion and the presence of collaterals. They include flank pain, nephrotic syndrome, proteinuria, azotemia, and occasionally arterial hypertension. When therapeutical management is planned, indications and contraindications of anticoagulation or systemic fibrinolysis have to be considered. In patients with renal cell carcinoma, intravascular growth involving the renal vein and the IVC has been described in 21%–35% and 5%–10% of cases, respectively. The existence of tumor thrombus and the level of thrombus extension into the IVC, however, affects the survival rate far less than other factors such as tumor invasion of the capsule or lymphadenopathy (Cherrie et al. 1982). Nevertheless, surgical intervention is indicated in patients with large tumor thrombus which may induce vascular complications or pulmonary embolism. Successful removal of intraluminal tumor requires accurate preoperative delineation of the superior tumor extent, as this determines the operative approach.

Ultrasonography

Noninvasive color-coded duplex Doppler US and dynamic CE CT have been established as the mainstays of vascular evaluation in renal cell carcinoma, while invasive conventional angiography may provide additional information in unclear cases of suspected tumor thrombus. With US, echogenic thrombus material can be detected more reliably in the right than in the left renal vein. The reported sensitivities and specificities range from 18% to 95% and 76% to 100%, respectively (Schwerk et al. 1985; Giuliani et al. 1987; London et al. 1989).

Computed Tomography

More reliably, CE CT can provide evidence of tumor thrombus in the renal veins when luminal enlargement is seen, and to delineate tumor thrombus directly when an intraluminal filling defect is found, with a sensitivity and specificity of 66%–100%

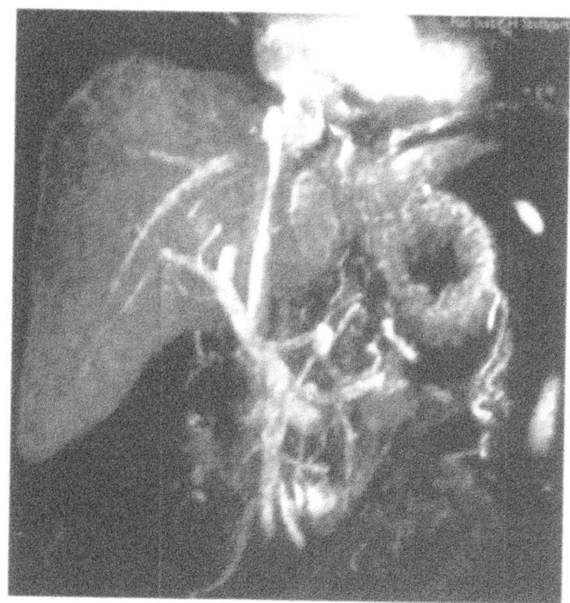

a

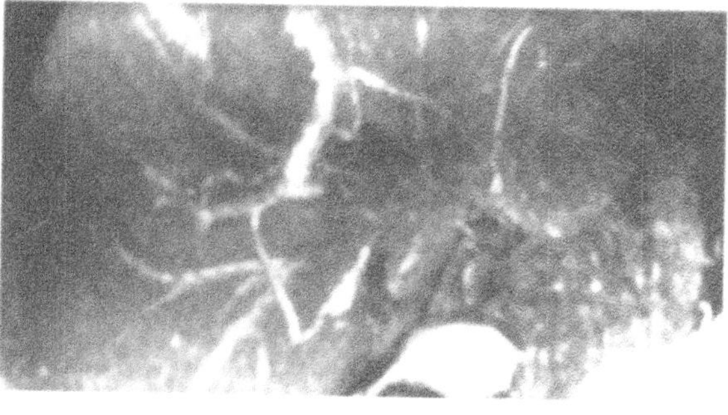

b

Fig. 20.9a, b. A 55-year-old male patient with cirrhotic disease of the liver before TIPS implantation. Indirect CE MR venography in subtraction technique. In the coronal (**a**) and transverse (**b**) plane reformatted images show the course of the hepatic and the portal veins and the distance between the branches suitable for a TIPS procedure

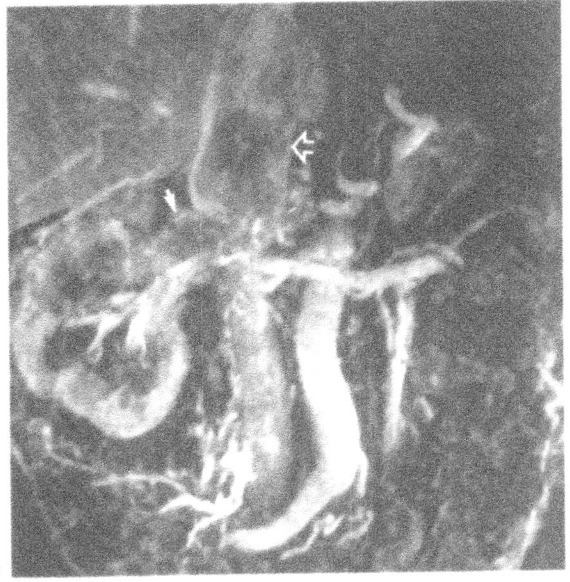

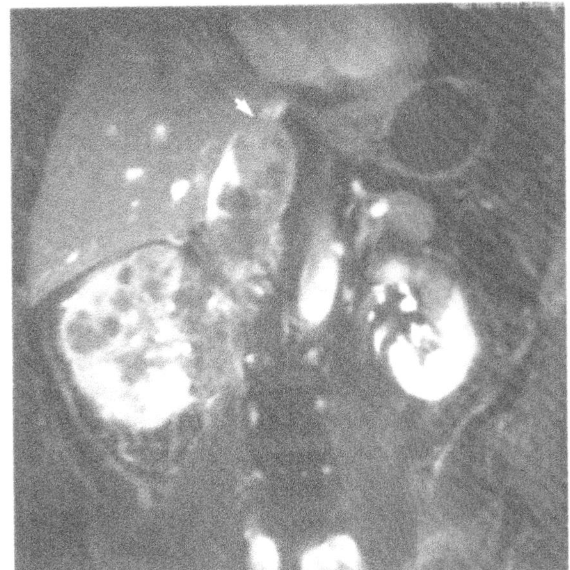

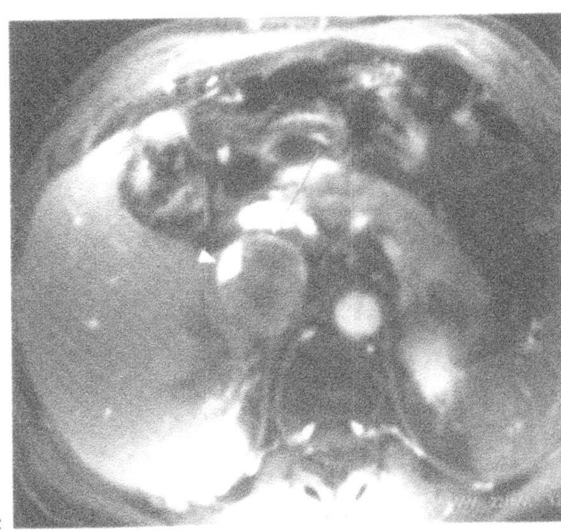

Fig. 20.10a–c. A 63-year-old male patient right side renal carcinoma invading the renal vein and the IVC up to the hepatic inflow. **a** Indirect CE MR venography, thrombus in the renal vein (*arrow*), and tumor thrombus the distended IVC (*open arrow*). **b** T1 FS FSPGR BH post-CE image showing the renal carcinoma with thrombus head (*arrow*) in the IVC. **c** T1 FS FSPGR BH post-CE image demonstrating thrombus (*long arrow*) and remaining perfusion (*arrowhead*) of the IVC

and 76%–100%, respectively (Giuliani et al. 1987; Hietala et al. 1988; London et al. 1989; Kallman et al. 1992).

MR Venography

Renal veins and their confluence into the IVC can be visualized by coronal and transverse MR imaging in many cases. Using a conventional T1-weighted SE sequence, a sensitivity and specificity of 65% and 81%, respectively, have been reported in the evaluation of tumor extension within the renal vein (Horan et al. 1989). A sensitivity of up to 100% has been reported (Goldfarb et al. 1990; Kallman et al. 1992; Roubidoux et al. 1992; Arlart et al. 1992) when additional 2D inflow GRE MR venography has been used to differentiate slow flow from thrombus material, particularly when 2D MR venographic sections were acquired in both coronal and transverse planes. Still there is the possibility of misdiagnosis when thrombus material includes methemoglobin, which appears bright on TOF acquisition and may mimic a patent lumen. CE 3D MR angiographic techniques have overcome this problem (Kaufman et al. 1995). Staging of renal cell carcinoma can be performed including this technique by displaying the renal arteries in a first step, the renal veins in a second step, and the renal parenchyma in a third step using additionally postcontrast fat-saturated T1-weighted imaging. Although CT is the preferred technique for staging renal cell carcinoma, CE 3D MR angiography in its venous phase can show the existence and the extension of tumor thrombus into the renal veins and IVC better, and, most importantly, the involvement of hepatic veins or tumor extension through the diaphragm.

20.3.2.2.5
Acute Thrombosis of the Ovarian Veins

Septic puerperal ovarian vein thrombosis (SPOVT) is a potentially life-threatening condition in the postpartum period that may have fatal consequences in the absence of adequate treatment of additional anticoagulation for approximately 3 weeks (Mintz et al. 1987; Cohen et al. 1986), (Fig. 20.11a, b). Puerperal sepsis occurs in only 2%–3% of cases after vaginal delivery but in up to 50% following cesarean section. There are many underlying causes such as endometritis, infected hematoma, pelvic abscesses, pyelonephritis, and septic thrombophlebitis of the ovarian veins in 5%–20% of cases. Characteristic symptoms are fever, lower abdominal or flank pain, and occasionally a palpable tender linear-shaped pelvic mass. The symptoms are consistent with parametritis, and the lack of response to antibiotic therapy. In up to 90% of cases, SPOVT occurs on the right side, since venous drainage here is more important and a common dextrotorsion of the enlarged uterus may lead to subsequent compression of the right ureter and right ovarian vein leading to venous stasis and superinfection in a state of hypercoagulability with some elevated clotting factors.

CT Angiography

Color-coded duplex Doppler US has limitations for the assessment of SPOVT due to overlying distended bowel structures in the majority of these patients. Thus, the best imaging method for the diagnosis of SPOVT before the era of MR angiography was CE CT, which shows a thickened inflamed vessel wall and the relatively hypodense thrombus of 1–2.5 cm in diameter within the lumen extending from the uterus cornua to the level of the renal veins.

a

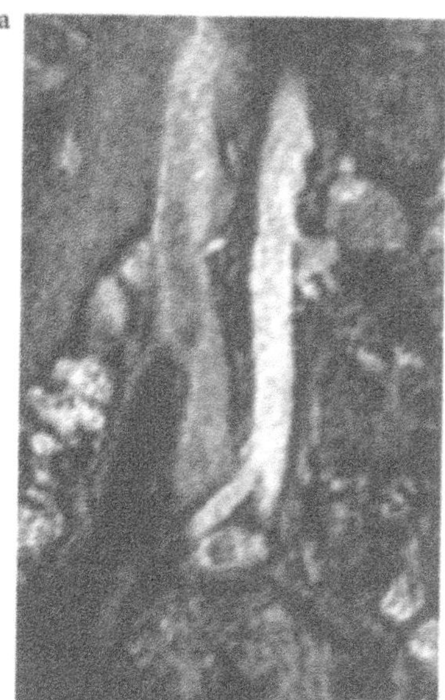

b

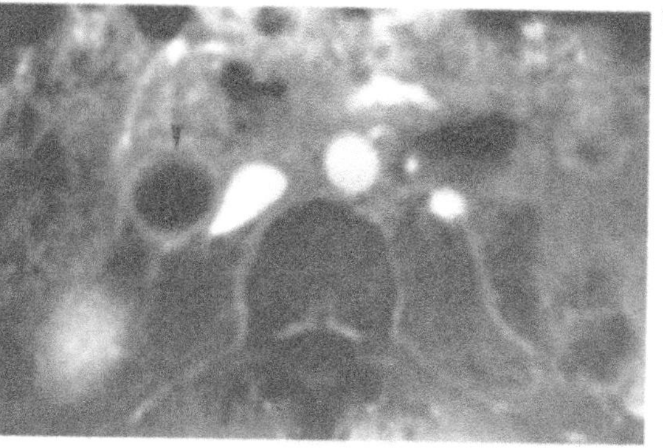

c

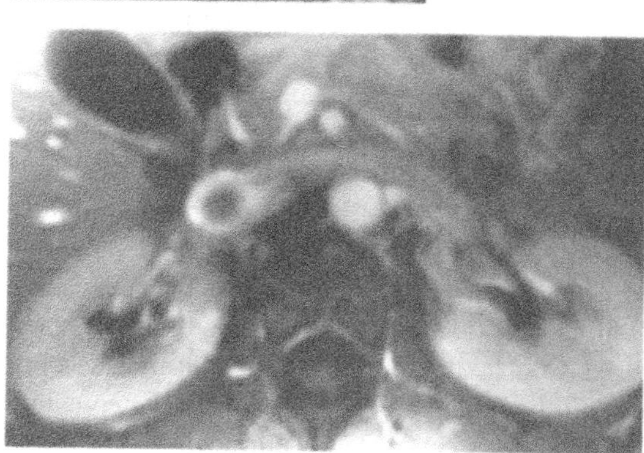

d

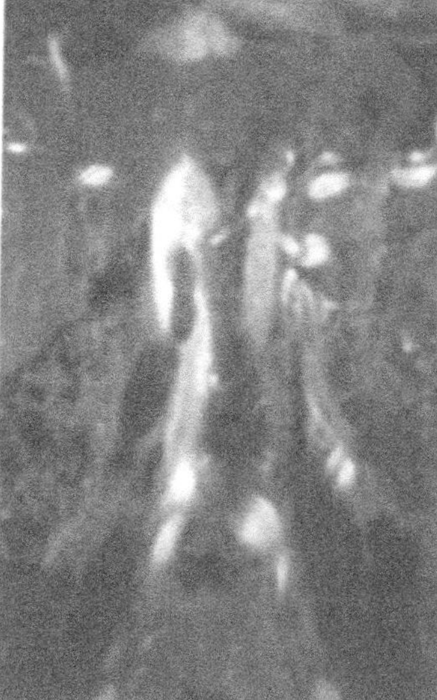

Fig. 20.11a–d. A 36-year-old female patient 8 days postpartum presenting with a thrombosis of the right ovarian vein. **a** Source image of a CE 3D angiogram showing thrombus in the IVC and thickened ovarian vein with signal loss. **b** CE FSPGR TRA image with fat saturation below the kidneys demonstrating thrombus in the ovarian vein and **c** at the level of the kidneys showing thrombus in the IVC. **d** CE FSPGR coronal image

MR Venography

Flow-sensitive 2D MR venography has been shown to be an accurate method for the evaluation of postpartal ovarian veins. These vessels can be depicted due to their increased diameter. In a prospective comparative study, TOF MR venography has been proved to be superior to CE CT and duplex Doppler US, demonstrating that SPOVT could be detected sonographically in only 50% of cases compared with MR venography, whereas CE CT provided two false-negatives and one false-positive result (Salvader et al. 1988). Indirect CE 3D MR venography might be even more useful than 2D inflow MR venography in detecting ovarian vein thrombosis, although to date, there are no representative studies (Fig. 20.11a–d).

20.3.2.3
Lower Extremity Veins

Conventional ascending contrast venography of the lower extremities is indicated in a number of different diseases, and has to provide answers to many pretherapeutic questions. Indications of venography include the exclusion of deep vein thrombosis, monitoring of postthrombotic changes, depiction of venous intraluminal spurs and malformations, preoperative imaging prior to saphenous venous stripping in varicose disease, and the determination of the suitability of the saphenous vein to serve as a coronary bypass vessel.

20.3.2.3.1
Acute Deep Venous Thrombosis

Deep venous thrombosis (DVT) is the third most common cardiovascular disease after myocardial infarction and cerebrovascular stroke. The clinical relevance of DVT results from the high risk of pulmonary embolism.

More than 90% of pulmonary emboli originate from the lower extremities or the pelvic area, and therefore early diagnosis of DVT and prevention of pulmonary embolism has to focus on this region. Between 100,000 and 300,000 hospitalizations each year are caused or complicated by acute DVT in the United States. In patients with verified DVT, radionuclide lung scans may reveal pulmonary embolism in up to 50% of cases. Ten to 30,000 deaths per year are attributed to pulmonary embolism. DVT may occur spontaneously due to a variety of intrinsic and extrinsic factors such as hypercoagulopathies, paraneoplastic states, immobilization, surgical interventions, traumatic events, and compression syndromes at different levels (Baker's cyst, popliteal aneurysm, groin hernias, or lymphadenopathy). As an additional cause of lower extremity DVT, occlusion of pelvic veins may play a role due to tumor masses, iliac lymphadenopathy, pregnancy, states after delivery, and iliac venous spurs, leading to descending femoropopliteal thrombosis. Postoperative DVT is a risk factor for lower extremity orthopedic surgery which may occur in 50% or more of patients, with pulmonary emboli occurring in 1%–10% of these patients when prophylaxis is absent (Davidson et al. 1996). However, despite prophylaxis approximately 10% of patients who undergo hip or knee surgery will develop DVT. Clinical diagnosis of DVT is difficult since only half of the patients will have characteristic symptoms. On the other hand, in patients with clinically suspected DVT, thrombosis is present in only 50% of cases (Huisman et al. 1989). The accurate diagnosis of acute DVT allows for optimal treatment, including anticoagulation therapy and systemic or catheter-directed thrombolysis (Bjarnason et al. 1997), thereby reducing the risk of subsequent complications associated with DVT and with needless anticoagulation therapy.

Conventional Venography

In the diagnostic work-up, conventional contrast venography and US have been shown to be the most reliable modalities for the detection of acute DVT (Naidich et al. 1988; Redman 1988; Cronan 1993; Stephen and Feied 1995). The gold standard contrast venography may demonstrate opacified patent vessels and thrombotic lesions in the deep veins of the calf, knee, thigh, and pelvis (Kälebo et al. 1997). Typical signs of thrombosis are the lack of opacification of single veins or groups of vessels, the presence of filling defects, and augmented flow in collaterals. Morphologic assessment of the age of a thrombus is difficult and only possible to a certain degree. Fresh clots usually are separated from the vessel wall and are surrounded by a thin layer of flowing blood. Within 48 h, increasing adherence will occur, and the areas with flow will disappear. Finally, complete occlusion may result. On the other hand, shrinking and retraction of the thrombus may produce increased areas of normal blood flow (Naidich et al. 1988; Redman 1988). Although the indirect signs of nonopacification and flow diversion are highly suggestive of DVT, they can occasionally be caused by edema, cellulitis, hematoma, and muscle fiber rupture, or may even be due to technical problems at the puncture site and supramalleolar bandage. Contrast venography is an invasive technique with the risk of adverse reactions to contrast material and a 2%–6%

rate of unsuccessful studies. Therefore, over recent years there has been a call for less invasive and more reliable techniques (CRONAN 1991).

Ultrasonography

US including its various techniques such as real-time compression US, duplex US, and color-coded Doppler US, provides highly promising results today (CRONAN 1991; YUCEL et al. 1991; CORNUZ et al. 1999), and these techniques are accepted as accurate and cost-effective methods for determining the presence of symptomatic DVT in the lower extremity. Although the positive predictive value of US for the above-the-knee DVT approaches 100% when modern technologies are used, the yield for below-the-knee DVT remains an unresolved tissue, resulting in a sensitivity ranging from 88% to 95% as reported in the literature (CORNUZ et al. 1999).

Nevertheless, in patients without risk factors for DVT, a negative venous US study can help exclude the presence of clinically important DVT if the examination includes careful evaluation of the calf veins. A DVT prevalence has been found in the US study of CORNUZ et al. (1999) which was restricted to below-the-knee veins in 15% of all patients with DVT. The incidence of overlooked DVT has been reported as being 0%. Thus, color-coded duplex Doppler US is commonly the method of first choice because it is readily available and avoids the potential morbidity associated with venography, although it has been shown that US is not as sensitive as venography in asymptomatic patients (WELLS et al. 1995).

CT Angiography

More recently, CE helical CT has been shown to be useful in depicting venous thrombosis of the iliofemoropopliteal region when performed consecutively after the examination of pulmonary arteries for exclusion of pulmonary embolism. In the study of BALDT et al. (1996), correlation was excellent between CT venography and conventional venography, and the sensitivity and specificity in detecting DVT has been reported to be 100% and 96%, respectively.

MR Venography

Noninvasive, inflow 2D MR venography has been shown to be a reliable and accurate approach for diagnosing DVT in the femoropopliteal and pelvic region (Fig. 20.12). It allows simultaneous visualization of the veins in both lower extremities and the pelvis. Typical MR venographic signs of thrombosis are the complete lack of bright signal of flowing blood in the region of a venous trunk, irregularly shaped flow void, eccentric filling defects with smooth margins in venous structures on transverse images, and the depiction of collateral vessels in chronic thrombosis (GEHL et al. 1990; SIEWERT et al. 1992; RICHTER et al. 1993), (Fig. 20.13). Several reports in the literature have described the value of MR imaging and MR venography in the detection of DVT. Even SE sequences have been shown to provide a high diagnostic accuracy (ERDMANN et al. 1990). However, in comparison, 2D GRE flow images with bright signal have been proved to be clearly superior to SE images in venous imaging (TOTTERMAN et al. 1990; EVANS et al. 1993; SOSTMAN et al. 1993) and detecting of DVT (ERDMANN et al. 1990; SPRITZER et al. 1998; LANZER et al. 1991), resulting in a sensitivity and specificity of up to 100% in the veins above the knee (EVANS et al. 1993; LAISSY et al. 1996). In their comparative study, LAISSY et al. (1996) found that MR venography was 100% sensitive and 100% specific in the diagnosis of DVT above the knee, whereas color Doppler US had a sensitivity and specificity of 87% and 83%, respectively. Moreover, in evaluating the extension of DVT, MR venography had a sensitivity of 95% and a specificity of 99% compared with 46% and 100%, respectively, for color Doppler US. In the majority of published reports, MR venographic data acquisition has been performed in the transverse plane to utilize maximum inflow effects of venous structures. Furthermore, image interpretation has not been limited on MIP reconstructions in the diagnosis of DVT, but has included the additional analysis of source images (SIEWERT et al. 1992; RICHTER et al. 1993). However, when using flow-sensitive MR venography, limitations have been reported particularly in the evaluation of calf veins. Thus, some authors did not consider MR angiography as reliable enough for below the knee (LANZER et al. 1991; SIEWERT et al. 1992; EVANS et al. 1993).

The evaluation of veins in the calf has remained challenging, reflecting the low velocity of blood flow within these veins. Improved imaging strategies have been developed that should allow a complete visualization of calf veins under conditions of increased flow velocity with increased signal intensity. Compression of the calf leading to an occlusion of superficial veins and a diameter reduction of deep veins yielded a sensitivity and specificity for detecting calf vein thrombosis of 87% and 90%, respectively (EVANS et al. 1993). Limitations of this technique are the possibility of overcompression, the poor patient tolerance of applied pressure, the reduced image quality when patient motion cannot be avoided, the necessity of using different

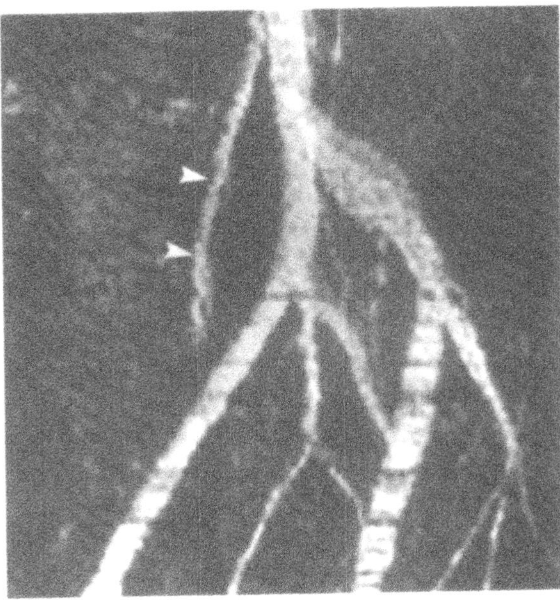

Fig. 20.12. Normal 2D TOF MRA of the pelvic veins in a 30° LAO projection showing the external and internal iliac veins, the branches of the internal iliac veins (superior and inferior gluteal posteriorly and the internal pudendal anteriorly), the common iliac veins and their confluence in the inferior vena cava, and the distal part of the superior mesenteric vein (*arrowheads*)

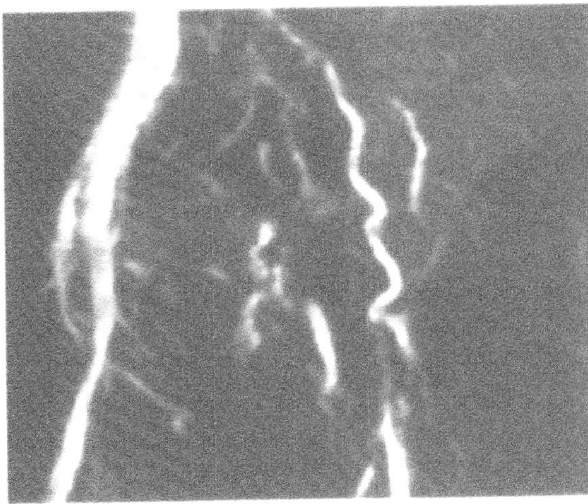

Fig. 20.13. Postthrombotic syndrome of the left iliac axis 6 months after acute DVT. There are some tortuous collaterals on the left and some enlarged branches of the internal iliac vein, but still complete occlusion of the external and common iliac veins on the left

planes for acquisition with relatively long imaging time, the phenomenon of in-plane saturation, and the insufficient signal within collapsed veins. Although flow augmentation techniques (compression and decompression) have shown some promising preliminary results in this difficult region (Holtz et al. 1996), flow-sensitive MR techniques have remained of only limited clinical value in the calf region.

Introduction of direct CE 3D MR venography might solve the problem of MR venography of the calf. This approach, based on the acquisition of 3D data sets during direct contrast filling of the venous system, is able to visualize even small muscle veins draining into the deep veins of the calf (Li et al. 1998; Ruehm et al. 2000). Compared with the 2D TOF technique, the acquisition time of low-dose CE 3D MR venography was much shorter, images looked sharper, more veins could be visualized, the technique was not affected by in-plane saturation, and the examination could be performed repeatedly because of the low dose of contrast (Li et al. 1998). Thus, direct CE 3D MR venography has been suggested as the MR modality of choice for detecting DVT and other disorders in the lower extremity (Li et al. 1998). However, pitfalls have been reported, such as signal void due to T2-effects by insufficient dilution of the contrast material, lack of signal due to incomplete coverage of venous structures for acquisition, and insufficient signal due to delayed venous filling. More experience has to be gained in order to provide a definitive evaluation of this promising MR angiographic modality (Fig. 20.14a, b, Fig. 20.15a, b).

20.3.2.3.2
Varicose and Postthrombotic Venous Disease

Primary varicose disease may be due to multiple causes such as genetic predisposition, obesity, and pregnancy. Typically, the extrafascial superficial saphenous venous system is involved including insufficient valves at the venous junction, whereas the deep veins are normal, and the communicating veins may be opacified from the superficial to the deep system. The cause of secondary varicose disease in the majority of cases is an abnormality of the deep veins with incompetent or absent valves, or a severe functional obstruction of the intrafascial venous system as a part of postthrombotic syndrome (PTS). In secondary varicose veins, the varicosities opacify via incompetent perforating veins that are typically located over the medial aspect of the leg. Other causes of varicose disease include arteriovenous malformations and congenital venous anomalies. Varicose veins typically appear redundant, dilated, and tortuous, and are deficient in

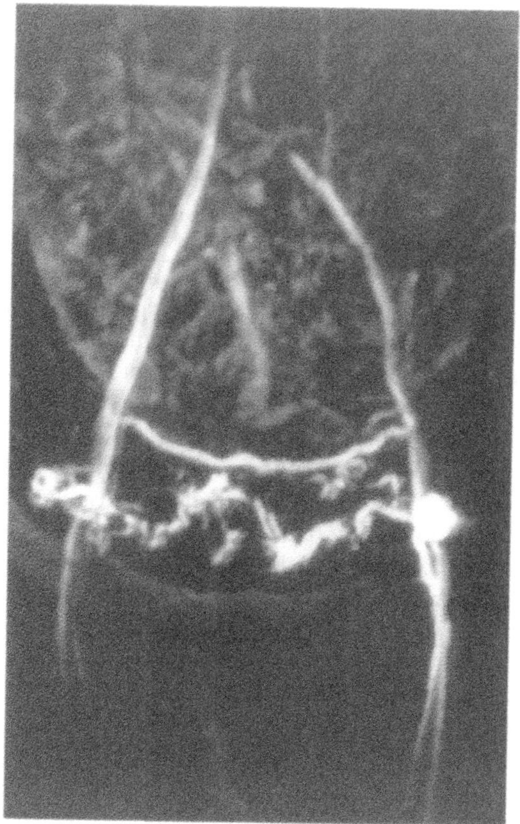

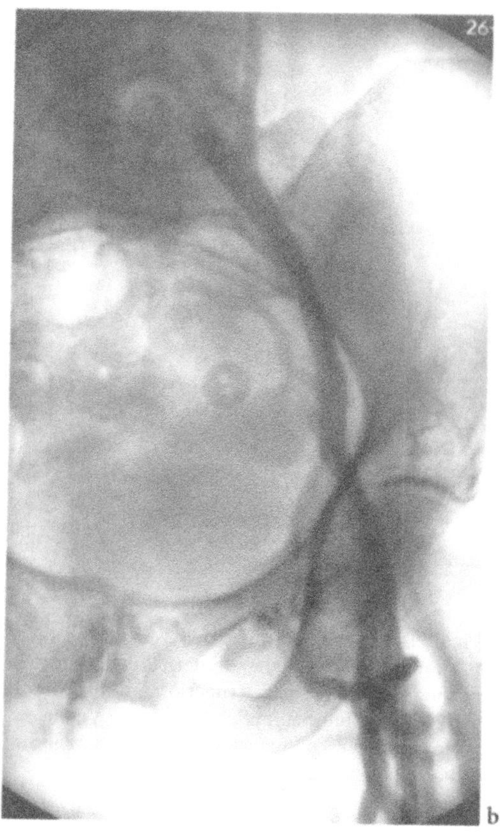

Fig. 20.14a, b. A 63-year-old female patient with a postthrombotic syndrome of the left common iliac vein. **a** Low-dose direct 3D CE MR venography both feet being punctured showing an occlusion of the left common iliac vein and collaterals supra- and prepubic. **b** Good correlation with conventional contrast venography

competent valves. Therapeutic regimen of varicose disease includes sclerosing therapy and surgical stripping techniques. A prerequisite of surgical intervention is the intact and patent deep venous system, which has to be evaluated before any invasive treatment.

Permanent damage in the veins after healing of acute DVT may result in chronic venous insufficiency and PTS. Typically, cutaneous ulcers may develop in up to 20% of patients within 5 years and in more than 50% within 10 years. A history of previous DVT can be obtained in only half of the cases since DVT may have been clinically silent. Residual anomalies in patients with PTS may include narrowing or occlusion of deep veins, multiple superficial or deep collateral veins, irregular vessel margins, inconstant vessel diameter, focal venous dilatation, deficiency of venous valves, and intraluminal fibrous septa.

MR Venography

In clinical routine, 2D TOF MR venography has never been used in assessing varicose veins. Limitations are reduced spatial resolution, potential in-plane flow saturation preventing reliable depiction of perforating veins, and the inability to present signal-intense information in slow or retrograde flow conditions.

Compared with TOF imaging, direct CE 3D MR venography permits the assessment of both postthrombotic and varicose changes as well as the bypass suitability of the saphenous vein. In a recently published study by Ruehm et al. (2000) using a comparative scoring that included segmental analysis of vessel visualization at conventional and MR venograms, varicose changes of the great and small saphenous veins were assessed with a 94% sensitivity and a 96% specificity. Postthrombotic changes were depicted with a sensitivity and specificity of 100% and 98%, respectively. Thus, this technique seems to be a promising approach in diagnosing distinct changes of the deep and superficial venous system of the lower extremity.

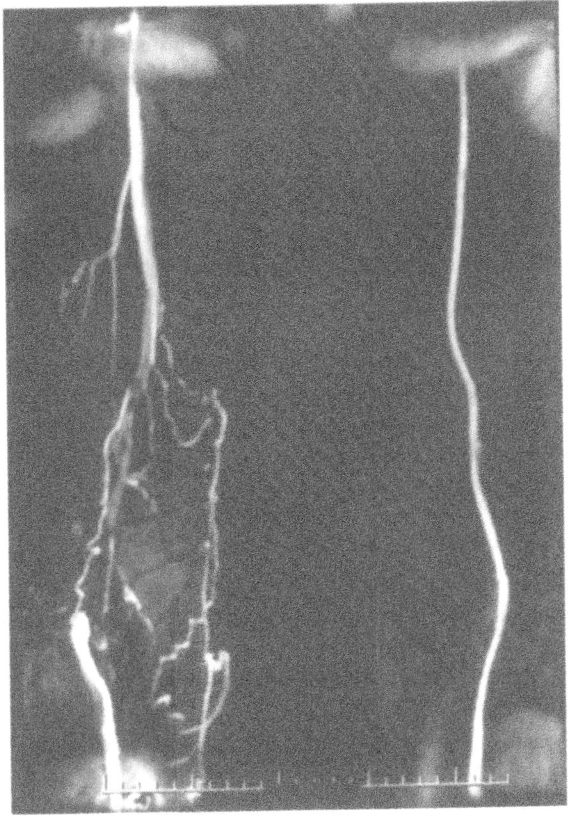

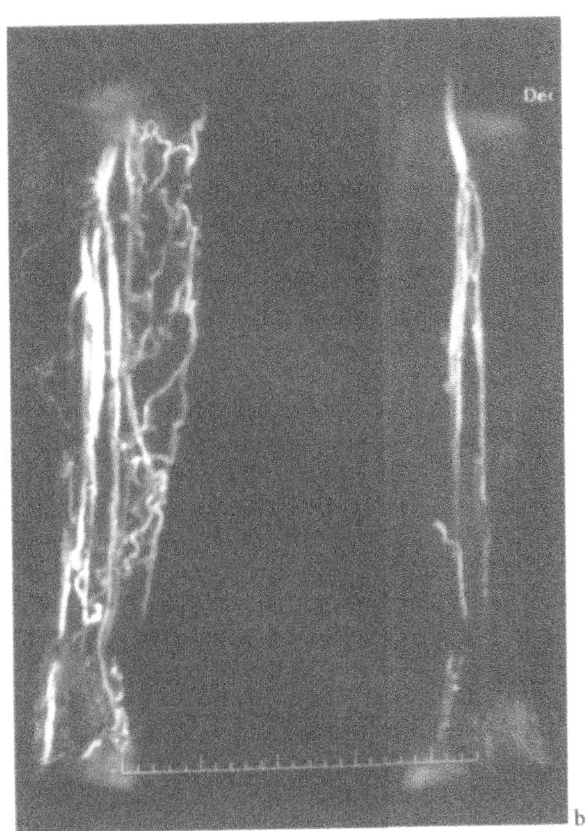

Fig. 20.15a, b. A 55-year-old male patient with suspicion of deep venous thrombosis of the right lower extremity. Normal venogram of the left side. Low-dose direct CE 3D MR venography of calf and thigh veins of both extremities with table stepping. **a** Veins above the right knee demonstrating thrombosis femoropopliteal with collaterals. **b** Veins below the knees with patent deep veins and filling of superficial collaterals on the right

20.3.2.3.3
Congenital Vascular Malformations

Congenital venous malformations can be classified into venous dysplasia including phlebangiomas, aplasia or hypoplasia of deep venous trunks, aplasia of venous valves, vessel duplication, anomalies of vessel course and ostial junction, mixed angiodysplasias such as arteriovenous fistulae, and combined arteriovenous dysplasias with or without fistulae. Congenital vascular malformations that most frequently occur in the lower extremities may include simple and cavernous hemangiomas, arteriovenous malformations with macro- and microfistulas, and venous angiomas. All these lesions originate from the abnormal development of the primitive vascular system. A typical appearance is seen in the Klippel-Trenaunay-Weber syndrome, which is characterized by dilated bulbous-appearing abnormal veins, absent valves, angiomatous or plexiform lesions, and occasionally an absent deep venous system. The clinical manifestations may vary extremely and extend from hardly visible, small strawberry-like birthmarks to clusters of massively enlarged vascular channels that may deform the whole extremity. The malformation can affect the venous system alone or can manifest itself clinically by enlarged venous structures fed by arteriovenous macro- or microfistulas (Malan and Puglionisi 1965; Szilagyi et al. 1976). Regardless of the type, vascular malformations present a difficult therapeutic challenge. Therefore, management of the disease requires detailed knowledge of the location and extent of the lesion, and precise delineation of its relationship to the surrounding anatomical and functional structures.

Color-coded duplex Doppler US, CE CT as well as conventional venography and arteriography have all been advocated for the evaluation of these lesions, but each has significant limitations.

Conventional Angiography

Conventional venograms generally allow only the detection of draining vessels, whereas arteriography can demonstrate suspected feeding arteries and arteriovenous fistulae. However, simple ascending venography can show a normal deep venous system in these cases, and visualization of purely venous superficial anomalies is possible only after direct puncture of the superficial venous channels.

MR Imaging and MR Angiography

MR imaging may be a valuable additional tool in the management of congenital vascular malformations of the lower limb (Cohen et al. 1986), providing important complementary information concerning the location and extent of the lesion and may even replace conventional venography. An imaging protocol, which includes both MR imaging and 2D MR venography, is useful in demonstrating the relationships to surrounding deep anatomical structures, especially the joints, and in visualizing large draining veins or tortuous venous anomalies. In order to depict arterial feeding vessels of arteriovenous malformations, 2D TOF MR angiography is merely of limited value, whereas fat-saturated CE 3D MR angiography is able to visualize the involved arteries in an early 3D data set and the venous malformations in a second delayed 3D data set that may compete with conventional angiography, having the potential to provide the complete desired information. CE MR venograms allow a more accurate assessment of most of the draining veins and their connections to vascular anomalies than flow-sensitive MR venography (Krestin et al. 1992). The results of direct low-contrast MR venography, which appear to be similar to those of conventional venograms (Ruehm et al. 2000), may be promising for improving the delineation of vascular patterns in venous malformation.

20.4 Conclusions

MR venography is able to provide vascular and perivascular information. It is well established in evaluating the large veins of the chest and trunk. 2D TOF angiographic imaging is still the preferred technique for the abdomen. CE 3D spoiled GRE sequences subtracting the arterial phase from the venous phase data set (indirect technique) are promising in the chest and abdomen including the renal and hepatic veins, the portomesenteric system, and the inferior vena cava. This technique is flow-independent, background suppression is excellent, and by utilizing MIP reconstruction and reformatting techniques, pure venograms can be obtained. Additionally, pre- and postcontrast conventional T1-weighted sequences allow the depiction of perivascular disease. The introduction of new contrast materials such as blood pool agents will yield a further improvement of the results.

Direct CE 3D GRE MR venography using diluted contrast material can be considered as the modality of choice in evaluating the upper extremity veins and the central chest veins. However, this approach to the lower extremities is still in discussion.

TOF techniques are time consuming and bear the risk of false interpretation of hyperintense thrombi. Direct CE 3D MR venography yields good results but is as invasive as conventional venography, except for the better acceptance of the contrast material, and it is more time consuming in preparing the patient.

There are limitations in inflow and CE MR venography including specific artifact patterns and reduced spatial resolution of images leading to the inability to detect distinct postthrombotic abnormalities which are important for therapeutic planning of anticoagulation as well as for expert witness. Furthermore, functional imaging comparable to US or press-venography in order to evaluate valve function in varicose disease is not possible. Thus, the effectiveness and clinical relevance of MR venography of the lower extremities remains to be established.

Acknowledgements. The authors thank Mrs. Tanja Endres for assistance with data acquisition and preparation of image material.

References

Abrams HL (1983) The vertebral and azygos veins. In: Abrams HL (ed) Abrams' angiography, vascular and interventional radiology, 3rd edn. Little, Brown, Boston, pp 895–922

Arlart IP (1997) MR angiography: veins of the abdomen. Radiologe 37:554–565

Arlart IP, Guhl L, Fauser L, Edelman RR, Kim D, Laub G (1991) Magnetic resonance angiography (MRA) of the abdominal veins. Radiologe 31:192–201

Arlart IP, Guhl L, Edelman RR (1992) MRA of renal veins and inferior vena cava for staging of renal cell carcinoma. Fortschr Roentgenstr 157:584–590

Arrive L, Menu Y, Dessart I, et al (1991) Diagnosis of abdominal venous thrombosis by means of spin-echo and gradient-echo MR imaging: analysis with receiver operating characteristic curves. Radiology 181:661–668

Baldt MM, Zontsich T, Stümpflen A, Fleischmann D, Schneider B, Minar E, Mostbeck GH (1996) Deep venous thrombosis of the lower extremity: efficacy of spiral CT venography compared with conventional venography in diagnosis. Radiology 200:423–428

Baxter GM, Kincaid W, Jeffrey RF, Millar GM, Porteous C, Morely P (1991) Comparison of colour Doppler ultrasound with venography in the diagnosis of axillary and subclavian vein thrombosis. Br J Radiol 64:777–781

Benenati JF, Becker GJ, Mail JT, Holden RW (1986) Digital subtraction venography in central venous obstruction. AJR Am J Roentgenol 147:685–688

Bettmann MA, Steinberg I (1983) The superior vena cava. In: Abrams HL (ed) Abrams'angiography, vascular and interventional radiology, 3rd edn. Little, Brown, Boston, pp 923–938

Bjarnason H, Kruse JR, Asinger DA, et al (1997) Iliofemoral deep venous thrombosis: safety and efficacy outcome during 5 years of catheter-directed thrombolytic therapy. J Vasc Interv Radiol 8:405

Bluemke DA, Wolf RL, Tani I, Tachiki S, McVeigh ER, Zerhouni EA (1997) Extremity veins: evaluation with fast-spin-echo MR venography. Radiology 204:562–565

Catalano C, Pavone P, Laghi A, Scipioni A, Fanelli F, Assael FG, Grossi A, Venosi S, Passariello R (1997) Role of MR venography in the evaluation of deep venous thrombosis. Acta Radiol 38:907

Cherrie RJ, Goldman DG, Lindner A, de Kernion JB (1982) Prognostic implications of vena caval extension of renal cell carcinoma. J Urol 128:910–912

Cohen JM, Weinreb JC, Redman HC (1986) Arteriovenous malformations of the extremities: MR imaging. Radiology 158:475–479

Cornuz J, Pearson SD, Polak JF (1999) Deep venous thrombosis: complete lower extremity venous US evaluation in patients without known risk factors – outcome study. Radiology 211:637–641

Cronan JJ (1991) Contemporary venous imaging. Cardiovasc Intervent Radiol 14:87–97

Cronan JJ (1993) Venous thrombembolic disease: the role of US. Radiology 186:619–630

Davidson HC, Mazzu D, Gage BF, et al (1996) Screening for deep venous thrombosis in asymptomatic postoperative othopedic patients using color Doppler sonography: analysis of prevalence and risk factors. AJR Am J Roentgenol 166:659

Debatin JF, Wildermuth S, Leung DA, Botnar R, Felbinger J, McKinnon GC (1995) Flow quantification with echo-planar phase-contrast velocity mapping: in vitro and in vivo evaluation. J Magn Reson Imaging 5:656–662

Derchi LE, Crespi G, Pretolesi F, Cecchini G, Oliva L (1991) Congenital anomalies and anatomical variants of the inferior vena cava and left renal vein: noninvasive diagnosis with duplex Doppler sonography. Eur Radiol 1:46–50

Dumoulin CL, Yucel EK, Vock P, Souza SP, Terroer F, Steinberg FL, Wegmueller H (1990) Two- and three-dimensional phase-contrast MR angiography of the abdomen. J Comput Assist Tomogr 14:779–784

Edelman RR, Wentz KU, Mattle H, Zhao B, Liu C, Kim D, Laub G (1989) Projection arteriography and venography: initial clinical results with MR. Radiology 172:351–357

Erdmann WA, Jayson HAT, Redman HC, Miller GL, Parkey RW, Peshock RW (1990) Deep venous thrombosis of extremities; role of MR imaging in the diagnosis. Radiology 174:425–431

Evans AJ, Sostman HD, Knelson MH, Coleman RE, Grist TM, MacFall JR (1993) Detection of deep venous thrombosis: prospective comparison of MR imaging with contrast venography. AJR Am J Roentgenol 161:131–139

Ferris EJ (1983) The inferior vena cava. In: Abrams HL (ed) Abrams' angiography, vascular and interventional radiology, 3rd edn. Little, Brown, Boston, p 939

Ferris EJ (1990) Deep venous thrombosis and pulmonary embolism: correlative evaluation and therapeutic implications. AJR Am J Roentgenol 159:1149–1152

Finn JP, Zisk JHS, Edelman RR, Wallner BK, Hartnell GG, Stokes KR, Longmaid HE (1993) Central venous occlusion: MR angiography. Radiology 187:245–251

Fishman EK, Feffrey RB Jr (1998) Spiral CT: principles, techniques, and clinical applications, 2nd edn. Lippincott-Raven, Philadelphia

Friedland GW, deVries PA, Nino-Murcio M, King BF, Leder RA, Stevens S (1992) Congenital anomalies of the inferior vena cava: embryogenesis and MR features. Urol Radiol 13:237–248

Gehl HB, Bohndorf K, Günther RW (1990) MR Angiographie (MRA) der tiefen Bein- und Beckenvenenthrombose: Vergleich mit der Phlebographie. Fortschr Roentgenstr 153:654–657

Giuliani L, Giberti C, Martorana G, Iserta A, Neumaier CE (1987) Value of computerized tomography and ultrasonography in the preoperative diagnosis of renal cell carcinoma extending into the inferior vena cava. Eur J Radiol 13:26–30

Goldfarb DA, Novick AC, Lorig R, et al (1990) Magnetic resonance imaging for assessment of vena caval tumor thrombi: a comparative study with vana cavography and computerized tomography scanning. J Urol 144:1100–1104

Gross CM, Krämer J, Waigand J, Uhlich E, Schröder G, Thalhammer C, Dechend R, Gulba DC, Dietz R (1997) Stent implantation in patients with superior vena cava syndrome. AJR Am J Roentgenol 169:429–432

Haire WD, Lynch TG, Lund GB, Liebermann RP, Edney JA (1991) Limitations of magnetic resonance imaging and ultrasound directed (duplex) scanning in the diagnosis of subclavian vein thrombosis. J Vasc Surg 13:391–397

Hansen ME, Spritzer CE, Sostman HD (1990) Assessing the patency of mediastinal and thoracic inlet veins: value of MR imaging. AJR Am J Roentgenol 155:1177–1182

Harris RD (1976) The etiology of inferior vena caval obstruction and compression. Crit Rev Clin Radiol Nucl Med 8:57–86

Hartnell GG, Hughes LA, Finn JP, Longmaid III HE (1995) Magnetic resonance angiography of the central chest veins: a new gold standard? Chest 107:1053–1057

Hayt DB, Binkert BL (1990) An overview of noninvasive methods of deep vein thrombosis detection. Clin Imaging 14:179–197

Hietala SO, Ekelund L, Ljungberg B (1988) Venous invasion in renal cell carcinoma: a correlative clinical and radiological study. Urol Radiol 9:210–216

Hirsh J, Hull RD, Raskob GE (1986) Epidemiology and pathogenesis of venous thrombosis. J Am Coll Cardiol 8:104–113

Holtz DJ, Debatin JF, McKinnon GC, et al (1996) MR venography of the calf: value of flow-enhanced time-of-flight echoplanar imaging. AJR Am J Roentgenol 166:663–668

Horan JJ, Robertson CN, Choyke PL, Frank JA, Miller DL, Pass HI, Linehan WM (1989) The detection of renal cell carcinoma extension into the renal vein and inferior vena cava: a prospective comparison of venography and magnetic resonance imaging. J Urol 142:943–948

Hosoki T, Kuroda C, Tokunaga K, Marukawa T, Masuike M, Kozuka T (1989) Hepatic venous outflow obstruction: evaluation with pulsed duplex sonography. Radiology 170:733–737

Huisman MV, Vuller HR, ten Cate JW, Van Rojen EA, Vreeken J, Kersten MJ, Bakx R (1989) Unexpected high prevalence of silent pulmonary embolism in patients with deep venous thrombosis. Chest 95:498–502

Kadir S (1986) Diagnsostic angiography. Saunders, Philadelphia

Kälebo P, Anthmyr B-A, Erikson BI, et al (1997) Optimization of ascending phlebography of the leg for screening of deep vein thrombosis in thromboprophylactic trials. Acta Radiol 38:320–326

Kallman DA, King BF, Hattery RR, Charboneau JW, Ehman RL, Guthman DA, Blute ML (1992) Renal vein and inferior vena cava tumor thrombus in renal cell carcinoma. J Comput Assist Tomogr 16:240–247

Kaufman JA, Waltman AC, Rivitz SM, Geller SC (1995) Anatomical observations on the renal veins and inferior vena cava at magnetic resonance angiography. Cardiovasc Intervent Radiol 18:153–157

Kee ST, Kinoshita L, Razavi MK, Nyman URO, Semba CP, Dake MD (1998) Superior vena cava syndrome: treatment with catheter-directed thrombolysis and endovascular stent placement. Radiology 206:187–193

König CW, Kaiser WA (1997) MR venography of the deep leg veins: signal enhancement by volume infusion. Fortschr Roentgenstr 166:206–209

Krestin GP, Bino M, Duewell S, Hauser M, Brennan RP, Brunner U (1992) Fat-saturated contrast-enhanced MR imaging and MR angiography of vascular malformations in the lower limb. Radiology 185:132

Laissy J-P, Cinqualbre A, Loshkajian A, Henry-Feugeas M-C, Crestani B, Riquelme C, Schouman-Claeys E (1996) Assessment of deep venous thrombosis in the lower limbs and pelvis: MR venography versus duplex Doppler sonography. AJR Am J Roentgenol 167:971–975

Lanzer P, Gross GM, Keller FS, Pohost GM (1991) Sequential 2D inflow venography: initial clinical observations. Magn Reson Med 19:470–476

Lebowitz JA, Rofsky NM, Kinsky GA, Weinreb JC (1997) Gadolinium-enhanced body MR venography with subtraction technique. AJR Am J Roentgenol 169:755–758

Li W, David V, Kaplan R, Edelman RR (1998) Three- dimensional low dose gadolinium-enhanced peripheral MR venography. J Magn Reson Imaging 8:630–633

London NLM, Messios N, Kinder RB, Smart JG, Osborn DE, Watkin EM, Flynn JT (1989) A prospective study of the value of conventional CT, dynamic CT, ultrasonography, and arteriography for staging renal cell carcinoma. Br J Urol 64:209–217

Longley DG, Yedlicka JW, Molina EJ, Schwabacher S, Hunter DW, Letourneau JG (1992) Thoracic outlet syndrome: evaluation of the subclavian vessels by color duplex sonography. AJR Am J Roentgenol 158:623–630

Lutterbey G, Gieseke J, Sommer T, Keller E, Kuhl C, Schild HH (1998) Rational examination of greater abdominal veins with 2D TOF- and turbo spin-echo sequences. Fortschr Roentgenstr 169:17–21

Malan E, Puglionisi A (1965) Congenital angiodysplasias of the extremities. J Cardiovasc Surg 6:255–345

Marchal G, Bosmans H, Van Hecke P et al (1990) MR angiography with gadopentate-dimeglumine polysine: evaluation in rabbits. AJR Am J Roentgenol 155:407–411

Menu Y, Alison D, Lorphelin JM, Valla D, Belghiti J, Nahum H (1985) Budd-Chiari syndrome: US evaluation. Radiology 157:761–764

Merritt CRB (1992) Doppler color imaging: abdomen. Churchill Livingstone, New York

Mintz MC, Levy DW, Axel L, Kressel HY, Arger PH, Coleman BG, Mennuti M (1987) Puerperal ovarian vein thrombosis: MR diagnosis. AJR Am J Roentgenol 149:1273–1274

Mohiaddin RH, Wann SL, Underwood R, Firmin DN, Rees S, Longmore DB (1990) Vena caval flow: assessment with cine MR velocity mapping. Radiology 177:537–541

Naidich JB, Feinberg AW, Karp-Harman H, Karmel MI, Tyma CG, Stein HL (1988) Contrast venography: reassessment of its role. Radiology 168:97–100

Nazarian GK, Foshager MC (1995) Color Doppler sonography of the thoracic inlet syndrome. Radiographics 15:1357–1371

Nicholson AA, Ettles DF, Arnold A, et al (1997) Treatment of malignant superior vena cava obstruction: metal stents or radiation therapy? J Vasc Interv Radiol 8:781

Patel MC, Berman LH, Moss HA, McPherson SJ (1999) Subclavian and internal jugular veins at Doppler US: abnormal cardiac pulsatility and respiratory phasicity as a predictor of complete central occlusion. Radiology 211:579–583

Prince MR, Yucel EK, Kaufman JA, Harrison DC, Geller SC (1993) Dynamic Gd-DTPA-enhanced 2D TOF abdominal MR angiography. J Magn Reson Imaging 3:877–881

Prince MR, Grist TM, Debatin JF (1999) 3D contrast MR venography. In: 3D contrast MR angiography. Springer, Berlin Heidelberg New York, pp 163–171

Qanadli SD, El Hajjam M, Bruckert F, Judet O, Barre O, Chagnon S, Lacombe P (1999) Helical CT phlebography of the superior vena cava: diagnosis and evaluation of venous obstruction. AJR Am J Roentgenol 172:1327–1333

Rabinov K, Paulin S (1983) Venography of the lower extremities. In: Abrams HL (ed) Abrams' angiography, vascular and interventional radiology, 3rd edn. Little, Brown, Boston, pp 1835–1922

Redman HC (1988) Deep venous thrombosis: is contrast venography still the diagnsotic "gold standard"? Radiology 168:277–278

Richter CS, Duewell S, Krestin GP, Vesti B, Franzeck UK, Bollinger A, von Schulthess GK, Fuchs WA (1993) Dreidimensionale Darstellung der Beckenvenen mit Magnetresonanz-Angiographie. Fortschr Roentgenstr 159:161–166

Rose SC, Gomes AS, Yoon HC (1996) MR angiography for mapping potential central venous access sites in patients with advanced venous occlusive disease. AJR Am J Roentgenol 166:1181–1187

Roubidoux MA, Dunnick NR, Sostman HD, Leder RA (1992) Renal carcinoma: detection of venous extension with gradient-echo MR imaging. Radiology 182:269–272

Ruehm SG, Wiesner W, Debatin JF (2000) Pelvic and lower extremity veins: contrast-enhanced three-dimensional MR venography with a dedicated vascular coil – initial experience. Radiology 215:421–427

Ruehm SG, Zimny K, Debatin JF (2001) Direct contrast-enhanced 3D MR venography. Eur Radiol 11:102–112

Salvader SJ, Ottero RR, Salvader BL (1988) Puerperal ovarian vein thrombosis: evaluation with CT, US, and MR imaging. Radiology 167:637–639

Schwerk WB, Schwerk WN, Rodeck G (1985) Venous renal tumor extension: prospective US evaluation. Radiology 156:491–495

Sheeran SR, Hallisey MJ, Murphy TP, et al (1997) Local thrombolytic therapy as part of a multidisciplinary approach to acute axillosubclavian vein thrombosis (Paget-Schroetter syndrome). J Vasc Interv Radiol 8:253–260

Shinde TS, Lee VS, Rofsky NM, Weinreb JC (1999) Three-dimensional gadolinium-enhanced MR venographic evaluation of patency of central veins in the thorax: initial experience. Radiology 213:555–560

Siewert B, Kaiser WA, Layer G, Träber F, Kania U, Hartlapp J (1992) MR-Venographie bei tiefen Bein- und Beckenvenenthrombosen. Fortschr Roentgenstr 156:549–554

Sonin AH, Mazer MJ, Powers TA (1992) Obstruction of the inferior vena cava: a multi-modality demonstration of causes, manifestations, and collatera pathways. Radiographics 12:309–322

Sostman HD, Debatin JF, Spritzer CE, Coleman RE, Grist TM, MacFall JR (1993) MRI in venous thromboembolic disease. Eur Radiol 3:53–61

Spritzer CE, Trotter P, Sostman DH (1998) Deep venous thrombosis: gradient-recalled-echo MR imaging changes over time – experience in 10 patients. Radiology 208:631–639

Stark DD, Hahn PF, Trey C, Clouse MR, Ferrucci JT (1986) MRI of Budd-Chiari syndrome. AJR Am J Roentgenol 146:1141–1148

Stephen JM, Feied CF (1993) Venous thrombosis: lifting the clouds of misunderstanding. Postgrad Med 97:36–42

Szilagyi DE, Smith RF, Elliott JP, Hageman JH (1976) Congenital arteriovenous anomalies of the limbs. Arch Surg 111:423–429

Tavares NJ, Auffermann W, Brown JJ, Gilbert TJ, Sommerhoff C, Higgins CB (1989) Detection of thrombus by using phase-image MR scans: ROC curve analysis. AJR Am J Roentgenol 153:173 –178

Tello R, Scholz E, Finn JP, Costello P (1993) Subclavian vein thrombosis detected with spiral CT and three-dimensional reconstruction. AJR Am J Roentgenol 160:33–34

Thornton MJ, Ryan R, Varghese JC, Farell MA, Lucey B, Lee MJ (1999) A three-dimensional gadolinium-enhanced MR venography technique for imaging central veins. AJR Am J Roentgenol 173:999–1003

Tottermann S, Francis CW, Foster TH, Brenner B, Marder VJ, Bryant RG (1990) Diagnosis of femoropopliteal venous thrombosis with MR imaging: a comparison of four MR pulse sequences. AJR Am J Roentgenol 154:175–178

Trigaux J-P, Vandroogenbroek S, De Wispelaere J-F, et al (1998) Congenital anomalies of the inferior vena cava and left renal vein: evaluation with spiral CT. J Vasc Interv Radiol 9:339–345

Vesely TM, Hovsepian DM, Pilgram TK, Coyne DW, Shenoy S (1997) Upper extremity central venous obstruction in hemodialysis patients: treatment with Wallstants. Radiology 204:343–348

Vorwerk D, Guenther RW, Wendt G, et al (1996) Iliocaval stenosis and iliac venous thrombosis in retroperitoneal fibrosis: percutaneous treatment by use of hydrodynamic thrombectomy and stenting. Cardiovasc Intervent Radiol 19:40

Weinreb JC, Mootz A, Cohen JM (1986) MRI evaluation of mediastinal and thoracic inlet venous obstruction. AJR Am J Roentgenol 146:679–684

Wells PS, Lensing AWA, Davidson BL, Prins MH, Hirsh J (1995) Accuracy of ultrasound for the diagnosis of deep venous thrombosis in asymptomatic patients after orthopedic surgery. Ann Intern Med 122:47–53

White CS, Baffa JM, Haney PJ, Pace ME, Campbell AB (1997) MR imaging of congenital anomalies of the thoracic veins. Radiographics 17:595

Yoshizako T, Sugimura K, Kawamitsu H, et al (1996) Two-dimensional time-of-flight MR venography: assessment with detection of chronic deep venous thrombosis in combination with magnetization transfer contrast. JCAT 20:957

Yucel EK, Fisher JS, Egglin TK, Geller SC, Waltman AC (1991) Isolated calf venous thrombosis: diagnosis with compression US. Radiology 179:443–446

21 The Splenoportal Venous System

JOCHEN GAA

CONTENTS

21.1 Introduction

Reliable and precise delineation of the splenoportal venous system is essential before liver transplantation, tumor resection, and transjugular portosystemic shunting (TIPS). In addition, adequate visualization of the splenoportal venous system is useful in the evaluation of patients with liver cirrhosis, portal hypertension, ascites of unknown etiology, and before portosystemic shunt surgery.

Since its introduction in the early 1950s, conventional catheter angiography has been the primary method of evaluating the splenoportal venous anatomy and portal hemodynamics. Since the mid-1970s, ultrasound (US) and computed tomography (CT) have been of considerable value in the evaluation of the abdominal vasculature. Currently, noninvasive evaluation is usually performed by US including duplex Doppler imaging and color Doppler flow imaging. These techniques allow for the visualization of the splenoportal venous system and provide important information about hepatic arterial and hepatic portal venous hemodynamics, such as velocity and flow direction.

In the past, magnetic resonance angiography (MRA), including time-of-flight (TOF) and phase-contrast (PC) techniques, was successfully applied as a noninvasive modality for the evaluation of vascular pathologies in the head and neck. In contrast, MRA of the abdominal vasculature has been of limited value due to technical challenges such as respiratory motion artifacts and the saturation effects of flowing spins. Recently, a new MRA technique – contrast-enhanced (CE) MRA – has been developed which overcomes many of the problems that have degraded conventional MR angiograms. When used in conjunction with high power gradient MR systems, images similar in appearance to conventional catheter angiography can be obtained.

21.2 Technical Considerations

MR angiographic techniques make use of flow effects to highlight the blood signal. "Bright-blood" imaging is divided into TOF and PC methods, depending on whether the predominant contrast mechanism is flow enhancement or flow-induced phase shifts. Both TOF and PC angiograms are produced using gradient echo sequences.

21.2.1 TOF MRA

TOF MRA relies on unsaturated flowing blood to generate a signal which appears bright in relation to

J. GAA, MD
Privat-Dozent, Institut für Klinische Radiologie, Universitätsklinikum Mannheim, Fakultät für Klinische Medizin der Universität Heidelberg, Theodor-Kutzer-Ufer 1-3, 68167 Mannheim, Germany

the adjacent saturated, relatively dark stationary tissues. TOF techniques employ flow-refocussing gradient pulses to rephase flow. On short repetition time (TR) sequences, regular bursts of radiofrequency energy saturate stationary spins, whereas blood flowing into the slice between phase-encoding steps is fully relaxed. The inflow of this relaxed blood results in reliable signal enhancement on gradient echo images (Axel 1980; Edelman et al. 1993).

The degree of flow enhancement is influenced by many factors, including the slice thickness, flow velocity, repetition time, flip angle, and T1 of stationary tissue. Enhancement is increased with thinner slices, higher flow velocity, longer repetition times, larger flip angles, and flow that is perpendicular to the image ("through-plane flow"). If the vessel runs a long course in the plane of the image ("in-plane flow"), the inflow effect becomes less effective and reduces the intravascular signal. Thus, potential difficulties in TOF MRA may arise in situations where larger sections of vessels lie within a section, and in situations where turbulent flow is present, as this suppresses bright intravascular signal.

TOF MR angiograms can be acquired as single slices (2D) or as a volume (3D). Although TOF MRA in the abdomen has most commonly been performed using 2D acquisitions, volume acquisition has also been successfully used (Lewin et al. 1991). While 2D techniques offer a high vessel-background contrast, the vessel-background contrast in 3D techniques is typically lower, and it progressively decreases when spins penetrate through the imaging volume. The slab thickness or vessel coverage in 3D techniques is therefore limited to a distance at which blood signal approaches a steady state signal. Typically, 3D TOF techniques are applicable in combination of fast flow situations, while 2D TOF techniques may be applied for the visualization of slower flow.

Flowing blood appears bright on TOF MRA regardless of the direction of flow. Hence, arteries and veins cannot be differentiated. Additional radiofrequency pulses, termed presaturation pulses, must be used to obtain selective TOF arteriograms or venograms.

21.2.2 PC MRA

Phase-contrast (PC) MRA techniques use velocity-induced phase shifts to distinguish flowing blood from stationary tissue. Although several pulse sequence variations are possible, nearly all are gradient echo techniques that use bipolar (flow-encoding) gradients along one or more axes. The fundamental flow principle underlying this strategy is that stationary spins experience no net phase shift by this combination of positive and negative gradients, whereas spins moving with constant velocity experience a phase shift proportional to flow velocity, amplitude of the bipolar gradient, and the time interval between the gradient lobes. The amplitude of the bipolar gradient determines the degree of velocity encoding (VENC). By adjusting VENC, it is possible to sensitize the sequence to slow or fast flows.

To generate optimal images, some a priori knowledge of the velocities to be encountered within the imaging volume must be used to set up appropriate flow sensitivity. Since each data set acquisition is considerably longer than TOF data sets, considerable time involvement may be necessary before optimal images are obtained in any particular clinical setting. In addition, PC techniques require high levels of machine performance, and are sensitive to errors from several non-flow-related sources such as eddy currents, gradient instabilities and magnetic field inhomogeneity. Like TOF techniques, phase-contrast can generate images as volume (3D) or as single-slice images (2D). In either case, the composite information can be post-processed to generate 3D angiograms.

21.2.3 Contrast-Enhanced 3D MRA

Contrast-enhanced 3D MRA (CE MRA) significantly differs from TOF and PC techniques in that it is not dependent on flow. In CE MRA, the use of a paramagnetic extracellular contrast agent (such as gadolinium-DTPA) increases the blood signal. This is due to shortening of the T1 relaxation time of blood after contrast injection. Depending on the actual concentration of gadolinium-DTPA, the arterial blood T1 can be as short as 50–100 ms and thus substantially shorter than T1 of fat. Therefore, blood produces the largest signal, and thus the vessel lumen will be picked up with the maximum intensity projection (MIP) to create an MR angiogram (Prince et al. 1999; Gaa et al. 2000).

The timing of the contrast medium injection must be chosen to ensure the presence of a high concentration of contrast material within the vessels of interest during the acquisition of the central portions of k-space that are responsible for image contrast. Bolus timing is most critical for the arterial phase images. The bolus timing can be done empirically ("best guess technique"), by using an automated sequence (MR Smart Prep), or by imaging very rapidly using k-space TRICKS ("time resolved imaging on contrast kinetics"). Bolus timing is not as important for the splenoportal venous system since the portal venous phase is longer than the arterial phase. Acquiring multiple phases guarantees visualization of the portal vein, even if there is flow reversal.

Since most abdominal surgeons are interested in both the arterial as well as the venous system, we routinely perform the breath-hold dual-phase 3D MRA technique (Fig. 21.1). In this technique an arterial phase 3D data set is acquired, followed by a portal venous phase data set acquired 40–45 s after the start of contrast injection. A double dose (0.2 mmol/kg body weight) of gadolinium-DTPA injected at a rate of 2 ml/s is recommended because gadolinium will have undergone considerable dilution by the time it reaches the portal vein. In order to ensure delivery of the entire contrast dose, a saline flush of 20–30 ml is then administered. Images are routinely reconstructed by using MIPs. By subtracting the arterial phase from the portal-venous phase data set, "pure" MR venograms may be obtained (Fig. 21.2). Subvolume or "targeted" MIPs are also helpful in delineating the vascular region of interest without overlaying structures (Fig. 21.3). When displayed at different angles (e.g., 15°), the MIPs can be viewed stereoscopically. However, for diagnostic purposes careful analysis of the source images is recommended. A phased-array multicoil should be used for all abdominal vascular studies in order to enhance intravascular signal as well as image resolution.

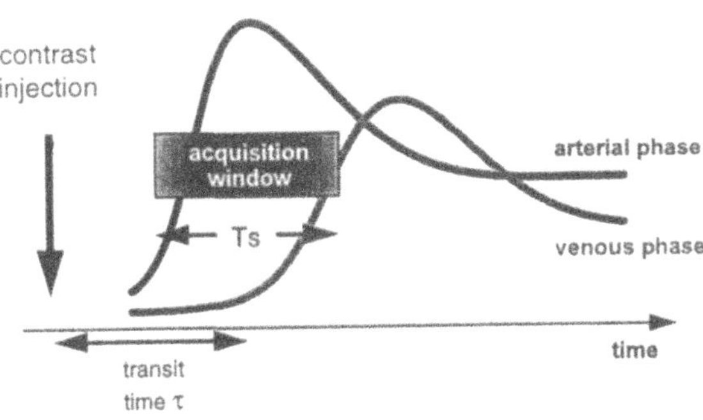

Fig. 21.1. Timing of contrast injection and data acquisition in dual-phase contrast-enhanced (CE) 3D MRA. Following the intravenous injection of the contrast agent, it is delivered to the vasculature of interest. Local blood signal is substantially enhanced due to the T1-shortening. This result is optimal when data collection (in particular the center of k-space) occurs just as the contrast agent arrives at the vessels being imaged

21.2.4 Flow Quantification

Flow direction and velocity can be derived directly from phase-contrast measurements, based on the measured phase shifts. Flow sensitivity is tailored to the expected velocity range, and slow flow can be detected with larger gradient moments. If the magnitude of the flow-sensitizing pulse is too great, however, velocity aliasing may occur.

Cine phase-contrast techniques have been shown to be highly accurate (Burkhart et al. 1992, 1993) and practicable for the evaluation of flow rates in the splenoportal venous system. However, phase-contrast techniques are time consuming since phase encoding must be done in all three gradient directions to obtain accurate results.

Bolus tracking (Edelman et al. 1989, 1990; Tamada et al. 1989; Finn et al. 1991) refers to a group of breath-hold 2D TOF techniques whereby flowing spins are tagged at one position in a vessel and imaged later at a downstream position. Two broad categories are excitation bolus tracking (Shimizu et al. 1986) and presaturation bolus tracking (Edelman et al. 1989). The displacement of the bolus between the time of tagging and the time of imaging allows direct visualization of the motion of the fluid (Fig. 21.4). The velocity of the bolus can be calculated as the ratio of bolus displacement and time delay between two corresponding images.

21.3 Applications of MRA to the Splenoportal Venous System

21.3.1 Normal Anatomy

The portal vein normally supplies 70% of the blood flow to the liver parenchyma. The portal vein receives almost all the blood flow from the digestive tract between the proximal stomach and upper rectum, as well as the spleen, pancreas, and gallbladder. The splenic and superior mesenteric veins join behind the pancreas to form the portal vein. The splenic vein sits in a groove of the pancreas and receives the short gastric veins, the pancreatic veins, the left gastroepiploic vein, and the inferior mesenteric vein. The portal vein receives the superior pancreaticoduodenal vein and the left gastric vein. The superior mesenteric vein receives the inferior pancreaticoduo-

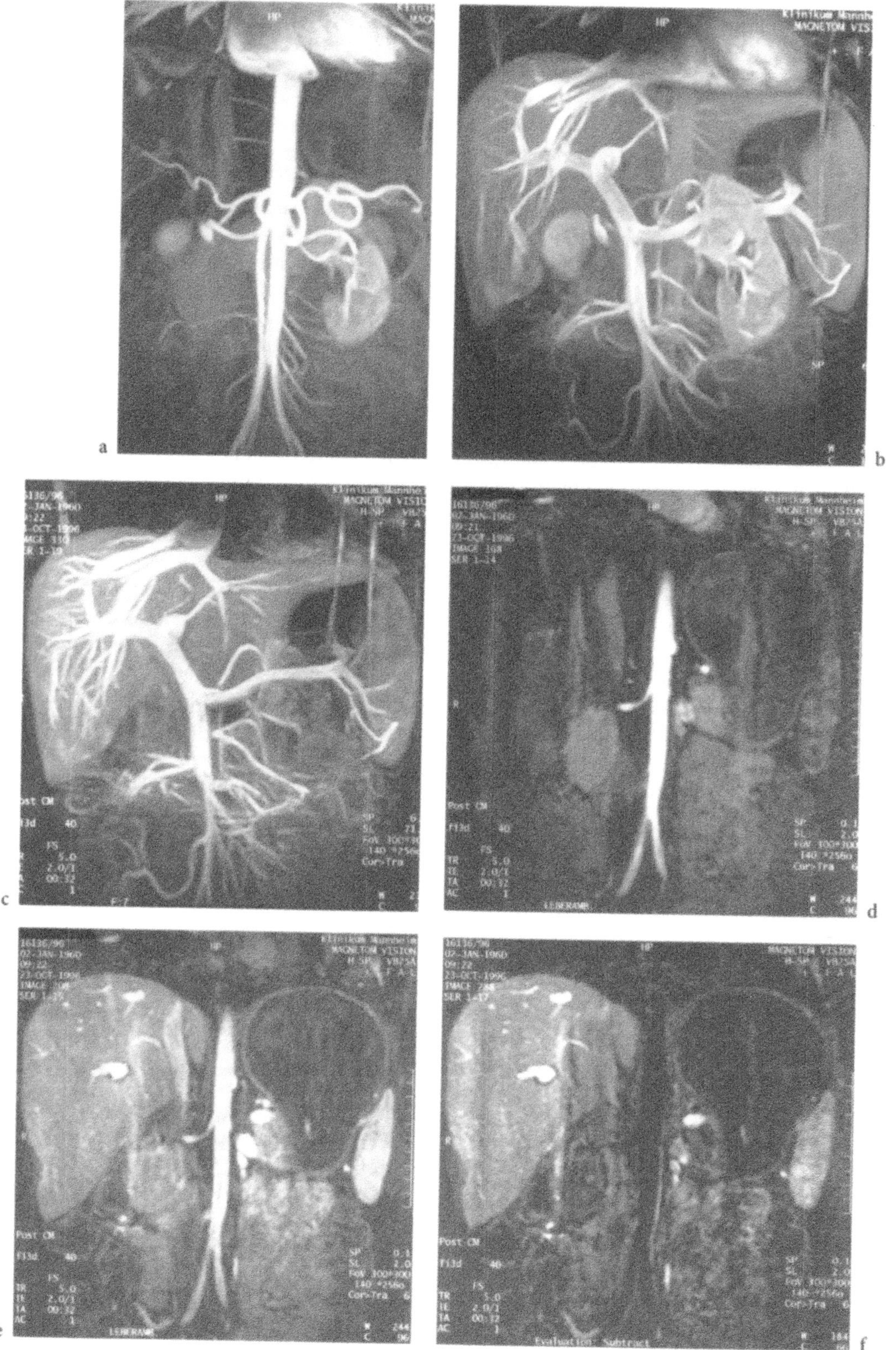

Fig. 21.2. Arterial phase (**a**) and portal-venous phase (**b**) MIP reconstructions of dual-phase CE 3D MRA. By subtracting the arterial phase data set from the portal-venous data set a "pure" MR venogram (**c**) with excellent depiction of the splenoportal-venous system as well as hepatic veins may be obtained. Raw data image of arterial phase (**d**) and portal-venous phase (**e**). Subtracted image (**f**) with absent arterial vascular signal

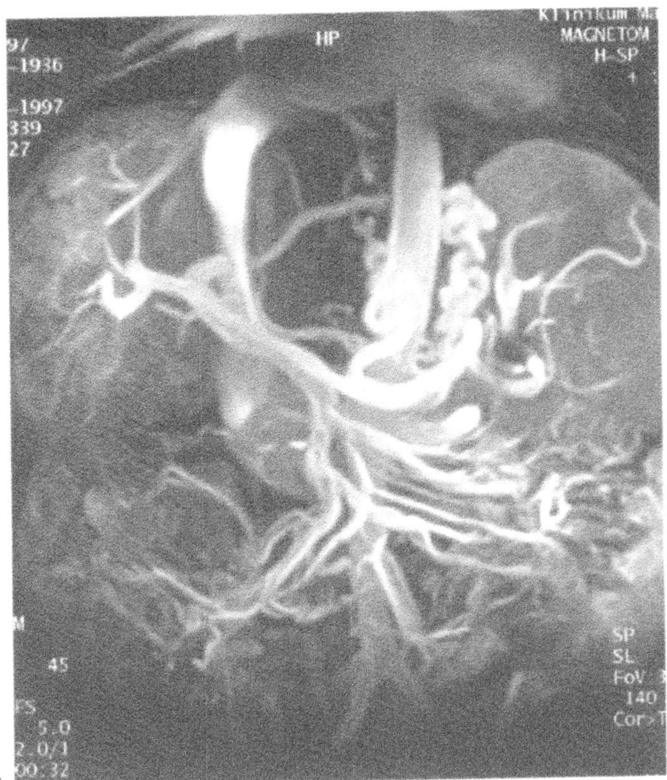

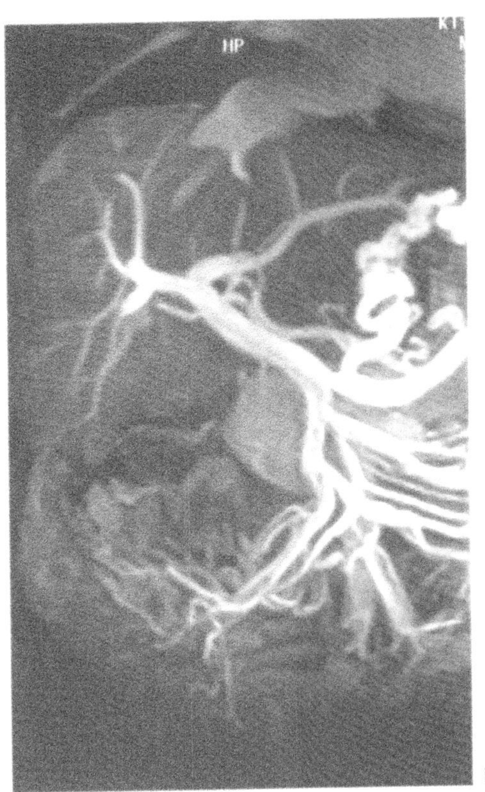

Fig. 21.3. Whole volume (**a**) and subvolume (**b**) MIP of CE 3D MRA in a patient with portal hypertension due to alcoholic liver cirrhosis. The subvolume ("targeted") MIP allows for excellent depiction of the splenoportal venous system without overlaying structures

denal vein and the right gastroepiploic vein. There is some variation in the veins draining into the portal system.

There are three main hepatic veins. The middle and left veins join before entering the vena cava in 80% of individuals. The major veins divide at acute angles into branches of equal diameter to form an axial tree that receives smaller tributaries at right angles. Anastomoses are commonly found between branches of the hepatic veins. Several additional veins drain directly into the vena cava, including those from the caudate lobe. The caudate veins usually remain patent when thrombosis affects the main hepatic veins in Budd-Chiari syndrome, allowing the caudate lobe to undergo compensatory hyperplasia.

21.3.2 Anomalies of the Portal Venous System

Anomalies of the portal venous system are uncommon. A portion of the right liver may be supplied by a branch of the left portal vein. The ductus venosus usually closes shortly after birth. Persistent ductus venosus prevents the normal development of the portal vein, leading to hypoplasia of the intrahepatic branches, nodular hyperplasia of the liver, and hyperammonemia. Atresia or agenesis of the portal vein may be congenital or a result of neonatal omphalitis or portal vein thrombosis. Portal vein thrombosis may lead to remodeling of the liver, recognized as nodular hyperplasia or atrophy of the left lobe.

21.3.3 Portal Venous Collateral Circulation

When portal vein blood flow is impeded by cirrhosis or thrombosis of portal and hepatic veins, dilated collateral veins are found at many sites (Fig. 21.5). These collateral vessels are prone to rupture, especially in the submucosa of the esophagus and stomach and less often in the colon. The surgeon encounters collateral veins at additional sites, especially in various hepatic ligaments, retroperitoneal attachments of other abdominal organs, both sides of the diaa

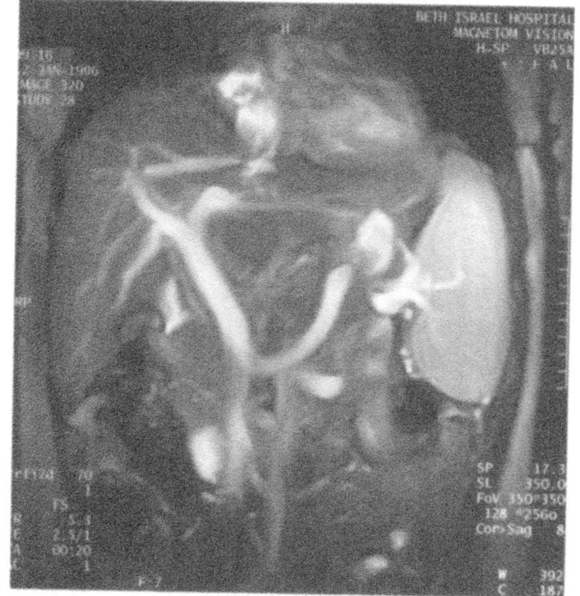

b

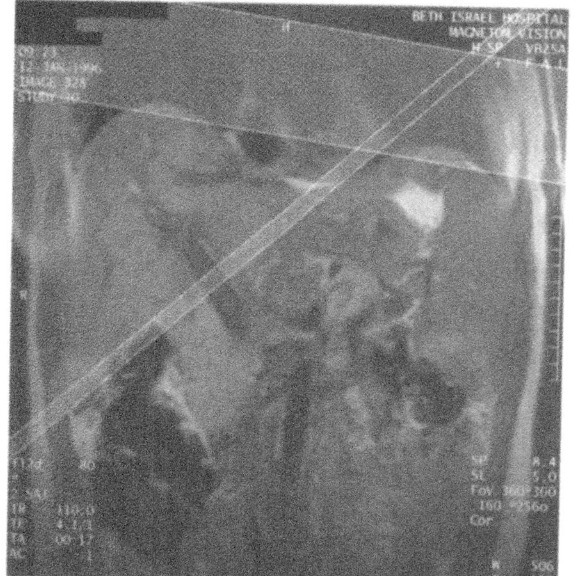

c

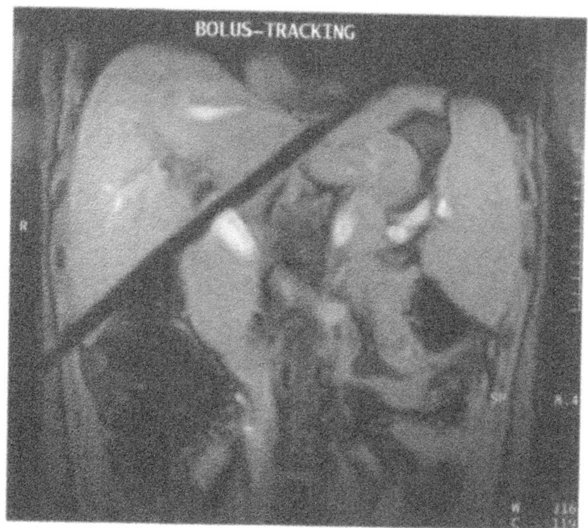

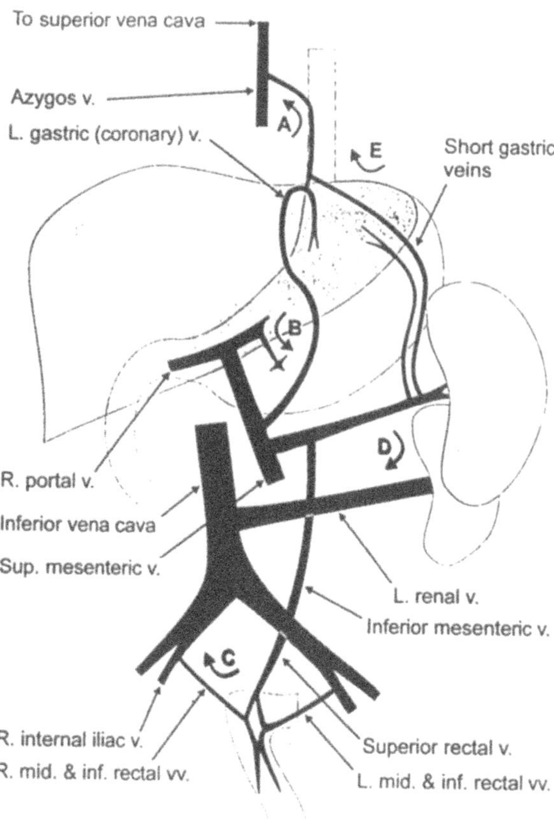

Fig. 21.5. Diagram of portal circulation with portosystemic collateral pathways. The most important sites for the potential development of portosystemic collateral vessels are shown. *A*, Esophageal submucosal veins, supplied by the left gastric vein and draining into the superior vena cava through the azygos vein; *B*, paraumbilical veins, supplied by the umbilical portion of the left portal vein and draining into abdominal wall veins near the umbilicus; *C*, rectal submucosal veins, supplied by the inferior mesenteric vein through the superior rectal vein and draining into the internal iliac veins through the middle rectal veins; *D*, splenorenal shunts, created spontaneously or surgically; *E*, short gastric veins communicate with the esophageal plexus

Fig. 21.4a–c. A 35-year-old patient with liver cirrhosis. Coronal 2D True-FISP image (**a**) and bolus-tracking technique (**b**). Bolus-tracking image (**c**) shows hepatopedal blood flow

phragm, the lesser omentum, and near the bladder and rectum. These veins drain into the systemic circuit mainly through the azygous, renal, adrenal, and inferior hemorrhoidal veins. Dilated periumbilical veins arise from the umbilical portion of the left portal vein, extend to the umbilicus by means of the round ligament, and connect with epigastric and internal mammary veins to produce umbilical and abdominal wall varices. Within the cirrhotic liver there is significant collateral flow in small veins that connect branches of the portal and hepatic veins.

21.3.4 Portal Hypertension

Cirrhosis, usually caused by alcohol ingestion or chronic viral hepatitis, is the most common cause of portal hypertension in Western populations, but there are many other causes, most of which are noncirrhotic. Schistosomiasis is a particularly prevalent cause of portal hypertension in developing countries. Knowledge of the pathology of these conditions has confirmed the existence of resistance to portal flow at a variety of different anatomic levels in the pathogenesis of portal hypertension. This is reflected in the conventional classification of the causes of portal hypertension according to the localization of the site of maximal resistance to portal flow (Table 21.1). Regarding the three major categories of prehepatic, intrahepatic, and posthepatic portal hypertension, the site of increased resistance is usually obvious. Thus, portal vein thrombosis exemplifies prehepatic portal hypertension, whereas inferior vena caval web typifies posthepatic portal hypertension. For intrahepatic causes, the site of resistance is conventionally further subdivided into presinusoidal, sinusoidal, and postsinusoidal portal hypertension.

The initial clinical presentation of portal hypertension may be with gastrointestinal hemorrhage or with other signs of liver disease. Congestive gastropathy may present with iron deficiency anemia. An initial presentation with acute bleeding in an otherwise healthy-appearing individual is typical in patients with prehepatic portal hypertension caused by portal vein thrombosis. Patients with cirrhosis or postsinusoidal portal hypertension (e.g., Budd-Chiari syndrome) more often present with other signs of advanced liver disease, including ascites, hepatic encephalopathy, jaundice, spider angiomata, or coagulopathy.

In most patients, portal hypertension is due to alcoholic liver cirrhosis. The physiologic diagnosis of portal hypertension is based on a direct pressure measurement of at least 6 mmHg more than that in the inferior vena cava. These measurements are obtained using hepatic wedge venography. With increasing portal pressure, blood is shunted away from the liver into systemic veins. The most common pathway is the left gastric vein-esophageal plexus pathway. Other collaterals include gastrosplenic, splenorenal, retroperitoneal, and periumbilical pathways (Fig. 21.6).

The initial techniques for the evaluation of patients with suspected portal hypertension – ultrasound including duplex Doppler and color Doppler flow imaging – accurately demonstrate reversed flow in the portal vein as well as other changes associated with portal hypertension such as ascites and splenomegaly. The advantages of MRA over ultrasound are largely related to its unrestricted field of view and its insensitivity to bowel gas and the patient's habitus.

Table 21.1. Causes of portal hypertension

Primary Increased Flow
Arterioportal venous fistula
Intrahepatic
Intrasplenic
Splanchnic
Splenic capillary hemangiomatosis
Primary Increased Resistance
Prehepatic
Thrombosis/cavernous transformation of the portal vein
Splenic vein thrombosis
Intrahepatic
Presinusoidal
Schistosomiasis
Sarcoidosis
Myeloproliferative diseases/myelofibrosis
Congenital hepatic fibrosis
Idiopathic portal hypertension (hepatoportal sclerosis)
Chronic arsenic hepatotoxicity
Azathioprine hepatotoxicity
Vinyl chloride hepatotoxicity
Early primary biliary cirrhosis
Early primary sclerosing cholangitis
Sinusoidal/mixed
Cirrhosis secondary to chronic hepatitis
Alcoholic cirrhosis
Cryptogenic cirrhosis
Methotrexate
Alcoholic hepatitis
Hypervitaminosis A
Incomplete septal fibrosis
Nodular regenerative hyperplasia
Postsinusoidal
Veno-occlusive disease
Hepatic vein thrombosis (Budd-Chiari syndrome)
Posthepatic
Inferior vena caval web
Constrictive pericarditis
Tricuspid insufficiency
Severe right heart failure

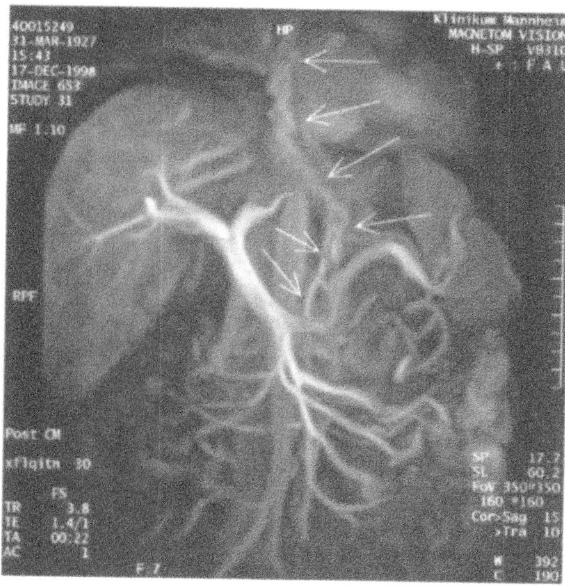

a

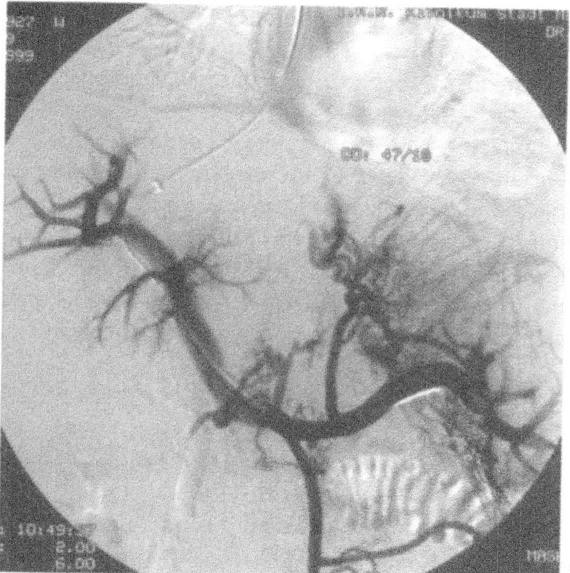
b

Fig. 21.6a, b. A 71-year-old patient with extensive submucosal and periesophageal varices. CE 3D MRA (**a**), direct splenoportogram during TIPS (**b**)

FINN et al. (1993) have shown that 2D TOF MRA was better than sonography for detecting varices and assessing shunt patency. Esophageal and deep abdominal varices frequently escaped detection on ultrasonography, and gastric varices were undergraded compared with findings on MRA and surgery (Fig. 21.7). In addition, MRA is able to show more varices than endoscopy (JOHNSON et al. 1991). This discrepancy can be explained by the fact that endoscopy only detects submucosal varices (BURCHARTH 1991), whereas in MRA both submucosal and periesophageal varices can be visualized.

The use of high power gradients in conjunction with breath-hold gadolinium-enhanced 3D GRE pulse sequences has dramatically enhanced the visualization of the splenoportal venous system compared with PC and TOF MRA techniques. Yamashita et al. (1996) successfully visualized the portal vein in 24 patients by using a gadolinium-enhanced rapid acquisition gradient echo sequence. LEUNG et al. (1996) acquired high-resolution images of the portal vein by using a 3D breath-hold fat-suppressed gradient echo technique. SHIRKHODA et al. (1997) reported excellent depiction of the entire mesenteric system by using a breath-hold fat-saturated multiecho 3D gradient echo sequence. We have had similar positive experiences with CE MRA in our own clinical setting over the past years (GAA et al. 1998). Thus, CE 3D MRA has replaced diagnostic catheter angiography in the abdomen in most cases and catheter angiography is only performed for interventional procedures.

21.3.5 Transjugular Intrahepatic Portosystemic Shunt and Surgical Shunts

Transjugular intrahepatic portosystemic shunt (TIPS) is a well-accepted nonsurgical method for decompressing portal hypertension in patients with esophageal variceal bleeding unresponsive to sclerotherapy or in patients with intractable ascites. Before performing a TIPS procedure, patency of the hepatic and portal veins as well as a normal hepatic arterialization should be demonstrated (Fig. 21.8). The shortest way to perform a stented communication between a hepatic vein and an intrahepatic branch of the portal vein can be estimated before beginning the intervention. Thus, the procedure can be performed within a shorter time and the number of needle punctures can be reduced (MUELLER et al. 1994). STAFFORD-JOHNSON et al. (1998) successfully used 3D gadolinium-enhanced portal venous MRA as part of the pre-TIPS evaluation or after unsuccessful attempts at creating a TIPS.

MRA has a limited role in assessing patients after TIPS because of the artifacts caused by the metallic stents placed in the shunt (Fig. 21.9). This may change once nitinol or other nonmagnetic materials are used to create these shunts. Rare complications of TIPS, such as arterioportal fistulae, may be detected using CE 3D MRA (Fig. 21.10).

Surgical shunts are rare today, but when they must be assessed, MRA is highly advantageous because of its 3D nature (Fig. 21.11). Often a stenosis is obscured

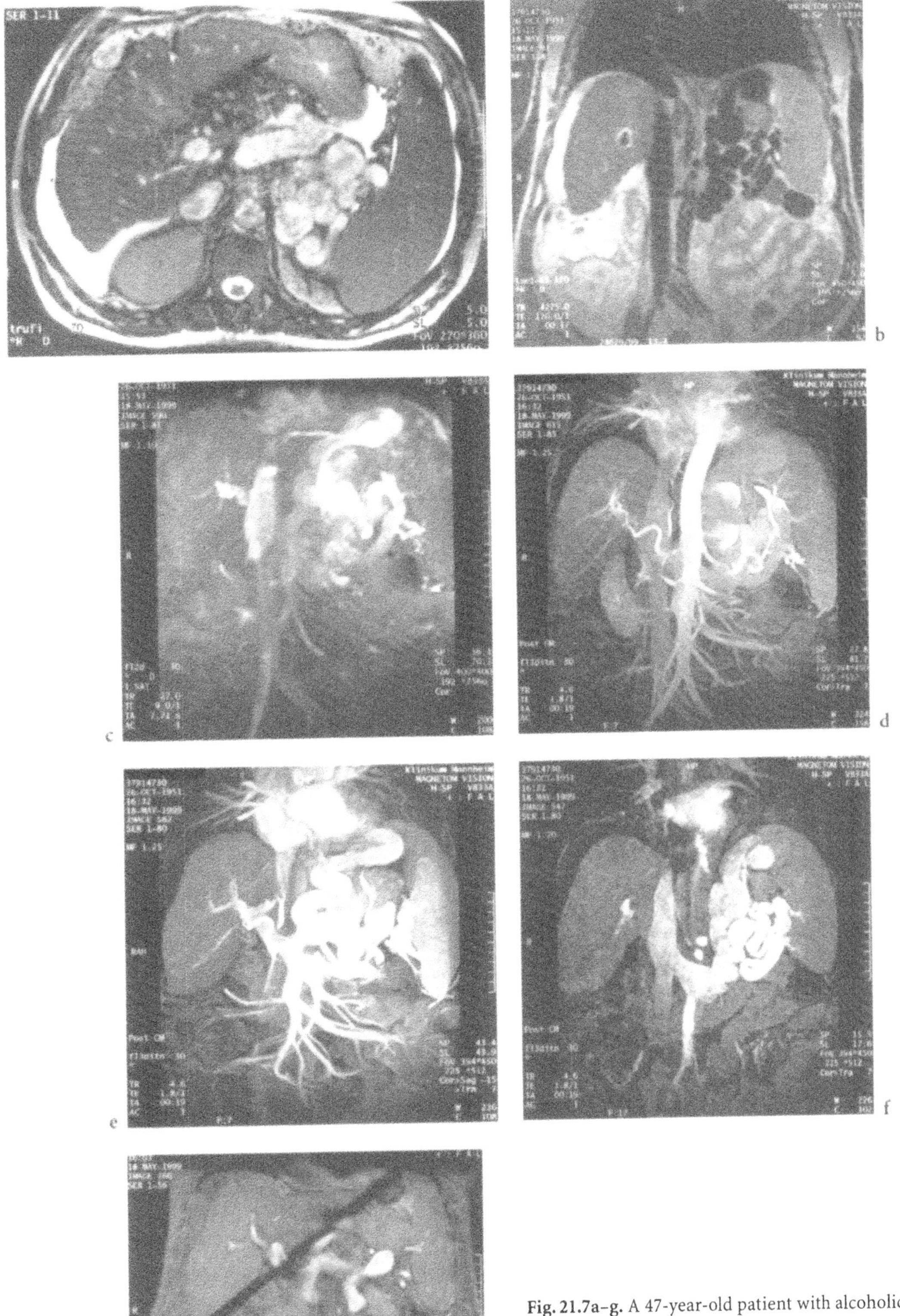

Fig. 21.7a–g. A 47-year-old patient with alcoholic liver cirrhosis (Child C). Transverse T2*-weighted True-FISP (**a**), coronal T2-weighted HASTE (**b**) coronal 2D TOF-MIP (**c**), coronal CE 3D MRA MIP (whole volume MIP **d**, targeted MIP **e**). The extensive varices are best seen using CE 3D MRA. A spontaneous splenorenal shunt is demonstrated using a "targeted" MIP of the 3D MRA (**f**). Bolus-tracking shows hepatofugal blood flow within the portal vein (**g**)

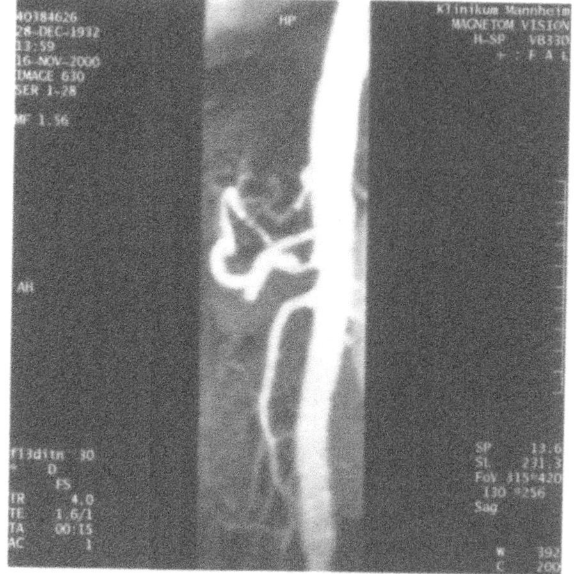

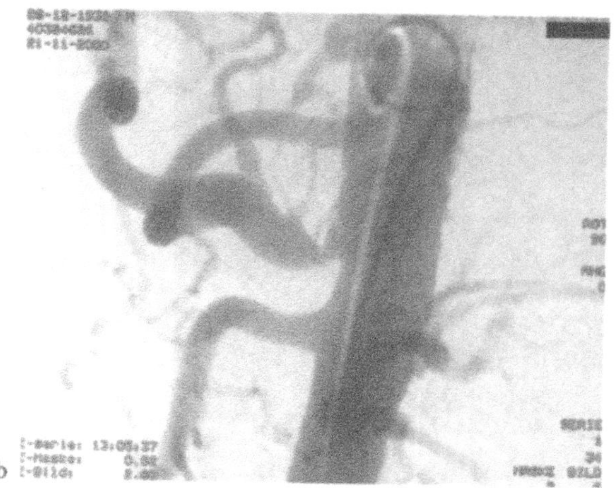

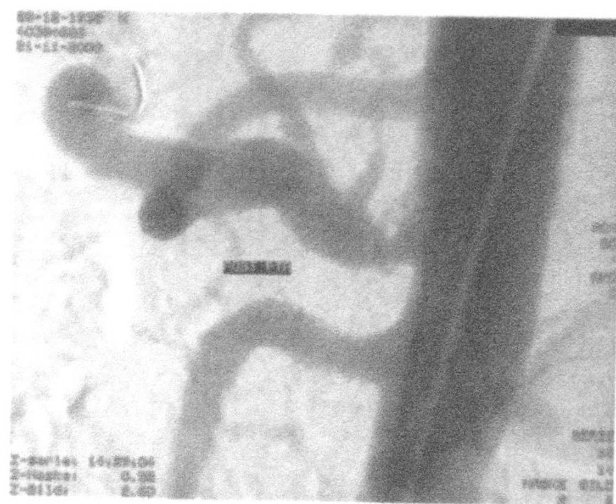

Fig. 21.8a–c. A 67-year-old patient with liver cirrhosis. Pre-TIPS evaluation using 3D MRA (arterial phase, **a**) shows high-grade stenosis of the celiac trunk. Correlation with intra-arterial DSA is shown in **b**. After percutaneous angioplasty (**c**) of the celiac trunk a TIPS was performed

by overlapping structures or an inadequate projection on conventional angiography. After a decompressive portosystemic shunt operation, assessment of shunt patency is required when the patient develops recurrent bleeding or ascites. While portacaval shunts can usually be evaluated by duplex ultrasound (Finn et al. 1987), this method is of limited value for the assessment of patency of the more commonly used spenorenal shunt, and especially the distal splenorenal (Warren) shunt because of bowel gas (Warren et al. 1982). In a study by Finn et al. (1991), MRA showed promising results in the follow-up of surgical shunt patency. In all shunt types, size and patency of the anastomotic area could be estimated by a presaturation or bolus tracking technique. Occasionally, metallic artifact from surgical clips may limit shunt evaluation by MRA.

21.3.6 Liver Transplantation

The major goal of the preoperative evaluation of liver transplant candidates is to provide the pertinent information needed to plan the transplant surgery and to exclude patients for whom surgery is not feasible or will be of no benefit. The direction and velocity of portal vein flow are generally not important for transplant patient selection. Portal vein thrombosis is no longer considered an absolute contraindication to transplantation because several methods of revascularization are now available (Stieber et al. 1991). Prior knowledge of the hepatic arterial supply is useful, as aberrant hepatic arterial anatomy is common (Fig. 21.12). In addition, preoperative arterial assessment is useful in identifying patients with celiac axis stenosis, who will then be predisposed to posttransplant ischemia.

Several studies reported that both TOF and PC techniques are accurate methods for determining portal venous patency. Finn et al. evaluated 30 patients before liver transplantation by using a breath-hold TOF technique and reported a sensitivity and specificity of 100% and 96%, respectively, in identifying portal vein occlusion (Finn et al. 1991). Hughes et al. compared 2D TOF of the portal venous system with ultrasound, computed tomography, and conventional angiography and reported an overall agreement of 98% (Hughes et al. 1996). Nghiem et al. (1995) evaluated 24 patients with portal hypertension by using a breath-hold PC technique (Nghiem et al. 1995). In this study, PC MRA accurately evaluated the status of the portal vein, superior mesenteric vein, and splenic vein, as well as identi-

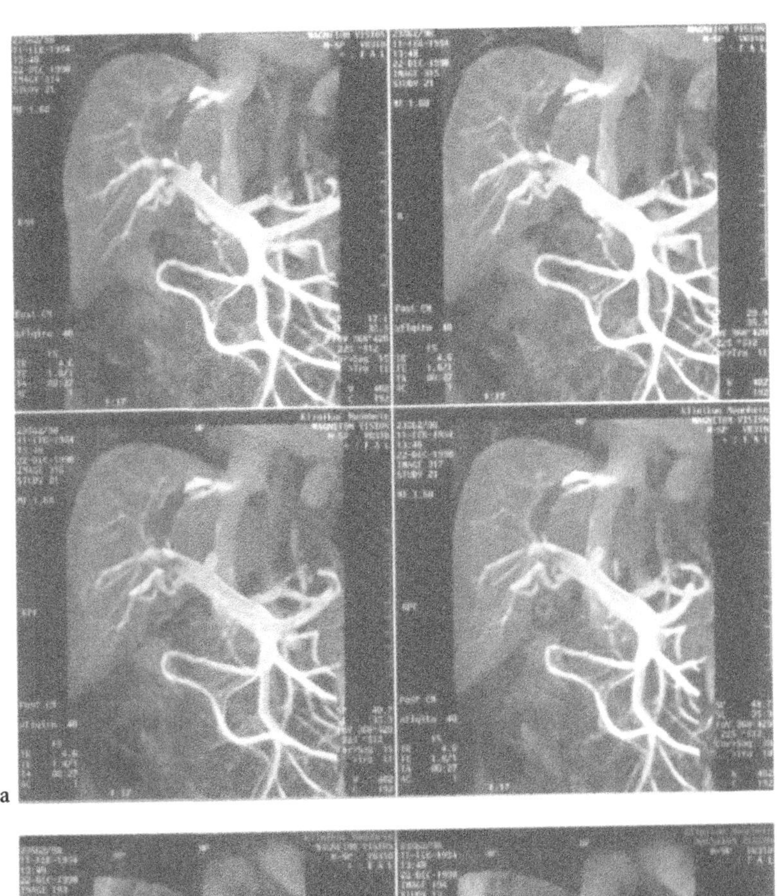

a

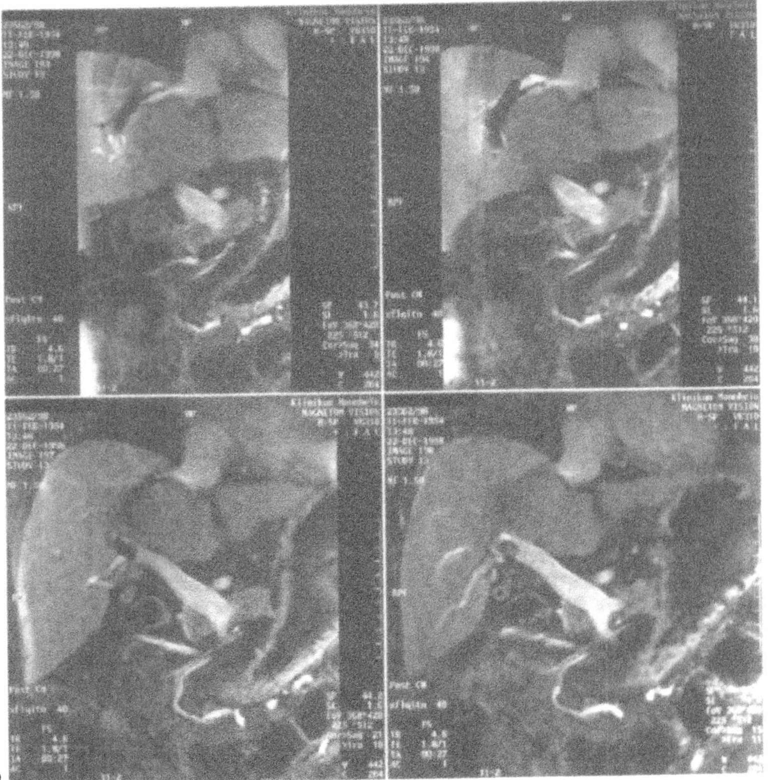

b

Fig. 21.9a, b. CE 3D MRA. (MIP reconstruction, **a**; multiplanar reformation; **b**) demonstrating signal loss within the TIPS tract due to susceptibility artifacts from Palmaz and Wallstent

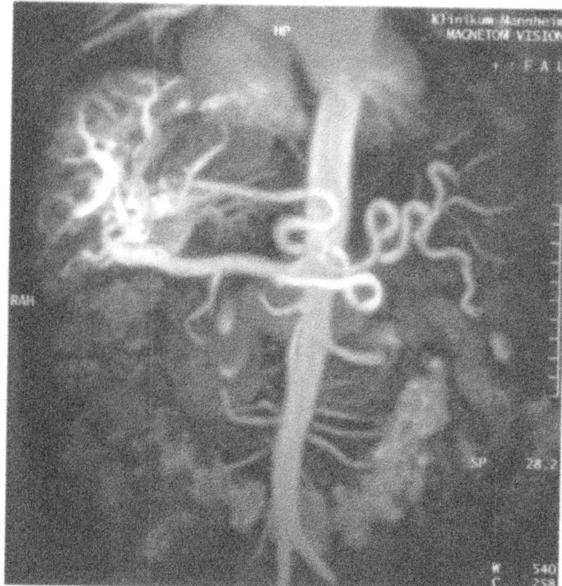

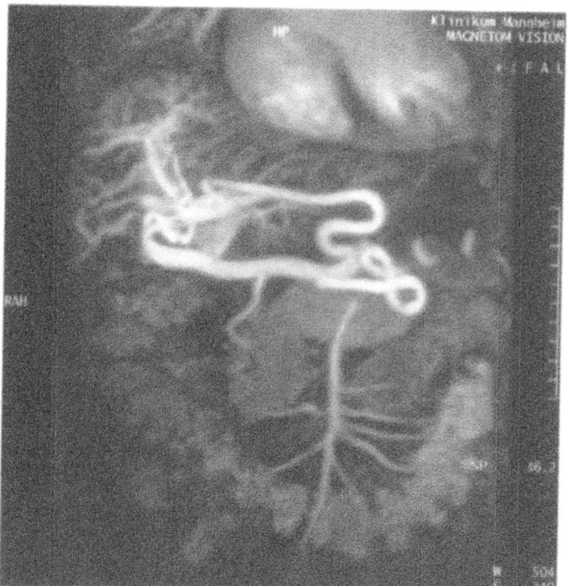

Fig. 21.10a, b. Arterioportal fistulae as a rare complication of TIPS demonstrated on 3D MRA. (whole volume MIP, **a**; targeted MIP, **b**)

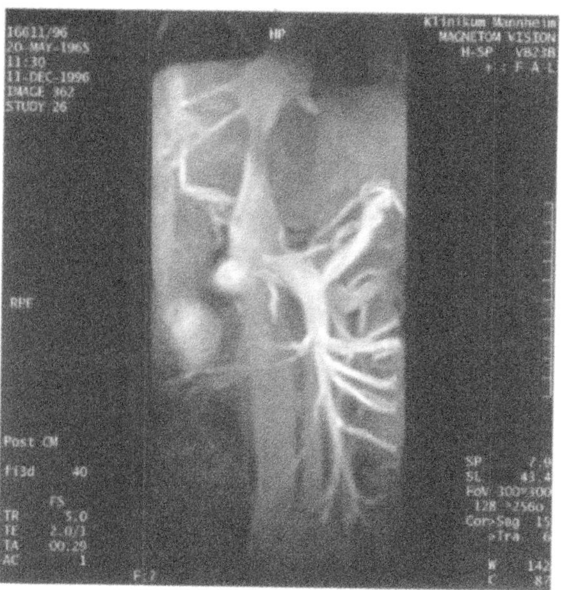

Fig. 21.11. CE 3D MRA of a patent surgical porto-caval end-to-side shunt

fying the presence of varices and assessing the patency of surgically placed shunts in patients with portal hypertension. Applegate et al. showed in their study that quantitative PC MRA provides rapid assessment of portal vein patency, flow direction, and velocity (Applegate et al. 1993).

Compared with TOF and PC techniques, visualization of the portal venous system has been greatly improved by using gadolinium-enhanced 3D MRA. Shirkoda et al. reported excellent depiction of the entire mesenteric system in a series of 16 patients by using a breath-hold fat-saturated multiecho 3D gradient echo sequence (Shirkoda et al. 1997). Yamashita et al. and Leung et al. acquired high-resolution images of the portal vein by using breath-hold 3D gradient echo sequences after gadolinium administration (Yamashita et al. 1996; Leung et al. 1996).

Vascular complications after liver transplantation most commonly involve the hepatic artery. Doppler ultrasound is the initial imaging technique for evaluating vascular complications after liver transplantation. However, when ultrasound is positive or inconclusive, MRA is recommended at some institutions for further evaluation. Stafford-Johnson et al. reported on the utility of breath-hold CE 3D MRA in the detection of vascular complications in 13 liver transplant patients (Stafford-Johnson et al. 1998). In their study, gadolinium-enhanced 3D MRA detected hepatic artery stenosis/thrombosis, portal vein stenosis/thrombosis, and inferior vena cava stenosis with an accuracy similar to conventional angiography. They concluded that the role of MRA is likely to be in patients for whom ultrasound examination is technically limited or for whom there is a discrepancy between the clinical status and the reported ultrasound findings.

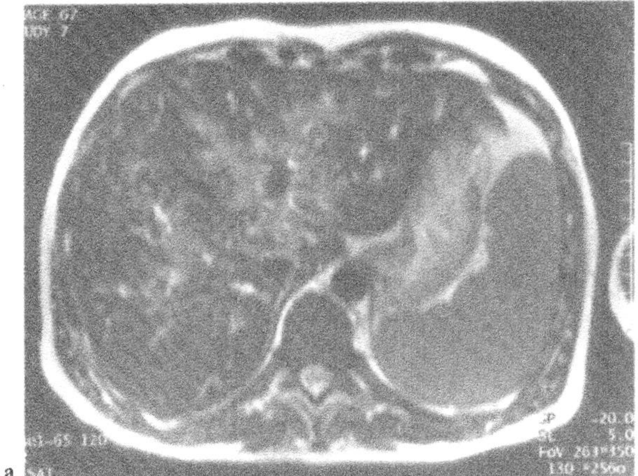

a

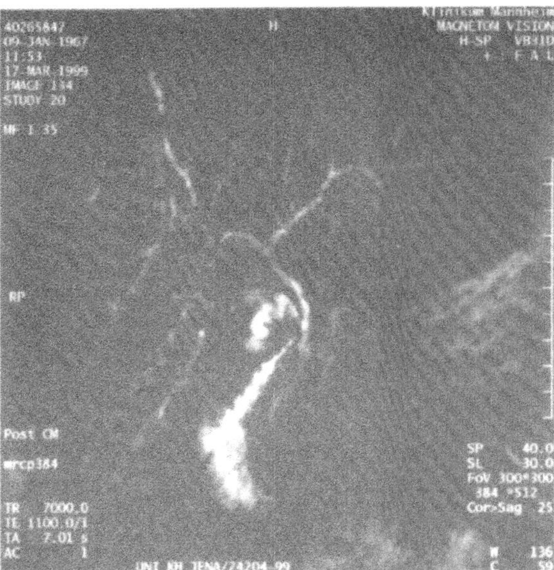

b

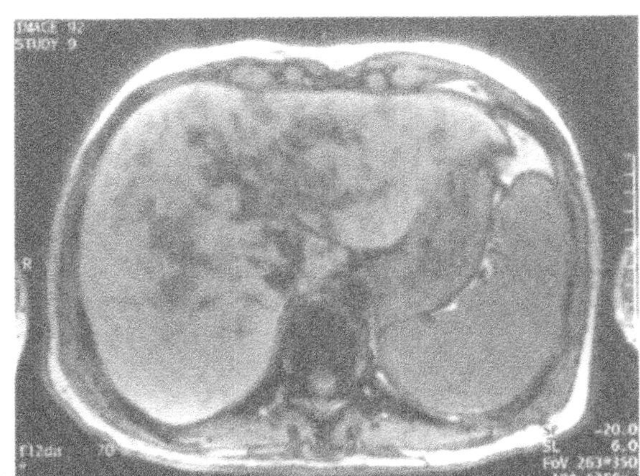

c

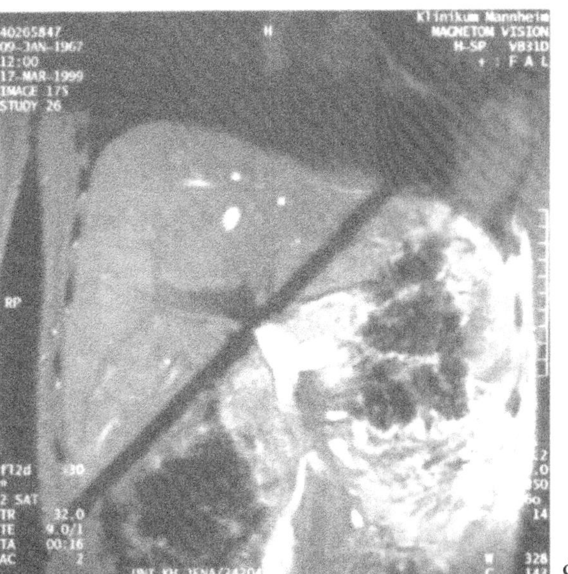

d

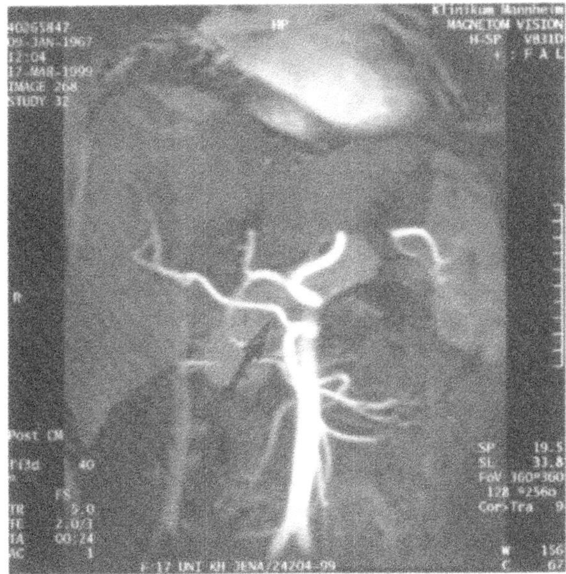

e

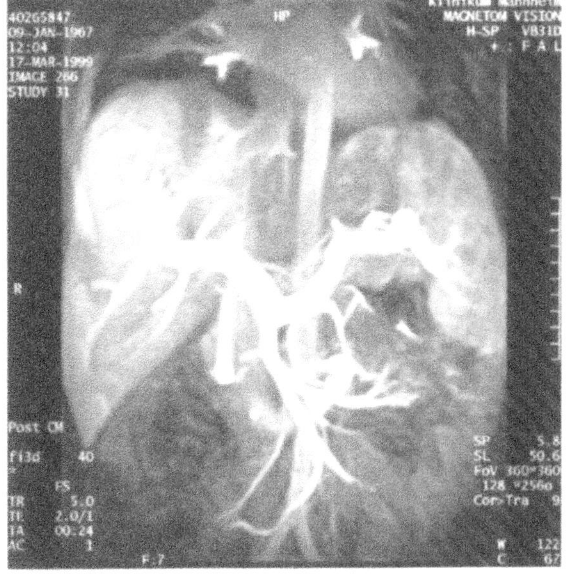

f

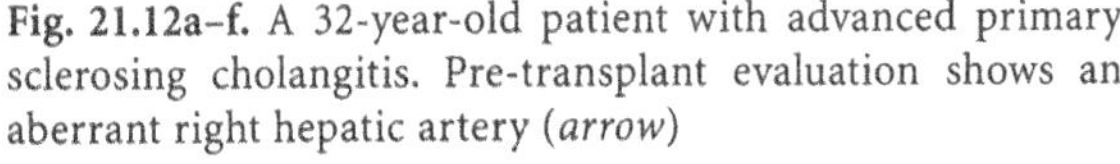

Fig. 21.12a–f. A 32-year-old patient with advanced primary sclerosing cholangitis. Pre-transplant evaluation shows an aberrant right hepatic artery (*arrow*)

21.3.7 Portal and Mesenteric Vein Thrombosis

Thrombosis of the portal vein can result from slow flow secondary to cirrhosis, direct invasion by cancer, obstruction by porta hepatis lymphadenopathy, inflammatory changes secondary to pancreatitis, abdominal infections, trauma, dehydration, oral contraceptives, polycythemia vera, and, in infants, umbilical vein cannulation (Table 21.2). Physical findings include abdominal tenderness, splenomegaly, and variceal bleeding. Patients with liver cirrhosis may additionally present with ascites and encephalopathy.

Ultrasound is effective at measuring portal vein flow and is usually sufficient to rule out complete thrombosis. B-mode imaging shows echogenic thrombus in the lumen of the main portal vein. Duplex Doppler imaging is helpful in determining whether the portal vein is thrombosed completely or partially. In patients with chronic portal vein thrombosis, multiple small collateral vessel develop in the porta hepatis. This result is termed cavernous transformation of the portal vein (Fig. 21.13). Duplex Doppler imaging is accurate for detecting thrombosis of the main portal vein with a sensitivity of 100% and a specificity of 93% (Lewis et al. 1989). However, diagnosing thrombosis of the intrahepatic portal branches is more difficult because of the background echogenicity of the liver. In addition, ultrasound cannot reliably examine the splenic and superior mesenteric vein tributaries for thrombosis. If overlying gas or surgical dressings preclude adequate evaluation, then CT or MRA using 2D TOF and True-FISP sequences or CE 3D gradient echo sequences provide a more

Table 21.2. Causes of portal vein thrombosis

Hypercoagulable States
Antiphospholipid syndrome
Factor V mutations
Paroxysmal nocturnal hemoglobinuria
Myeloproliferative diseases
Oral contraceptives
Polycythemia rubra vera
Pregnancy
Protein S deficiency
Sickle cell disease
Inflammatory Diseases
Behçet's disease
Crohn's disease
Pancreatitis
Ulcerative colitis
Complications of Medical Intervention
Alcohol injection
Ambulatory dialysis
Chemoembolization
Islet cell injection
Liver transplantation
Partial hepatectomy
Sclerotherapy
Splenectomy
Transjugular intrahepatic portosystemic shunt
Umbilical catheterization
Infections
Actinomycosis
Appendicitis
Candida albicans infection
Diverticulitis
Miscellaneous
Cirrhosis
Bladder cancer
Nodular regenerative hyperplasia

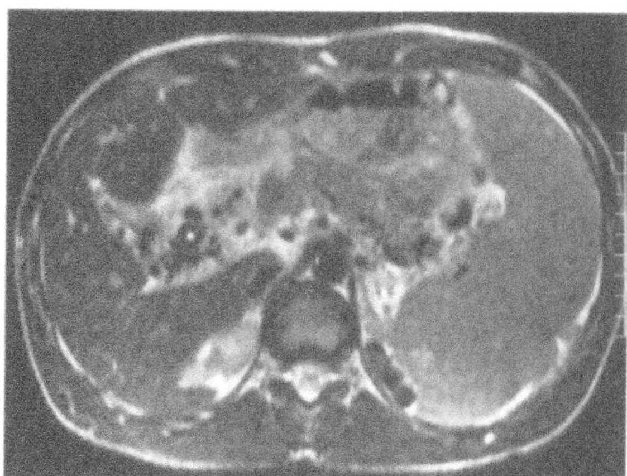
a

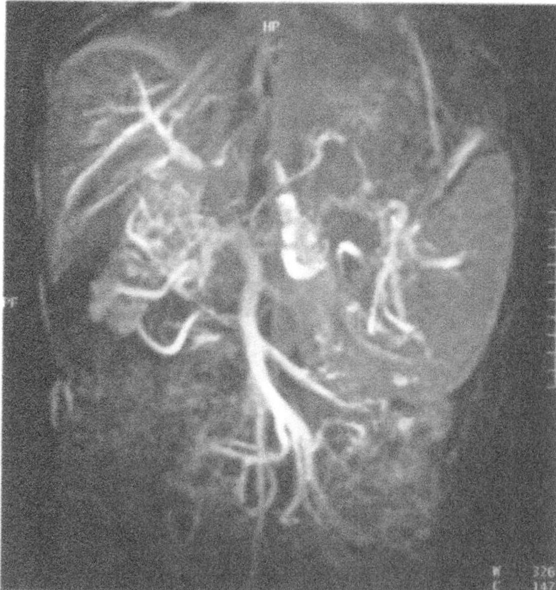
b

Fig. 21.13a, b. Cavernous transformation of the portal vein with multiple small collateral vessels within the porta hepatis. T2-weighted TSE-sequence (**a**), CE 3D MRA (**b**). There is also splenic vein thrombosis

comprehensive examination, allowing one to evaluate the liver and pancreas for malignancy and the abdomen for infection (Fig. 21.14). When using CE MRA, careful analysis of the source images as well as multiplanar reformations are most helpful for correct diagnosis.

21.3.8 Tumor Encasement

Vascular encasement may involve an artery, vein, or both. Narrowing of the splenic, superior mesenteric, or portal vein is a common finding in patients with pancreatic adenocarcinoma. MRA plays a significant role in the preoperative evaluation of tumors of the liver, bile ducts, and particularly the pancreas. McFarland et al. (1996) reported on the use of a CE breath-hold 2D TOF sequence in the preoperative assessment of vascular encasement in 20 patients with pancreatic carcinoma. In this study, MRA correctly identified all 11 resectable tumors but only five of nine unresectable tumors. In a prospective study (Trede et al. 1997) comparing dual-phase 3D MRA with conventional catheter angiography in 58 patients with pancreatic tumors, sensitivity, specificity, and overall accuracy of MRA in the assessment of vascular infiltration were 81.9%, 96.0%, and 89.1%, respectively. Conventional angiography yielded a sensitivity, specificity, and overall accuracy of 442.9%, 100%, and 68.8% (Figs. 21.15, 21.16).

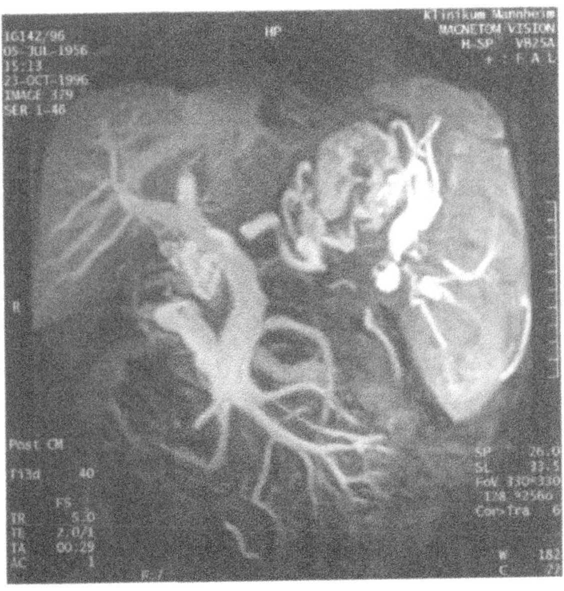

Fig. 21.14. CE 3D MRA in a 40-year-old patient with splenic vein thrombosis due to chronic pancreatitis

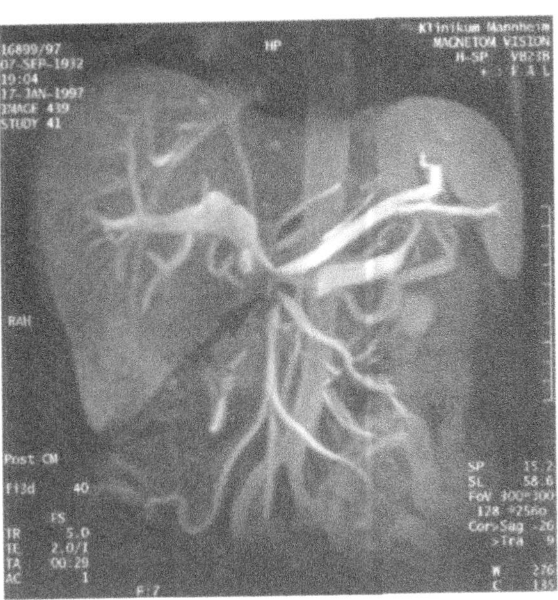

Fig. 21.15. CE 3D MRA in a patient with unresectable pancreatic head adenocarcinoma due to tumor infiltration of the venous confluence

21.3.9 Budd-Chiari Syndrome

The Budd-Chiari syndrome (BCS) comprises a collection of anatomic and physiologic changes brought about by a reduction of hepatic venous outflow. The reduction can be caused by impediments to flow anywhere from the right atrium to small radicles of the hepatic veins, thus sharing features with veno-occlusive disease (VOD).

In its classic form, BCS is an almost complete obstruction to flow by the acute formation of blood clot at the opening of the hepatic veins into the inferior vena cava. This sudden event is followed by the onset of hepatomegaly, pain, ascites, and liver failure. Early mortality in untreated patients with this classic form of the syndrome is very high. Improved methods of imaging the hepatic vasculature have resulted in recognition of more subtle forms of BCS. In Western countries, the leading cause is "idiopathic", accounting for 40% of collected cases. One fourth of cases are due to hematologic disorders, primarily polycythemia rubra vera. Tumors, infections, and pregnancy each cause about 10% of cases (Table 21.3).

The presentation of BCS can be fulminant, acute or chronic. Fulminant BCS is seen most often in women with pregnancy-related BCS. Severe pain, hepatomegaly, jaundice, ascites, and rapid deterioration of hepatic function are characteristic. Few of these

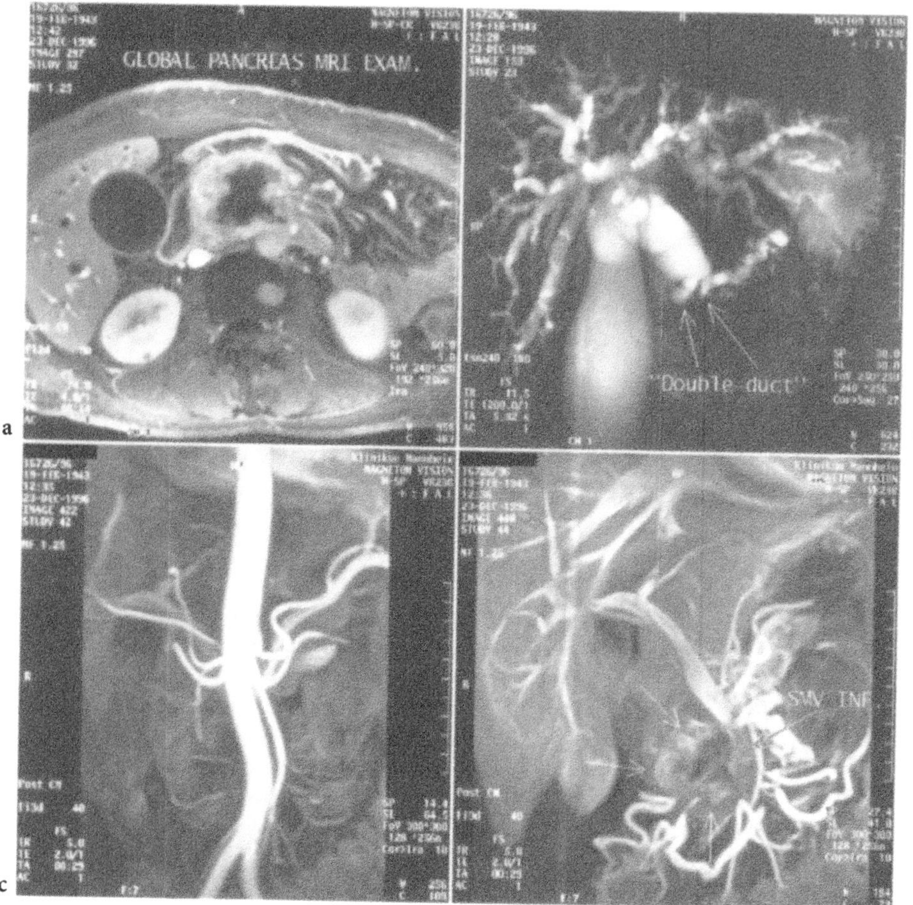

Fig. 21.16a–d. Global ("One-stop-shop") MRI examination in a 46-year-old patient with unresectable adenocarcinoma of the pancreatic head. T1-weighted fat-suppressed gradient echo with fat-suppression (**a**), MRCP (**b**), arterial (**c**) and portal-venous phase (**d**) 3D MRA

Table 21.3. Causes of Budd-Chiari syndrome

Hypercoagulable States
- Antiphospholipid syndrome
- Antithrombin III deficiency
- Essential thrombocytosis
- Factor V Leiden
- Lupus anticoagulant
- Myeloproliferative disorder
- Paroxysmal nocturnal hemoglobinuria
- Polycythemia rubra vera
- Postpartum thrombocytopenic purpura
- Protein C deficiency
- Protein S deficiency
- Sickle cell disease

Infections
- Amebic liver abscess
- Aspergillosis
- Filariasis
- Hepatic abscess
- Hydatid cysts
- Pelvic cellulitis
- Schistosomiasis
- Syphilis
- Tuberculosis

Cancer
- Adrenal cancer
- Bronchogenic carcinoma
- Fibrolamellar cancer
- Hepatoma
- Leiomyosarcoma
- Leukemia
- Renal cell cancer
- Rhabdomyosarcoma

Miscellaneous
- Behçet's disease
- Celiac disease
- Crohn's disease
- Laparoscopic cholecystectomy
- Membranous obstruction of vena cava
- Oral contraceptives
- Polycystic disease
- Pregnancy
- Sarcoidosis
- Trauma

patients survive without prompt intervention. Patients with chronic BCS have obviously survived the acute interruption of hepatic venous outflow. Prognosis depends on underlying disease, severity of liver failure, and the success of treatment.

Traditionally, catheterization of the inferior vena cava or percutaneous transhepatic venography has been needed to clearly establish the diagnosis of BCS. With duplex Doppler imaging and color Doppler imaging the diagnosis of BCS can be straightforward if the hepatic veins are filled with echogenic thrombus and Doppler evaluation shows no flow. However, the diagnosis can be more difficult in patients with underlying liver parenchymal disease or small-vein thrombosis. In these cases, CT and MRI are more effective in establishing the correct diagnosis. BCS most often results in atrophy of peripheral liver, which has especially severe venous obstruction, and hypertrophy of the caudate lobe and central liver, which are relatively spared. The absence of hepatic veins may be well shown by MR techniques in which flowing blood is signal void or by techniques in which flowing blood is high in signal, such as TOF techniques or gadolinium-enhanced gradient echo sequences (Fig. 21.17). In acute onset BCS the peripheral liver enhances less than central liver because of acute increased tissue pressure which results in diminished blood flow of both the hepatic arterial and portal venous system. Increased enhancement of peripheral liver may be seen in chronic BCS and may be due to a combination of decreased portal perfusion and dilatation of hepatic sinusoids.

21.3.10 Liver Tumors

As both hepatic arteries and liver/portal veins are displayed with dual-phase CE 3D MRA, this technique may be used as a tool for treatment planning in hepatic tumor surgery. Using multiplanar reconstructions, tumors can be allocated to the individual liver segments defined by these venous structures (Bismuth 1982; Couinaud 1957; Fig. 21.18). The dual-phase MRA protocol has the added advantage of essentially being a dynamic liver study. Thus, a hepatic mass can be evaluated dynamically provided it is included in the imaging volume (Figs. 21.19, 21.20).

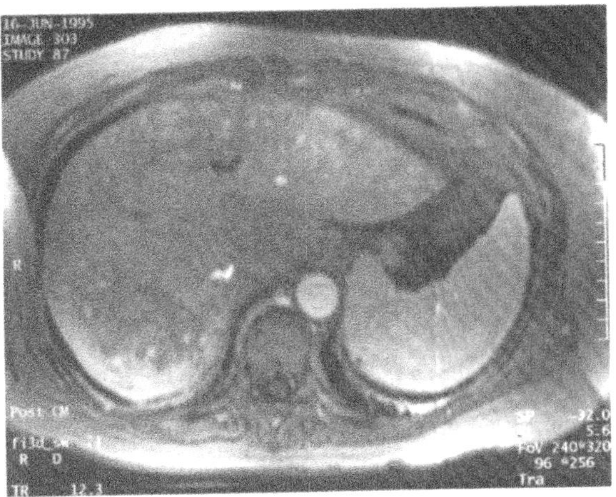
a

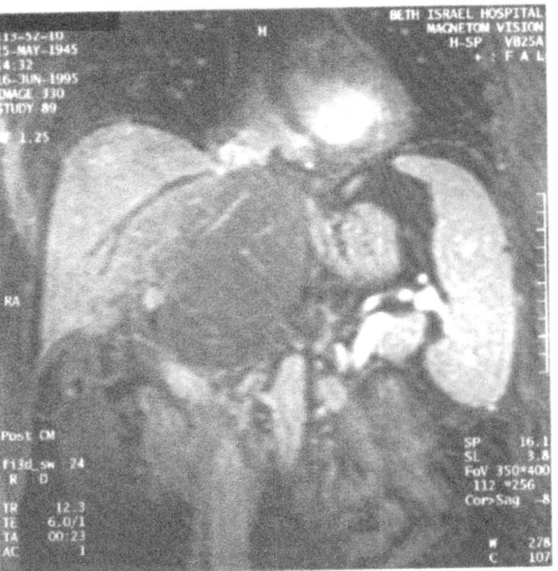

b

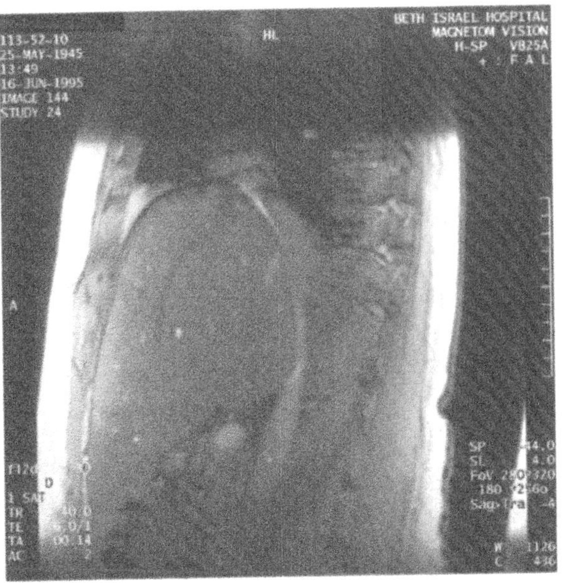

c

Fig. 21.17a–c. Acute Budd-Chiari syndrome. MRI shows patchy enhancement of liver parenchyma and absent vascular signal within hepatic veins. Gadolinium-enhanced fat-suppressed T1-weighted gradient echo images (transverse, **a**; coronal **b**) and sagittal 2D TOF gradient echo image (**c**)

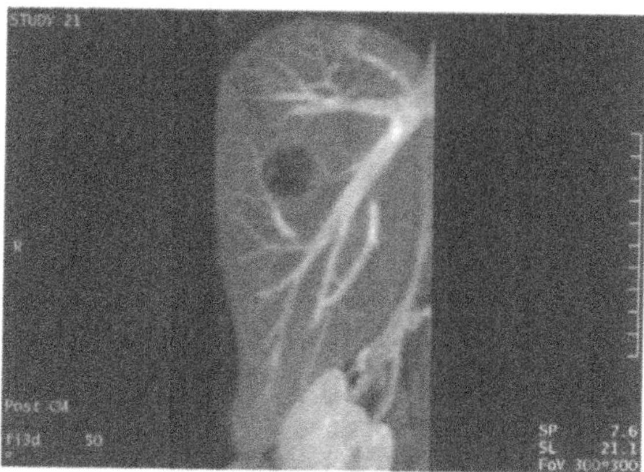

Fig. 21.18. CE 3D MRA (venous phase) showing relationship of hepatic metastasis and hepatic veins

a

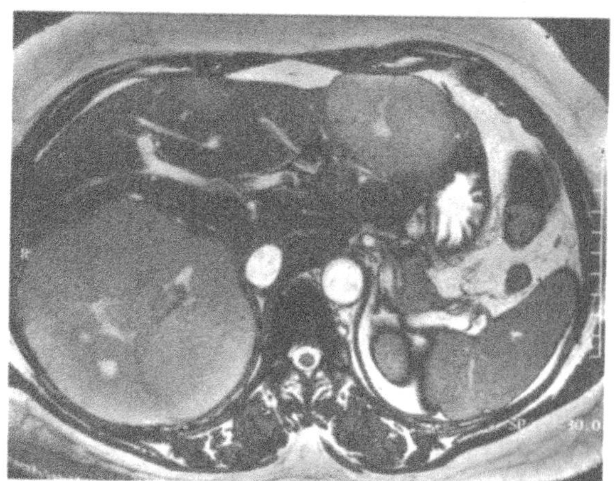

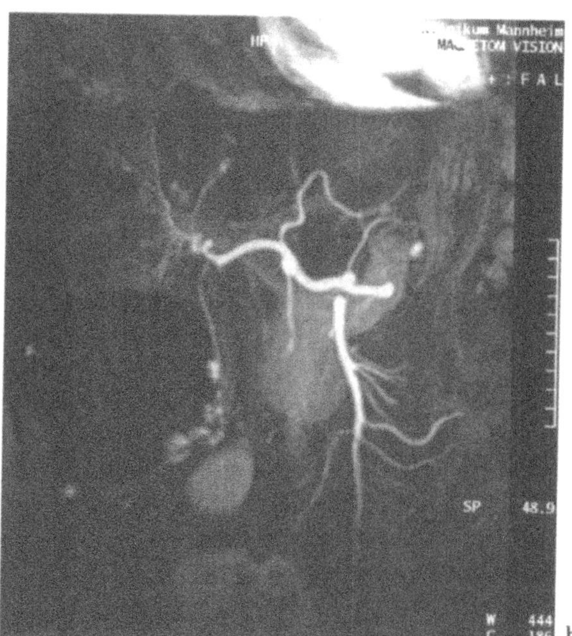

b

c

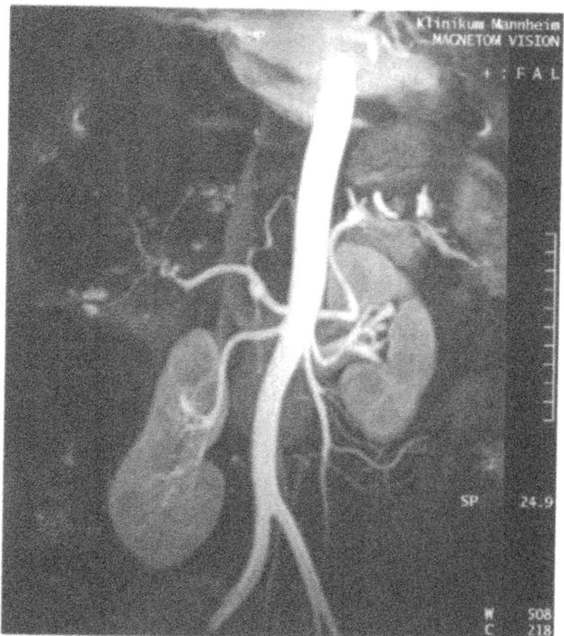

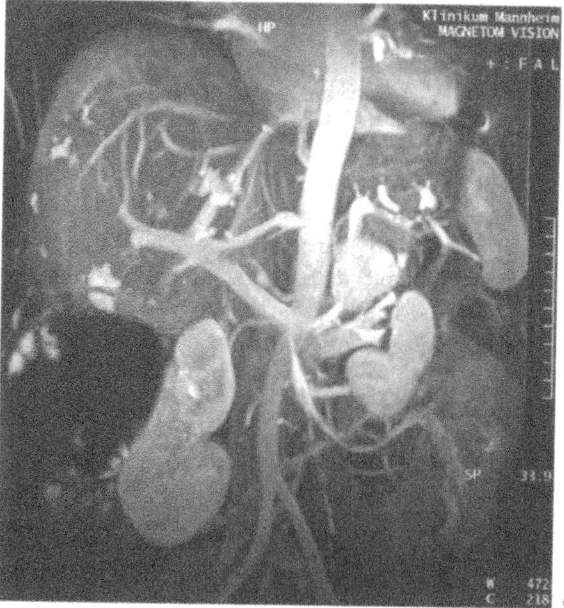

d

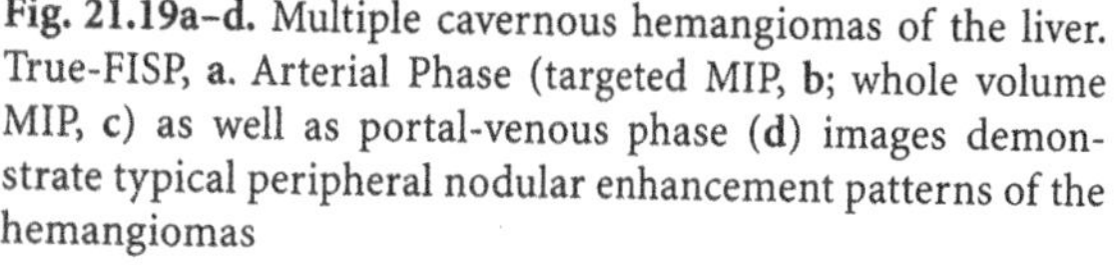

Fig. 21.19a–d. Multiple cavernous hemangiomas of the liver. True-FISP, **a.** Arterial Phase (targeted MIP, **b**; whole volume MIP, **c**) as well as portal-venous phase (**d**) images demonstrate typical peripheral nodular enhancement patterns of the hemangiomas

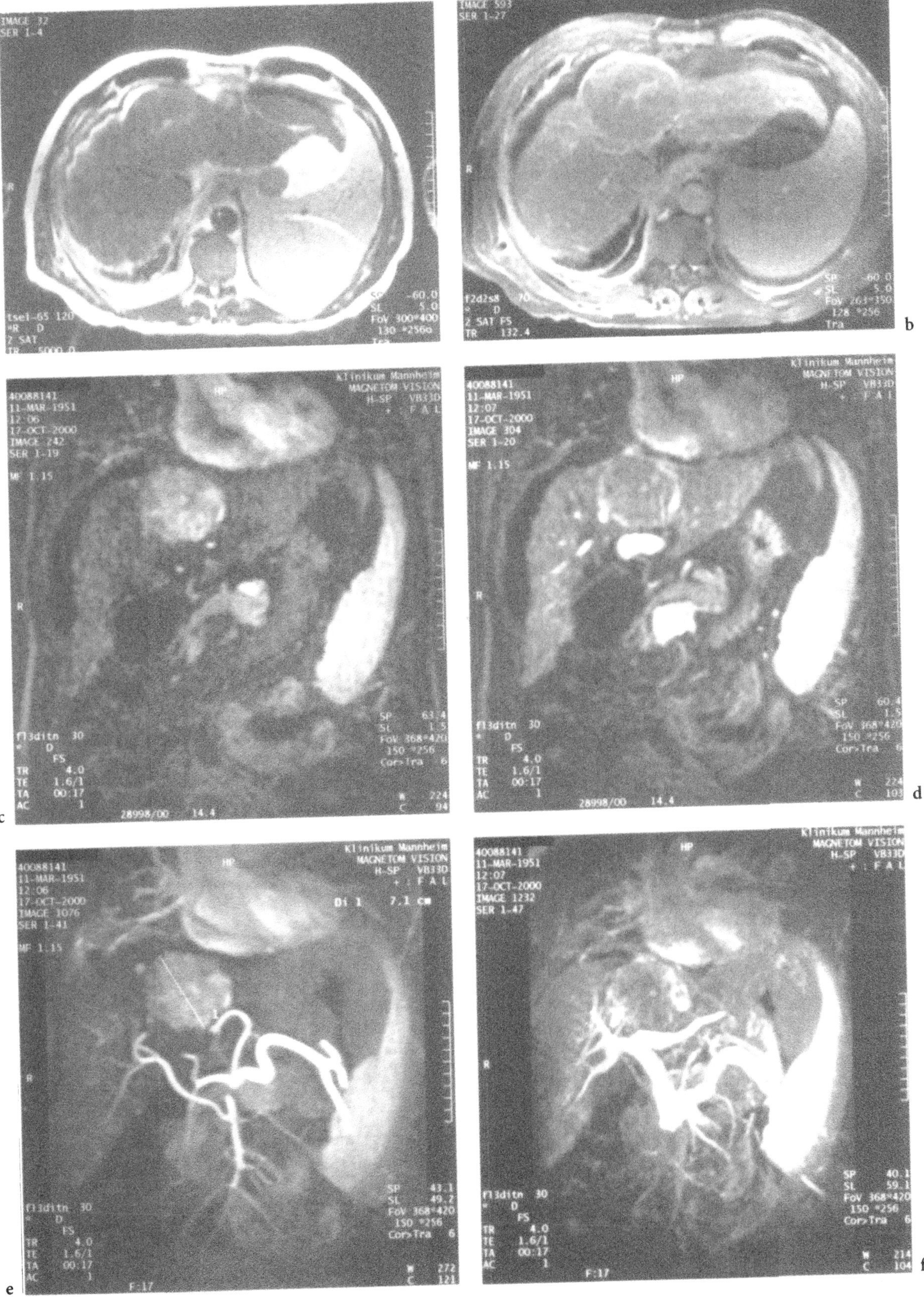

Fig. 21.20g–j. See next page

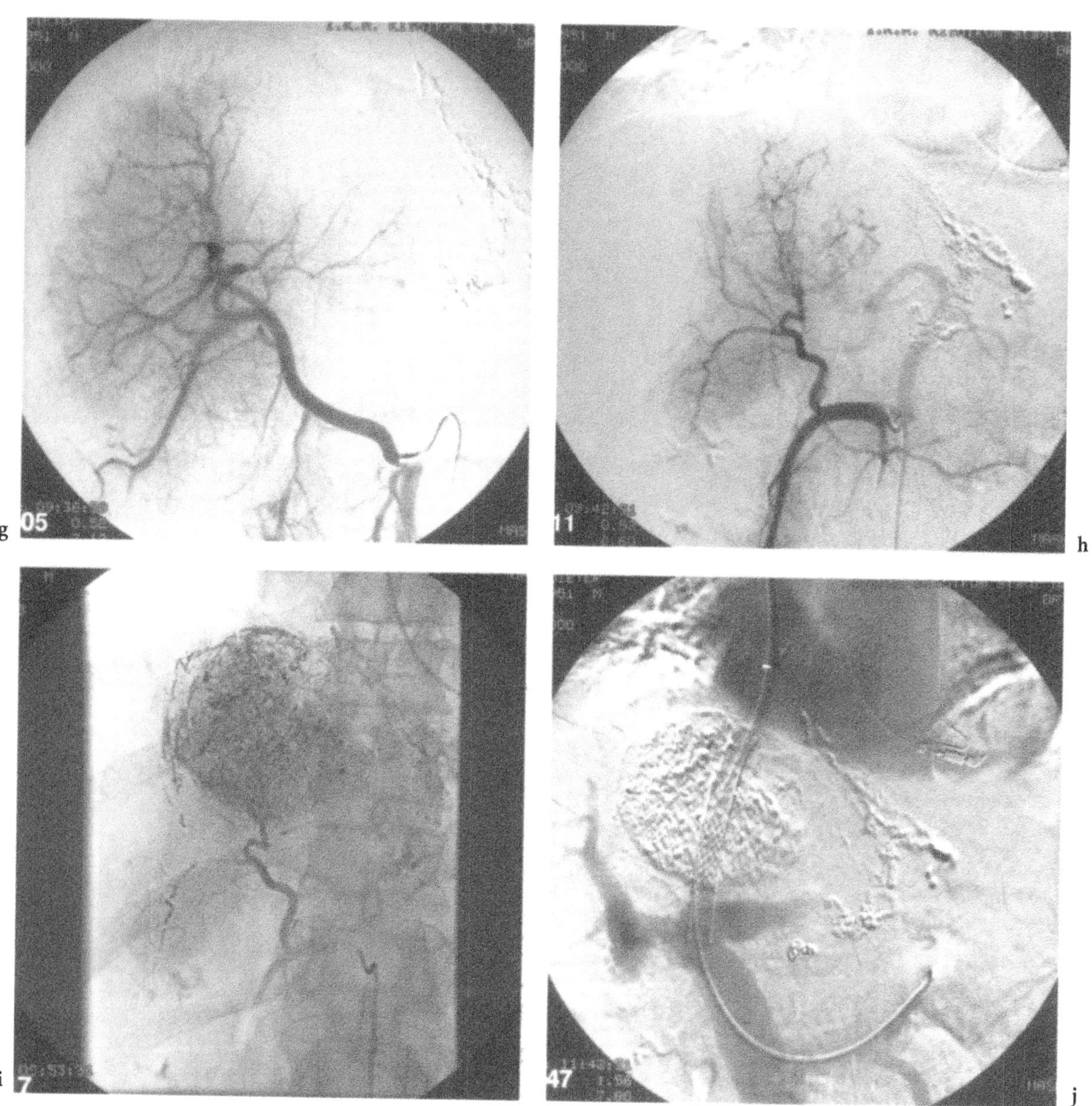

Fig. 21.20a–j. Continued
A 48-year-old patient with advanced liver cirrhosis complicated by recurrent upper gastrointestinal bleeding from esophageal and gastric varices. Pre-TIPS MR evaluation shows large hepatocellular carcinoma supplied by left hepatic artery. The right hepatic artery arises from the superior mesenteric artery (T2-weighted turbo spin-echo, **a**; T1-weighted gadolinium-enhanced fat-suppressed gradient echo, **b**; arterial and portal-venous phase CE 3D MRA with raw data (**c**, **d**) and MIP (**e**, **f**) images. Findings were confirmed by catheter angiogram (**g**, **h**). Subsequently, tumor embolization (**i**) and TIPS (**j**) procedure were performed within a single session (**g–j** courtesy of Dr. Tesdal, Friedrichshafen)

21.4 Conclusions

MRA allows for an accurate evaluation of the splenoportal system and may be considered as the non-invasive imaging modality of choice for the abdomen. In our own experience, breath-hold CE 3D MRA provides more information than TOF and PC techniques and may be superior to conventional indirect catheter splenoportograms in many clinical situations. Thus, CE 3D MRA has replaced diagnostic catheter angiography in the abdomen in most cases, and catheter angiography is only performed for interventional procedures (Fig. 21.21) As the technique becomes more widely available, the clinical significance of breath-hold CE MRA is expected to grow continuously.

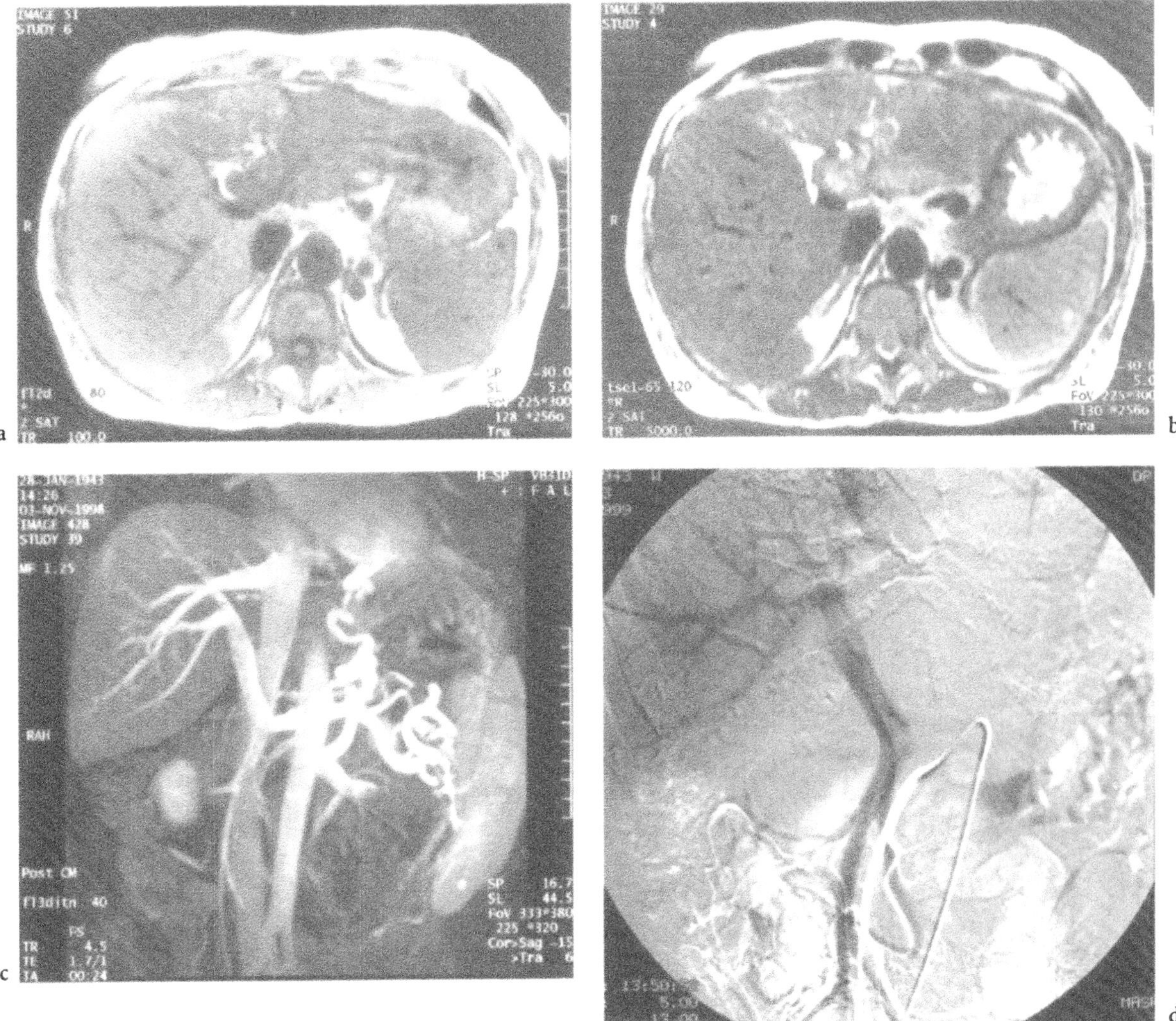

Fig. 21.21a–d. A 45-year-old patient with hepatocellular carcinoma and tumor infiltration of left portal vein branch. T1-weighted gradient echo image (**a**), T2-weighted turbo spin-echo image (**b**), CE 3D MRA (**c**). The findings were confirmed by catheter angiogram (**d**) and subsequently the tumor was embolized

References

Applegate GR, Thaete FL, Meyers SP, et al (1993) Blood flow in the portal venous system before liver transplantation: velocity quantitation with phase-contrast MR angiography. Radiology 187:253–256

Axel L (1984) Blood flow effects in magnetic resonance imaging. AJR Am J Roentgenol 143:1157–1166

Bismuth H (1992) Surgical anatomy and anatomical surgery of the liver. World J Surg 6:3–9

Burkhart DJ, Johnson CD, Morton MJ, Wolf RL, Ehman RL (1992) Volumetric flow rates in the portal venous system: measurement with cine phase-contrast MR imaging. AJR Am J Roentgenol 160:1113–1118

Burkhart DJ, Johnson CD, Ehman RL, Weaver AL, Ilstrup DM (1993) Evaluation of portal venous hypertension with cine phase-contrast MR flow measurements: high association of hyperdynamic portal flow with variceal hemorrhage. Radiology 188:643–648

Couinaud C (1957) Le foie: études anatomiques et chirurgicales. Masson, Paris, pp 9–12

Edelman RR, Mattle HP, Kleefield J, Silver MS (1989) Quantification of blood flow with dynamic MR imaging and presaturation bolus tracking. Radiology 171:551–556

Edelman RR, Zhao B, Liu C, Wentz KU, Mattle HP, Finn JP, McArdle C (1989) MR angiography and dynamic fow evaluation of the portal venous system. AJR Am J Roentgenol 153:755–760

Edelman RR, Mattle HP, Atkinson D, Hoogewoud HM (1990) MR angiography. AJR Am J Roentgenol 154:937–946

Finn JP, Edelman RR, Jenkins RL, et al (1991) Liver transplantation: MR angiography with surgical validation. Radiology 179:265–269

Finn JP, Kane RA, Edelman RR, et al (1993) Imaging of the portal venous system in patients with cirrhosis: MR angi-

ography vs duplex Doppler sonography. AJR Am J Roentgenol 161:989–994
Gaa J, Laub G, Edelman RR, Georgi M (1998) First clinical results of ultrafast contrast-enhanced dual-phase 3D MR angiography in the abdomen. Fortschr Röntgenstr 169:135–139
Gaa J, Lehmann KJ, Georgi M (2000) MR-angiography and electron-beam CT-angiography. Thieme, Stuttgart
Hughes LA, Hartnell GG, Finn JP, et al (1996) Time-of-flight MR angiography of the portal venous system: value compared with other imaging procedures. AJR Am J Roentgenol 166:375–378
Leung DA, McKinnon GC, Davis CP, Pfammater T, Krestin GP, Debatin JF (1996) Breath-hold contrast-enhanced. three-dimensional MR angiography. Radiology 200:569–571
Lewin JS, Laub G, Hausmann R (1991) Three-dimensional time-of-flight MR angiography: applications in the abdomen and thorax. Radiology 179:261–264
Lewis BD, James EM (1989) Current applications of Duplex and color Doppler ultrasound imaging: abdomen. Mayo Clin Proc 64:1158–1169
Mathieu D, Vasile N, Menu Y, Van Beers B, Lorphelin JM, Pringot J (1997) Budd-Chiari syndrome: dynamic CT. Radiology 165:409–413
Miller WJ, Federle MP, Straub WH, Davis PL (1993) Budd-Chiari syndrome: imaging with pathologic correlation. Abdom Imaging 18:329–335
Mueller MF, Siewert B, Kim D, Edelman RR, Stokes KR, Finn JP (1994) The role of MR angiography before transjugular placement of a portosystemic stent shunt (TIPS). Fortschr Röntgenstr 160:312–318
Nghiem HV, Winter TC III, Mountford MC, et al (1995) Evaluation of the portal vein: velocity quantitation with phase-contrast MR angiography. AJR Am J Roentgenol 164:871–878
Prince MR, Grist TM, Debatin JF (1999) 3D Contrast MR angiography. Springer, Berlin Heidelberg New York
Shimizu K Matsuda T, Sakurai T, et al (1986) Visualization of moving fluid: quantitative analysis of blood flow velocity using MR imaging. Radiology 159:195
Shirkoda A, Konez O, Shetty AN, Bis KG, Ellwood RA, Kirsch MJ (1997) Mesenteric circulation: three-dimensional MR angiography with a gadolinium-enhanced multiecho gradient-echo technique. Radiology 202:257–261
Stafford-Johnson DB, Chenevert TL, Cho KJ, Prince MR (1998) Portal venous magnetic resonance angiography: a review. Invest Radiol 33:628–636
Stieber AC, Zetti G, Todo S, et al (1991) The spectrum of portal vein thrombosis in liver transplantation. Ann Surg 213:199–206
Tamada T, Moriyasu F, Shigeki O, et al (zzzz) Portal blood flow: measurement with MR imaging. Radiology 173:639
Trede M, Rumstadt B, Wendl K, et al (1997) Ultrafast magnetic resonance imaging improves the staging of pancreatic tumors. Ann Surg 226:393–407
Yamashita YY, Mitsuzaki K, Miyazaki T, et al (1996) Gadolinium-enhanced breath-hold three-dimensional MR angiography of the portal vein: value of the magnetization-prepared rapid acquisition gradient-echo sequence. Radiology 201:283–288

22 Guidance of Intravascular Therapeutic Procedures: Current Status and Future Prospects

Mark E. Ladd and Jörg F. Debatin

CONTENTS

22.1 Introduction

For most of its short history, the clinical utilization of magnetic resonance (MR) has been largely confined to the area of diagnostic imaging. However, excellent soft tissue contrast and multiplanar imaging capabilities have motivated several groups to explore the possibility of using MR to guide simple interventional procedures. These were primarily biopsies (Mueller et al. 1986; Lufkin et al. 1987; VanSonnenberg et al. 1988; Orel et al. 1994), but interest has also been shown regarding vascular interventions (Rubin et al. 1990; Kochli et al. 1994; Bakker et al. 1996, 1997). Insufficient patient access afforded by the long magnet tunnel limited initial success.

With the advent of new, open-configuration magnet designs, the interest in performing interventional procedures under MR guidance has received new impetus. These magnets have either a horizontal (Lenz and Drobnitzky 1997) or a vertical gap (Schenck et al. 1995), which allows access to the imaging volume. Alternatively, the length of the magnet tunnel has been shortened to such an extent that the imaging volume is accessible from the ends of the tunnel (Van Vaals 1997).

The excellent soft tissue discrimination inherent to MR procedures, combined with the availability of a wide variety of pulse sequences to optimize image appearance, provides a unique alternative to fluoroscopy for guidance of vascular interventions. Magnetic resonance imaging (MRI) is not restricted to imaging only the lumen of the vascular tree, but can be used to examine surrounding structures or the vessel wall itself. Another advantage of MR is the ability to provide functional information in addition to morphologic information - flow measurements can provide immediate feedback as to the success of a vascular intervention.

Prerequisite to the safe and successful performance of any intervention is not only the collection of relevant anatomic information, but also the reliable visualization of the interventional instruments in relation to the surrounding tissue morphology. In contrast to ultrasound, X-ray fluoroscopy, or computed tomography (CT), visualization of interventional instruments in MR has proven to be difficult.

22.2 Guidance Objectives

Ideally, a technique used to render vascular instruments visible in MR would be characterized by high spatial and temporal resolution. It should also provide a high-contrast instrument signature, making it easy to pick out the instrument in the MR image. MR is, unfortunately, characterized by comparatively low spatial and temporal resolution, although it is possible to trade off one form of resolution with respect

M.E. Ladd, PhD
Zentralinstitut für Röntgendiagnostik, Universitätsklinikum Essen, Hufelandstrasse 55, 45122 Essen, Germany
J.F. Debatin, MD
Professor, Zentralinstitut für Röntgendiagnostik, Universitätsklinikum Essen, Hufelandstrasse 55, 45122 Essen, Germany

to the other. Recently, faster gradient hardware and innovative pulse sequence designs have even made real-time imaging a reality. The biggest challenge is therefore to generate adequate instrument contrast.

There are also some secondary considerations for an MR-based vascular guidance system. Since MR is not a projection technique like fluoroscopy, but relies rather on the acquisition of sections, control of the scan plane based on instrument position is a desirable feature. Furthermore, complex interventions requiring the use of several instruments in close proximity to one another mandate a means for distinguishing the different instruments.

A number of approaches have been developed for depicting vascular instruments in an MR environment. They can be broadly grouped into two categories: passive and active visualization. The passive techniques are the familiar approach taken in ultrasound, X-ray fluoroscopy, and CT: the material properties of the instrument are manipulated so that the instrument appears with adequate contrast in the image itself. No additional hardware or instrument modifications are required. The active techniques rely on additional hardware and postprocessing to achieve instrument localization.

22.3 Passive Guidance Techniques

22.3.1 Signal Voids

An interventional instrument composed of solids will displace a certain amount of tissue, blood, or other signal source as it is inserted through the body. Since solids produce no signal because of their short transverse relaxation times, the contrast between the signal void of the instrument and the signal of the surrounding tissue will allow the instrument to be seen in the MR image. Visibility of the instrument is determined solely by image resolution. Low in-plane resolution or thick sections will reduce the contrast between the instrument and the local surroundings, since the instrument will occupy a smaller percentage of the volume element (voxel) corresponding to a particular pixel within the image. This represents the familiar partial voluming effect.

To provide interactive guidance, the MR image must be rapidly updated as the instrument is manipulated, preferably at a rate of at least one image per second. High imaging speeds are traditionally obtained by sacrificing in-plane image resolution, which leads to poorer instrument contrast. Furthermore, to ensure that the instrument is contained within the imaging plane a thick image section is often required. Otherwise, multiple contiguous images must be collected, leading to a considerable increase in total image acquisition time.

Thus, instrument visualization based on signal voids will work well only with large-diameter instruments. Thin instruments are poorly visualized, reflecting limited in-plane and through-plane image resolution.

22.3.2 Contrast Agents

An alternate approach to passive visualization is to render the instrument brighter than its surroundings. Paramagnetic contrast agents can be used to shorten the longitudinal relaxation time, T1, of fluids. Normally, as the repetition time of an imaging sequence is reduced, the longitudinal magnetization becomes saturated and the available signal decreases. By decreasing T1, the signal of the contrast-enhanced fluid is maintained when using very short repetition times.

The contrast effect can be put to use by filling an instrument with a contrast-doped solution and imaging with a short repetition and echo time, and a relatively high flip angle. This combination saturates the longitudinal magnetization in the non-contrast-enhanced tissue outside the instrument. In the resultant images, the instrument is displayed with high contrast relative to the background.

Figure 22.1 shows a 6-F catheter imaged with a gradient echo sequence with a section thickness of 4 cm. The guidewire lumen has been filled with a Gd-based contrast agent. Use of a thick section during guidance is important to ensure continuous visualization of the entire catheter length within the same section. Despite the 4-cm thickness, the catheter is still well seen in this in vivo experiment thanks to the addition of a slice selection dephaser which dephases any signal from thick objects while maintaining the phase coherence of thin objects such as the catheter (Unal et al. 1998).

Rather than filling the lumen of the catheter with liquid contrast solution, another approach is to treat the surface of the catheter with Gd^{3+} ions (Frayne et al. 1999). As a consequence, the T1 of blood in the immediate vicinity of the catheter is shortened, making the catheter visible.

Recently, new contrast agents with a prolonged intravascular presence lasting up to several hours

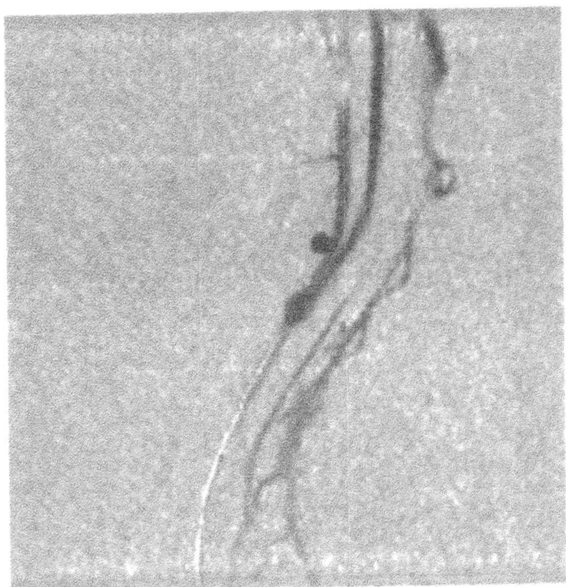
a

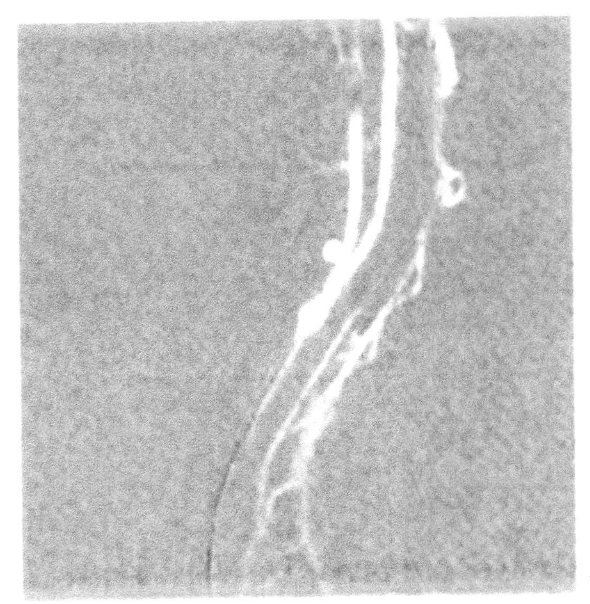
b

Fig. 22.1. A temporal snapshot of a 6 French Gd-DTPA-filled catheter obtained with projection dephaser during movement through the common carotid artery of a canine is shown superimposed onto a road map image using (**a**) bright catheter image (**b**) inverted catheter image. Scan parameters are TR/TE/Flip = 4.8/1.4 ms/60°, acquisition matrix = 160×256, reconstruction matrix = 256×256, FOV=20 cm×20 cm, slice thickness = 4 cm, and temporal frame rate is 3 images/s. [Courtesy of Dr. O. Unal et al., University of Wisconsin, Madison, WI, USA (UNAL et al. 1998)]

have been developed (ANZAI et al. 1997; LAUFFER et al. 1998). Several of these agents are currently undergoing clinical testing. These blood pool agents will likely be invaluable for guiding vascular interventions, since they allow repetitive, high-resolution three-dimensional (3D) imaging of the vascular morphology. Unfortunately, these contrast agents reduce the longitudinal relaxation time of the blood surrounding the catheter to a value comparable to the contrast solution inside the catheter, thus eliminating any contrast. One approach for getting around this problem with certain classes of blood pool agents has been suggested by NANZ and coworkers (NANZ et al. 1999). One of the newer blood pool agents, NC100150 (Clariscan, Nycomed Amersham Imaging, Wayne, Pennsylvania) (ANZAI et al. 1997), is based on starch-coated ultrasmall particles of superparamagnetic iron oxide which cause not only a substantial T1-shortening effect, but also a substantial T2*-shortening effect. The vascular system and instruments can be visualized separately with a double-echo gradient echo sequence. The image based on the short-TE echo renders both the vasculature and the catheter bright, while the image based on the long-TE echo renders only the catheter bright. The T2* decay of the blood eliminates any signal within the vascular system (Fig. 22.2). The catheter-only image (second echo) can be thresholded and overlaid in color on the vascular image (first echo).

22.3.3 Susceptibility Artifacts

Some of the most common artifacts encountered in MRI are due to magnetic susceptibility differences. Differences in magnetic susceptibility cause local inhomogeneities in the static magnetic field, which in turn lead to geometric distortion and intra-voxel dephasing (LUDEKE et al. 1985; BAKKER et al. 1993). The human body is filled with areas of nonuniform magnetic susceptibility, the most obvious of which can be found at tissue–air boundaries in the paranasal sinuses, the lungs, or the bowel.

To date, exploitation of the susceptibility artifact has been the most common method of making interventional instruments visible in MR images. The artifact has been employed for visualization of needles for MR-guided biopsies (MUELLER et al. 1986; LUFKIN et al. 1987; VANSONNENBERG et al. 1988; OREL et al. 1994; SILVERMAN et al. 1995; FRAHM et al. 1996; LEWIN et al. 1996) as well as catheters and guidewires for vascular interventions (RUBIN et al. 1990; KOCHLI et al. 1994; BAKKER et al. 1996, 1997; LENZ

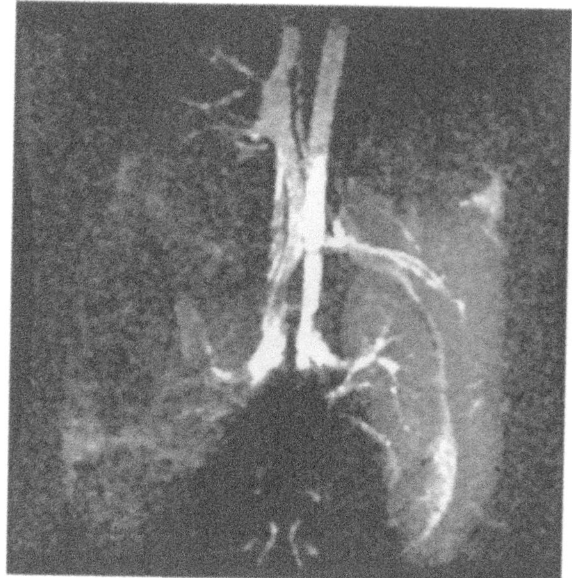
a

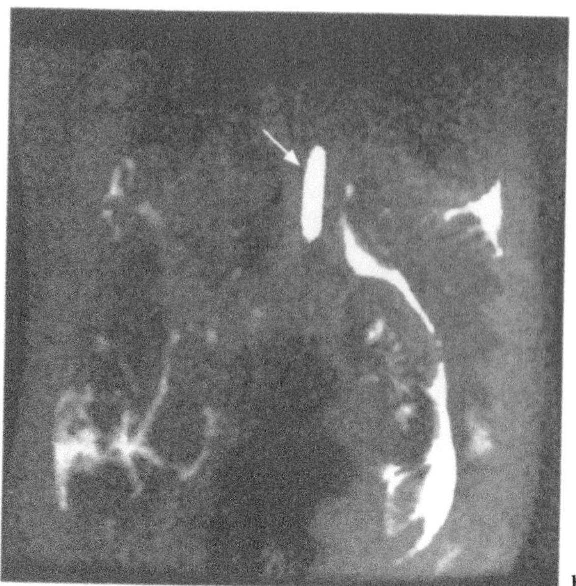
b

Fig. 22.2a, b. In vivo spoiled gradient-echo images of the abdomen of a pig with a 12-mm balloon catheter inserted into the abdominal aorta. (**a**) TE=1.2 ms, short-echo. (**b**) TE=9.0 ms, long-echo. Note the bright signal intensity of both vascular system and catheter balloon in the short-echo image. With TE=9 ms, only the balloon (*arrow*) is visible. [Courtesy of Dr. D. Nanz, et al., University Hospital, Zurich, Switzerland (Nanz et al. 1999)]

et al. 1996). Unfortunately, the effect is highly dependent on a number of factors, including field strength, pulse sequence parameters, and device orientation within the magnetic field. These dependencies prevent a consistent portrayal of instruments. Additionally, although a large artifact is required for easy detection of the instrument, the same large artifact inherently distorts the local anatomy and reduces the obtainable targeting accuracy (Langen et al. 1997).

The orientation dependency can be ameliorated by using shapes other than cylindrical. Spherical objects, for example, show less dependency due to their symmetry. This fact has been exploited in catheters by incorporating multiple rings of paramagnetic dysprosium oxide (Dy_2O_3) along the catheter tip, allowing the catheter to be consistently visualized independent of orientation (Bakker et al. 1996, 1997).

22.4 Active Guidance Techniques

All passive techniques are confronted with the challenge of generating sufficient contrast between the instrument and its surroundings without distorting the anatomic information. Unlike X-ray projections, the instrument can easily disappear as the MR section thickness is increased. If a thick section cannot be used and the instrument position cannot be predicted, a series of contiguous images must be collected and searched. For display of a significant length of the instrument, the additional acquisition of oblique sections will be required. During the course of an intervention, the plane of the instrument can change, and the search process must begin anew. Several active guidance alternatives have been developed which overcome these difficulties inherent to passive visualization.

22.4.1 MR Tracking

MR tracking relies on the incorporation of a miniature radiofrequency (RF) coil into the instrument (Ackerman et al. 1986; Dumoulin et al. 1993). The RF coil provides a robust signal, identifying the instrument location with high contrast. The built-in coil, usually a short solenoid, has limited spatial extent in all axes and allows determination of the 3D spatial position of a single point of the instrument in near real time.

If a nonselective RF pulse is applied, followed by a gradient read-out along a particular axis (i.e., a projection along the gradient axis), the localized spatial sensitivity of the small coil leads to a peak in the

Fourier-transformed signal. The location of the peak provides the location of the coil along that particular axis. If this experiment is repeated along all three spatial axes, the full 3D position of the coil can be found in three MR repetition times. In practice, four excitations are applied, using a Hadamard encoding scheme for the gradients to compensate for off-resonance effects (DUMOULIN et al. 1993). Typically, repetition times of 25 ms are used, rendering an update rate of ten positions per second.

The location of the point is typically projected as a color-coded icon onto a separately acquired image providing a road map of the anatomy. Since the 3D position of the coil is known, its position can be projected onto any arbitrary plane as well as onto multiple images delineating the vascular morphology in multiple planes simultaneously, without incurring any loss in temporal resolution. Biplanar or triplanar tracking is therefore possible (LEUNG et al. 1995a). The actively available 3D spatial coordinates can also be used to prescribe an imaging section passing through the tracking point, allowing for 2D imaging updates at the exact location of the coil.

MR tracking has been demonstrated to be feasible and highly accurate in vitro as well as in vivo for catheters (LEUNG et al. 1995b) and guidewires (LADD et al. 1998b). Complex vascular interventions, including the transjugular intrahepatic portosystemic shunt (TIPS) procedure, have been performed in animal experiments under MR guidance and control (WILDERMUTH et al. 1997; KEE et al. 1999).

Aside from the instrument complexity, one drawback of this technique is that only the position of a single point on the instrument is provided. The orientation remains undetermined. In order to derive more information about the orientation of the instrument, multiple coils need to be incorporated (LIU et al. 1997). Each coil can be connected to a separate receiver and a uniquely colored icon can be chosen for each individual coil.

22.4.2 MR Profiling

For most interventions employing flexible instruments such as catheters or guidewires, depiction of the full instrument curvature is of critical importance. One way to obtain the curvature information missing with the MR tracking technique is to elongate the RF coil in the instrument. Because instruments such as catheters and guidewires are long and thin, initial attempts to outline these instruments have been based on electrically-coupled, loopless antennas (dipoles or stubs) (MCKINNON et al. 1996; BURL et al. 1997; OCALI and ATALAR 1997). The acquisition of a conventional MR image with these antennas leads to an outline or "profile" of the instrument due to the localized sensitivity of these "surface coils". Figure 22.3 shows a balloon angioplasty being monitored with a guidewire equipped with a loopless antenna. The loopless antenna consists of a coaxial cable with an extended inner conductor. The guidewire is thin enough to fit through the regular guidewire lumen of the catheter, and the penetration depth of the signal surrounding the antenna is adequate to visualize the expansion of the balloon and the concomitant elimination of the vessel stenosis.

One of the potential drawbacks of these types of antennas is that the rendered instrument outline generally exceeds the size of the instrument itself. To limit the width of the coil profile to the width of the instrument, magnetically coupled antennas, the traditional loop antennas of MR, can be used. The coils are simply wound very thin and extended over a length of several centimeters (Fig. 22.4a) (LADD et al. 1997, 1998c; BURL et al. 1999). These antennas generate an outline of limited extent, which sharply delineates the instrument.

Just as with MR tracking, the localization information can be projected onto a separately acquired anatomic road map (Fig. 22.4b). Compared to MR tracking, MR profiling is more limited in temporal resolution, since data for a full image must be col-

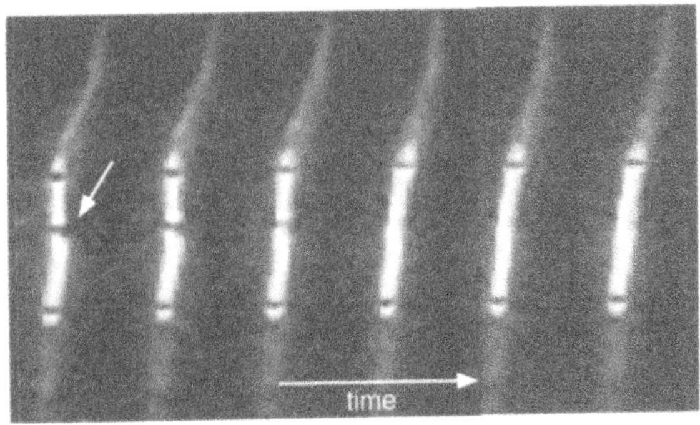

Fig. 22.3. Balloon angioplasty in a rabbit aorta monitored with a guidewire equipped with a loopless antenna. The top and bottom signal voids are markers on the angioplasty balloon. The center void (*arrow*) is an artificially-created stenosis. The stenosis is progressively eliminated as the balloon is expanded. Scan parameters are spoiled gradient echo, TR=5.0 ms, acquisition matrix = 256×128, FOV=24×12 cm, no slice selection, acquisition time = 320 ms. [Courtesy of Dr. E. Atalar, et al., Johns Hopkins University, Baltimore, MD, USA (YANG et al. 1998)]

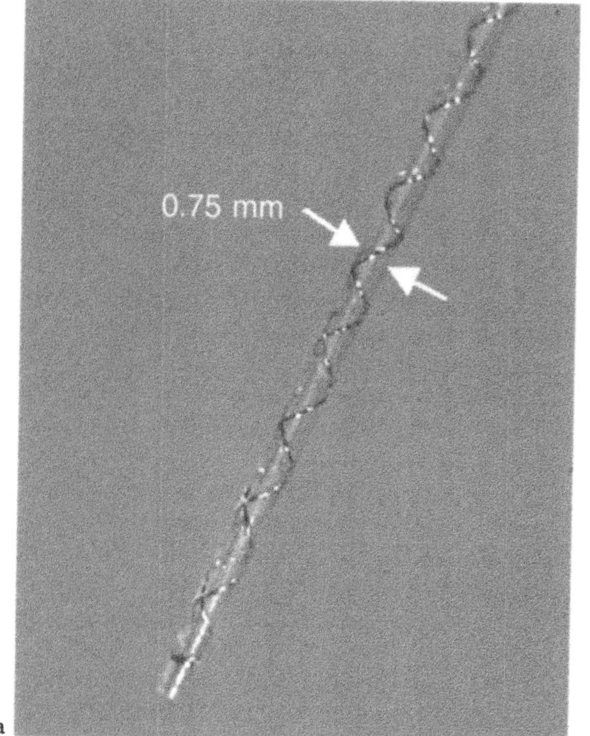

a

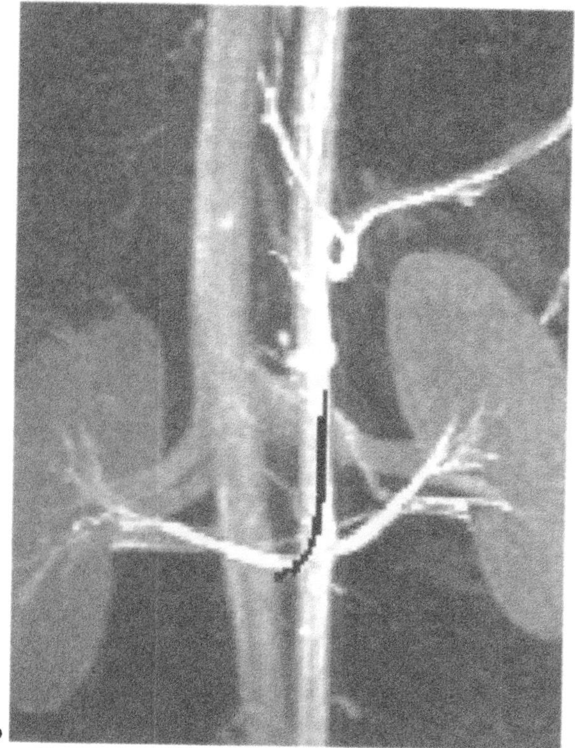

b

Fig. 22.4. (**a**) Close-up of an MR profiling coil in the tip of a 0.035-inch guidewire. (**b**) MR profiling in a swine, showing the curvature of the guidewire as it is steered into the right renal artery

lected. However, the instrument curvature information gained is often worth the trade-off, and fast data acquisition strategies can provide update rates of several frames per second (Atalar et al. 1998).

MR profiling overcomes the partial voluming problems associated with passive techniques. Because the instrument coil is only sensitive to spins in its immediate vicinity, the localization images can be collected with the slice selection gradient disabled, resulting in true projections through the entire patient, just as in X-ray fluoroscopy.

If projections from two slightly distinct perspectives are acquired – no problem given the multiplanar capabilities of MR – then an impression of the 3D depth of the instrument inside the body can be achieved (Atalar et al. 1998). If a limited number of additional projections are acquired, then the full 3D position of the catheter or guidewire within the body can be reconstructed (Solaiyappan et al. 1999; Vaara et al. 1999).

22.5 Hybrid Guidance Techniques

22.5.1 Active Field Inhomogeneity

An additional guidance technique has been developed which shares characteristics of both passive and active techniques. By including a small coil in the instrument, with a cable connected to the outside, a small direct or low-frequency current can be passed through the instrument (Glowinski et al. 1997; Adam et al. 1998; Buecker et al. 1998). The current creates an adjustable inhomogeneity in the magnetic field of the MR imager. The artifact is similar to that produced by susceptibility differences, since both disturb the local magnetic field. The technique relies on making the instrument visible in the MR image itself, which is similar to the passive techniques, but now the artifact can be actively turned on and off and adjusted in size (Fig. 22.5). For rough maneuvering and easy instrument localization, the artifact can be enlarged; for fine placement, the artifact can be reduced.

The advantage of this technique is that the instrument appears directly in the image itself, so there is no distinction between image collection and instrument localization. However, as with passive techniques, there is no control over the scan plane, and there is a trade-off between instrument visibility and image distortion.

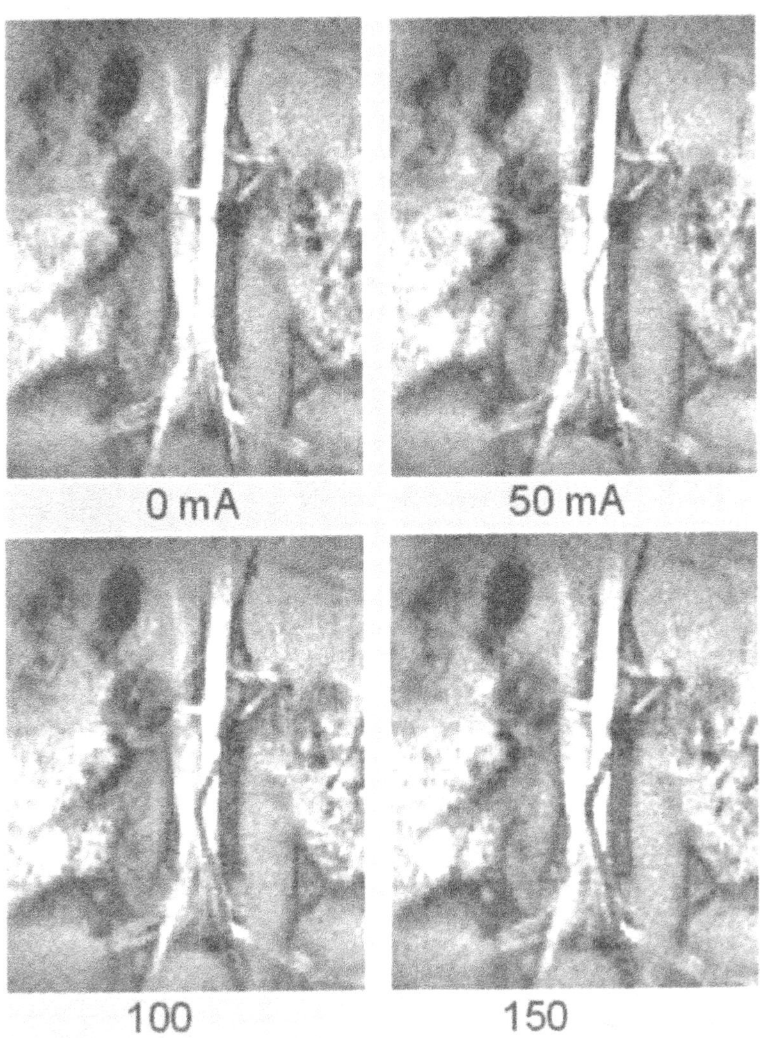

Fig. 22.5. Field inhomogeneity catheter scanned with radial k-space trajectories. The catheter is visualized using four different current strengths [Courtesy of A. Glowinski, et al., Aachen University of Technology, Aachen, Germany (GLOWINSKI et al. 1997)]

22.6 Safety

The primary consideration when performing any intervention is ensuring the safety of the patient. Any instrument which is introduced inside the patient must fulfill a number of stringent requirements. Instruments designed to be used under MR guidance must, in addition, satisfy many considerations unique to the MR environment. A comprehensive treatment of all of these factors is outside the scope of this chapter, but a couple are worthy of mention, as they relate particularly to the presented guidance techniques.

Passive guidance techniques and the active field inhomogeneity technique rely on making the interventional instrument visible in the MR image itself. Since the anatomic information and positioning information are collected simultaneously using the same imaging process, the error in instrument positioning is minimized, with the caveat that if the size of the instrument is artifactually enhanced to make instrument localization easier, the enhanced visibility is achieved at the cost of lower positional accuracy.

The active techniques often separate in time the acquisition of the instrument position information from the acquisition of the anatomic vascular road map information. Both the MR tracking and MR profiling techniques customarily rely on the collection of morphologic vascular road maps on which the positioning information is superimposed. Any change in patient position is not accounted for. The most obvious source of error is respiratory motion. Associated displacement of thoracic or abdominal structures can considerably complicate catheterization of small vessels. While the implementation of navigator echoes for real-time position feedback (EHMAN and FELMLEE

1989) may solve the issue of respiratory motion, gross patient movement over time can only be compensated for by periodic updates of the road map itself.

As an alternative, the instrument position information and the anatomic information can be collected simultaneously. With MR tracking, this can be achieved by using projection reconstruction acquisition rather than traditional Fourier acquisition (Buecker et al. 1999). The same projections can be used to locate the tracking coil and reconstruct an anatomical image, whereby the anatomical image is collected with a conventional body or surface coil. For MR profiling, use of an electrically coupled antenna gives a poorly defined instrument profile, but the increased penetration depth may be adequate to visualize enough of the surrounding anatomy to allow guidance.

A major concern in interventional MR is the possibility of localized increases in the RF specific absorption rate (SAR) near interventional instruments. The local electric field can be amplified if the instruments are conducting, making the peak SAR difficult to predict. The MR tracking, MR profiling, and active field inhomogeneity techniques all involve incorporation of a long, electrically conducting cable and a small coil. The small coil, if properly detuned, will not couple with the transmit energy of the body coil. The coupling to the coaxial cable is more difficult to reduce. The cable is basically a long antenna sensitive to the transmit electric field of the body coil. Significant temperature increases have been demonstrated in high-field imagers (1.5 T) near the tips of MR tracking and MR profiling instruments when using RF-intense imaging sequences such as fast spin echo (Maier et al. 1995; Ladd et al. 1998a; Wildermuth et al. 1998). Incorporation of coaxial baluns can reduce the electric-field coupling and prevent excessive heating (Atalar 1999; Ladd and Quick 1999).

22.7 Future Directions

Much research has been devoted to solving the problems of instrument visualization in MR, but these are not the only problems to be solved in order to render MR practical as a guidance modality for vascular interventions. Although there has been much progress in making magnets more open, access to the patient is still an issue for certain procedures. Furthermore, vascular work demands very high image quality, which can only be realized at high field strengths. Most of the current open designs are low-field or mid-field systems. A more conventional, high-field system (>1.0 T) with a very short magnet bore might be satisfactory for certain vascular work, since the interventionalist can stand at the puncture site at the groin and still image at the target site (Van Vaals 1997). Even shorter magnets are being developed by the major manufacturers.

Real-time imaging, reconstruction, and display capabilities are also becoming rapidly available, driven primarily by interest in cardiac and functional imaging, as well as interventional guidance. For interventional guidance, interactive control of the scan plane and scan parameters is just as important as real-time imaging. As the intervention progresses, the scan plane and scan parameters must often be adjusted. While there are already systems which offer scan plane and limited scan parameter (FOV, slice thickness) control, it is still cumbersome to switch pulse sequences, for instance, from a spin echo to a gradient echo. A true MR guidance scanner will have to offer an interface for fast and flexible modification of all scanning parameters, much like an ultrasound machine.

One of the biggest challenges facing interventional MR is ambient acoustic noise due to gradient switching. For diagnostic imaging, the primary concern has been ensuring that the noise level does not exceed short-term exposure limits. In an MR guidance suite, where physicians and nurses will be exposed to the gradient noise over long periods, and where communication between the team members is critical, the noise levels of most currently available scanners is unacceptable. Noise reduction will become an active area of research and development for this reason.

The guidance of vascular therapeutic procedures with MR could open a range of possibilities not available with X-ray fluoroscopy. With antennas (surface coils) inside the vessel, high-quality images of the vessel wall are possible (Correia et al. 1997; Quick et al. 1999b; Zimmermann Paul et al. 1999). Intravascular images can be used to characterize various plaque components, and may prove valuable for predicting which plaques are prone to restenosis. While intravascular ultrasound can currently be used to characterize plaques, the advantages of MR imaging lie in its superior soft tissue contrast, its ability to see behind calcified plaques and the struts of intravascular stents, and the ease with which tomographic or 3D data with a known relation to other anatomic landmarks can be generated.

It is also possible to use an intravascular stent itself as a form of intravascular antenna (Quick et al. 1999a). The stent antenna can be used to guide the placement of the stent; it might also be used for repeated imaging post-placement to monitor the development of endothelial hyperplasia, which can lead to stenosis or even occlusion.

One of the most exciting fields of endeavor on the horizon is the transvascular delivery of therapeutic drugs and genes (THOMAS et al. 1998; VOSS and KRUSKAL 1998). For instance, vascular endothelial growth factor can be deployed on the surface of an angioplastic balloon (ISNER et al. 1996). Magnetic resonance imaging offers a unique opportunity for both guidance of gene delivery and monitoring of gene expression (WEISSLEDER et al. 1997; MOORE et al. 1998).

22.8 Conclusion

Passive guidance techniques rely on visualization of the instrument directly as part of the image. Since the positional information of the instrument is not actively available, it is difficult to determine the exact imaging plane and it is difficult to distinguish different instruments from one another. These aspects make passive visualization of instruments precarious. Signal voids and susceptibility effects emanating from multiple instruments are difficult to separate from one another when in close proximity, particularly problematic for combinations such as a guidewire and catheter.

Given the challenges involved with passive imaging, it is likely that a combination of active and passive approaches will find application in the MR interventional suite of the future. Some techniques can even be combined in the same instrument. For example, the same instrument can be used for MR profiling and active field inhomogeneity if the coil is designed properly. Combination of MR with other interventional guidance modalities is also a possibility. A hybrid system consisting of a 1.5-T MR imager and a mono-planar X-ray fluoroscopy suite has already been developed and demonstrated successfully (VAN VAALS 1997).

Interventional MR imaging has the potential to revolutionize intravascular therapy, and is currently a fertile ground for research. Not only is there the potential to duplicate the success of procedures currently performed with X-ray fluoroscopy in an environment free of ionizing radiation, but new applications including vessel wall characterization and delivery and visualization of gene therapy may also be possible. Certainly the promise warrants further investment in developing this burgeoning field.

References

Ackerman JL, Offutt MC, Buxton RB, et al (1986) Rapid 3D tracking of small RF coils. In: Proceedings of the Society for Magnetic Resonance in Medicine, 5th Annual Meeting, Montreal, p 1131

Adam G, Glowinski A, Neuerburg J, et al (1998) Visualization of MR-compatible catheters by electrically induced local field inhomogeneities: evaluation in vivo. J Magn Reson Imaging 8:209–213

Anzai Y, Prince MR, Chenevert TL, et al (1997) MR angiography with an ultrasmall superparamagnetic iron oxide blood pool agent. J Magn Reson Imaging 7:209–214

Atalar E (1999) Safe coaxial cables. In: Proceedings of the International Society for Magnetic Resonance in Medicine, 7th Scientific Meeting and Exhibition, Philadelphia, p 1006

Atalar E, Kraitchman DL, Carkhuff B, et al (1998) Catheter-tracking FOV MR fluoroscopy. Magn Reson Med 40:865–872

Bakker CJ, Bhagwandien R, Moerland MA, et al (1993) Susceptibility artifacts in 2DFT spin-echo and gradient-echo imaging: the cylinder model revisited. Magn Reson Imaging 11:539–548

Bakker CJ, Hoogeveen RM, Weber J, et al (1996) Visualization of dedicated catheters using fast scanning techniques with potential for MR-guided vascular interventions. Magn Reson Med 36:816–820

Bakker CJ, Hoogeveen RM, Hurtak WF, et al (1997) MR-guided endovascular interventions: susceptibility-based catheter and near-real-time imaging technique. Radiology 202:273–276

Buecker A, Adam G, Neuerburg JM, et al (1998) [Real-time MRI with radial k-radial scanning technique for control of angiographic interventions]. Rofo Fortschr Geb Röntgenstr Neuen Bildgeb Verfahr 169:542–546

Buecker A, Adam G, Neuerburg JM, et al (1999) MR-guided PTA applying radial k-space filling and active tip tracking: simultaneous real-time visualization of the catheter tip and the anatomy. In: Proceedings of the International Society for Magnetic Resonance in Medicine, 7th Scientific Meeting and Exhibition, Philadelphia, p 575

Burl M, Young IR, Herlihy AH, et al (1997) Comparison of two approaches to transmit/receive RF systems for intravascular use. In: Proceedings of the International Society for Magnetic Resonance in Medicine, 5th Scientific Meeting and Exhibition, Vancouver, p 1519

Burl M, Coutts GA, Herlihy DJ, et al (1999) Twisted-pair RF coil suitable for locating the track of a catheter. Magn Reson Med 41:636–638

Correia LC, Atalar E, Kelemen MD, et al (1997) Intravascular magnetic resonance imaging of aortic atherosclerotic plaque composition. Arterioscler Thromb Vasc Biol 17:3626–3632

Dumoulin CL, Souza SP, Darrow RD (1993) Real-time position monitoring of invasive devices using magnetic resonance. Magn Reson Med 29:411–415

Ehman RL, Felmlee JP (1989) Adaptive technique for high-definition MR imaging of moving structures. Radiology 173:255–263

Frahm C, Gehl HB, Weiss HD, et al (1996) [Technique of MRT-guided core biopsy in the abdomen using an open low-field scanner: feasibility and initial clinical results]. Rofo Fortschr Geb Röntgenstr Neuen Bildgeb Verfahr 164:62–67

Frayne R, Wehelie A, Yang Z, et al (1999) MR evaluation of signal-emitting coatings. In: Proceedings of the International Society for Magnetic Resonance in Medicine, 7th Scientific Meeting and Exhibition, Philadelphia, p 580
Glowinski A, Adam G, Bucker A, et al (1997) Catheter visualization using locally induced, actively controlled field inhomogeneities. Magn Reson Med 38:253–258
Isner JM, Walsh K, Symes J, et al (1996) Arterial gene transfer for therapeutic angiogenesis in patients with peripheral artery disease. Hum Gene Ther 7:959–988
Kee ST, Rhee JS, Butts K, et al (1999) MR-guided transjugular portosystemic shunt placement in a swine model. Cardiovasc Intervent Radiol 10:529–535
Kochli VD, McKinnon GC, Hofmann E, et al (1994) Vascular interventions guided by ultrafast MR imaging: evaluation of different materials. Magn Reson Med 31:309–314
Ladd ME, Quick HH (1999) A 0.7 mm triaxial cable for significantly reducing RF heating in interventional MR. In: Proceedings of the International Society for Magnetic Resonance in Medicine, 7th Scientific Meeting and Exhibition, Philadelphia, p 104
Ladd ME, Erhart P, Debatin JF, et al (1997) Guidewire antennas for MR fluoroscopy. Magn Reson Med 37:891–897
Ladd ME, Quick HH, Boesiger P, et al (1998a) RF heating of actively visualized catheters and guidewires. In: Proceedings of the International Society for Magnetic Resonance in Medicine, 6th Scientific Meeting and Exhibition, Sydney, p 473
Ladd ME, Zimmermann GG, McKinnon GC, et al (1998b) Visualization of vascular guidewires using MR tracking. J Magn Reson Imaging 8:251–253
Ladd ME, Zimmermann GG, Quick HH, et al (1998c) Active MR visualization of a vascular guidewire in vivo. J Magn Reson Imaging 8:220–225
Langen HJ, Kugel H, Heindel W, et al (1997) [Localization of puncture needles in MRI: experimental studies on precision using spin-echo sequences at 1.0 T]. Rofo Fortschr Geb Röntgenstr Neuen Bildgeb Verfahr 167:501–508
Lauffer RB, Parmelee DJ, Dunham SU, et al (1998) MS-325: albumin-targeted contrast agent for MR angiography. Radiology 207:529–538
Lenz G, Drobnitzky M (1997) Interventional MRI with an open low-field system. In: Debatin JF, Adam G (eds) Interventional magnetic resonance imaging. Springer, Berlin Heidelber New York, pp 3–9
Lenz G, Drobnitzky M, Dewey C (1996) MR-visible catheters for intra-vascular interventional MRI procedures. In: Proceedings of the International Society for Magnetic Resonance in Medicine, 4th Scientific Meeting and Exhibition, New York, p 901
Leung DA, Debatin JF, Wildermuth S, et al (1995a) Real-time biplanar needle tracking for interventional MR imaging procedures. Radiology 197:485–488
Leung DA, Debatin JF, Wildermuth S, et al (1995b) Intravascular MR tracking catheter: preliminary experimental evaluation. AJR Am J Roentgenol 164:1265–1270
Lewin JS, Duerk JL, Jain VR, et al (1996) Needle localization in MR-guided biopsy and aspiration: effects of field strength, sequence design, and magnetic field orientation. AJR Am J Roentgenol 166:1337–1345
Liu H, Truwit CL (1997) A comprehensive interventional device tracking method. In: Proceedings of the International Society for Magnetic Resonance in Medicine, 5th Scientific Meeting and Exhibition, Vancouver, p 1921
Ludeke KM, Roschmann P, Tischler R (1985) Susceptibility artefacts in NMR imaging. Magn Reson Imaging 3:329–343
Lufkin R, Teresi L, Hanafee W (1987) New needle for MR-guided aspiration cytology of the head and neck. AJR Am J Roentgenol 149:380–382
Maier SE, Wildermuth S, Darrow RD, et al (1995) Safety of MR tracking catheters. In: Proceedings of the Society for Magnetic Resonance, 3rd Scientific Meeting and Exhibition, Nice, p 497
McKinnon GC, Debatin JF, Leung DA, et al (1996) Towards active guidewire visualization in interventional magnetic resonance imaging. MAGMA 4:13–18
Moore A, Basilion JP, Chiocca EA, et al (1998) Measuring transferrin receptor gene expression by NMR imaging. Biochim Biophys Acta 1402:239–249
Mueller PR, Stark DD, Simeone JF, et al (1986) MR-guided aspiration biopsy: needle design and clinical trials. Radiology 161:605–609
Nanz D, Weishaupt D, Quick HH, et al (1999) TE-switched double-contrast enhanced visualization of vascular system and instruments for MR-guided interventions. In: Proceedings of the International Society for Magnetic Resonance in Medicine, 7th Scientific Meeting and Exhibition, Philadelphia, p 581
Ocali O, Atalar E (1997) Intravascular magnetic resonance imaging using a loopless catheter antenna. Magn Reson Med 37:112–118
Orel SG, Schnall MD, Newman RW, et al (1994) MR imaging-guided localization and biopsy of breast lesions: initial experience. Radiology 193:97–102
Quick HH, Ladd ME, Nanz D, et al (1999a) Vascular stents as RF antennas for intravascular MR guidance and imaging. Magn Reson Med 42:738–745
Quick HH, Ladd ME, Zimmermann-Paul GG, et al (1999b) Single-loop coil concepts for intravascular MR imaging. Magn Reson Med 41:751–758
Rubin DL, Ratner AV, Young SW (1990) Magnetic susceptibility effects and their application in the development of new ferromagnetic catheters for magnetic resonance imaging. Invest Radiol 25:1325–1332
Schenck JF, Jolesz FA, Roemer PB, et al (1995) Superconducting open-configuration MR imaging system for image-guided therapy. Radiology 195:805–814
Silverman SG, Collick BD, Figueira MR, et al (1995) Interactive MR-guided biopsy in an open-configuration MR imaging system. Radiology 197:175–181
Solaiyappan M, Lee J, Atalar E (1999) Depth reconstruction from projection images for 3D visualization of intravascular MRI probes. In: Proceedings of the International Society for Magnetic Resonance in Medicine, 7th Scientific Meeting and Exhibition, Philadelphia, p 483
Thomas JW, Kuo MD, Chawla M, et al (1998) Vascular gene therapy. Radiographics 18:1373–1394
Unal O, Korosec FR, Frayne R, et al (1998) A rapid 2D time-resolved variable-rate k-space sampling MR technique for passive catheter tracking during endovascular procedures. Magn Reson Med 40:356–362
Vaara TJ, Tanttu JI, Taivalkoski S, et al (1999) Catheter RF-coil profile reconstruction from 2D-projections. In: Proceedings of the International Society for Magnetic Resonance

in Medicine, 7th Scientific Meeting and Exhibition, Philadelphia, p 1952

VanSonnenberg E, Hajek P, Gylys Morin V, et al (1988) A wire-sheath system for MR-guided biopsy and drainage: laboratory studies and experience in 10 patients. AJR Am J Roentgenol 151:815–817

Van Vaals JJ (1997) Interventional MRI with a hybrid high-field system. In: Debatin JF, Adam G (eds) Interventional magnetic resonance imaging. Springer, Berlin Heidelberg New York, pp 19–32

Voss SD, Kruskal JB (1998) Gene therapy: a primer for radiologists. Radiographics 18:1343–1372

Weissleder R, Simonova M, Bogdanova A, et al (1997) MR imaging and scintigraphy of gene expression through melanin induction. Radiology 204:425–429

Wildermuth S, Debatin JF, Leung DA, et al (1997) MR imaging-guided intravascular procedures: initial demonstration in a pig model. Radiology 202:578–583

Wildermuth S, Dumoulin CL, Pfammatter T, et al (1998) MR-guided percutaneous angioplasty: assessment of tracking safety, catheter handling and functionality. Cardiovasc Intervent Radiol 21:404–410

Yang X, Bolster BD, Jr., Kraitchman DL, et al (1998) Intravascular MR-monitored balloon angioplasty: an in vivo feasibility study. J Vasc Interv Radiol 9:953–959

Zimmermann Paul GG, Quick HH, Vogt P, et al (1999) High-resolution intravascular magnetic resonance imaging: monitoring of plaque formation in heritable hyperlipidemic rabbits. Circulation 99:1054–1061

23 Intravascular Implants: Safety and Artifacts

PAUL R. HILFIKER, DOMINIK WEISHAUPT, JÖRG F. DEBATIN

CONTENTS

23.1 Introduction

Magnetic resonance angiography (MRA) is emerging as a credible noninvasive alternative to digital subtraction angiography (DSA) and computer tomography (CT) for the assessment of the entire arterial system (HANY et al. 1997; LEUNG et al. 1996; PRINCE et al. 1993; QUINN et al. 1993, 1998; ROGG et al. 1999). Beyond being used to identify vascular disease, contrast-enhanced three-dimensional (3D) MRA can also be employed to monitor therapeutic effectiveness following percutaneous angioplasty, stent placement (HILFIKER et al. 1998b), as well as arterial bypass grafting.

The consideration of magnetic resonance imaging (MRI) safety and artifacts in the presence of metallic intravascular devices has gained increased importance in light of the wide use of these devices and the continuing evolution of MRA. Metallic implants are of concern during MRI because theoretically they can move or dislodge, induce electrical currents, heat tissues, or produce image-degrading artifacts (NEW et al. 1983; SOULEN et al. 1985). A number of studies have outlined means of protecting the patient (SHELLOCK and KANAL 1998a; SHELLOCK et al. 1993; SHELLOCK and MORISOLI 1994b; TEITELBAUM et al. 1988, 1989). Prior to imaging a patient with an implant, several factors have to be carefully considered, especially if the device is located in a potentially dangerous area of the body, such as vascular and neural tissue, where dislodgment could substantially injure the patient. These factors include the strength of the static and gradient magnetic fields, the degree of ferromagnetism of the object, the mass of the object, the geometry and orientation of the object, the location within the body, and the length of time the object has been in place.

Numerous studies have assessed the ferromagnetic qualities of various implants, materials, and devices by measuring deflection forces and interaction with the magnetic field. In general, these studies demonstrated that MRI may be performed in patients harboring non- or minimally ferromagnetic objects which are only minimally deflected by the static magnetic field (i.e., the associated deflection force or attraction is insufficient to move or dislodge the implant in situ) (SHELLOCK et al. 1993). Therefore, prior knowledge of the relative degree of ferromagnetism characterizing a specific metallic implant or device is essential for proper screening of patients before performing MRI.

While hazardous thermal effects have been associated with monitoring equipment, surface coils, and interventional including actively guided catheters, guidewires and needles (LADD et al. 1998; MAIER et al. 1995; QUICK et al. 1997), no such effects have been associated with any of the examined metallic implants and devices (DAVIS et al. 1981; SHELLOCK et al. 1993). To date, there are no reports of injury to patients as a result of heat developing in an implant

P.R. HILFIKER, MD
Institute of Diagnostic Radiology, University Hospital Zurich, Raemistrasse 100, 8091 Zurich, Switzerland
D. WEISHAUPT, MD
Institute of Diagnostic Radiology, University Hospital Zurich, Raemistrasse 100, 8091 Zurich, Switzerland
J.F. DEBATIN, MD
Professor, Zentralinstitut für Röntgendiagnostik, Universitätsklinikum Essen, Hufelandstrasse 55, 45122 Essen, Germany

or device. The only exceptions are burns that have occurred as a result of induced current in electrically conductive devices. Nevertheless, all new implants and devices should be evaluated for heat production in a controlled in vitro setting prior to use in patients subjected to MRI.

Metallic implants are known to cause various degrees of artifacts on MR images. The signal distortion is caused by a disruption of the local magnetic field that perturbs the relationship between position and frequency on which image reconstruction is based. The effects of bioimplants on MR images can be grouped into two categories: displacement of water by the implant itself, and artifacts created by magnetic susceptibility differences between implants and human tissue. The former is virtually negligible as it merely results in a signal void corresponding to the exact size of the implant. Artifacts caused by susceptibility differences, on the other hand, are highly variable and depend on a number of different object- and scanning-related factors. Factors influencing image distortion and therefore the artifact size include magnetic susceptibility, orientation of the device in the B0 field, device material, quantity and shape of the device, as well as field strength, type of MR sequence and the particular imaging parameters employed (Bellon et al. 1986; Pusey et al. 1986). Differences in magnetic susceptibility cause local inhomogeneities in the static magnetic field B0. These inhomogeneities in turn lead to geometric distortion and intra-voxel dephasing. The resultant artifacts can become manifest as local or regional distortions or as complete signal voids. Nonferromagnetic objects tend to be associated with less severe artifacts compared to ferromagnetic objects. Artifacts caused by nonferromagnetic implants result from eddy currents that can be generated in the objects by gradient magnetic fields used for MRI that, in turn, disrupt the local magnetic field and distort the image.

To minimize device- or implant-related artifacts on MR images, the following rules should be observed:

1. Devices should be manufactured from MR-compatible, nonferromagnetic materials such as titanium instead of stainless steel
2. Spin echo (SE) sequences should be employed instead of gradient recalled echo (GRE) sequences
3. The echo time (TE) should be kept as short as possible to minimize the time during which dephasing can occur. Therefore fast (turbo) spin echo (FSE or TSE) sequences are generally preferable to conventional SE sequences
4. Increasing the bandwidth reduces the effective echo time, thereby reducing dephasing artifacts

23.2 Aneurysm and Hemostatic Clips

Aneurysm clips have been used for more than two decades as the principal tools for surgical treatment of intracranial aneurysms and arteriovenous malformations. The examination of patients with nonferromagnetic intracranial aneurysm clips with MR systems is no longer absolutely contraindicated (Becker et al. 1988; Davis et al. 1981; Piepgras et al. 1995; Shellock and Crues 1988; Shellock and Curtis 1991; Shellock et al. 1993). As a result, postoperative MRI of these patients is possible.

Safety and Artifacts. MRI remains contraindicated in patients in whom aneurysm clips that display ferromagnetic qualities have been used. Studies have demonstrated that there is a real hazard of subjecting ferromagnetic aneurysm clips to static magnetic fields, as these clips may be displaced with serious consequences for the patient (Becker 1994; Dujovny et al. 1984; Shellock 1988; Shellock and Crues 1988, Shellock and Curtis 1991; Shellock et al. 1993). In fact, a patient death has been attributed to displacement of a ferromagnetic aneurysm clip during an MR examination (Klucznik et al. 1993).

Patients with nonferromagnetic or weakly ferromagnetic clips have, however, been studied safely with MRI (Becker et al. 1988; Shellock 1996; Shellock et al. 1993). The term "weakly ferromagnetic" refers to metal that may demonstrate extremely low ferromagnetic qualities as assessed with highly sensitive measurement equipment. Therefore, these materials may not be technically referred to as nonferromagnetic. Technically, all metals possess some degree of magnetism, and thus no metal is considered totally nonferromagnetic (Shellock and Kanal 1998a).

Because of the profound safety implications related to performing an MR examination on patients with aneurysm clips, every clip should be identified (specific manufacturer, model number and type) and then compared to the recent literature on safety evaluation (Kanal and Shellock 1993; Kanal et al. 1996; Shellock 1988, 1996; Shellock and Kanal 1998a, 1998b; Shellock et al. 1993; Shellock and Morisoli 1994a, 1994b; Shellock and Shellock 1998; Teitelbaum et al. 1988). To prevent such accidents with patients who have a ferromagnetic implant, Shellock (1996) proposes a system similar to that used to indicate a severe allergy in a chart.

All commonly used intracranial aneurysm clips induce artifacts which can distort the diagnostically important areas of interest. The artifacts caused by the metallic clips consist of a central signal void, referred to as the black-hole artifact (TEITELBAUM et al. 1988), which is surrounded by a high-signal rim and an area of spatial distortion, extending well beyond the high-signal rim (Fig. 23.1). While the central signal void is caused by an off-resonance condition during excitation (LUDEKE et al. 1985), the high-signal rim and the surrounding spatial distortion result from smaller local magnetic field variations leading to ill-positioned signals along the frequency-encoding direction.

23.3 Intravascular Devices

Increasingly, transcatheter interventional procedures are being used to treat vascular diseases with various types of intravascular coils, filters, stents, and stent-grafts. Many of them have been evaluated for their MR compatibility (LAISSY et al. 1995; SHELLOCK et al. 1993; TEITELBAUM et al. 1988, 1989). Since these devices typically become firmly incorporated in the vessel wall after approximately 6 weeks, even ferromagnetic stents are unlikely to be dislodged by attraction to magnetic fields up to 1.5 T (SHELLOCK et al. 1993; TEITELBAUM et al. 1988). As long as there is a possibility that the intravascular coil, filter, or stent is not firmly positioned, MR examination should not be performed. No such precautions are required if the intravascular device is known to be non- or only minimally ferromagnetic.

23.3.1 Aortic Stent Grafts

Bifurcated aortic stent grafts are being increasingly used for treatment of abdominal aortic aneurysms. In contrast to surgery, aneurysmal stenting requires long-term imaging follow-up (ROZENBLIT et al. 1995). Contrast-enhanced 3D MRA appears well suited for assessing the abdominal and pelvic vasculature following aortic stent implantation (ENGELLAU et al. 1998; HILFIKER et al. 1998a).

Safety and Artifacts. In vitro evaluation of a commonly used aortic stent graft (Vanguard; Boston Scientific, Oakland, NJ) did not reveal any heating or

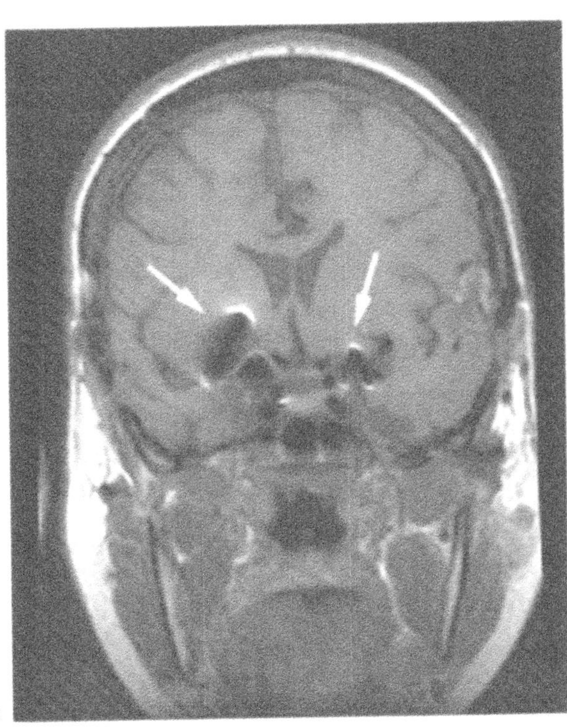

a

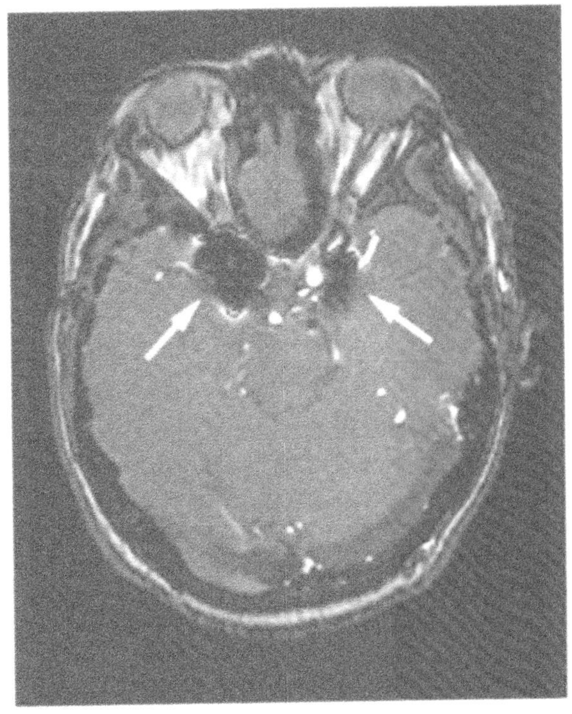

b

Fig. 23.1a, b. A 45-year-old female patient with nonferromagnetic intracranial aneurysm clips (middle cerebral artery on both sides). (**a**) Coronal SE T1-weighted image. The artifacts (*arrows*) caused by the metallic clips consist of a central signal void, referred to as the black-hole artifact, which is surrounded by a high-signal rim and an area of spatial distortion. (**b**) The artifact size is increased on the axial gradient recalled echo (GRE) image (*arrows*)

movement in a 1.5-T MR environment (Hilfiker et al. 1998a). This self-expanding endoprosthesis is composed of a nitinol frame annealed into a tubular zigzag configuration by a 7–0 polypropylene thread (Cragg et al. 1993) and covered with a 0.1-mm woven-polyester fabric. The stent graft is tagged with platinum markers allowing proper device positioning under fluoroscopic guidance. The very short echo time of less than 2 ms, inherent in the fast 3D GRE acquisition employed for contrast-enhanced 3D MRA, limits stent-related magnetic susceptibility artifacts, which have been associated with other sequences (New et al. 1983; Teitelbaum et al. 1988, 1989). A recent study demonstrated that as with CT, MR images tended to slightly overestimate the width of the stent graft wall. Based on measurements, the degree of wall thickness overestimation and associated underestimation of luminal stent diameters was no more pronounced for MRA than CTA (Hilfiker et al. 1998a). In fact, artifacts emanating from the platinum markers were considerably less severe on the MR images. A wider area of signal loss was seen only at the insertion of the iliac stent leg into the aortic stent portion (Fig. 23.2). This reflects the overlap of two radio-opaque platinum markers. It is important to recognize this artifact and not confuse it with a stenosis (Fig. 23.3).

It is crucial to point out that the favorable results documented with the Vanguard bifurcated stent graft cannot be generalized to other devices. Both artifact and safety characteristics are dependent on the composition of the individual stent graft. In view of considerable similarities between the different models, similarly favorable results can, however, be expected.

23.3.2 Peripheral Stents and Stent Grafts

Intravascular stents are being widely used to improve vessel patency rates following balloon angioplasty (Cragg et al. 1993; Palmaz et al. 1992). Peripheral arteries stented with metallic endoprosthesis are subject to intimal hyperplasia and thrombus formation both of which threaten vascular patency. Driven by a need for close follow-up, several techniques have been employed to monitor vessel patency following stent placement (Long et al. 1991; Vorwerk et al. 1996). Contrast-enhanced 3D MRA would constitute an ideal noninvasive alternative for the close follow-up required after implantation of selected MR-compatible stents.

Safety and Artifacts. In a phantom study of six commercially available stents, differences in stent characteristics became evident (Table 23.1, 23.2) (Hilfiker et al. 1998b). The stainless steel Palmaz stent as well as the cobalt-based alloy Easy Wallstent caused large signal voids on 3D MRA images (Fig. 23.4). Assessment of the stent lumen and thus stent patency was not possible. The covered Corvita stent is constructed from the same cobalt based alloy as the Wallstent. However, it also contains a tantalum core. Addition of this core reduced the associated artifact, thereby maintaining the possibility to assess the stent's luminal patency. The artifacts were too extensive, however, to exclude the presence of even a significant (>50%) stenosis.

Stents made of nitinol on the other hand (Cragg stent, Cragg EndoPro system 1 stent, Passager stent) caused only minor artifacts. With these stents the luminal diameter was artifactually reduced by merely 0%–20%. The nitinol frame filaments of the stent grafts were identifiable on the individual sections and reformations as distinct areas of signal void,

Table 23.1. Evaluated peripheral stents

Non-covered stents	Easy Wallstent (Schneider Worldwide, Bülach, Switzerland)
	Cragg stent (Mintec, Bahamas Islands)
	Palmaz stent (Cordis/Johnson and Johnson, New Jersey, USA)
Covered stents	Cragg EndoPro system 1 stent (Mintec, Bahamas Islands)
	Corvita stent (Schneider Worldwide, Bülach, Switzerland)
	Passager stent (Medi-Tech/Boston Scientific, Natick, USA)

Table 23.2. Underlying stent materials

Stent types	Material
Easy Wallstent	Cobalt based alloy
Cragg stent	Nitinol wire
Palmaz stent	Stainless steel
Cragg EndoPro system 1 stent	Nitinol wire, Dacron covering
Corvita stent	Cobalt alloy with tantalum core, polycarbonate elastomere
Passager stent	Nitinol wire, platinum markers, woven-polyester fabric

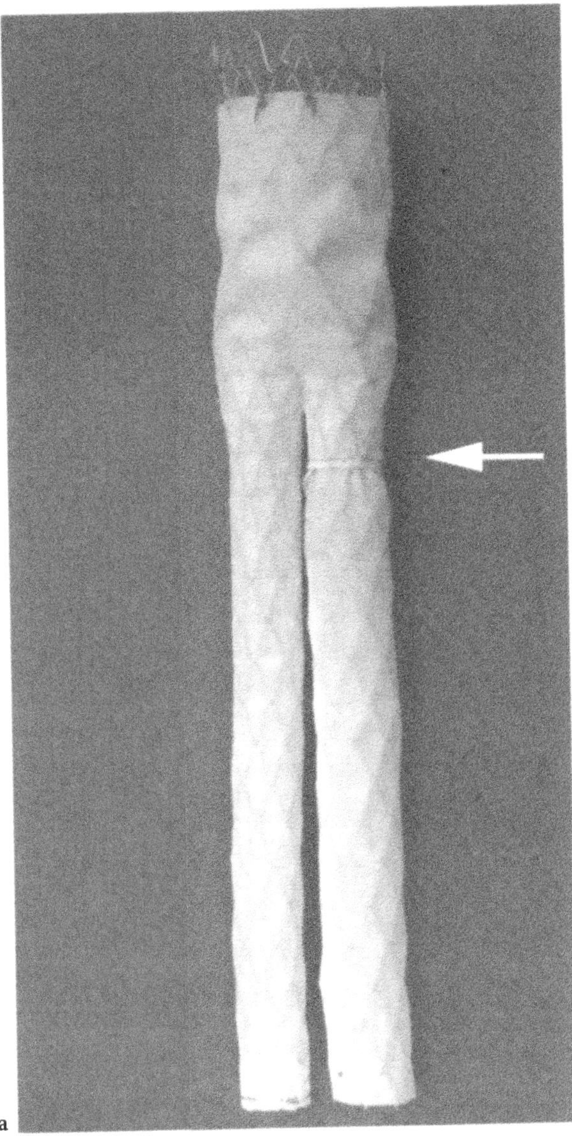

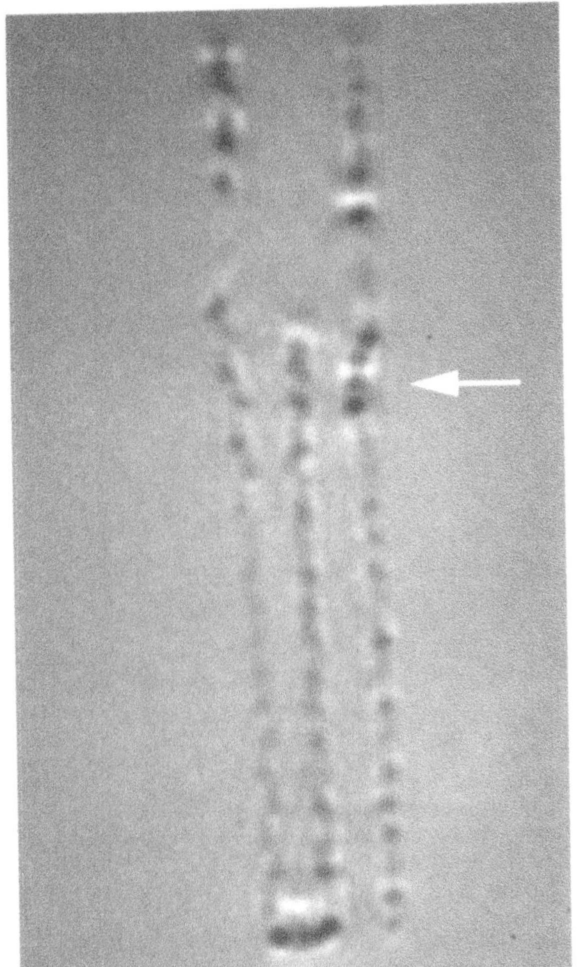

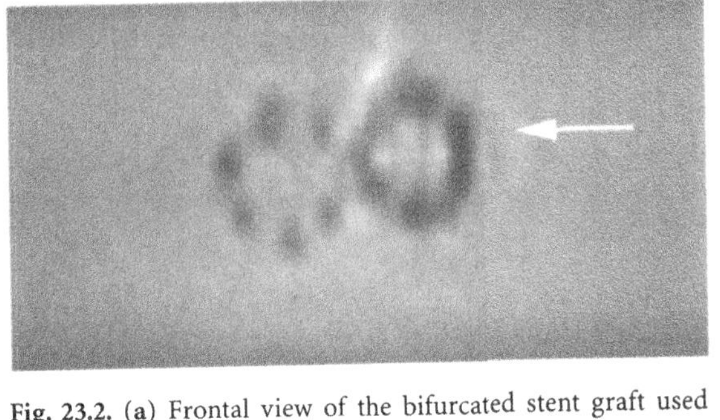

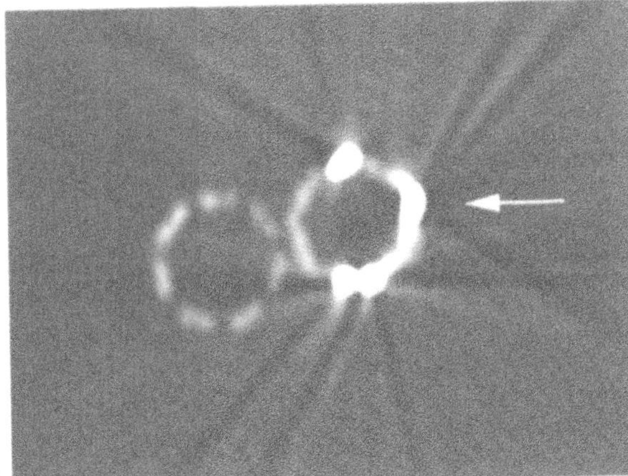

Fig. 23.2. (**a**) Frontal view of the bifurcated stent graft used for the endoluminal treatment of intrarenal aortic aneurysms (Vanguard, Boston Scientific, Oakland, New Jersey). The graft has two components that are inserted separately and subsequently joined: the primary component consists of an aortic and iliac stent graft with an attachment site for the secondary component, which is placed in the contralateral iliac artery. Junction of the two stent components (*arrow*). (**b**) Coronal 3D MRA source image of the stent graft which is embedded in agar gel. The woven wires of the stent graft are well visualized on the image against the contrast-enhanced agar gel. Platinum markers at the junction of the two stent components (*arrow*). CT image (**c**) and axial 3D MRA reconstruction (**d**) of the stent graft obtained at identical location traversing the platinum marker (*arrow*) at the junction of the two stent components in the proximal iliac portion. The platinum markers induce a starburst pattern on CT images, whilst the platinum-induced signal voids simulated a widening of the stent wall on MR images

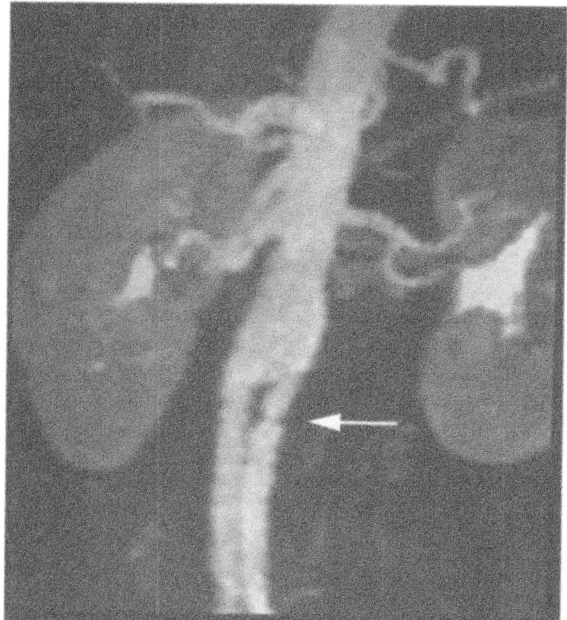

Fig. 23.3. Most intensity projection image (MIP) of a coronal 3D MRA data set acquired in a patient 3 months after aortic stent grafting. The overlap of platinum markers at the junction of the two stent components in the proximal right iliac artery causes a widened signal void (*arrow*), which should not be confused with a stenosis

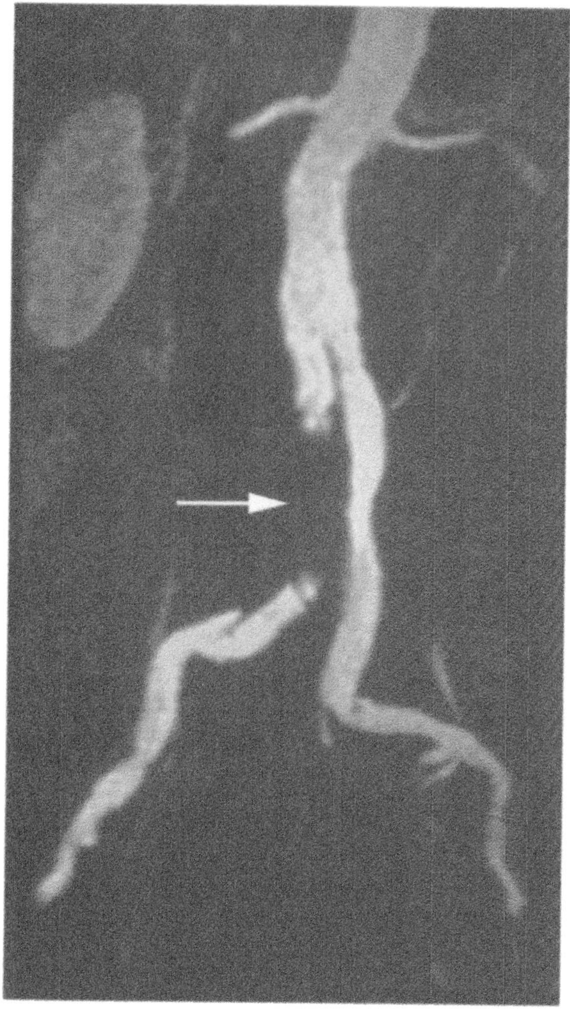

Fig. 23.4. MIP image of a coronal 3D MRA data set after implantation of a Wallstent in the right iliac leg of a bifurcated aortic stent graft. The Wallstent (material: cobalt based alloy) causes a large signal void (*arrow*), whereas the lumen of the bifurcated aortic stent graft (material: nitinol wire) remained well visible

allowing for a detailed assessment of stent structure. The stented lumen can be evaluated with ease. Luminal patency can be established and hemodynamically significant stenosis, causing more than 50% luminal narrowing, excluded with certainty. Intimal hyperplasia causing less than 50% luminal narrowing would likely remain undetected, however (Hilfiker et al. 1998b).

23.3.3 Coronary Stents

The use of intracoronary stents has dramatically increased. Because of the increased indications for intracoronary stent implantation, which include bail-out therapy, nonelective treatment of suboptimal angiographic results, and elective stenting of primary lesions, there is a rapidly expanding population of patients with coronary stents in situ who need to undergo MRI procedures for various diagnostic reasons (Kotsakis et al. 1997).

Safety and Artifacts. The most commonly used coronary stents are made of stainless steel or tantalum. In vitro experiments by Scott and Pettigrew (1994) demonstrated no deflection among the most widely used stents. In vitro experiments in dogs revealed no evidence of stent migration after repeated MRI (Matsumoto et al. 1989). However, it is well known, that coronary stents typically become endothelialized and firmly incorporated into the vessel wall approximately 6 weeks after implantation, so it is highly unlikely any of them would become dislodged by attraction to magnetic fields. Furthermore, the deflection forces on ferromagnetic coronary stents caused by magnetic field in routine MRI procedures are considered to be less than the force exerted on them by the beating heart (Kotsakis et al. 1997).

Stainless steel stents create a significant "black hole" MR susceptibility artifact, whereas tantalum stents produce negligible magnetic susceptibility artifacts (DUERINCKX 1995; DUERINCKX et al. 1995, 1998; MATSUMOTO et al. 1989).

23.4 Ligating and Marking Clips

To date, DSA and X-ray angiography are considered the standard of reference in the assessment of bypass graft stenosis. A 12% incidence of bypass graft stenosis within the first postoperative year (BERKOWITZ et al. 1981) mandates frequent imaging of these patients. For these patients, noninvasive contrast-enhanced MRA provides a most attractive alternative to the invasive DSA examinations. Thus, contrast-enhanced MRA can be employed to monitor the therapeutic effectiveness following arterial bypass grafting. The assessment of vascular grafts can be complicated by the presence of vascular clips, used for either vessel ligation or tissue marking, mainly due to susceptibility artifacts of varying magnitude which may simulate graft stenosis (BENDIB et al. 1997) (Fig. 23.5).

Safety and Artifacts. Almost all commercially available vascular clips are made either of chemically pure titanium metal, or of the absorbable polymer polydioxanon (GREISLER et al. 1988). Clips are available in different sizes ranging from 3.4 mm0.7 mm (long axis × short axis) up to 12.3 mm×1.7 mm. In vitro evaluations have shown that these clips are unequivocally safe in a high field 1.5-T MR environment with regard to heating and field-induced mechanical clip motion (SHELLOCK 1998; WEISHAUPT et al. 1999). Lack of any measurable heating, even under extreme scanning conditions, supports the hypothesis that the induction of electrical currents is indeed negligible for small implants at clinically used magnetic field strengths (SHELLOCK 1998). The small longitudinal extension of the clips in relation to the wavelength of the RF radiation at 1.5 T impedes the build-up of resonant oscillating currents that could lead to heating. The lack of any field-induced clip motion reflects the titanium or polymer basis of the clips. The size and appearance of the clip-induced artifact are primarily related to the underlying material. Biodegradable polydioxanon clips cause virtually no susceptibility artifacts. In contrast, all titanium-based clips are associated with typical artifacts on spoiled 3D GRE images as described above.

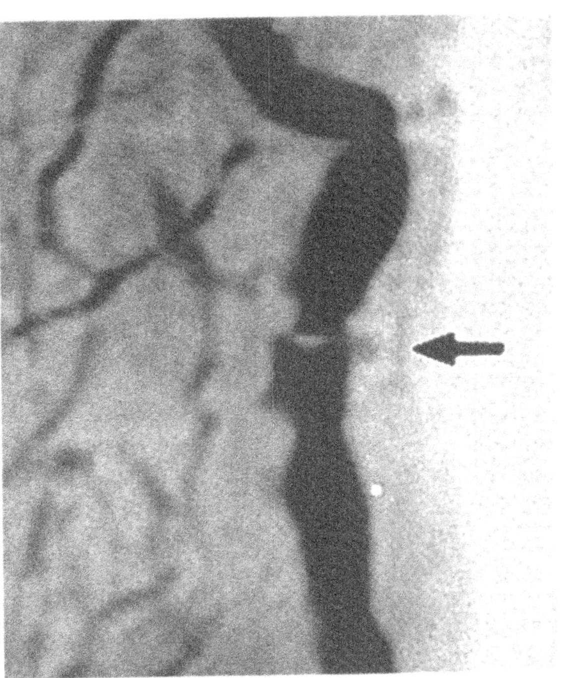

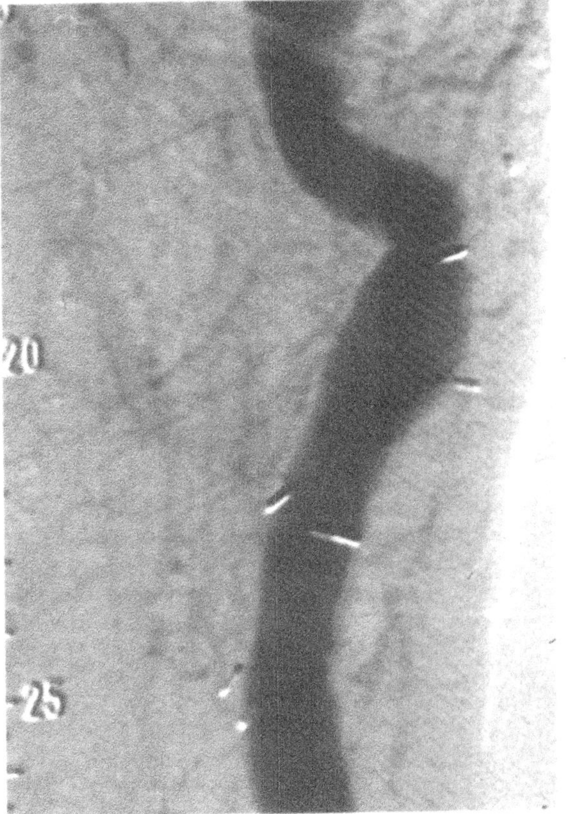

Fig. 23.5. 3D MRA (**a**) and digital subtraction angiography (DSA) (**b**) of a 58-year-old male patient with an arterialized autologous saphenous vein graft. 3D MRA suggests a stenosis of the in situ femoropopliteal graft due a ligating clip (*arrow*). Corresponding DSA reveals patency of the graft. Note dilatation of the entire in situ graft on both images

The magnitude of underlying susceptibility artifacts is dependent on various parameters. Recent in vitro evaluations of 15 different titanium clips at 1.5 T using a 3D spoiled GRE sequence have shown that a direct relationship exists between the length of the clip long axis and the associated artifact size. The most pronounced artifacts were present when the long axis of the clip was oriented perpendicular to the main magnetic field. Other parameters influencing artifact size which can be adjusted relate to the imaging experiment itself. Thus the magnitude of susceptibility effects is known to be directly proportional to the magnetic field strength (Farahani et al. 1990). Since most scanners operate at a given strength, the choice of imaging parameters such as echo time and k-space coverage is a more practical means of adjusting artifact size (Shellock and Kanal 1998a; Shellock and Shellock 1998). Since the magnitude of the susceptibility effect is directly dependent on the TE length, 3D image data sets should be acquired with partial echo techniques (Weishaupt et al. 1999). In addition, artifact size is also dependent on the degree of k-space coverage. Thus, imaging with 0.5 excitations results in significantly more clip-related signal distortion along the phase-encoded direction due to the lack of measured data and a different reconstruction algorithm in fractional-echo, partial k-space images. Hence, in the presence of metallic vascular clips, fast 3D data sets should be collected with partial echo techniques and reconstruction should be based on a complete set of k-space data.

23.5 Heart Valve Prosthesis

Prosthetic heart valves were initially believed to constitute a contraindication to MRI. Recent studies have now indicated that patients with modern types of valves may be examined without risk.

Safety and Artifacts. Many heart valves, evaluated for deflection forces, displayed measurable attraction to the static magnetic field (Hassler et al. 1986; Shellock and Crues 1988; Soulen et al. 1985). However, because the deflection forces of these valves were minimal compared with the force exerted by the beating heart, an MR procedure is not considered to be hazardous for patients with a heart valve as described in the following references (Hassler et al. 1986; Shellock 1996; Shellock and Crues 1988; Shellock et al. 1993; Soulen et al. 1985). There is no report in the literature of a patient incidence during an MR procedure related to the presence of a heart valve prosthesis.

GRE imaging of 13 different heart valve prostheses consisting of pyrolytic carbon and titanium produced only a mild degree of distortion of the MR image (Shellock and Morisoli 1994b). The relatively minor artifact should therefore not affect the diagnostic quality of an MRI examination in those patients.

23.6 Cardiac Occluders

Patients with patent ductus arteriosus (PDA), atrial septal defect (ASD), or ventricular septal defect (VSD) can be treated with metallic cardiac occluders. These implants are generally stable as long as a proper size is used. Eventually, tissue overgrowth covers the cardiac occluder (Dupuy et al. 1993; Shellock and Morisoli 1994a).

Safety and Artifacts. In vitro evaluations of cardiac occluders demonstrated either minor or total lack of ferromagnetism. Patients with minor ferromagnetic occluders may undergo MRI approximately 6 weeks after placement of the device, whereas patients with nonferromagnetic occluders can be imaged any time after placement of the occluder (Shellock 1996; Shellock and Morisoli 1994a).

23.7 Vascular Access Ports and Catheters

Patients with vascular access ports frequently undergo serial MR exams for assessment of therapeutic effectiveness against a plethora of underlying diseases. Therefore it is of paramount importance that these devices are MR compatible. These implants are typically placed in subcutaneous pockets with the catheter in the jugular, subclavian, or cephalic vein.

Safety and Artifacts. Shellock et al. (1993) tested 38 implantable vascular access ports. Three of them showed measurable deflection forces, but the forces were believed to be minor in relation to the in vivo application of these implants (Shellock et al. 1995; Shellock and Shellock 1996). Nonmetal devices produce the least amount of artifact whereas metal ones have the greatest amount of artifacts. However, the danger of piercing a device made of nonmetal due to the repeated needle access of a plastic reservoir is much higher than in a device consisting of metal (Shellock 1996). Therefore, harder materials or metal may be more acceptable for use in patients with vascular access ports with reservoirs (Shellock et al. 1995). Future developments will include vascular access ports that are electronically activated and regulated. Based on currently employed technology, these types of vascular access ports would not be MR compatible.

23.8 Safety Information About Implants

The safety and artifact size characteristics of various vascular implants have been evaluated in numerous publications. However, the value of these reports regarding the MR compatibility of certain vascular implants was itself an issue for publication (Kanal and Shellock 1994). Any list is incomplete to some degree because either only certain sequences were performed or only certain devices were tested. Furthermore, any list of devices is outdated when published as new devices rapidly become available on the market. Furthermore, manufactures are permitted to change components within their devices without being required to notify authorities as long as the device function remains the same and the effectiveness is not substantially altered. Therefore, periodically it is necessary to make sure that there are no alterations in the device components by contacting the manufacturers. Of course, this is more important in devices like aneurysm clips which are implanted in more sensitive regions than other devices.

Most of the data published in the current literature were gathered at a field strength not exceeding 1.5 T. However, with the propagation of high field units (2 T and more), safety concerns have to be addressed. Mild ferromagnetism in a 1.5-T MR system can be more serious in a higher field unit and pose a hazard to patients undergoing an MR procedure.

23.9 Conclusion

Patients with intravascular implants may not undergo MRI unless the implanted clip has been demonstrated to be unaffected by the MR environment. Devices which are electrically or magnetically activated should be excluded from MR procedures. For guidance with respect to the safety of performing MR procedures in patients with an implant or device, MR users may rely on an extensive foundation of peer-reviewed literature.

References

Becker GJ (1994) Should metallic vascular stents be used to treat cerebrovascular occlusive diseases? [editorial; comment]. Radiology 19:309–312

Becker RL, Norfray JF, Teitelbaum GP, et al (1988) MR imaging in patients with intracranial aneurysm clips. AJNR Am J Neuroradiol 9:885–889

Bellon EM, Haacke EM, Coleman PE et al (1986) MR artifacts: a review. AJR Am J Roentgenol 147:1271–1281

Bendib K, Berthezene Y, Croisille P, et al (1997) Assessment of complicated arterial bypass grafts: value of contrast-enhanced subtraction magnetic resonance angiography. J Vasc Surg 26:1036–1042

Berkowitz HD, Hobbs CL, Roberts B, et al (1981) Value of routine vascular laboratory studies to identify vein graft stenosis. Surgery 90:971–979

Cragg AH, De Jong SC, Barnhart WH, et al (1993) Nitinol intravascular stent: results of preclinical evaluation. Radiology 189:775–778

Davis PL, Crooks L, Arakawa M, et al (1981) Potential hazards in NMR imaging: heating effects of changing magnetic fields and RF fields on small metallic implants. AJR Am J Roentgenol 137:857–860

Duerinckx AJ (1995) MR angiography of the coronary arteries. Top Magn Reson Imaging 7:267–285

Duerinckx AJ, Atkinson D, Hurwitz R, et al (1995) Coronary MR angiography after coronary stent placement. AJR Am J Roentgenol 165:662–664

Duerinckx AJ, Atkinson D, Hurwitz R (1998) Assessment of coronary artery patency after stent placement using magnetic resonance angiography. J Magn Reson Imaging 8:896–902

Dujovny M, Kossovsky N, Kossowsky R, et al (1984) Intracranial clips: an examination of the devices used for aneurysm surgery. Neurosurgery 14:257–267

Dupuy DE, Hartnell GG, Lipsky M (1993) MR imaging of a patient with a ferromagnetic foreign body (letter). AJR Am J Roentgenol 160:893

Engellau L, Larsson EM, Albrechtsson U, et al (1998) Magnetic resonance imaging and MR angiography of endoluminally treated abdominal aortic aneurysms. Eur J Vasc Endovasc Surg 15:212–219

Farahani K, Sinha U, Sinha S, et al (1990) Effect of field strength on susceptibility artifacts in magnetic resonance imaging. Comput Med Imaging Graph 14:409–413

Greisler HP, Endean ED, Klosak JJ, et al (1988) Polyglactin 910/polydioxanone bicomponent totally resorbable vascular prostheses. J Vasc Surg 7:697–705

Hany TF, Debatin JF, Leung DA, et al (1997) Evaluation of the aortoiliac and renal arteries: comparison of breath-hold, contrast-enhanced, three-dimensional MR angiography with conventional catheter angiography. Radiology 204:357–362

Hassler M, Le Bas JF, Wolf JE, et al (1986) Effects of the magnetic field in magnetic resonance imaging on 15 tested cardiac valve prostheses. J Radiol 67:661–666

Hilfiker PR, Pfammatter T, Hany TF, et al (1998a) 3D MRA in patients with abdominal aortic aneurysm post stent-grafting. In: Proceedings of the International Society for Magnetic Resonance in Medicine, 6th Scientific Meeting and Exhibition, Sydney, p 175

Hilfiker PR, Quick HH, Pfammatter T, et al (1998b) In vitro evaluation of 3D MRA imaging characteristics of plain and covered stent grafts. In: Proceedings of the International Society for Magnetic Resonance in Medicine, 6th Scientific Meeting and Exhibition, Sydney, p 104

Kanal E, Shellock FG (1993) MR imaging of patients with intracranial aneurysm clips [editorial; comment]. Radiology 187:612–614

Kanal E, Shellock FG (1994) The value of published data on MR compatibility of metallic implants and devices. AJNR Am J Neuroradiol 15:1394–1396

Kanal E, Shellock FG, Lewin JS (1996) Aneurysm clip testing for ferromagnetic properties: clip variability issues [see comments]. Radiology 200:576–578

Klucznik RP, Carrier DA, Pyka R, et al (1993) Placement of a ferromagnetic intracerebral aneurysm clip in a magnetic field with a fatal outcome [see comments]. Radiology 187:855–856

Kotsakis A, Tan KH, Jackson G (1997) Is MRI a safe procedure in patients with coronary stents in situ? [editorial]. Int J Clin Pract 51:349

Ladd ME, Quick HH, Boesiger P, et al (1998) RF heating of actively visualized catheters and guidewires. In: Proceedings of the International Society for Magnetic Resonance in Medicine, 6th Scientific Meeting and Exhibition, Sydney, p 473

Laissy JP, Grand C, Matos C, et al (1995) Magnetic resonance angiography of intravascular endoprostheses: investigation of three devices. Cardiovasc Intervent Radiol 18:360–366

Leung DA, McKinnon GC, Davis CP, et al (1996) Breath-hold, contrast-enhanced, three-dimensional MR angiography. Radiology 200:569–571

Long AL, Page PE, Raynaud AC, et al (1991) Percutaneous iliac artery stent: angiographic long-term follow-up. Radiology 180:771–778

Ludeke KM, Roschmann P, Tischler R (1985) Susceptibility artefacts in NMR imaging. Magn Reson Imaging 3:329–343

Maier SE, Wildermuth S, Darrow RD, et al (1995) Safety of MR tracking catheters. In: Proceedings of the Society of Magnetic Resonance, 3rd Annual Meeting and Exhibition, Nice, p 497

Matsumoto AH, Teitelbaum GP, Barth KH, et al (1989) Tantalum vascular stents: in vivo evaluation with MR imaging. Radiology 170:753–755

New PF, Rosen BR, Brady TJ, et al (1983) Potential hazards and artifacts of ferromagnetic and nonferromagnetic surgical and dental materials and devices in nuclear magnetic resonance imaging. Radiology 147:139–148

Palmaz JC, Laborde JC, Rivera FJ, et al (1992) Stenting of the iliac arteries with the Palmaz stent: experience from a multicenter trial. Cardiovasc Intervent Radiol 15:291–297

Piepgras A, Guckel F, Weik T, et al (1995) [Titanium aneurysm clips and their advantages in diagnostic imaging]. Radiologe 35:830–833

Prince MR, Yucel EK, Kaufman JA, et al (1993) Dynamic gadolinium-enhanced three-dimensional abdominal MR arteriography. J Magn Reson Imaging 3:877–881

Pusey E, Lufkin RB, Brown RK, et al (1986) Magnetic resonance imaging artifacts: mechanism and clinical significance. Radiographics 6:891–911

Quick HH, Ladd ME, Von Schulthess GK, et al (1997) Heating effects of an intravascular maging catheter. In: Proceedings of the European Society for Magnetic Resonance in Medicine and Biology, 14th Annual Meeting and Exhibition, Geneva, p 563

Quinn SF, Demlow TA, Hallin RW, et al (1993) Femoral MR angiography versus conventional angiography: preliminary results. Radiology 189:181–184

Quinn SF, Sheley RC, Semonsen KG, et al (1998) Aortic and lower-extremity arterial disease: evaluation with MR angiography versus conventional angiography. Radiology 206:693–701

Rogg JM, Smeaton S, Doberstein C, et al (1999) Assessment of the value of MR imaging for examining patients with angiographically negative subarachnoid hemorrhage. AJR Am J Roentgenol 172:201–206

Rozenblit A, Marin ML, Veith FJ, et al (1995) Endovascular repair of abdominal aortic aneurysm: value of postoperative follow-up with helical CT. AJR Am J Roentgenol 165:1473–1479

Scott NA, Pettigrew RI (1994) Absence of movement of coronary stents after placement in a magnetic resonance imaging field. Am J Cardiol 73:900–901

Shellock FG (1988) MR imaging of metallic implants and materials: a compilation of the literature. AJR Am J Roentgenol 151:811–814

Shellock FG (1996) Magnetic Resonance: bioeffects, safety and patient management, 2nd edn. Lippincott-Raven, Philadelphia

Shellock FG (1998) Pocket guide to MR procedures and metallic objects: update 1998. Raven, New York

Shellock FG, Crues JV (1988) High-field-strength MR imaging and metallic biomedical implants: an ex vivo evaluation of deflection forces. AJR Am J Roentgenol 151:389–392

Shellock FG, Curtis JS (1991) MR imaging and biomedical implants, materials, and devices: an updated review. Radiology 180:541–550

Shellock FG, Morisoli SM (1994a) Ex vivo evaluation of ferromagnetism and artifacts of cardiac occluders exposed to a 1.5-T MR system. J Magn Reson Imaging 4:213–215

Shellock FG, Morisoli SM (1994b) Ex vivo evaluation of ferromagnetism, heating, and artifacts produced by heart valve prostheses exposed to a 1.5-T MR system. J Magn Reson Imaging 4:756–758

Shellock FG, Shellock VJ (1996) Vascular access ports and catheters: ex vivo testing of ferromagnetism, heating, and artifacts associated with MR imaging. Magn Reson Imaging 14:443–447

Shellock FG, Shellock VJ (1998) Spetzler titanium aneurysm clips: compatibility at MR imaging. Radiology 206:838–841

Shellock FG, Kanal E (1998a) Aneurysm clips: evaluation of MR imaging artifacts at 1.5 T. Radiology 209:563–566

Shellock FG, Kanal E (1998b) Yasargil aneurysm clips: evaluation of interactions with a 1.5-T MR system. Radiology 207:587–591

Shellock FG, Morisoli S, Kanal E (1993) MR procedures and biomedical implants, materials, and devices: 1993 update. Radiology 189:587–599

Shellock FG, Nogueira M, Morisoli S (1995) MR imaging and vascular access ports: ex vivo evaluation of ferromagnetism, heating, and artifacts at 1.5 T. J Magn Reson Imaging 5:481–484

Soulen RL, Budinger TF, Higgins CB (1985) Magnetic resonance imaging of prosthetic heart valves. Radiology 154:705–707

Teitelbaum GP, Bradley WG Jr, Klein BD (1988) MR imaging artifacts, ferromagnetism, and magnetic torque of intravascular filters, stents, and coils. Radiology 166:657–664

Teitelbaum GP, Raney M, Carvlin MJ, et al (1989) Evaluation of ferromagnetism and magnetic resonance imaging artifacts of the Strecker tantalum vascular stent. Cardiovasc Intervent Radiol 12:125–127

Vorwerk D, Gunther RW, Schurmann K, et al (1996) Aortic and iliac stenoses: follow-up results of stent placement after insufficient balloon angioplasty in 118 cases. Radiology 198:45–48

Weishaupt D, Quick HH, Nany D, et al (1999) In vitro evaluation of ligating clips for 3D MRA at 1.5 T. Proceedings of the International Society for Magnetic Resonance in Medicine, 7th Scientific Meeting and Exhibition, Philadelphia, p 20

Subject Index

List of Contributors

INGOLF P. ARLART, PhD, MD
Professor, Ärztlicher Direktor
Radiologisches Institut Stuttgart
Katharinenhospital
Kriegsbergstrasse 60
70174 Stuttgart
Germany

MICHAEL BOCK, PhD
Forschungsschwerpunkt Radiologische Diagnostik
und Therapie Deutsches Krebsforschungszentrum
Heidelberg (dkfz)
Universitätsklinik Heidelberg
Im Neuenheimer Feld 280
69120 Heidelberg
Germany

JAN BOGAERT, MD, PhD
Department of Radiology
University Hospital K.U.L.
Herestraat 49
3000 Leuven
Belgium

GEORG M. BONGARTZ, PhD, MD
Professor, Department of Radiology
University Hospital, Kantonsspital
Petersgraben 4
4031 Basel
Switzerland

MATTHIAS BOOS, MD
IRN – Institute of Radiology
and Nuclearmedicine Ltd.
Krankenhausstraße 70
85276 Pfaffenhofen
Germany

HILDE BOSMANS, PhD
MR Physicist
Department of Radiology
University Hospitals K.U. Leuven
Herestraat 49
3000 Leuven
Belgium

JÖRG F. DEBATIN, MD
Professor, Zentralinstitut für Röntgendiagnostik
Universitätsklinikum Essen
Hufelandstrasse 102
45122 Essen
Germany

CURT DIEHM, MD
Professor, Innere Abteilung
Klinikum Karlsbad-Langensteinbach
Guttmannstrasse 1
76307 Karlsbad
Germany

ANDRÉ J. DUERINCKX, MD, PhD
Professor of Radiology and Medicine
The University of Texas Southwestern Medical
Center and Chief of Radiology Service
VA North Texas Healthcare System
4500 South Lancaster Road
Dallas, TX 75216
USA
e-mail: andrejd@earthlink.net

STEVEN DYMARKOWSKI, MD
Department of Radiology
University Hospital K.U.L.
Herestraat 49
3000 Leuven
Belgium

Jochen Gaa, MD
Privat-Dozent, Institut für Klinische Radiologie
Universitätsklinikum, Fakultät für Klinische Medizin
der Universität Heidelberg
Theodor-Kutzer-Ufer 1-3
68167 Mannheim
Germany

Anna Gerlach, MD
Radiologisches Institut Stuttgart
Katharinenhospital
Kriegsbergstrasse 60
70174 Stuttgart
Germany

Richard Hausmann, PhD
Med. Solution CT, Siemens AG
Siemensstrasse 1
91301 Forchheim
Germany

Paul R. Hilfiker, MD
Institute of Diagnostic Radiology
University Hospital Zurich
Raemistrasse 100
8091 Zürich
Switzerland

Gabriel P. Krestin, MD
Department of Radiology
University Hospital Rotterdam
P.O. Box 2040
3000 CA Rotterdam
The Netherlands

Mark E. Ladd, PhD
Zentralinstitut für Röntgendiagnostik
Universitätsklinikum Essen
Hufelandstrasse 102
45122 Essen
Germany

Gerhard Laub, PhD
Siemens AG, Medizinische Technik
Henkestrasse 127
91052 Erlangen
Germany

Guy Marchal, MD, PhD
Professor, Department of Radiology
University Hospitals K.U.L.
Herestraat 49
3000 Leuven
Belgium

Peter Reimer, MD
PD, Zentrale Röntgendiagnostik
Städtisches Klinikum
Moltkestrasse 14
76133 Karlsruhe
Germany

Klaus Scheffler, PhD
Radiologische Universitätsklinik Freiburg
Bildgebende & Funktionelle Medizinische Physik
Hugstetterstrasse 55
79106 Freiburg
Germany

Stefan Sonnet, MD
Department of Radiology
University Hospital, Kantonsspital
Petersgraben 4
4031 Basel
Switzerland

Johan Van Cleynenbreugel, PhD
Radiology ESAT
University Hospitals K.U.L.
Herestraat 49
3000 Leuven
Belgium

Rolf Vosshenrich, MD
Zentrum Radiologie der Universität
Röntgendiagnosik I
Robert-Koch-Strasse 40
37083 Göttingen
Germany

Stephan Wetzel, MD
Abteilung für Neuroradiologie
Universitätsklinik Basel
Petersgraben 4
4031 Basel
Switzerland

Guido Wilms, MD
Professor, Department of Radiology
University Hospitals K.U.L.
Herestraat 49
3000 Leuven
Belgium

MEDICAL RADIOLOGY

Diagnostic Imaging and Radiation Oncology

Titles in the series already published

DIAGNOSTIC IMAGING

Innovations in Diagnostic Imaging
Edited by J. H. Anderson

Radiology of the Upper Urinary Tract
Edited by E. K. Lang

The Thymus - Diagnostic Imaging, Functions, and Pathologic Anatomy
Edited by E. Walter, E. Willich, and W.R. Webb

Interventional Neuroradiology
Edited by A. Valavanis

Radiology of the Pancreas
Edited by A. L. Baert, co-edited by G. Delorme

Radiology of the Lower Urinary Tract
Edited by E. K. Lang

Magnetic Resonance Angiography
Edited by I. P. Arlart, G. M. Bongartz, and G. Marchal

Contrast-Enhanced MRI of the Breast
S. Heywang-Köbrunner and R. Beck

Spiral CT of the Chest
Edited by M. Rémy-Jardin and J. Rémy

Radiological Diagnosis of Breast Diseases
Edited by M. Friedrich and E.A. Sickles

Radiology of the Trauma
Edited by M. Heller and A. Fink

Biliary Tract Radiology
Edited by P. Rossi

Radiological Imaging of Sports Injuries
Edited by C. Masciocchi

Modern Imaging of the Alimentary Tube
Edited by A. R. Margulis

Diagnosis and Therapy of Spinal Tumors
Edited by P. R. Algra, J. Valk, and J. J. Heimans

Interventional Magnetic Resonance Imaging
Edited by J. F. Debatin and G. Adam

Abdominal and Pelvic MRI
Edited by A. Heuck and M. Reiser

Orthopedic Imaging
Techniques and Applications
Edited by A. M. Davies and H. Pettersson

Radiology of the Female Pelvic Organs
Edited by E. K.Lang

Magnetic Resonance of the Heart and Great Vessels
Clinical Applications
Edited by J. Bogaert, A. J. Duerinckx, and F. E. Rademakers

Modern Head and Neck Imaging
Edited by S. K. Mukherji and J. A. Castelijns

Radiological Imaging of Endocrine Diseases
Edited by J. N. Bruneton in collaboration with B. Padovani and M.-Y. Mourou

Trends in Contrast Media
Edited by H. S. Thomsen, R. N. Muller, and R. F. Mattrey

Functional MRI
Edited by C. T. W. Moonen and P. A. Bandettini

Radiology of the Pancreas
2nd Revised Edition
Edited by A. L. Baert
Co-edited by G. Delorme and L. Van Hoe

Emergency Pediatric Radiology
Edited by H. Carty

Spiral CT of the Abdomen
Edited by F. Terrier, M. Grossholz, and C. D. Becker

Liver Malignancies
Diagnostic and Interventional Radiology
Edited by C. Bartolozzi and R. Lencioni

Medical Imaging of the Spleen
Edited by A. M. De Schepper and F. Vanhoenacker

Radiology of Peripheral Vascular Diseases
Edited by E. Zeitler

Diagnostic Nuclear Medicine
Edited by C. Schiepers

Radiology of Blunt Trauma of the Chest
P. Schnyder and M. Wintermark

Portal Hypertension
Diagnostic Imaging-Guided Therapy
Edited by P. Rossi
Co-edited by P. Ricci and L. Broglia

Recent Advances in Diagnostic Neuroradiology
Edited by Ph. Demaerel

Virtual Endoscopy and Related 3D Techniques
Edited by P. Rogalla, J. Terwisscha Van Scheltinga, and B. Hamm

Multislice CT
Edited by M. F. Reiser, M. Takahashi, M. Modic, and R. Bruening

Pediatric Uroradiology
Edited by R. Fotter

Radiology of AIDS
A Practical Approach
Edited by J.W.A.J. Reeders and P.C. Goodman

CT of the Peritoneum
Armando Rossi and Giorgio Rossi

Magnetic Resonance Angiography
2nd Revised Edition
Edited by I. P. Arlart, G. M. Bongratz, and G. Marchal

Pediatric Chest Imaging
Edited by Javier Lucaya and Janet L. Strife

Applications of Sonography in Head and Neck Pathology
Edited by J. N. Bruneton in collaboration with C. Raffaelli and O. Dassonville

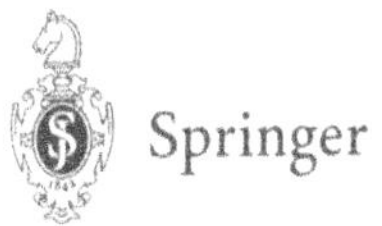

Medical Radiology
Diagnostic Imaging and Radiation Oncology

Titles in the series already published

Radiation Oncology

Lung Cancer
Edited by C.W. Scarantino

Innovations in Radiation Oncology
Edited by H. R. Withers and L. J. Peters

Radiation Therapy of Head and Neck Cancer
Edited by G. E. Laramore

Gastrointestinal Cancer – Radiation Therapy
Edited by R.R. Dobelbower, Jr.

Radiation Exposure and Occupational Risks
Edited by E. Scherer, C. Streffer, and K.-R. Trott

Radiation Therapy of Benign Diseases
A Clinical Guide
S.E. Order and S. S. Donaldson

Interventional Radiation Therapy Techniques – Brachytherapy
Edited by R. Sauer

Radiopathology of Organs and Tissues
Edited by E. Scherer, C. Streffer, and K.-R. Trott

Concomitant Continuous Infusion Chemotherapy and Radiation
Edited by M. Rotman and C. J. Rosenthal

Intraoperative Radiotherapy – Clinical Experiences and Results
Edited by F. A. Calvo, M. Santos, and L.W. Brady

Radiotherapy of Intraocular and Orbital Tumors
Edited by W. E. Alberti and R. H. Sagerman

Interstitial and Intracavitary Thermoradiotherapy
Edited by M. H. Seegenschmiedt and R. Sauer

Non-Disseminated Breast Cancer
Controversial Issues in Management
Edited by G. H. Fletcher and S.H. Levitt

Current Topics in Clinical Radiobiology of Tumors
Edited by H.-P. Beck-Bornholdt

Practical Approaches to Cancer Invasion and Metastases
A Compendium of Radiation Oncologists' Responses to 40 Histories
Edited by A. R. Kagan with the Assistance of R. J. Steckel

Radiation Therapy in Pediatric Oncology
Edited by J. R. Cassady

Radiation Therapy Physics
Edited by A. R. Smith

Late Sequelae in Oncology
Edited by J. Dunst and R. Sauer

Mediastinal Tumors. Update 1995
Edited by D. E. Wood and C. R. Thomas, Jr.

Thermoradiotherapy and Thermochemotherapy
Volume 1:
Biology, Physiology, and Physics
Volume 2:
Clinical Applications
Edited by M.H. Seegenschmiedt, P. Fessenden, and C.C. Vernon

Carcinoma of the Prostate
Innovations in Management
Edited by Z. Petrovich, L. Baert, and L.W. Brady

Radiation Oncology of Gynecological Cancers
Edited by H.W. Vahrson

Carcinoma of the Bladder
Innovations in Management
Edited by Z. Petrovich, L. Baert, and L.W. Brady

Blood Perfusion and Microenvironment of Human Tumors
Implications for Clinical Radiooncology
Edited by M. Molls and P. Vaupel

Radiation Therapy of Benign Diseases
A Clinical Guide
2nd Revised Edition
S. E. Order and S. S. Donaldson

Carcinoma of the Kidney and Testis, and Rare Urologic Malignancies
Innovations in Management
Edited by Z. Petrovich, L. Baert, and L.W. Brady

Progress and Perspectives in the Treatment of Lung Cancer
Edited by P. Van Houtte, J. Klastersky, and P. Rocmans

Combined Modality Therapy of Central Nervous System Tumors
Edited by Z. Petrovich, L. W. Brady, M. L. Apuzzo, and M. Bamberg

Age-Related Macular Degeneration
Current Treatment Concepts
Edited by W. A. Alberti, G. Richard, and R. H. Sagerman

The manufacturer's authorised representative in the EU is Springer Nature Customer Service Centre GmbH, Europaplatz 3, 69115 Heidelberg, Germany. If you have any concerns regarding our products, please contact ProductSafety@springernature.com

Printed and bound by CPI Group (UK) Ltd, Croydon, CR0 4YY
28/04/2026
02098462-0007